Anesthesia Unplugged

NOTICE

Medicine is an ever-changing science. As new research and clinical experience broaden our knowledge, changes in treatment and drug therapy are required. The authors and the publisher of this work have checked with sources believed to be reliable in their efforts to provide information that is complete and generally in accord with the standards accepted at the time of publication. However, in view of the possibility of human error or changes in medical sciences, neither the authors nor the publisher nor any other party who has been involved in the preparation or publication of this work warrants that the information contained herein is in every respect accurate or complete, and they disclaim all responsibility for any errors or omissions or for the results obtained from use of the information contained in this work. Readers are encouraged to confirm the information contained herein with other sources. For example and in particular, readers are advised to check the product information sheet included in the package of each drug they plan to administer to be certain that the information contained in this work is accurate and that changes have not been made in the recommended dose or in the contraindications for administration. This recommendation is of particular importance in connection with new or infrequently used drugs.

Anesthesia Unplugged

SECOND EDITION

Editors

Christopher Gallagher, MD
Professor of Anesthesiology
Residency Program Director
Department of Anesthesiology
Stony Brook University Medical Center
Stony Brook, New York

Steven H. Ginsberg, MD
Associate Professor of Anesthesiology
Division of Cardiac Anesthesia
Program Director Cardiothoracic Anesthesia
  Fellowship
Medical Director Pre Admission Testing Clinic
Robert Wood Johnson University Hospital
University of Medicine and Dentistry of New Jersey
Robert Wood Johnson Medical School
New Brunswick, New Jersey

Michael C. Lewis, MD
Professor Anesthesiology
Senior Associate Dean for Graduate
  Medical Education
University of Miami
Miller School of Medicine
Miami, Florida

Christine Park, MD
Assistant Professor of Anesthesiology
Northwestern University
Feinberg School of Medicine
Chicago, Illinois

Deborah Schwengel, MD
Residency Program Director
Anesthesiology and Critical Care Medicine
The Johns Hopkins Hospital
Department of Anesthesiology and
  Critical Care Medicine
Johns Hopkins University School of Medicine
Baltimore, Maryland

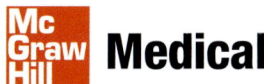

New York Chicago San Francisco Lisbon London Madrid Mexico City
Milan New Delhi San Juan Seoul Singapore Sydney Toronto

Anesthesia Unplugged, Second Edition

Copyright © 2012 by The McGraw-Hill Companies, Inc. All rights reserved. Printed in China. Except as permitted under the United States Copyright Act of 1976, no part of this publication may be reproduced or distributed in any form or by any means, or stored in a data base or retrieval system, without the prior written permission of the publisher.

1 2 3 4 5 6 7 8 9 0 CTP/CTP 17 16 15 14 13 12

ISBN 978-0-07-176717-0
MHID 0-07-176717-7

This book was set in Slimbach by Thomson Digital.
The editors were Brian Belval and Brian Kearns.
The production supervisor was Sherri Souffrance.
Project management was provided by Aakriti Kathuria, Thomson Digital.
The cover design and illustration was by Todd Radom Design.
China Translation & Printing, Ltd. was printer and binder.

Library of Congress Cataloging-in-Publication Data

Anesthesia unplugged / editors, Christopher Gallagher ... [et al.]. — 2nd ed.
  p. ; cm.
  Includes bibliographical references and index.
  ISBN 978-0-07-176717-0 (pbk.)
  ISBN 0-07-176717-7 (pbk.)
  I. Gallagher, Christopher
  [DNLM: 1. Anesthesia. WO 200]
  617.9'6—dc23

2012011451

McGraw-Hill books are available at special quantity discounts to use as premiums and sales promotions, or for use in corporate training programs. To contact a representative please e-mail us at bulksales@mcgraw-hill.com.

DEDICATION

The authors dedicate this book to their patients.
"We hope to do right by you."

ACKNOWLEDGMENTS

The authors wish to acknowledge their teachers.
"Thank you for bringing us here."

CONTENTS

CONTRIBUTORS / xi

PART I
VENOUS ACCESS / 1

CHAPTER 1
PERIPHERAL INTRAVENOUS (IV) ACCESS / 3
Obianuju Okocha

CHAPTER 2
THE INTERNAL JUGULAR (IJ) LINE / 9
Al Solina and Bo-Lu Zhou

CHAPTER 3
SUBCLAVIAN VEIN CATHETERIZATION / 23
Jessica Brodt and Christian Diez

CHAPTER 4
CENTRAL VENOUS ACCESS IN THE PEDIATRIC PATIENT / 29
Lydia M. Jorge, Amanda Saab, and Richard Elf

CHAPTER 5
FEMORAL VENOUS ACCESS—THE THUNDER DOWN UNDER: THE FEMORAL VEIN / 43
Rose Alloteh and Arlene Lamba

CHAPTER 6
PICC LINES—JUST REALLY, REALLY LONG IVS / 49
Justin Hamrick and Deborah Schwengel

PART II
ARTERIAL ACCESS / 55

CHAPTER 7
THE RADIAL A-LINE: A VERSATILE AND ESSENTIAL TOOL / 57
Julian B. Kertsman and Vincent DeAngelis

CHAPTER 8
THE BRACHIAL A-LINE / 67
Edgar Pierre and Jordan Taylor

CHAPTER 9
STAND BY ME: THE FEMORAL ARTERIAL LINE / 75
Sylviana Barsoum

CHAPTER 10
THE BEAT-TO-BEAT FAUCET DOWN YONDER: THE PEDAL A-LINE / 81
Artemus Flagg and Deborah Schwengel

PART III
AIRWAY / 85

CHAPTER 11
MASK VENTILATION: THE MASK OF ZORRO / 87
Kimberly Schinnerer Cover and Lauren Berkow

CHAPTER 12
"GOODNIGHT, SLEEP TIGHT": SETUP AND MASK INDUCTION FOR PEDIATRIC PATIENTS / 95
Peggy Seidman and Kathleen Dubrow

CHAPTER 13
LARYNGEAL MASK AIRWAY AND OTHER SUPRAGLOTTIC AIRWAY DEVICES / 101
Meltem Yilmaz and Rena Beckerly

CHAPTER 14
LARYNGOSCOPY / 113
Fouad Souki and Michael C. Lewis

CHAPTER 15
AWAKE INTUBATION / 119
Sarah LaSalle, Geza K. Kiss, and John Denny

CHAPTER 16
WHIZ-BANG INTUBATION GIZMOS / 129
Katherine S.L. Gil

CHAPTER 17
FIRE! FIRE! IN THE OPERATING ROOM / 141
Lalitha Sundararaman, Carlos Mijares, and Michael C. Lewis

CHAPTER 18
KIDDIE AIRWAY / 145
Jamie Wingate, Mark Rossberg, and Deborah Schwengel

CHAPTER 19
SURGICAL AIRWAY / 153
Wendy Daley, John Denny, George P. Batsides, and Neil Stockmaster

CHAPTER 20
SMOOTH AWAKENING / 169
Michael Wong and Renu Chhokra

CHAPTER 21
SHOW ME THE MYCOBACTERIUM!—TB PROTECTION / 175
Raina Lourens and Theresa L. Hartsell

CHAPTER 22
INTUBATIONS OUTSIDE THE OPERATING ROOM / 181
Heather Nixon

CHAPTER 23
NASOGASTRIC TUBE PLACEMENT: THE AGONY AND THE ECSTASY / 189
Asher Emanuel, Thomas Corrado, and Christopher Gallagher

PART IV
BACK / 195

CHAPTER 24
SPINAL ANESTHESIA / 197
Alexander M. DeLeon and Amreesh Mahil

CHAPTER 25
EPIDURAL, LUMBAR / 207
Sofia Geralemou, Rany Makaryus, Robert Kyureghian, Robin J. Schiller, and Joy Schabel

CHAPTER 26
THORACIC EPIDURALS—WHAT'S THE BIG DEAL? / 223
Jonathan Kraidin, Kristoffer de Lara, and John Langenfeld

CHAPTER 27
MENDING FENCES—THE BLOOD PATCH / 231
Dennis Hall and Anjana Sahani Panjwani

CHAPTER 28
KIDDIE CAUDAL EPIDURAL AND PENILE BLOCKS / 239
Zvi Jacob and Rebecca Sangster

CHAPTER 29
BLADDER EXSTROPHY—KIDDIE CAUDAL WITH TUNNEL / 247
Shivani Patel and Sabine Kost-Byerly

PART V
REGIONAL / 255

CHAPTER 30
REGIONAL BLOCK OF THE UPPER EXTREMITY / 257
Geza K. Kiss, Ahdev Kuppasamy, and Sarah LaSalle

CONTENTS

CHAPTER 31
LOWER EXTREMITY NERVE BLOCKS / 279
Andres Missair, Carlos de La Hoz, and Ralf E. Gebhard

CHAPTER 32
ABDOMINAL PAIN BE GONE: THE TAP BLOCK / 293
Brandon Togioka, Jean-Pierre Ouanes, and Richard Elliott

CHAPTER 33
NERVE BLOCKS FOR ABDOMINAL SURGERY / 301
Joni Maga and Luis Narciso

CHAPTER 34
PERIPHERAL NERVE CATHETERS— COMFORTABLY NUMB / 309
Joseph C. Hung and Marie Hanna

CHAPTER 35
KIDDIE NERVE BLOCKS / 317
J. Gabriel Tsang and Richard Elliott

CHAPTER 36
CHRONIC PAIN BLOCKS / 325
Brian Durkin

CHAPTER 37
INSIGHTS ON OPHTHALMIC ANESTHESIA / 335
Steven Gayer

PART VI
CHEST / 345

CHAPTER 38
"THE LUNG'S NOT DOWN, YOU IDIOT!"— LUNG ISOLATION / 347
Lebron Cooper and Adam Sewell

CHAPTER 39
PACING: "KEEPING THE PACE" / 365
Christian McDonough, Deepak Saluja, Jonathan Kraidin, and Asad Khan

CHAPTER 40
TEE LOOK! IT'S A BIRD...IT'S A PLANE...NO, IT'S TEE MAN! / 375
Khuram Khan and Enrique Pantin

CHAPTER 41
THE SWAN SONG / 395
Jochen Steppan, Mary Beth Brady, and Nanhi Mitter

CHAPTER 42
ANESTHESIA FOR THE CARDIAC CATHETERIZATION LAB / 407
William Grubb and Danny Chaung

CHAPTER 43
PORT ACCESS SURGERY: ALL FEAR MINIMUS MAXIMUS—MINIMALLY INVASIVE PORT ACCESS HEART SURGERY / 413
Jonathan Kraidin, Mark Anderson, and Steven H. Ginsberg

PART VII
BRAINIACS / 425

CHAPTER 44
ICP MONITORING / 427
Mark R. Ettinger and Adam Schiavi

CHAPTER 45
CEREBRAL OXIMETRY—BRAIN POWER / 439
Rebecca Reeves and Eugenie Heitmiller

CHAPTER 46
MRI—DO'S AND DONUTS / 445
Anastassia Grigorieva and Deborah Schwengel

PART VIII

ROOMSMANSHIP / 451

CHAPTER 47
GETTING STARTED / 453
Nicholas B. Nedeff, Justin Thampi, and Travis Lee

CHAPTER 48
ROOMSMANSHIP / 461
Rachel M. Kacmar and Christine Park

CHAPTER 49
POSITIONING 101 / 471
Tejal Mehta and Christine Hunter

CHAPTER 50
HANDOFF IN THE OR / 479
Luke S. Theilken

CHAPTER 51
DON'T DROP THE BALL: A STANDARDIZED HANDOFF / 485
Jana Janco, Margit Kaufman, Steven H. Ginsberg, and Jonathan Kraidin

CHAPTER 52
ANESTHESIA INFORMATION MANAGEMENT SYSTEMS: GEEK SQUAD TO THE OR STAT! / 491
Justin Long and Rafael M. Richards

CHAPTER 53
DECODING SURGEON SPEAK / 499
Sarah Olson Reck and Christine Park

PART IX

FAR FROM THE MADDENING CROWD / 505

CHAPTER 54
PREADMISSION TESTING / 507
Mark Slomovits and Steven H. Ginsberg

CHAPTER 55
OFF-SITE ANESTHESIA / 517
Christian Altman

CHAPTER 56
TRANSPORTING A PATIENT, OR DON'T GET CAUGHT IN THE ELEVATOR UNPREPARED / 523
Sarah Olson Reck and Christine Park

CHAPTER 57
INTENSIVE CARE UNIT / 529
Nishant Gandhi and Theresa L. Hartsell

CHAPTER 58
HIGHWAY TO THE DANGER ZONE: HAZMAT / 541
James A. Rothschild, Bradford Winters, and Kelly Brenan-Rothschild

CHAPTER 59
SIMULATION / 551
Christine Park and Olya Polishchuk

CHAPTER 60
FIGHTING AN UPHILL BATTLE: ANESTHESIA FOR THE OBESE PATIENT AND WEIGHT-LOSS SURGERY / 561
Emmett Whitaker and Owen Halloran

INDEX / 569

CONTRIBUTORS

Rose Alloteh, Mb.Chb
Assistant Professor of Anesthesiology
Robert Wood Johnson University Hospital
University of Medicine and Dentistry of New Jersey
Robert Wood Johnson Medical School
New Brunswick, New Jersey
Chapter 5

Christian Altman, MD
Assistant Professor
Department of Anesthesiology
Northwestern University Feinberg School of Medicine
Chicago, Illinois
Chapter 55

Mark Anderson, MD, FACS
Professor of Surgery, Division of Cardiothoracic Surgery
University of Medicine and Dentistry of New Jersey
Robert Wood Johnson School of Medicine
New Brunswick, New Jersey
Chapter 43

Sylviana Barsoum, MD
Associate Professor of Anesthesiology
Robert Wood Johnson University Hospital
University of Medicine and Dentistry of New Jersey
Robert Wood Johnson Medical School
New Brunswick, New Jersey
Chapter 9

George P. Batsides, MD
Assistant Professor of Cardiothoracic Surgery
Robert Wood Johnson University Hospital
University of Medicine and Dentistry of New Jersey
Robert Wood Johnson Medical School
New Brunswick, New Jersey
Chapter 19

Rena Beckerly, MD
Assistant Professor of Anesthesiology
Northwestern University
Feinberg School of Medicine
Chicago, Illinois
Chapter 13

Lauren Berkow, MD
Associate Professor
Anesthesia and Critical Care Medicine
Johns Hopkins School of Medicine
Baltimore, Maryland
Chapter 11

Mary Beth Brady, MD, FASE
Director, Intraoperative Transesophageal
 Echocardiography Program
Anethesiology and Critical Care Medicine
Johns Hopkins School of Medicine
Baltimore, Maryland
Chapter 41

Kelly Brenan-Rothschild, MD
Illustrator
Johns Hopkins University School of Medicine
Department of Anesthesiology and Critical Care Medicine
Baltimore, Maryland
Chapter 58

Jessica Brodt, MBBS
Anesthesiology Resident
Department of Anesthesiology, Perioperative
 Medicine and Pain Management
University of Miami/Jackson Health System
Miami, Florida
Chapter 3

Danny Chaung, DO
Anesthesia Resident
Robert Wood Johnson University Hospital
University of Medicine and Dentistry of New Jersey
Robert Wood Johnson Medical School
New Brunswick, New Jersey
Chapter 42

Renu Chhokra, MD
Assistant Professor of Anesthesiology
Robert Wood Johnson University Hospital
University of Medicine and Dentistry of New Jersey
Robert Wood Johnson Medical School
New Brunswick, New Jersey
Chapter 20

Lebron Cooper, MD
Assistant Professor of Clinical Anesthesiology
Chief of Anesthesiology, Co-Medical Director for
  Perioperative Services
University of Miami Hospital
Anesthesiology, Perioperative Medicine, and
  Pain Management
University of Miami
Miller School of Medicine
Miami, Florida
Chapter 38

Thomas Corrado, MD
Assistant Professor
Stony Brook University Medical Center
Stony Brook, New York
Chapter 23

Kimberly Schinnerer Cover, MD
Resident, Anesthesiology and Critical Care Medicine
Johns Hopkins University School of Medicine
Baltimore, Maryland
Chapter 11

Wendy Daley, MD, MPH
Anesthesia Resident
Robert Wood Johnson University Hospital
University of Medicine and Dentistry of New Jersey
Robert Wood Johnson Medical School
New Brunswick, New Jersey
Chapter 19

Kristoffer de Lara, MD
Chief Resident
Department of Anesthesiology
Robert Wood Johnson University Hospital
University of Medicine and Dentistry of New Jersey
Robert Wood Johnson Medical School
New Brunswick, New Jersey
Chapter 26

Vincent DeAngelis, MD
Associate Professor
Department of Anesthesiogy
Robert Wood Johnson University Hospital
University of Medicine and Dentistry of New Jersey
Robert Wood Johnson Medical School
New Brunswick, New Jersey
Chapter 7

Alexander M. DeLeon, MD
Assistant Professor
Associate Chair for Education
Department of Anesthesiology
Northwestern University Feinberg School of Medicine
Chicago, Illinois
Chapter 24

John Denny, MD
Associate Professor
Anesthesia
Robert Wood Johnson University Hospital
University of Medicine and Dentistry of New Jersey
Robert Wood Johnson Medical School
New Brunswick, New Jersey
Chapters 15, 19

Christian Diez, MD
Assistant Professor/Associate Program Director
Department of Anesthesiology
University of Miami
Jackson Health System
Miami, Florida
Chapter 3

Kathleen Dubrow, MD
Chief Resident
Stony Brook University Medical Center
Stony Brook, New York
Chapter 12

Brian Durkin, DO
Assistant Professor of Clinical Anesthesiology
Anesthesiology
Stony Brook University Medical Center
Stony Brook, New York
Chapter 36

Richard Elf, MD
Fellow in Pediatric Anesthesiology
Voluntary Professor of Anesthesiology
University of Miami
Miami, Florida
Chapter 4

Richard Elliott, MD
Assistant Professor
Department of Anesthesiology and Critical Care Medicine
Johns Hopkins University School of Medicine
Baltimore, Maryland
Chapters 32, 35

Asher Emanuel, MD, MPH
Resident Physician
Department of Anesthesiology
Stony Brook University Medical Center
Stony Brook, New York
Chapter 23

Mark R. Ettinger, MD
Resident, Anesthesiology and Critical Care Medicine
Johns Hopkins University School of Medicine
Baltimore, Maryland
Chapter 44

CONTRIBUTORS

Artemus Flagg, MD
Chief Resident, Anesthesiology and Critical Care Medicine
The Johns Hopkins Hospital
Johns Hopkins University School of Medicine
Baltimore, Maryland
Chapter 10

Christopher Gallagher, MD
Professor of Anesthesiology
Residency Program Director
Department of Anesthesiology
Stony Brook University Medical Center
Stony Brook, New York
Chapter 23

Nishant Gandhi, DO
Resident
Anesthesiology and Critical Care Medicine
Johns Hopkins University School of Medicine
Baltimore, Maryland
Chapter 57

Steven Gayer, MD, MBA
Professor of Clinical Anesthesiology
Chief of Anesthesiology
Bascom Palmer Eye Institute
University of Miami
Miller School of Medicine
Miami, Florida
Chapter 37

Ralf E. Gebhard, MD
Division Chief
Professor, Department of Anesthesiology
Division of Regional Anesthesia and Acute Pain
University of Miami
Miller School of Medicine
Miami, Florida
Chapter 31

Sofia Geralemou, MD
Assistant Professor
Stony Brook University Medical Center
Stony Brook, New York
Chapter 25

Katherine S.L. Gil, MD
Assistant Professor of Anesthesiology & Neurological Surgery
Anesthesiology Clerkship Coordinator
Northwestern University Feinberg School of Medicine
Chicago, Illinois
Chapter 16

Steven H. Ginsberg, MD
Associate Professor of Anesthesiology
Division of Cardiac Anesthesia
Program Director Cardiothoracic Anesthesia Fellowship
Medical Director Pre Admission Testing Clinic
Robert Wood Johnson University Hospital
University of Medicine and Dentistry of New Jersey
Robert Wood Johnson Medical School
New Brunswick, New Jersey
Chapters 43, 51, 54

Anastassia Grigorieva, MD
Resident, Department of Anesthesia
Sinai Hospital
Baltimore, Maryland
Chapter 46

William Grubb, MD, DDS
Associate Professor of Anesthesiology
Program Director Pain Fellowship
Robert Wood Johnson University Hospital
University of Medicine and Dentistry of New Jersey
Robert Wood Johnson Medical School
New Brunswick, New Jersey
Chapter 42

Dennis Hall, MD
Associate Professor of Anesthesiology
Robert Wood Johnson University Hospital
University of Medicine and Dentistry of New Jersey
Robert Wood Johnson Medical School
New Brunswick, New Jersey
Chapter 27

Owen Halloran, MD
Clinical Associate
Department of Anesthesia and Critical Care Medicine
Johns Hopkins University Bayview Medical Center
Baltimore, Maryland
Chapter 60

Justin Hamrick, MD
Fellow
Pediatric Anesthesia and Critical Care Medicine
Johns Hopkins University-School of Medicine
Baltimore, Maryland
Chapter 6

Marie Hanna, MD
Assistant Professor
Anesthesiology and Critical Care Medicine
The Johns Hopkins Hospital
Johns Hopkins University School of Medicine
Baltimore, Maryland
Chapter 34

Theresa L. Hartsell, MD, PhD
Assistant Professor, Anesthesiology and
 Critical Care Medicine
Program Director, Critical Care Anesthesiology Fellowship
Johns Hopkins University School of Medicine
Baltimore, Maryland
Chapters 21, 57

Eugenie Heitmiller, MD
Associate Professor of Anesthesiology and Pediatrics
Anesthesiology and Critical Care Medicine
Johns Hopkins School of Medicine
Baltimore, Maryland
Chapter 45

Carlos De La Hoz, MD
Senior Resident
Department of Anesthesiology
University of Miami/Jackson Memorial Hospital
Miami, Florida
Chapter 31

Joseph C. Hung, MD
Chief Resident
Johns Hopkins Hospital
Department of Anesthesiology and Critical Care Medicine
Johns Hopkins University School of Medicine
Baltimore, Maryland
Chapter 34

Christine Hunter, MD
Associate Professor of Anesthesiology
Chair, Department of Anesthesia
Robert Wood Johnson University Hospital
University of Medicine and Dentistry of New Jersey
Robert Wood Johnson Medical School
New Brunswick, New Jersey
Chapter 49

Jana Janco, MD
Anesthesia Resident
Robert Wood Johnson University Hospital
University of Medicine and Dentistry of New Jersey
Robert Wood Johnson Medical School
New Brunswick, New Jersey
Chapter 51

Zvi Jacob, MD
Assistant Professor
Stony Brook University Medical Center
Stony Brook, New York
Chapter 28

Lydia M. Jorge, MD
Assistant Professor of Clinical Anesthesiology
Department of Pediatric Anesthesiology
University of Miami
Miami, Florida
Chapter 4

Rachel M. Kacmar, MD
Chief Resident
Department of Anesthesiology
Northwestern University
Feinberg School of Medicine
Chicago, Illinois
Chapter 48

Margit Kaufman, MD
Chief Resident
Department of Anesthesia
UMDNJ-Robert Wood Johnson Medical School
New Brunswick, New Jersey
Chapter 51

Julian B. Kertsman, MD
Pediatric Anesthesiology Fellow
Anesthesiology
St. Christopher's Children's Hospital
Philadelphia, Pennsylvania
Chapter 7

Asad Khan, MD, FAAP
Anesthesia Resident
Robert Wood Johnson University Hospital
University of Medicine and Dentistry of New Jersey
Robert Wood Johnson Medical School
New Brunswick, New Jersey
Chapter 39

Khuram Khan, DO
Anesthesia Resident
Robert Wood Johnson University Hospital
University of Medicine and Dentistry of New Jersey
Robert Wood Johnson Medical School
New Brunswick, New Jersey
Chapter 40

Geza K. Kiss, MD
Associate Professor
Director of Regional Anesthesia and Acute Pain Management
Robert Wood Johnson University Hospital
University of Medicine and Dentistry of New Jersey
Robert Wood Johnson Medical School
New Brunswick, New Jersey
Chapters 15, 30

CONTRIBUTORS

Sabine Kost-Byerly, MD
Associate Professor
Anesthesiology and Critical Care Medicine, Pediatric Division
Johns Hopkins University School of Medicine
Department of Anesthesiology and Critical Care Medicine
Baltimore, Maryland
Chapter 29

Jonathan Kraidin, MD
Associate Professor of Anesthesiology
Chief, Section of Thoracic Anesthesia
Robert Wood Johnson University Hospital
University of Medicine and Dentistry of New Jersey
Robert Wood Johnson Medical School
New Brunswick, New Jersey
Chapters 26, 39, 43, 51

Ahdev Kuppasamy, MD
Anesthesia Pain Fellow
Robert Wood Johnson University Hospital
University of Medicine and Dentistry of New Jersey
Robert Wood Johnson Medical School
New Brunswick, New Jersey
Chapter 30

Robert Kyureghian, MD
Chief Resident
Department of Anesthesiology
Stony Brook University Medical Center
Stony Brook, New York
Chapter 25

Arlene Lamba, MD
Anesthesia Resident
Robert Wood Johnson University Hospital
University of Medicine and Dentistry of New Jersey
Robert Wood Johnson Medical School
New Brunswick, New Jersey
Chapter 5

John Langenfeld, MD
Associate Professor
Chief of Thoracic Surgery
Robert Wood Johnson University Hospital
University of Medicine and Dentistry of New Jersey
Robert Wood Johnson Medical School
New Brunswick, New Jersey
Chapter 26

Sarah LaSalle, DO
Anesthesia Resident
Robert Wood Johnson University Hospital
University of Medicine and Dentistry of New Jersey
Robert Wood Johnson Medical School
New Brunswick, New Jersey
Chapters 15, 30

Travis Lee, MD
Associate Professor
Department of Anesthesia
South Miami Hospital
South Miami, Florida
Chapter 47

Michael C. Lewis, MD
Professor Anesthesiology
Senior Associate Dean for Graduate Medical Education
University of Miami
Miller School of Medicine
Miami, Florida
Chapters 14, 17

Justin Long, MD
Resident
Anesthesiology and Critical Care Medicine
The Johns Hopkins Hospital
Baltimore, Maryland
Chapter 52

Raina Lourens, MD
Resident Physician
Department of Anesthesiology and Critical Care Medicine
Johns Hopkins Hospital
Baltimore, Maryland
Chapter 21

Joni Maga, MD
Assistant Professor
Department of Anesthesiology and
 Perioperative Pain Medicine
University of Miami
Miller School of Medicine
Miami, Florida
Chapter 33

Amreesh Mahil, MD
Resident in Anesthesiology
Northwestern University
Feinberg School of Medicine
Chicago, Illinois
Chapter 24

Rany Makaryus, MD
Assistant Professor
Department of Anesthesiology
Stony Brook University Medical Center
Stony Brook, New York
Chapter 25

Christian McDonough, MD
Instructor of Anesthesiology
Robert Wood Johnson University Hospital
University of Medicine and Dentistry of New Jersey
Robert Wood Johnson Medical School
New Brunswick, New Jersey
Chapter 39

Tejal Mehta, MD
Instructor
Department of Anesthesia
Robert Wood Johnson University Hospital
University of Medicine and Dentistry of New Jersey
Robert Wood Johnson Medical School
New Brunswick, New Jersey
Chapter 49

Carlos Mijares, MD
Assistant Professor of Anesthesiology
Anesthesiology
Miller Medical School
University of Miami
Miami, Florida
Chapter 17

Andres Missair, MD, DESRA
Assistant Professor
Anesthesiology and Acute Pain
University of Miami
Miller School of Medicine
Miami, Florida
Chapter 31

Nanhi Mitter, MD
Assistant Professor
Anesthesiology and Critical Care Medicine
Johns Hopkins Hospital
Baltimore, Maryland
Chapter 41

Luis Narciso, DO
Resident
Department of Anesthesiology
University of Miami
Miami, Florida
Chapter 33

Nicholas B. Nedeff, MD
Assistant Professor of Clinical Anesthesiology
Department of Anesthesiology
University of Miami
Miami, Florida
Chapter 47

Heather Nixon, MD
Assistant Professor
Department of Anesthesiology
University of Illinois at Chicago
Chicago, Illinois
Chapter 22

Obianuju Okocha, MD
Clinical Instructor
Department of Anesthesiology
Northwestern University
Feinberg School of Medicine
Chicago, Illinois
Chapter 1

Jean-Pierre Ouanes, DO
Assistant Professor
Anesthesia and Critical Care Medicine
Johns Hopkins University
Baltimore, Maryland
Chapter 32

Anjana Sahani Panjwani, MD
Resident, Department of Anesthesiology
Robert Wood Johnson University Hospital
University of Medicine and Dentistry of New Jersey
Robert Wood Johnson Medical School
New Brunswick, New Jersey
Chapter 27

Enrique Pantin, MD
Associate Professor of Anesthesiology
Division of Cardiac Anesthesia
Head, Section of Pediatric Anesthesia
Head, Section of Intraoperative Echocardiography
Robert Wood Johnson University Hospital
University of Medicine and Dentistry of New Jersey
Robert Wood Johnson Medical School
New Brunswick, New Jersey
Chapter 40

Christine Park, MD
Assistant Professor of Anesthesiology
Northwestern University
Feinberg School of Medicine
Chicago, Illinois
Chapters 48, 53, 56, 59

Shivani Patel, MBBS
Assistant Professor
Anesthesiology and Critical Care Medicine, Pediatric Division
Johns Hopkins University School of Medicine
Baltimore, Maryland
Chapter 29

CONTRIBUTORS

Edgar Pierre, MD
Assistant Professor
Department of Anesthesiology
University of Miami, Jackson Memorial Hospital
Miami, Florida
Chapter 8

Olya Polishchuk, MD
Resident in Anesthesiology
Northwestern University
Feinberg School of Medicine
Chicago, Illinois
Chapter 59

Sarah Olson Reck, MD
Assistant Professor
Department of Anesthesiology
Medical College of Wisconsin
Milwaukee, Wisconsin
Chapters 53, 56

Rebecca Reeves, DO
Anesthesiology and Critical Care Medicine
Johns Hopkins University School of Medicine
Department of Anesthesiology and Critical Care Medicine
Baltimore, Maryland
Chapter 45

Rafael M. Richards, MD, MS
Assistant Professor
Anesthesiology and Critical Care Medicine
Johns Hopkins University School of Medicine
Baltimore, Maryland
Chapter 52

Mark Rossberg, MD
Assistant Professor
Anesthesiology and Critical Care Medicine
The Johns Hopkins Hospital
Department of Anesthesiology and Critical Care Medicine
Johns Hopkins University School of Medicine
Baltimore, Maryland
Chapter 18

James A. Rothschild, MD
Chief Resident
Anesthesiology and Critical Care Medicine
Johns Hopkins University School of Medicine
Baltimore, Maryland
Chapter 58

Amanda Saab, MD
Fellow in Pediatric Anesthesiology
Department of Anesthesiology
University of Miami
Miami, Florida
Chapter 4

Deepak Saluja, MD
Assistant Professor Medicine in Cardiology
Robert Wood Johnson University Hospital
University of Medicine and Dentistry of New Jersey
Robert Wood Johnson Medical School
New Brunswick, New Jersey
Chapter 39

Rebecca Sangster, MD
Chief Resident
Department of Anesthesiology
Stony Brook University Medical Center
Stony Brook, New York
Chapter 28

Joy Schabel, MD
Associate Professor
Anesthesiology
Stony Brook University Medical Center
Stony Brook, New York
Chapter 25

Adam Schiavi, MD, PhD
Assistant Professor
Anesthesiology and Critical Care Medicine
Johns Hopkins University School of Medicine
Baltimore, Maryland
Chapter 44

Robin J. Schiller, DMD
Resident
Department of Anesthesia
Stony Brook University Medical Center
Stony Brook, New York
Chapter 25

Deborah Schwengel, MD
Residency Program Director
Anesthesiology and Critical Care Medicine
The Johns Hopkins Hospital
Department of Anesthesiology and Critical Care Medicine
Johns Hopkins University School of Medicine
Baltimore, Maryland
Chapters 6, 10, 18, 46

Peggy Seidman, MD
Associate Professor
Stony Brook University Medical Center
Stony Brook, New York
Chapter 12

Adam Sewell, MD
Resident
Johns Hopkins University School of Medicine
Baltimore, Maryland
Chapter 38

Mark Slomovits, MD
Resident, Department of Anesthesiology
Robert Wood Johnson University Hospital
University of Medicine and Dentistry of New Jersey
Robert Wood Johnson Medical School
New Brunswick, New Jersey
Chapter 54

Al Solina, MD
Professor, Vice Chairman
Chief of Cardiac Anesthesia
Anesthesia
Robert Wood Johnson Medical School
New Brunswick, New Jersey
Chapter 2

Fouad Souki, MD
Resident, Department of Anesthesiology
Jackson Memorial Hospital
Miami, Florida
Chapter 14

Jochen Steppan, MD
Resident, Anesthesiology and Critical Care Medicine
Johns Hopkins University
Baltimore, Maryland
Chapter 41

Neil Stockmaster, MD
Cardiothoracic Surgery Fellow
Department of Surgery, Division of Cardiothoracic Surgery
Robert Wood Johnson University Hospital
University of Medicine and Dentistry of New Jersey
Robert Wood Johnson Medical School
New Brunswick, New Jersey
Chapter 19

Lalitha Sundararaman, MBBS, MD
Resident
Department of Anesthesiology and Critical Care
University of Miami
Jackson Memorial Hospital
Miami, Florida
Chapter 17

Jordan Taylor, MD
Resident, Department of Anesthesiology
University of Miami
Jackson Memorial Hospital
Miami, Florida
Chapter 8

Justin Thampi, MD
Resident, Department of Anesthesiology
Jackson Memorial Hospital
University of Miami
Miami, Florida
Chapter 47

Luke S. Theilken, MD
Instructor
Department of Anesthesiology
Northwestern University
Feinberg School of Medicine
Chicago, Illinois
Chapter 50

Brandon Togioka, MD
Assistant Professor
Anesthesiology and Critical Care Medicine
Johns Hopkins Hospital
Baltimore, Maryland
Chapter 32

J. Gabriel Tsang, MBBS
Resident
Anesthesiology and Critical Care Medicine
Johns Hopkins Hospital
Baltimore, Maryland
Chapter 35

Emmett Whitaker, MD
Assistant Professor
Anesthesiology and Critical Care Medicine
Johns Hopkins Medical Institutions
Baltimore, Maryland
Chapter 60

Jamie Wingate, MD
Resident
Anesthesiology and Critical Care Medicine
Johns Hopkins
Baltimore, Maryland
Chapter 18

CONTRIBUTORS

Bradford Winters, PhD, MD
Assistant Professor
Anesthesiology and Critical Care Medicine
Johns Hopkins University School of Medicine
Baltimore, Maryland
Chapter 58

Michael Wong, MD
Anesthesia Resident
Department of Anesthesia
Robert Wood Johnson University Hospital
University of Medicine and Dentistry of New Jersey
Robert Wood Johnson Medical School
New Brunswick, New Jersey
Chapter 20

Meltem Yilmaz, MD
Assistant Professor of Anesthesiology
Northwestern University
Feinberg School of Medicine
Chicago, Illinois
Chapter 13

Bo-Lu Zhou, MD
Cardiothoracic Anesthesia Fellow
Robert Wood Johnson University Hospital
University of Medicine and Dentistry of New Jersey
Robert Wood Johnson Medical School
Department of Anesthesia
New Brunswick, New Jersey
Chapter 2

PART I

VENOUS ACCESS

CHAPTER 1
PERIPHERAL INTRAVENOUS (IV) ACCESS

OBIANUJU OKOCHA

"Before we get started, I just wanted to let you know, I have difficult veins and I want only the anesthesiologist to put in my IV."

Anonymous patient

INTRODUCTION

Why: It is the only route that ensures the easiest administration and fastest delivery of drugs and fluids into the systemic circulation.

When: In all adult cases requiring any anesthetic and in almost all pediatric procedures.

How: Now, here's where you get paid to do a proficient job and make it look easy. Especially when everyone else fails, you are the go-to person.

BACKGROUND

Intravenous cannulation has come a long way. The first recorded infusion of any sort dates back to 1492 when blood transfusion was done by anastomosing the donor and recipient veins. By the mid-1600s, injections were given through tiny silver tubes, and for almost two centuries that was all we had. The mid-1800s heralded the invention of hollow needles, but it was not until 1945 that the first plastic catheter was made. The major breakthrough in intravenous cannulation occurred in 1950, when an anesthesiology resident at the Mayo Clinic invented the Rochester plastic needle. (Yes, if it were not for anesthesiology, IV advancement would probably still be in the Stone Age.) This plastic needle prevented infiltration, prevented leaking at the IV site, and allowed patients to be mobile (much like we know IVs today). During this time, plastic tubing replaced rubber IV tubing.

IV 101

In thinking about the planned procedure, you have to decide what IV size is necessary. Putting a 24-gauge IV in a patient with visibly large veins for, say, a kidney transplant procedure, would be very poor form. If you anticipate significant, potentially rapid blood loss, a central line is indicated. (This does not necessarily have to occur while the patient is awake.) You would then perform a quick history and physical to assess potentially how difficult IV placement may be (as in IV drug addicts, patients with a history of chemotherapy, or patients with a history of difficult IV stick) or if there any contraindications, such as the breast cancer patient who has had lymph nodes resected or the patient with end-stage renal disease who has an arteriovenous (AV) fistula. These contraindications should go out the window in the event of an emergency. Now, gather your equipment:

- Gloves
- Tourniquet (absolutely contraindicated for the placement of an IV in the external jugular vein)
- Chloraprep wipe
- Tuberculin (TB) syringe/needle containing local anesthetic
- IV catheter (angiocatheter)
- IV fluid/tubing already set up for connection to the catheter or a Luer lock with saline flush
- Tegaderm and tape to secure IV (Figure 1-1)

TECHNIQUE

Talk with the patient as you place the IV; explain what you are doing as you do it. Use soothing descriptions, such as "You are going to feel a little pinch" instead of "You are going to feel a sharp stick, and then a burning sensation." Believe it or not, it helps. Patients are less likely to withdraw their arm or vocalize pain. The techniques for placing the IV are as follows (Figures 1-2 through 1-7):

- Place the tourniquet close to the vein of interest.
- Avoid making the tourniquet too tight, as this may prevent arterial flow, which in turn prevents the vein from filling up.
- Cannulation is easier at the junction where veins meet.
- Place a skin wheal of local anesthetic where you plan on sticking.
- Hold the limb such that, using your thumb, you can pull the skin taut.
- Stick the angiocatheter through the skin and into the vein with your angle parallel to the skin.
- Advance the angiocatheter until you see the flash of blood filling the hub of the needle.
- Keeping the skin still taut, advance the catheter over the needle into the vein.
- Undo the tourniquet and compress the vein just distal to where the tip of the catheter is placed (this prevents bleeding out of the catheter).
- Retract/remove the needle.
- Connect the Luer lock or the IV tubing and secure it to the catheter.
- Place a Tegaderm dressing over the catheter and use tape to secure the IV.
- Flush the Luer lock or open the IV and make sure the IV works and is not infiltrated.
- Put all sharps in the sharps container.
- If there is any blood on the floor, take the time to clean it up. Patients and their families will assume that the care and neatness you demonstrate with this procedure indicates how careful you are with your overall treatment. And they are right.

EXTERNAL JUGULAR

Equipment
- See the above list.

Technique

Think of the external jugular (EJ) as a central line. Place the patient in the Trendelenburg position to allow for engorgement of the EJ. The IV should be placed in the EJ only if the vein is visible; otherwise, the catheter could be placed anywhere, including the carotid. The technique is otherwise the same as putting an IV in a limb (reminder: there is no tourniquet used). It helps to keep your angle of approach almost flat with the plane of the skin, but that is not always easy to do. Also, since the EJ is highly collapsible, you may go through and through the vein and see a "flash" only upon the slow withdrawal of the needle.

The EJ is superficial! You can see it with your own eyes, right? Not too long ago, a patient suffered a pneumothorax after an IV was placed in the EJ vein (the catheter was advanced several centimeters). You should approach EJ vein cannulation as you would a central line, but not literally. Pneumothorax is never included as a complication when "consenting" a patient for placement of a peripheral IV.

PEDIATRICS

Pediatric patients, especially infants, can be difficult IV sticks for exactly the reason that they are so cute: their chubbiness. In most pediatric cases, the IV is placed once inhalation induction is achieved. This makes IV placement easier than when the patient is awake because the veins become dilated and the patient is immobile. In the awake patient, it is definitely a challenge. The key is making sure the skin is adequately topically anesthetized and that the patient is amenable (or "encourage" them to be amenable with oral/IM medications versus administering nitrous oxide where applicable). Keep in mind that sometimes, whether the patient has been induced or awake, you may need to bring in the "big guns" (see the "Pearls" section below).

Equipment
- Same as above, plus EMLA cream (for the awake patient), which should be applied at least 30 minutes prior.

Technique
- Same as above.

THERE ARE SABOTEURS EVERYWHERE

- Any IV that was placed by someone else should be scrutinized before use. Make sure it works well and is secured properly before proceeding to the operating room.
- When in doubt, place another IV.
- If you have asked your assistant to run the IV fluid to make sure the IV works, don't take their word for it, especially if there is no flow. Make sure there are no kinks in the tubing or that the tubing was not inadvertently clamped before pulling out the IV catheter that you just placed.
- Try to place IVs in veins that will be readily visible once the patient is positioned for the procedure.

This will allow you to easily troubleshoot an IV (especially if the IV becomes infiltrated).
- Similarly, make sure the IV runs after the patient is positioned. Once the drapes are on, life gets difficult.
- Simply because there are drugs/fluids infusing via the pump through an IV does not mean that the IV works. Depending on the rate of infusion, fluids can be pumped in the subcutaneous tissue. Briefly disconnect the infusion and flush the IV with 5 to 10 mL of saline. If resistance is encountered or swelling and pain are noted, place another IV.
- Peripherally inserted central catheter (PICC) lines are not your friend (somehow the surgeons don't understand why you are putting in another IV). Patients with a history of difficult IV sticks are most likely to have a PICC line. You may be able to induce anesthesia with the PICC line but not to give adequate fluids. Again, if you anticipate large volume shifts, place a central line.

PEARLS

- There are "standard" veins that may not be visible, but they are in the same spot for just about everyone, young and old: between the fourth and fifth metacarpal bones and the anatomical snuff box.
- Look at the upper arm past the antecubital fossa and consider the palmar surface of the wrist.
- Don't be afraid to place a peripheral IV in the lower extremity. If you have looked at both arms and the EJ and there is nothing visible or you have tried cannulating "hidden" veins in vain, take a look at the feet.

The saphenous vein is another one of those "hidden" veins; it lies just anterior to the medial malleolus.
- Keep in mind that if you do place a central line, the patient may be required to go to the ICU/Step-Down Unit as a result. Talk about penny wise, pound foolish! An IV in the foot can be a temporary IV pending placement of a PICC. Also, for outpatient procedures, placing a central line (due to a difficult stick) because you don't want to place an IV in the foot may be overkill, and cumbersome for ambulating patients.
- Bringing in the "big guns": You may need to use an ultrasound machine when you anticipate a difficult stick, but this is limited by how well you know how to use this equipment. Practice using the ultrasound when placing an IV in veins that are readily visible so that you will know what to look for with difficult sticks. The transilluminator is another piece of equipment that can be used for difficult sticks. It is mostly useful in pediatric patients since light easily penetrates their tissues (their bones are not fully calcified).

CONCLUSION

Placing an IV is the one skill you inevitably will have. You will likely place more IVs than you will do intubations. As an anesthesiologist, you will also likely place more difficult IVs than will the nurses, phlebotomists, or anyone else. Learn how to place IVs properly, and, as with driving a car (you know how you feel when you see bad drivers), your good technique will become second nature to you.

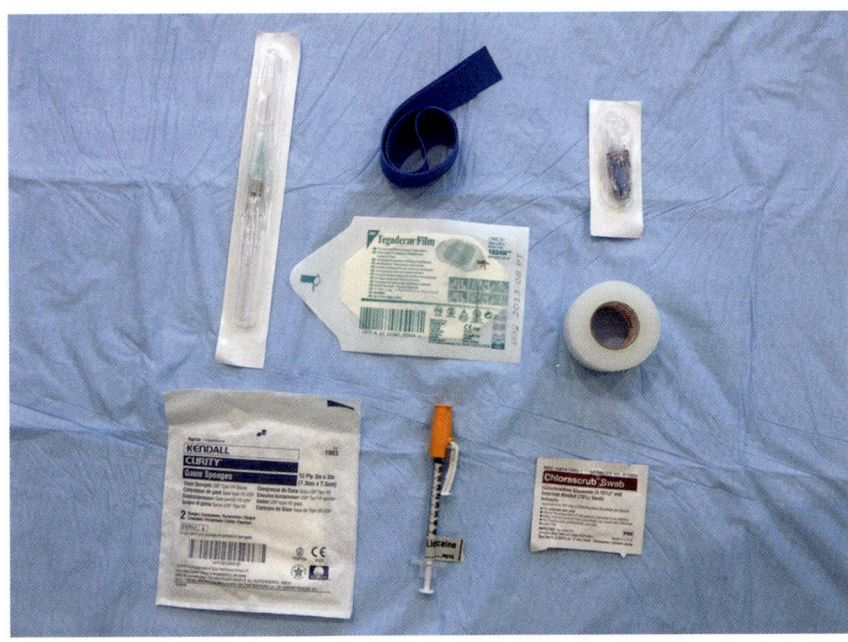

FIGURE 1-1 Equipment needed for IV placement.

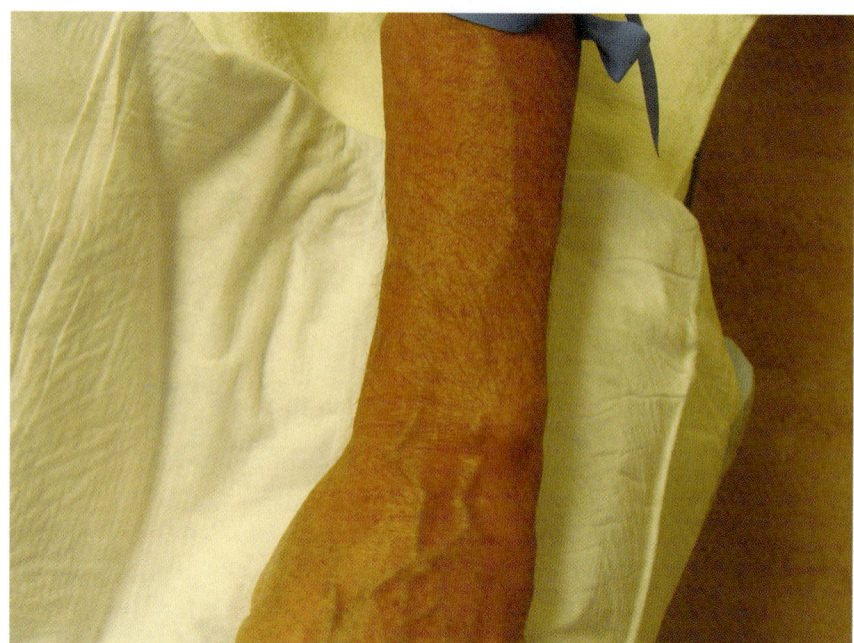

FIGURE 1-2 Notice the Y or even the X configuration that the veins form. Aim for the point where the veins meet.

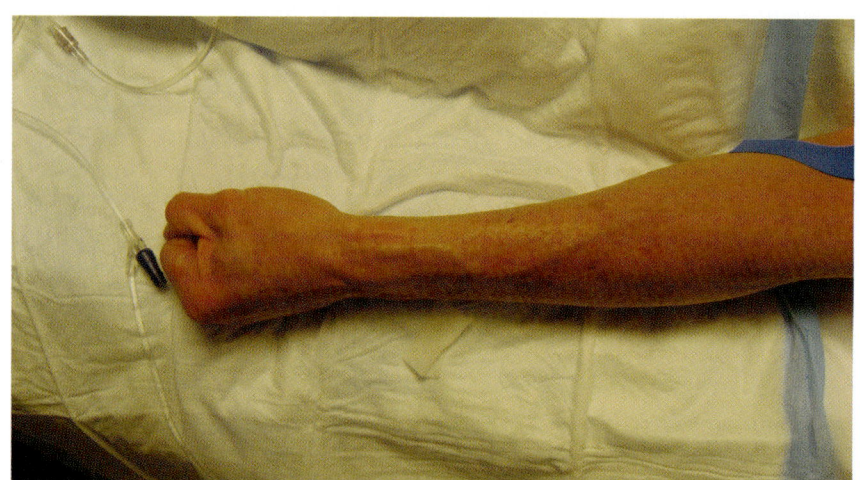

FIGURE 1-3 This is one of those straight veins that make for a good IV stick. Don't you wish all veins looked like this?

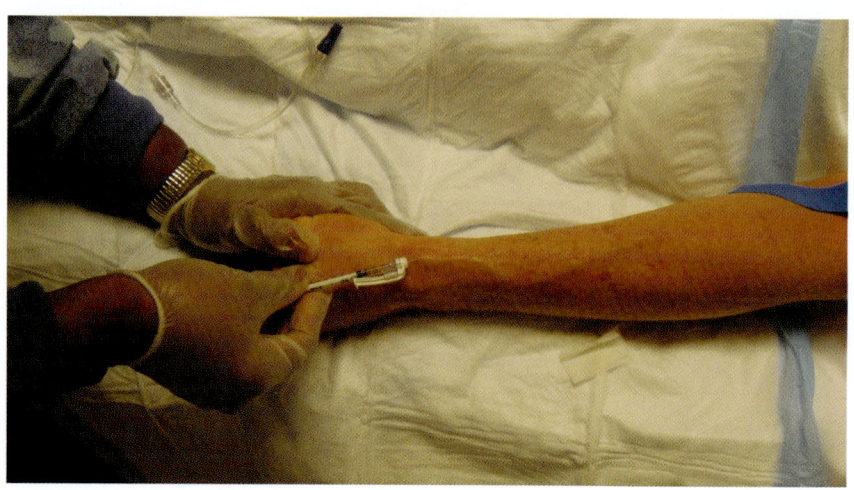

FIGURE 1-4 Place the local anesthetic superficially, forming a wheal.

Chapter 1 PERIPHERAL INTRAVENOUS (IV) ACCESS

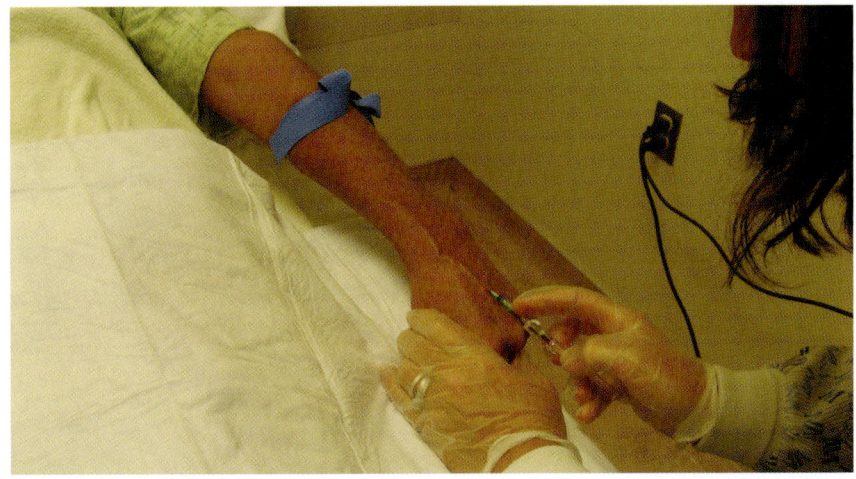

FIGURE 1-5 Aim for the vein, keeping the angle parallel to the skin. Remember to keep the skin taut while advancing the catheter.

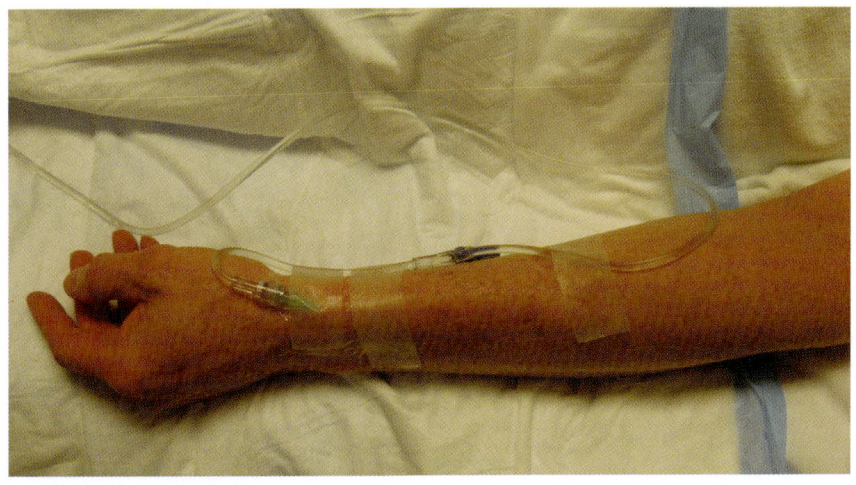

FIGURE 1-6 Once the IV is in place, tape it securely. Applying clear tape allows you see if the vein becomes infiltrated, if there is leakage, and the source of the leakage.

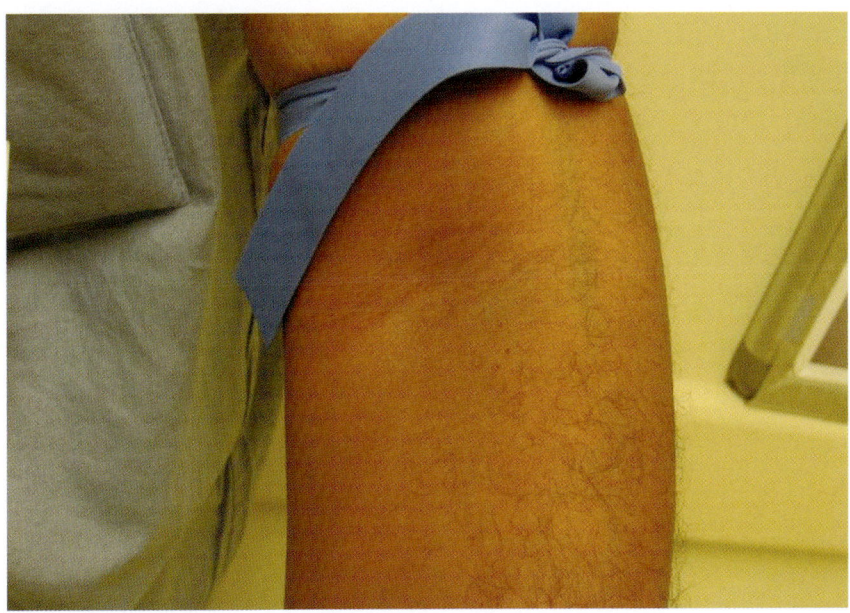

FIGURE 1-7 Veins in the antecubital fossa are readily visible; if not, they are usually palpable. Confirm it is a vein you are palpating by having the patient flex his/her arm (a tendon will feel firm even when the arm is flexed, but a vein will not).

SUGGESTED READING

Dutt-Gupta J, Bown T, Cyna AM. Effect of communication on pain during intravenous cannulation: a randomized controlled trial. *Br J Anaesth* 2007;99(6):871–875.
Talking with patient during IV placement helps create a better experience during this time.

Millam D. The history of intravenous therapy. *J Intravenous Nurs* 1996;19(1):5–14.
This article looks at the origins of intravenous therapy including IV cannulation.

Ortega R, Sekhar P, Song M, et al. Peripheral intravenuous cannulation. *N Engl J Med* 2008;359:e26.
This article provides a step-by-step approach to peripheral IV placement. It makes the procedure look so easy that even an internist can place an IV.

Rogers TL, Ostrow CL. The use of EMLA cream to decrease venipuncture pain in children. *J Pediatr Nurs* 2004;19(1):33–39.
Decreasing pain during pediatric IV cannulation will allow for easier placement.

Stein JC, Cole W, Kramer N, Quinn J. Ultrasound-guided peripheral intravenous cannulation in emergency department patients with difficult IV access. *Acad Emerg Med* 2004;11(5):581–582.
In patients with difficult IV access, ultrasound guidance helps identify vessels, thereby aiding cannulation.

CHAPTER 2

THE INTERNAL JUGULAR (IJ) LINE

AL SOLINA
BO-LU ZHOU

It is in men as in soils, where sometimes there is a vein of gold which the owner knows not.

Jonathan Swift

INTRODUCTION

There are certain skills that every good cardiac anesthesiologist must have. Efficiently and safely placing an IJ line is certainly one of them. You should be able to do this in your sleep, because you may have to!

The IJ is most often the final common pathway to the heart for the cardiac anesthesiologist. It is utilized as a volume line, a drug push line, a vasoactive substance drip line, and as a conduit through which to place other catheters. Acquiring the skill to place an IJ line safely and efficiently is of paramount importance. This skill involves knowledge of the relational anatomy of the vessel, the various types of catheters that are available, complications and their management, and the use of ultrasound (US) techniques as they are applied to line placement, as well as basic catheterization skills.

WHY IS THE RIGHT INTERNAL JUGULAR (RIJ) THE "FAVORITE SON"?

- The RIJ is frequently exposed to the anesthesiologist for cannulation, inspection, and manipulation purposes even after the drapes are set up.
- The RIJ provides a straight pathway to the heart, which facilitates the passage of catheters and wires to it.
- The RIJ frequently remains unscathed even after all the peripheral veins have been consumed or damaged beyond repair by non-anesthesiology sorts.
- The RIJ catheter runs nicely even when a sternal retractor is in place, a feat that a subclavian line is ill-prepared to perform.
- The RIJ is easy to interrogate by US.
- The RIJ is accessible far enough away from the pleura to render a pneumothorax misadventure less likely than when utilizing the subclavian approach.
- The RIJ is less likely to cause a chylothorax (by virtue of a thoracic duct injury) on the right than on the left.
- When time counts, it's a short distance for emergency epinephrine and other medications to travel to get into the heart.
- A good assortment of catheters accommodate the IJ.
- There is a high success rate for cannulation.
- Unlike with the subclavian approach, it is easy to compress the IJ site in the event of a "misadventure" resulting in bleeding.
- The RIJ provides good access to the right side of the heart for aspiration of air emboli.
- The RIJ is more reliably found at the apex of Sédillot's triangle than is the left internal jugular (LIJ).[1]

INDICATIONS: WHAT IS THE IJ LINE USED FOR?

- Rapid infusion of fluids
- Drug administration: vasoactive drip medication
- Hyperalimentation
- Chemotherapy
- Prolonged antibiotic therapy
- Central venous pressure monitoring
- Pulmonary artery catheterization
- Transvenous cardiac pacing
- Temporary hemodialysis
- Aspiration of air emboli

RELATIVE CONTRAINDICATIONS, OR "AT LEAST STOP, AND PROCEED WITH CAUTION!"

- Distorted anatomy
- Previous neck dissection
- Neck radiation
- Trauma
- Prior carotid surgery
- Superior vena cava (SVC) obstruction
- Significant coagulopathy
- Other in-situ lines/wires sharing the anatomy

LET'S TALK ANATOMY

- The vein originates at the jugular foramen and runs down in the neck to terminate behind the sternoclavicular joint (medial side of the clavicle), where it joins the subclavian vein.
- It lies alongside the carotid artery and the vagus nerve within the carotid sheath. The vein is initially posterior to, then lateral to, and then anterolateral to the carotid artery during its descent in the neck. The vein lies most superficially in the upper part of the neck.
- At the level of the thyroid cartilage the vein lies deep to the sternomastoid muscle. As it passes toward the thorax, it emerges from behind the muscle and comes to lie at the apex of the triangle between the sternal and clavicular insertions of the muscle.
- On both ends of the IJ vein there is a bulb (superior and inferior). The inferior jugular bulb contains a bicuspid valve that permits the flow of blood toward the heart.
- On the left side of the neck the IJ vein lies anterior to the thoracic duct. The right side is preferred to avoid the risk of thoracic duct injury. In addition, the right side offers a more direct access to the superior vena cava.
- If you go in on the right, you have a straight shot all the way, but on the left, the vessel takes a "right turn" once you enter the thorax, so a vigorous push with a dilator could tear through the vessel at this right turn and cause a hemothorax. Some manufacturers offer a "short sheath" catheter for use on the left side for just this reason.

PROCEDURE AND APPROACH: OK, HOW DO WE PLACE AN IJ LINE?

Before anything else, preparation is the key to success.
Alexander Graham Bell

- **Patient preparation**
  - Identify the patient and confirm the intended surgical procedure.
  - Review medical history for relative contraindications.
    - Coagulopathy
      - Bleeding from an IJ procedure is usually compressible, and many cardiac and vascular patients will be therapeutically anticoagulated.
    - Having simultaneous carotid/neck surgery that precludes using a particular side.
    - Presence of preexisting catheters/wires.
  - Obtain and document informed consent for the procedure.
  - "Do unto others as you would have others do unto you." If the line is to be placed while the patient is awake, sedation as tolerated is indicated, and much appreciated by the patient who knows that tachycardia is bad for myocardial supply and demand.
  - The patient should be appropriately monitored. Listen to the electrocardiogram (ECG) for arrhythmias incited by those pesky guidewires. A pulse oximeter is requisite.
  - Controlling your work space.
    - Ensure that you have adequate room around the patient so that your movement is not encumbered and sterility is not compromised.
  - Place the patient in a "universal lining position" that allows everyone who may help with the procedure (IV, A-line, etc.) to participate without having to move the patient or the bed/stretcher/table. Move the ECG leads that the floor or holding-area nurse infuriatingly may have placed right in your way, and tape the nasal oxygen tubing over the forehead to get it away from the field. Move the hanging IV tubing, which invariably tries to contaminate your field, out of the way. Lower the side rails (while you are in direct attendance), and remove the head board if it protrudes in your way. Place the patient in the Trendelenburg position if physiologically tolerated, as this increases the size of the IJ and reduces the risk of an air embolism.
  - Open your selected kit, place a Swan catheter and an US sleeve on your field if you will need them, so that you maximize your subsequent autonomy (and minimize waiting for your assistants to supply them later).
  - Make sure that you have immediate access to a garbage bin for contaminated materials and to a sharps container so that refuse can be appropriately and safely disposed.

- Neatness counts. Not only will you ingratiate yourself with the housekeeping staff, but you will help to create a safe work environment, and you will look professional at the same time. Real professionals leave the work area the way they found it. Throw out the garbage as you create it! Don't double-handle dirty and sometimes sharp refuse.
- "Cleanliness is next to godliness."
  - Wash your hands. Wear sterile gloves, a gown, a facemask, and protect your eyes, too!
  - Check the guidelines for sterility that are promulgated by the Joint Commission on Accreditation of Healthcare Organizations (JCAHO), the Centers for Disease Control and Prevention (CDC), and the Department of Health on a regular basis, as this is a bit of a moving target, especially in view of new "pay-for-performance" initiatives that are sure to increase in number and scope.[2]
- **Selecting a catheter and kit**
  - There are myriad kits and catheters to suit your needs. It behooves the users to familiarize themselves with the plethora of catheters and options that are available. Kits should contain chlorhexidine preparation sticks, sterile local anesthetic, and a see-through drape (patients feel less claustrophobic if they can see out) that covers a large part of the body. Typical catheters include:
    - Triple-lumen catheters: These catheters have relatively limited flow capacity, but they provide central access, enable central venous pressure (CVP) monitoring, and are tolerated postoperatively on the wards, without the need to switch the catheter out at the most inopportune moment (and without compensation in most cases).
    - Large-gauge "Cordis" (actually a brand, not a type, like "Scotch" tape) catheters: An 8.5-French (F) single-lumen catheter is most commonly used for routine applications. Double-lumen 9F and triple-lumen 9.5F (aka "Big Momma") are used when higher flow rates are required (e.g., for bloody trauma, redo hearts, deep circulation arrest cases, etc.).
    - Specialty catheters: There are specialty catheters that are used in specific situations (e.g., to place special "endovent" and "endoplegia" catheters for minimally invasive valve surgery) (Figure 2-1).
- **The anatomical landmark (i.e., "blind man's") approach**
  - Create a safe work space and construct a sterile field as delineated above.
  - Place the patient in the Trendelenburg position and rotate the head away from the side that you are attempting to place the line on. Don't over-rotate the neck; the lateral separation between the carotid artery and the IJ vein is maximized with something less than 45 degrees of rotation. We will discuss this again later in the section that describes the use of US for line placement.
  - Get the kit ready.
    - We have seen many IJ attempts fail because operators did not have the tray well prepared and they then required too much time and motion between steps, therefore allowing patient movement. Have everything prepared before you make your first move! Being and looking professional is all about preparation.
  - Delineate the anatomy
    - Anterior approach: We favor this approach, as your needle direction is away from the carotid artery.
      - ▲ Locate the triangle formed by the clavicle and the sternal and clavicular heads of the sternocleidomastoid muscle (Sédillot's triangle; it must be cool to have a triangle named after you!).
      - ▲ With an anterior approach, your target is near the top of the triangle, at least three finger breadths above the clavicle, if possible (this puts your needle further away from the pleura). This usually places you caudad to the external jugular vein, which sometimes crosses the neck near the apex of the triangle.
      - ▲ In cadaveric studies the apex of Sédillot's triangle accurately locates the IJ 97% of the time on the right, but only 79% on the left.[3]
      - ▲ The IJ is usually largest below the level of the cricoid cartilage.
      - ▲ You should be lateral to "Big Red" (the carotid artery), but you don't want to massage, push on, or poke the carotid too much for fear of disturbing the flow or the plaques inside of it.
      - ▲ You can't pull the carotid medially away from the IJ, as it is contained in the sheath.
      - ▲ You don't want to start too far lateral, because then in order to get into the IJ you would need to head back medially, which puts you into the trajectory of Big Red. Rather, make your primary attempt with the finder needle lateral to the carotid but close to it. Point in the lateral direction, toward where the nipple should be.

- Posterior approach
  ▲ Locate a point one third of the way from the clavicle on a line running from the sternal head of the clavicle to the mastoid process.
  ▲ Advance the needle through the skin at a 30- to 40-degree angle, in an inferior and medial direction until entering the IJ vein.
- Administer an adequate amount of local anesthetic.
  - Deposit the local anesthetic with a thin needle (e.g., 21 gauge [G]) of adequate length to reach the tissue within the intended trajectory.
  - Don't place so much local anesthetic subcutaneously so as to completely obscure your landmarks.
  - This should not be a torture session. Keep your patient comfortable.
- Finding the vessel
  - Use a thin (e.g., 21 G) 1.5- to 2.0-inch needle at about a 30-degree angle to the skin to find the IJ. If you don't get the IJ on the first pass, don't fret, and stay calm! It happens. Sometimes even highly experienced professionals need more than one pass with the finder! We suggest making an orderly sweep heading laterally, away from the carotid, thus giving yourself a chance to succeed without breaking the plane that heads you back medially toward Big Red. If that fails, then start fanning back medially. If that doesn't work, we recommend that you recheck your landmarks, and consider using an US!
  - When making the orderly sweep, progress from each attempt to the next without hesitation. Do not persevere with the same angle and depth that just led to failure. Move on! We see residents moving in and out of the same site/trajectory incessantly, as if not giving up will engender success! (Figure 2-2)
- The finder is now in the IJ. Now what?
  - Some professionals leave the finder in and place the larger needle or angiocatheter right next to it and approximate the same angle and direction that was successful. Others (like myself) feel that it is easier and more accurate to simply get that finder out of the way altogether.
  - Whatever you do, don't allow any movement now! Don't allow the anatomy to rotate on you.
  - Place the angiocatheter or long needle ("harpoon") in the vessel and obtain completely free blood flow.
  - Once you have free flow with the harpoon or angiocatheter, do not move them. We repeat, do not move them! More lines are lost at this time than at any other. You must be deliberate here. Keep that vessel secured. Don't move the fingers that are holding the angiocatheter or harpoon. Don't allow the patient's head to rotate either. Carefully remove the syringe, and advance the wire in to the vessel. Advance an angiocatheter into the vessel. If using an angiocatheter, instead of the harpoon, you may float the catheter into the vessel primarily, without the use of a wire, thus saving a step if you intend to replace the harpoon with an angiocatheter for the purpose of transducing the line (Figure 2-3).
- Confirm that you are in the IJ.
  - Confirm by "transducing" the vessel with the "poor man's technique," which entails connecting it to an IV tubing extension, and holding the free end above the level of the heart. If you are in Big Red territory, the blood keeps rising up the tube, all the way to the top, and spills over (assuming that the patient has a reasonable blood pressure). Of course, patients with high right heart pressures may have a column of blood that rises even if the catheter is properly placed in the low pressure (i.e., venous) system (Figure 2-4).
  - "Transduce" 100% of the time, even during an emergency! It only takes a couple of seconds.
  - Some operators favor confirmation of placement with an angiocatheter in place, rather than through the harpoon, because you may confirm placement with the harpoon, and then have the needle move through the vessel, before you exchange the harpoon for the final catheter. This error is harder to commit when you transduce through an angiocatheter, as the catheter tends not to migrate through the vessel as easily.
  - Be careful about using the color of the blood return to determine placement. Arterial blood could be fairly desaturated in some ill patients who need neck lines.
- Placement of the guidewire
  - Place the wire back into the vessel, being careful of precipitating arrhythmias. Mechanically induced arrhythmias are usually transient, but one must be careful.
  - "Moderation in all things." The wire should pass easily. **NEVER FORCE THE GUIDEWIRE!!**
  - Failure to pass the guidewire could be due to a turn in the vessel, an obstruction in the vessel, rotation of the head creating a temporary occlusion of the vessel, or the wire not being in an actual vessel.

- If it doesn't feel right, it probably isn't! Call for help, or ask for a "do over."
- How much wire?
  ▲ The wire has a flexible-J end, but has been known to inflict damage nonetheless (e.g., in arrhythmias, entrapment of other wires or devices, and perforation of vessels or the heart itself). Don't insert more wire than you need.
  ▲ RIJ to RA-SVC junction = 16 cm.[4]
  ▲ LIJ to RA-SVC junction = 19 cm.[4]
- **Don't lose the wire!** You lose big style points if you let the patient slurp up the wire. This requires a trip to the radiology suite and the help of an interventional radiologist, which can be very embarrassing (Figure 2-5).
- Make a skin nick to allow for passage of the dilator or dilator/catheter.
  - You don't need to bury the full length of the scalpel in the neck to accomplish this. A properly placed relatively shallow nick that gets through the skin will afford safe passage and not risk lacerating the vessel itself. We slide the blade down the wire at an angle, with the blade pointed away from the carotid artery. A single, shallow, properly placed incision will do the trick. When done thusly, you will obviate the need to butcher the insertion site (Figure 2-6).
- "This too, shall pass." Slide the catheter/dilator over the wire.
  - Don't kink the wire or you will need to start the whole process over.
  - The catheter should slide over the wire without the need for excessive force. You don't need to be strong to do this. It's all technique—just like golf. The catheter and dilator only need to be together to get through the skin and subcutaneous tissue (2 to 3 cm). Once you "pop" through this tissue, you should advance the catheter over the dilator. The dilator is stiff and sharp. It wants to "seek and destroy" anything in its path, including important bits of anatomy. If the catheter doesn't slide over the wire easily, then do the following:
    ▲ Make sure that the wire is not kinked and moves freely within the catheter.
    ▲ Ensure that the skin nick is adequate (i.e., no skin tags).
    ▲ Hold the skin taut when advancing the catheter.
    ▲ Make sure that the angle of catheter insertion is "anatomical" (i.e., parallel to the direction of the vessel).
    ▲ Place the head in a relatively neutral anatomical position.
    ▲ Make sure that the dilator is fully inserted in the catheter, so that there is a smooth and even surface at the distal end of the catheter as it pierces through the tissue.
    ▲ Make sure that catheter has not been damaged by previous attempts. It is difficult and dangerous to pass a catheter that has a burr on the end of it.
    ▲ "Pride cometh before the fall." Don't force the issue! Call for help. **If it doesn't feel right, it probably isn't!** (Figure 2-7)
- Once the catheter has been successfully placed, remove the dilator, and ensure good blood return.
  - If you don't have free return of blood, there are two distinct possibilities. The catheter lumen may be against the vessel wall, or you are not in the vessel! (Figure 2-8)
- Make sure that the catheter is placed at a proper depth.
  - Triple-lumen catheters inserted to a depth no greater than 12 cm are less likely to damage the right heart or precipitate arrhythmias. This places the catheter 3 to 4 cm above the atriocaval junction.
  - The RIJ is about 16 cm from the atriocaval junction.[4]
  - The LIJ is about 19 cm from the atriocaval junction.
  - Large-bore catheters should be completely inserted because they will kink if secured when partially out.
- Secure the catheter with heavy-gauge suture, as if someone's life may depend upon it. Consider using a purse-string suture around the insertion site for large-bore catheters (i.e., greater than 9F) (Figure 2-9).
- If not floating a pulmonary artery catheter through the catheter, remember to occlude the valved lumen with the provided cap.
- Place an antibacterial ring around the catheter site and dress the catheter appropriately.
- Aspirate the air in the line and flush the catheter.
- Many of the commercially available flush syringes are not actually sterile (check the packaging), so don't handle them until you are all done with your sterile work.
- **CLEAN UP YOUR MESS!**
- Immediate x-ray confirmation is recommended before use, but is frequently not done in the operating room setting, especially for a case involving sternotomy.

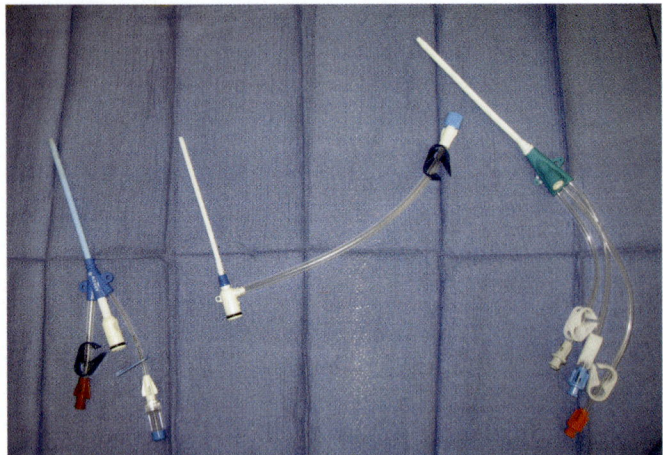

FIGURE 2-1 Large-bore central IV catheters. From left to right: a 9.0F double-lumen catheter, an 8.5-F single-lumen catheter, and a 9.5F triple-lumen "Big Mama" catheter.

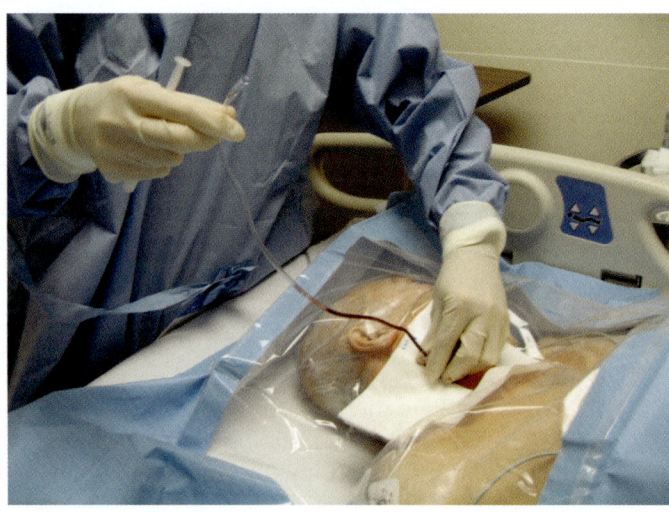

FIGURE 2-4 Transducing the catheter to confirm placement in the "low pressure system."

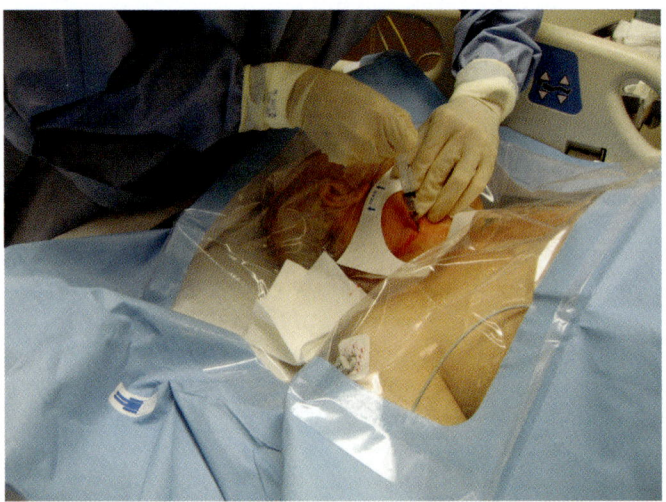

FIGURE 2-2 Finding the vessel.

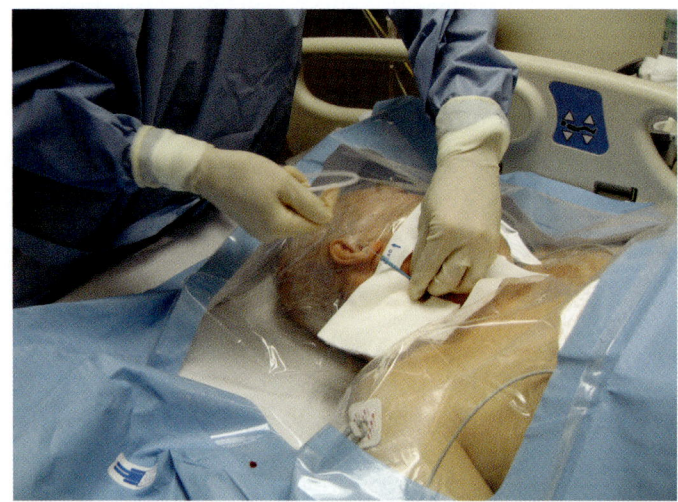

FIGURE 2-5 Advancing the wire.

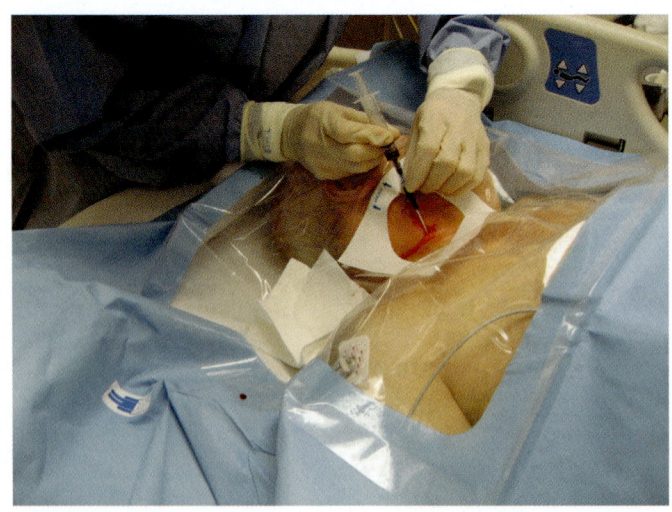

FIGURE 2-3 Advancing the angiocatheter.

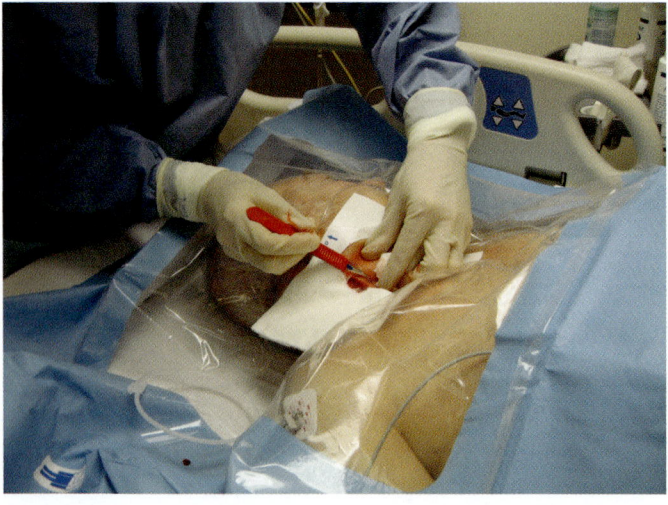

FIGURE 2-6 Making a skin nick.

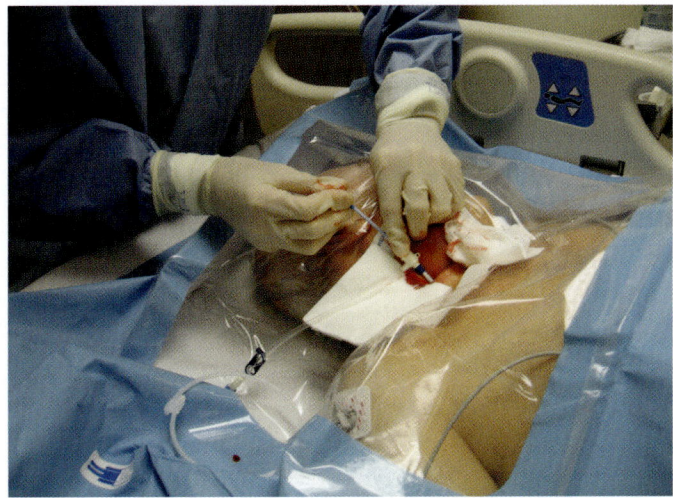

FIGURE 2-7 Advance the catheter over the dilator.

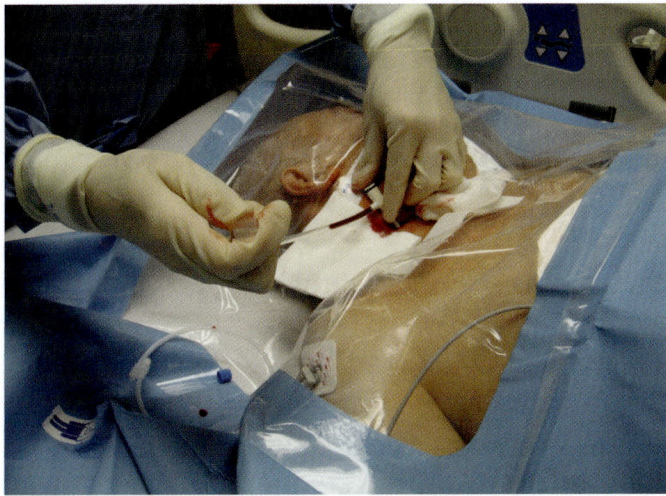

FIGURE 2-8 Confirm good blood return.

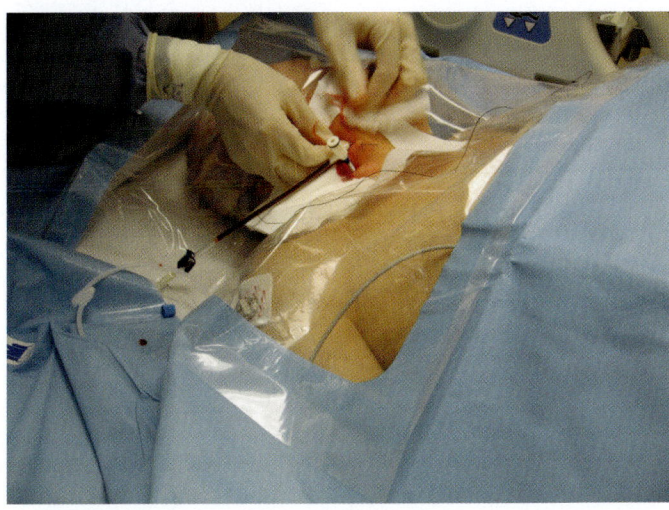

FIGURE 2-9 Secure the catheter.

- **The US-guided approach**
  - Let me introduce you to the US.
    - This is not a matter of pride. US-guided approaches have been found to be safer and more efficient. US reduces the number of attempts and time required to achieve successful cannulation, and also reduces the complication rate.[5-8] We have been practicing cardiac anesthesia for 20 years and have placed thousands of central lines, and we are not ashamed to admit that the US machine is our friend. We know that some of us old-timers will say, "I've been placing these dang things since you were in elementary school, Sonny, and I don't need that darn machine!" Well, they are wrong! Everyone needs to use the US machine. At the very least, you should use it before you even open the kit, to scan the neck and identify the target. You should definitely become facile with US-guided technique so that you can use it when you really need it (e.g., in obese patients, in patients who can't tolerate the Trendelenburg position, and in cases of neck pathology, significant coagulopathy, aberrant anatomy, etc.).
    - "Where is that pesky little critter?" Complications tend to occur more frequently when there is a poor anatomical target and operators persevere in searching for it.
      - ▲ The IJ is anterolateral to the carotid artery 92% of the time.[3]
      - ▲ The IJ may not lie in the path delineated by surface landmarks at all in up to 5% of patients.[3]
      - ▲ The IJ may actually be anteromedial to the carotid artery in 2% of patients.[3]
    - You save time and material and reduce patient risk involved with an unsuccessful attempt. Utilizing US for IJ catheterization results in fewer required attempts for successful cannulation, and a statistically less frequent occurrence of carotid puncture, hematoma, hemothorax, and pneumothorax.[9]
    - There is no excuse for not using an US.
    - A linear array 7.5- to 10.0-MHz transducer is usually used as it provides adequate tissue penetration and resolution.
    - We recommend using the US for continuous guidance throughout the procedure, as opposed to a simple vessel finder (Figure 2-10).
- Preparation
  - Prepare the patient and select the appropriate catheter as described above.
  - Position the US machine so that it may be viewed comfortably.

- Perform a quick nonsterile scan of the anatomy to ensure that there is a safe target IJ. If not, take a look on the other side.
- Adhere to sterile technique as delineated above.
- Once the sterile field has been created, and the kit has been prepared, take the probe from an assistant, who provides US conducting gel (used to provide acoustic coupling), and places the probe into the sterile sleeve. Place a sterile rubber band over the distal end of the US transducer, so as to contain the US gel (Figure 2-11).
- Finding the vessel with the US
  - You should attempt to locate the IJ at about the same location as described above for the anterior approach (i.e., Sédillot's triangle).
  - Place some sterile US gel in the correct anatomical area, and place the probe parallel to the clavicle, near the top of Sédillot's triangle. This provides a short-axis view of the IJ and carotid artery.
  - Ensure that the US probe is oriented appropriately by tapping on its lateral edges and determining its medial/lateral polarity.
  - Survey the anatomy of the neck. Locate the IJ and the relative anatomy, including the relational anatomy of the carotid artery. The IJ is frequently larger than, and lateral to, the carotid. However, the anatomy is highly variable. The carotid artery frequently demonstrates pulsatility, and the IJ should be easily compressible when pressure is applied to the US probe. Additionally, the IJ usually increases in size with maneuvers that increase preload.
  - Scan the area in a rostral-caudal axis to determine where the vessel presents itself most robustly (Figure 2-12).
  - Head/neck rotation changes the relative position of the IJ and the carotid artery. You want to gently rotate the patient's neck to maximize the lateral separation of the two vessels. Studies suggest there is significant overlap of the IJ and carotid artery, especially in older patients. The best angle of head rotation is a function of a patient's particular anatomy, but that the best angle of neck rotation is less than 45 degrees. Overlap of the vessels increases as the neck is more severely rotated[10,11] (Figures 2-13, 2-14, and 2-15).
  - Survey the IJ in the long axis to determine its patency and the presence of valves. The IJ has a demonstrable valve in 88% to 100% of cases, which is usually located distally in the retroclavicular space, near the jugular bulb, and can at times preclude passage of wires/catheters.[12]
- Placement of the local anesthetic
  - Once you have defined the anatomy, selected an insertion site, determined IJ vessel patency, and maximized lateral separation of the carotid artery and IJ by determining the correct neck/head rotation, place the US probe so that the IJ is in the center of your US viewing screen.
  - Ensure that you have the needle and probe properly lined up by pressing the needle against the skin without puncturing it. You will see the indentation on the top of your image and can make fine adjustments.
  - Place the local anesthetic only where it needs to be according to the US image. Deposit the local anesthetic along the intended path of your needle and catheter. Placing excessive local anesthetic may obscure the US image and distort the anatomy.
- Cannulate the vessel
  - Cannulate the IJ by slowly advancing the trocar needle under US guidance, and with negative pressure on the syringe, in a path defined by the US image. Once the needle has penetrated the skin, and the proper orientation of the needle has been achieved (see above), the operator should only look at the US screen, and avoid temptation to look at the operative field itself. Note that we are not utilizing a finder needle with US technique (Figure 2-16).
  - The operator should attempt to cannulate the vessel away from any overlap or proximity to the carotid artery.
  - It is not uncommon to see the anterior surface of the IJ indent as the needle is advanced to its surface. You need to "pop" through the vessel without running past its posterior wall, especially when there is overlap with the carotid artery (Figure 2-17 and 2-18).
- Once you have free blood return, you may place the US probe away from the insertion site, but keep it sterile so that you can use it to confirm wire placement.
- The guidewire is then placed through the trocar needle and advanced in the usual fashion as described above.
- Confirm wire placement within the IJ. Note that to visualize the wire, one needs to place the US probe caudal to the skin entry site (since the wire does not enter the vessel at the level of the skin penetration). You can rotate the US probe 90 degrees to view the wire/vessel in the long axis. US has a near 100% sensitivity and specificity for wire placement confirmation[13] (Figure 2-19).
- Once the wire position has been confirmed, the catheter is advanced utilizing Seldinger technique, and secured as described above.

Chapter 2   THE INTERNAL JUGULAR (IJ) LINE

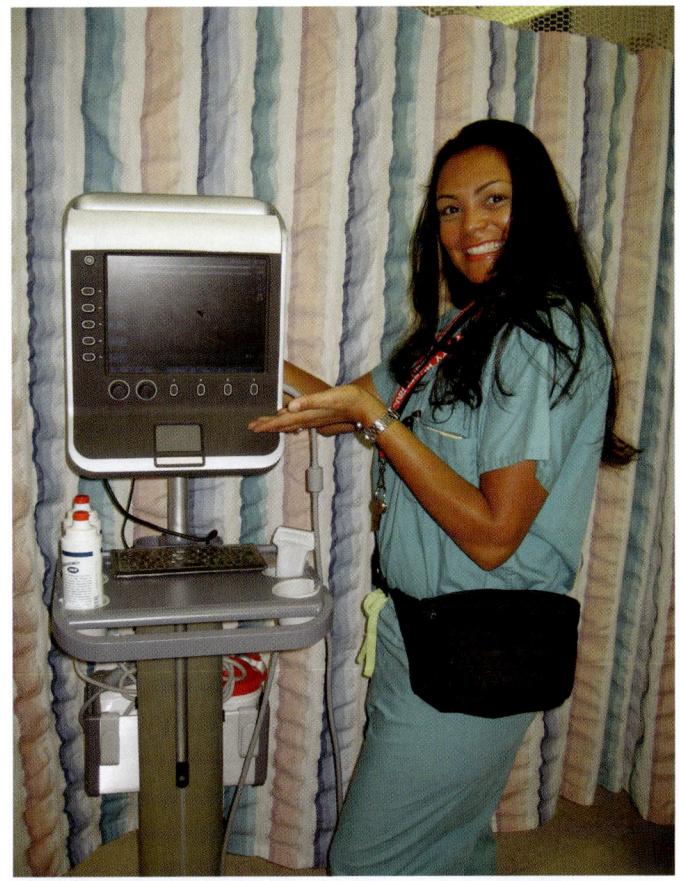

FIGURE 2-10 The ultrasound machine (model not included).

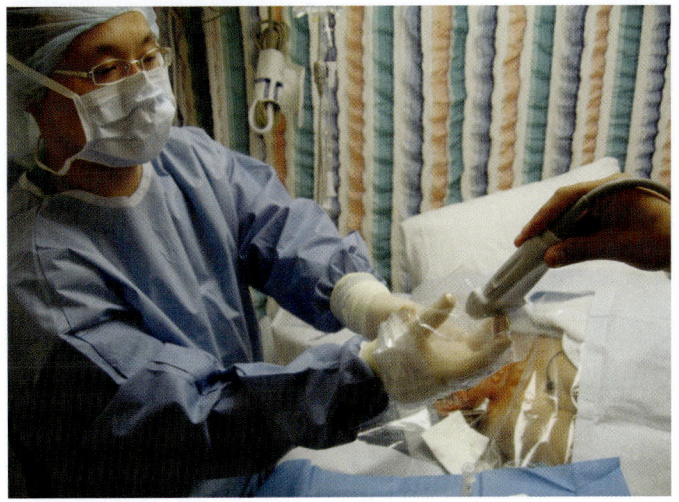

FIGURE 2-11 Placing the ultrasound probe in the sterile sleeve.

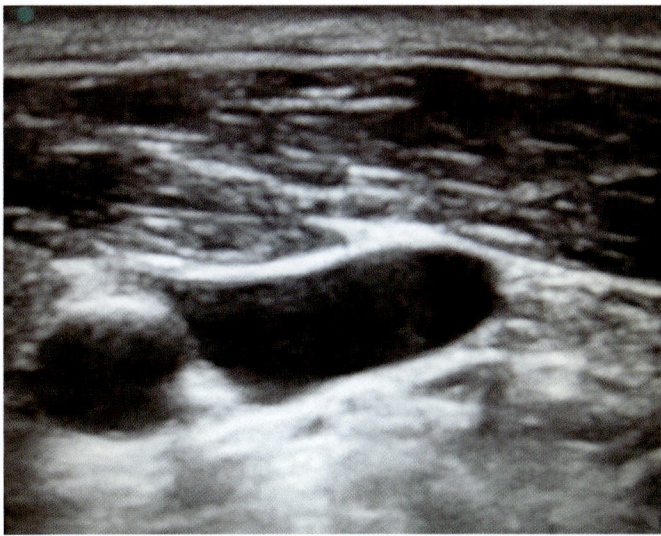

FIGURE 2-12 Ultrasound anatomy. The IJ is frequently lateral to the carotid artery, is compressible and nonpulsatile, and will change in size with maneuvers that effect preload. Note that the IJ (*right*), which is lateral to the round carotid artery (*left*), has been compressed and appears oblong.

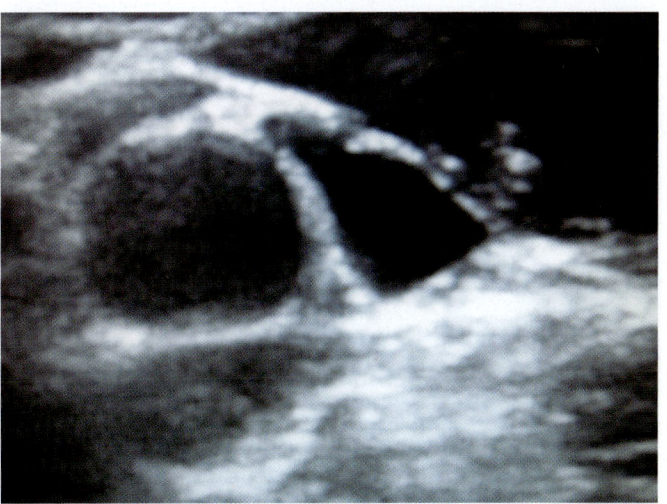

FIGURE 2-13 The relative anatomy of the IJ and carotid change as the neck is rotated. Shows the anatomy at 0 degrees rotation.

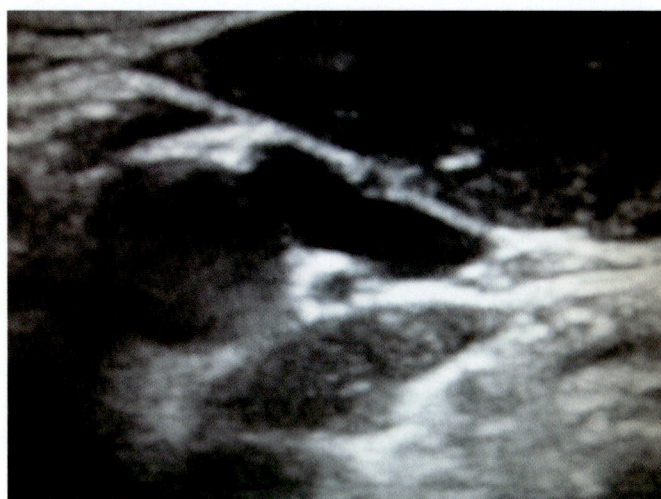

FIGURE 2-14 Shows the anatomy at 45 degrees of rotation.

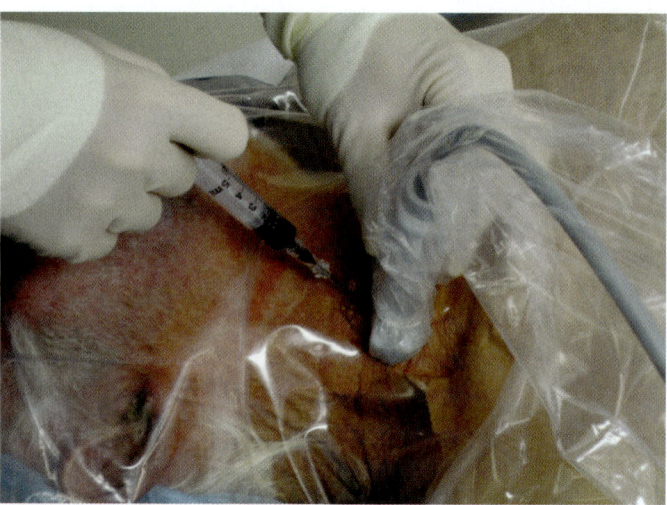

FIGURE 2-16 Advancing the trocar needle under continuous US guidance.

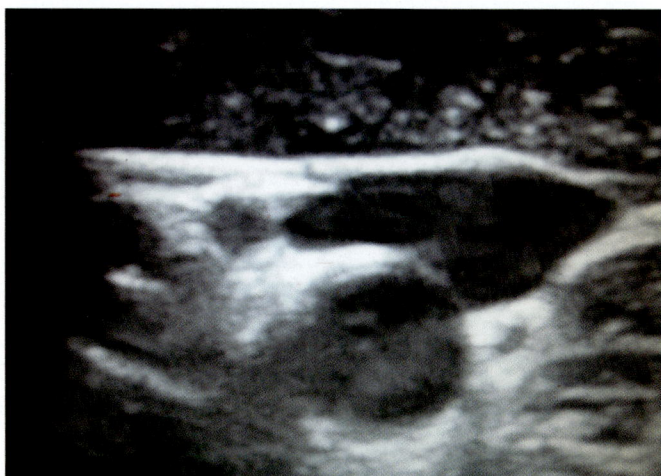

FIGURE 2-15 Shows the anatomy at 90 degrees of rotation. Note that there is the least overlap of the vessels at 0 degrees of rotation.

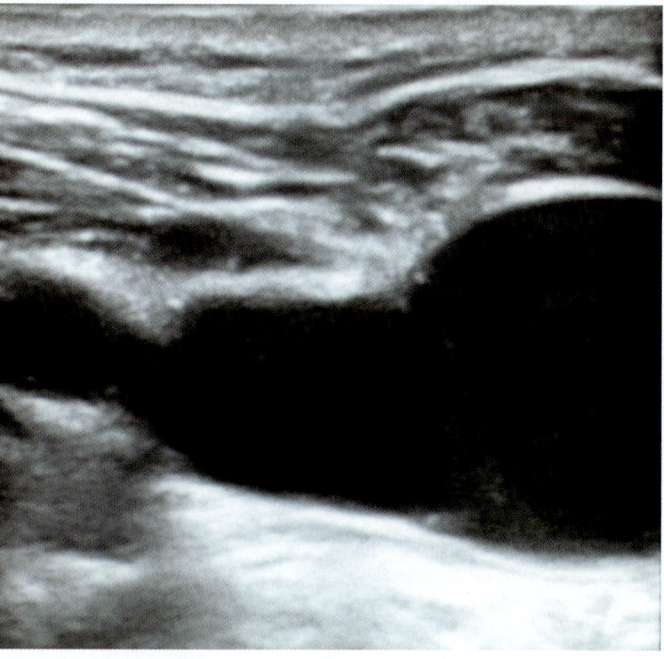

FIGURE 2-17 The trocar needle is indenting the anterior surface of the IJ vein.

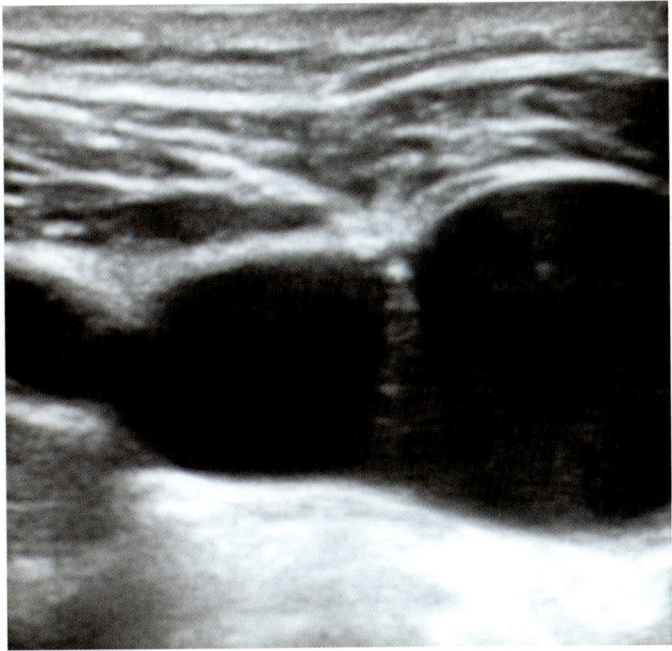

FIGURE 2-18 The trocar needle is within the IJ vein.

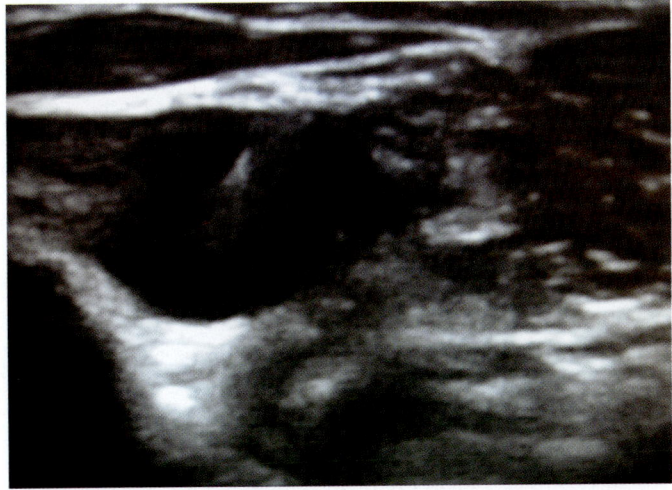

FIGURE 2-19 Confirming that the guidewire is within the IJ vein.

COMPLICATIONS

- **"Big Red"—carotid puncture/cannulation**
  - The IJ may significantly overlie the carotid artery in more than 50% of patients.[10,11]
    - This anatomical overlap increases with age, and occurs in almost 65% of patients 70 years of age or older.[10]
    - Puncture of the internal carotid artery has been reported to occur in up to 11.3% of attempts when not utilizing US guidance.[1] Cannulation of the carotid with a large-bore catheter occurs in 1 to 7 per 1000 attempts of IJ line placement.[14]
    - Puncture can obviously lead to bleeding, which can result in compression of anatomically related structures, not the least important of which is the airway!
    - Puncture of the carotid artery can also result in plaque disruption and migration.
    - Puncture caused by a finder needle does not usually lead to significant injury.
    - If you puncture the carotid with a large-bore needle, then you should apply *gentle* pressure over the site for several minutes, but be aware that this may represent critical cerebral blood flow for the patient.
    - When you find yourself in the situation where you have a large-bore (i.e., an actual central line) catheter in the carotid, remember to take your own pulse first. Don't panic. Don't just remove the catheter in an attempt to destroy the evidence. Although there is presently no standardized approach to this problem, a smaller catheter may be safely removed in a patient who has acceptable risk in terms of coagulation profile. However, when a large-bore catheter has been placed in the carotid in a patient who is coagulopathic, it is better to expeditiously seek the expertise of a vascular surgeon before removing the catheter. It is possible for a large-bore catheter to significantly interrupt flow in the carotid; don't forget to ask the patient how he/she is doing!
- **Brachial plexus injury**
  - This is a relatively rare complication that is more common when utilizing the posterior approach than the anterior one for IJ cannulation.
- **Phrenic nerve injury**
  - The phrenic nerve can be damaged by direct penetration or by compression due to hematoma formation.
- **Hoarseness**
  - Although rare, damage to the recurrent laryngeal branch of the vagus nerve can result in hoarseness.
- **Pneumothorax**
  - Although much less likely to occur than when using a subclavian approach, a pneumothorax can result when a needle is advanced too caudal when performing an IJ line insertion.
  - Pneumothorax is asymptomatic in about 22% of patients.[15]
  - An upright end-expiratory chest x-ray is best for detecting a pneumothorax.
  - Tension may develop after institution of positive pressure ventilation.

- **Chylothorax**
  - Although rare, damage to the thoracic duct when performing a LIJ line insertion can result in a chylothorax. (You'll know it when you hit it; the fluid is straw-colored.)
- **Hemothorax**
  - A penetrating injury to the IJ/subclavian vein juncture can lead to a hemothorax.

SHOW ME THE MONEY!

- **Pay-for-performance (P4P) Initiatives**
  - P4P initiatives attempt to incentivize health care providers to perform according to delineated guidelines for quality and efficiency. The Centers for Medicare and Medicaid Services (CMS) has already started P4P initiatives in certain locations. It has established certain Physician Quality Reporting Initiative (PQRI) indicators, which, when achieved according to guidelines, can result in supplemental payment to the institution and the individual health care provider.
  - Health care reform promises a large-scale proliferation of P4P initiatives. At present, these initiatives involve financial rewards. In the future they may take the form of penalties.
  - One of the present PQRI indicators (No. 76) is maintenance of sterility during central line insertion, in an effort to reduce catheter-related bloodstream infections.
    - The current billing code that is used to document that you complied with this particular PQRI indicator is 6030F.
  - This whole initiative (like most CMS policies) is a moving target. Your practice administrators will need to keep current with all the changes. A good starting point is the CMS Web site: http://www.cms.gov/pqri/.
- **US-guided central line insertion**
  - You can bill (and collect!) for real-time US-guided central line placement.
    - The US must be used continuously throughout the catheter placement, not just for vessel localization.
    - You must document the use of US.
      - Digitally record the US images on the US machine hard drive or print US images used in the process, and attach to the medical record.
    - The correct current code is 76937-26.
- **Placing lines in the operating room after induction of anesthesia—CMS rules**
  - You can't collect for time spent placing lines in a preoperative holding area.
  - You can collect for time spent placing catheters while in the operating room.

REFERENCES

1. Boon JM, Van Schoor AN, Abrahams PH, Meiring JH, Welch T. Central venous catheterization—an anatomical review of a clinical skill. *Clin Anat* 2008;21:15–22.
   A review of anatomy and complications relevant to IJ catheter placement.
2. McGee D, Gould M. Preventing complications of central venous catheterization. *N Engl J Med* 2003;348:1123–1133.
   An excellent review of techniques utilized to reduce complications encountered when placing and utilizing central venous catheters.
3. Botha R, Van Schoor AN, Boon JM, Becker JH, Meiring JH. Anatomical considerations of the anterior approach for central venous catheter placement. *Clin Anat* 2006;19:101–105.
   A review of the anatomy involved with the IJ.
4. Andrews R, Bova D, Venbrux A. How much guidewire is too much? *Crit Care Med* 2000;28(1):138–142.
   Direct measurement of the distance from the internal jugular vein access sites to the superior vena cava-atrial junction during central venous catheter placement.
5. Teodoro D, Bausano B, Lawrence L, Evanoff B, Kollef M. A descriptive comparison of ultrasound-guided central venous cannulation of the internal jugular vein to landmark-based subclavian vein cannulation. *Acad Emerg Med* 2010;17:416–422.
   Compares adverse event rates among operators using US IJ versus landmark subclavian vein approach without US.
6. Feller-Kopman D. Ultrasound-guided internal jugular access. *Chest* 2007;132:302–309.
   A proposed standardized approach and implications for training and practice.
7. Dunning J, Williamson J. Ultrasonic guidance and the complications of central line placement in the emergency department. *Emerg Med J* 2003;20:551–552.
   Compares efficiency and safety of US-guided technique to landmark-based technique for central line insertion.
8. Bailey P, Whitaker E, Palmer L, Glance L. The accuracy of the central landmark used for central venous catheterization of the internal jugular vein. *Anesth Analg* 2006;102:1327–1332.
   A prospective study that demonstrated that landmark-based technique for inserting IJ catheters would result in carotid puncture and failed attempts.
9. Karakitsos D, Labropoulos N, Groot E, et al. Real-time ultrasound-guided catheterisation of the internal jugular vein. *Crit Care* 2006;10(6):R162.
   A prospective comparison of ultrasound versus landmark based technique for IJ cannulation; demonstrates that ultrasound-based technique is safer and more efficient than landmark-based technique for IJ cannulation.

10. Troianos CA, Kuwik RJ, Pasqual JR, Lim AJ, Odasso DP. Internal jugular vein and carotid artery anatomic relation as determined by ultrasonography. *Anesthesiology* 1996;85(1):43–48.
    Elucidates the fact that the IJ significantly overlaps the carotid artery in a majority of patients.
11. Wang R, Snoey ER, Clements RC, Hern HG, Price D. Effect of head rotation on vascular anatomy of the neck: an ultrasound study. *J Emerg Med* 2006;31(3):283–286.
    Demonstrates that there is more overlap of the carotid artery and the IJ vein when the neck is rotated away from the neutral position toward the side contralateral to the cannulation attempt.
12. Fukazawa K, Aguina L, Pretto EA Jr. Internal jugular valve and central catheter placement. *Anesthesiology* 2010;112(4):979.
    Discusses the importance of the anatomy of valves in the IJ vein and relative importance during cannulation attempts.
13. Stone M, Nagdev A, Murphy M, Sisson C. Ultrasound detection of guidewire position during central venous catheterization. *Am J Emerg Med* 2010;28:82–84.
14. Parsons AJ, Alfa J. Carotid dissection: a complication of internal jugular vein cannulation with the use of ultrasound. *Anesth Analg* 2009;109(1):135–136.
15. Plewa M, Ledrick D, Sferra J. Delayed tension pneumothaorax complicating venous catheterization and positive pressure ventilation. *Am J Emerg Med* 1995;13:532–535.

CHAPTER 3

SUBCLAVIAN VEIN CATHETERIZATION

JESSICA BRODT
CHRISTIAN DIEZ

The blood is the life...and it shall be mine.
Dracula

INTRODUCTION

Subclavian lines typically have the same indications as any central line, though they are used far less frequently than the internal jugular (IJ) vein for central access in the perioperative setting that anesthesiologists frequent. However, there are distinct advantages of using the subclavian over the IJ (e.g., ease of positioning and identification of landmarks, and the surrounding connective tissue holds open the subclavian so it doesn't collapse as much with hypovolemia). There are also clear disadvantages (increased risk of bleeding and pneumothorax) that you must bear in mind when selecting patients for these lines.

PATIENT SELECTION

- In a patient in hypovolemic shock, you can't always feel a carotid pulse to outline the landmarks for an IJ, but landmarks for the subclavian will still be obvious. In addition, the subclavian vein is held open by attachments to the surrounding connective tissue, unlike the IJ, which tends to collapse with hypovolemia. A patient in code presents a similar scenario, but never forget the utility of a femoral line.
- Patients requiring multiple line changes (giving the IJ sites time to heal) or patients more cognizant of their surroundings are likely to complain. The subclavian site is generally better tolerated than the IJ. In addition, the subclavian is least likely to be associated with catheter-related bloodstream infections.
- In any morbidly obese patient or others with a short, fat neck, the landmarks for an IJ may be difficult to identify. The clavicle and sternal notch can usually still be palpated for placement of a subclavian line.
- In patients with cervical-spine injuries or with spine precautions in place, the head stays neutral with the collar in place without interfering with positioning or sterile precautions.
- In patients with no peripheral intravenous (IV) access coming in for carotid surgery, the IJ cannot be placed on the same side as the surgery, and you don't want to risk puncturing the contralateral carotid.

INDICATIONS

The indications are generally the same as for any central line:
- Delivery of volume
- Delivery of medications or nutrition that requires central access
- Central venous pressure (CVP) measurements
- IV access in a patient with poor or no peripheral access
- As a conduit for:
  - Swan-Ganz catheters
  - Hemodialysis catheters
  - Temporary pacemaker wires

CONTRAINDICATIONS (ABSOLUTE VERSUS RELATIVE)

Absolute
- Superior vena cava syndrome
- Thrombosis of the subclavian vein
- Infection at the site of entry
- Injury or fracture of the clavicle or proximal ribs

Relative
- Coagulopathy
- Chronic obstructive pulmonary disease (COPD) (higher risk of phrenic nerve palsy and pneumothorax than IJ)
- Contralateral pneumothorax (or recent attempt at contralateral subclavian line)
- High positive-end expiratory pressure (PEEP)
- Pending sternotomy (a subclavian line will be nonfunctional until the sternal edges are realigned)

EQUIPMENT

- Sterile gown, drapes and gloves, skin prep, protective hat, and face shield
- Trendelenburg-capable bed
- Monitors and oxygen
- Needle, guidewire, catheter of your choice, dilator
- Flush syringes (and normal saline for flushing)
- Suture and needle driver, dressing

CONSIDERATIONS

- The left subclavian vein provides a smoother approach to the right heart so it is preferable if you are planning to use a pulmonary artery (PA) catheter or pacing wires (this is the opposite of IJ anatomy, where the right IJ provides a better line to the right atrium).
- The first rib is very close to the clavicle and gets closer the more medial you are. If you insert your needle too medially, you might be able to thread the wire in, but when you advance the catheter it will get stuck between the bones.
- If there is any reason to suspect a coagulopathy, choose a different site. If you hit the subclavian artery, you cannot compress it no matter how hard you push.
- If you feel a bounding pulse right where you are planning on inserting the needle, reconsider your site. Subclavian arteries may become dilated and tortuous or can vary in their anatomical position, so, as with the IJ, avoid anything that is pulsatile.
- Don't forget: a large, short peripheral IV can provide better resuscitative capacity than some central lines.

PATIENT HISTORY AND PHYSICAL

- Aspects of the patient's history that suggest possible difficult subclavian line placement include a history of trauma to the clavicle (sports injury, motor vehicle accident), chest wall radiation therapy, or thrombosed subclavian veins (from previous central lines, dialysis catheters, or Port-a-Caths).
- A complete presubclavian physical is simple: look at and then palpate the clavicle. If the skin is infected or scarred, or the bone feels abnormal, review the patient's history to ascertain any risks for difficult line placement.
- Congenital disorders may affect the clavicle (such as craniocleidodystosis—congenital absence of the clavicles). Conversely, children who experienced a fractured clavicle during birth rarely have any residual deficit.

PREPARATION

- Make yourself comfortable: good lights, good workspace, and an appropriate table.
- Always remember the patient first. Do not compromise the ABCs for placement of a line.
- Identify the anatomy: clavicle ends and clavicular bend, suprasternal notch. The needle insertion site is 1 cm inferior and 1 cm lateral from the clavicular bend. Visualize the path of the vein and artery: the subclavian vein passes closest to the clavicle under the middle third of the clavicle, and the subclavian artery runs posteriorly and superiorly to the vein.
- Position the patient. The Trendelenburg position (10-15 degrees) reduces the risk of venous air embolism and engorges the vein. Pull the arm 5 cm caudally to counteract the effect of Trendelenburg positioning. A roll or IV bag between the scapulae may help move the humerus out of the way, though this is not essential. Keep the patient's head neutral. Position yourself on the same side as where you're placing the line and keep your equipment tray within easy reach of your dominant hand.
- If the patient is on a ventilator, place him or her on 100% oxygen and reduce the tidal volumes and PEEP where feasible.
- Don't bother with the ultrasound; you will find it quite difficult to visualize anything beneath the clavicle, though not impossible.

TECHNIQUE

- Position the patient and yourself (see Figures 3-1 and 3-2).
- Perform sterile preparation and drape the patient fully.

- Identify the landmarks and insertion site 1 cm inferior and 1 cm lateral to the clavicular bend. Inject local anesthetic at the insertion site; be generous (unless the patient is anesthetized or coding) (Figure 3-3).
- Prepare the line: flush and clamp all lumina but leave the distal port (usually brown) unclamped and uncapped; the guidewire will come out through here.
- Select the long needle (the finder needle will be too short, and the catheter often kinks).
- Insert the needle, aspirating continuously, aiming for the suprasternal notch (Figure 3-4).
- Keep the needle parallel to the ground. Don't point toward the head (you'll hit the artery). Don't point toward the ground (you'll drop the lung).
- If you hit the clavicle, walk off it by pushing down on the needle with the fingers on your free hand. Keep the needle parallel to the ground.
- You should enter the vein under the inner third of the clavicle. When you get blood, stop. Disconnect the syringe from the needle. Make sure the blood is venous (transduce the CVP with a short length of tubing or examine the waveform by connecting to your monitor) (Figure 3-5).
- Advance the guidewire through the needle. It should go in smoothly without any resistance. Watch for ectopy, and if any arrhythmia occurs, pull the wire back until it stops (Figure 3-6).
- Remove the needle, keeping the guidewire in place. Make a small incision at the skin, keeping the scalpel against the wire while inserting it (Figure 3-7).
- Using the Seldinger technique advance the dilator over the guidewire. Hold the dilator close to the skin and use a gentle twisting motion for a smoother insertion.
- Remove the dilator, keeping the guidewire in place, and then advance the catheter over the wire. Look for the guidewire to come out the distal port (usually brown). You may need to pull the wire back slightly in order to grasp it distally as it comes out of the port. Once you have the guidewire gripped distally, continue advancing the catheter as you remove the guidewire until the catheter is all the way in. The catheter should go in smoothly without resistance (Figure 3-8).
- Aspirate, flush, and then clamp all ports (Figure 3-9).
- Sew the line in place, apply a sterile dressing, take the patient out of the Trendelenburg position, and remove your equipment.
- Order a chest x-ray (and check it) to confirm appropriate line placement and absence of a pneumothorax.

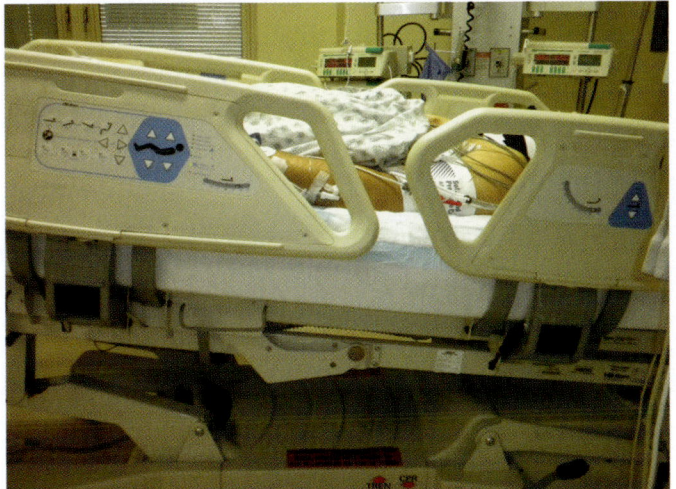

FIGURE 3-1 Position the patient in a 10- to 15-degree Trendelenburg position to prevent venous air embolism and engorge the vein for easier line placement.

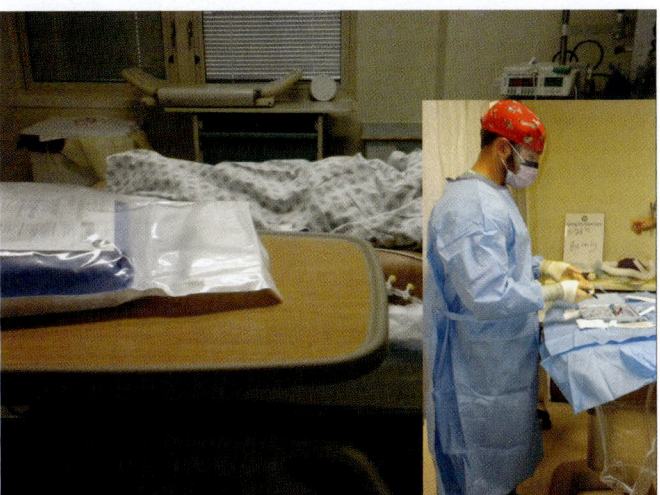

FIGURE 3-2 A good workspace is essential, with good lighting and clear access to the patient. Keep the catheter tray within easy reach of your dominant hand.

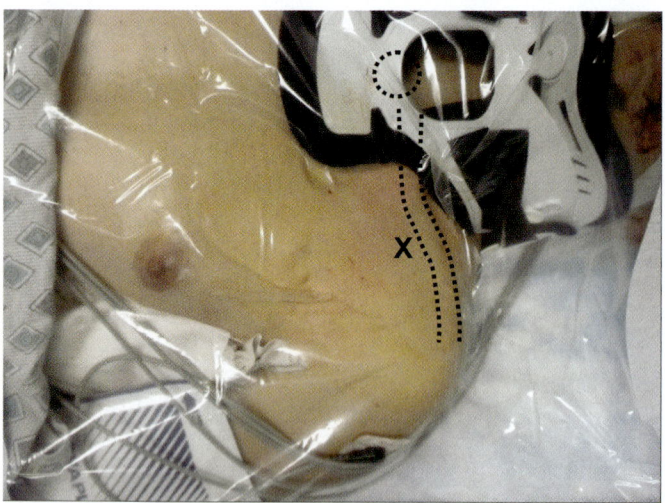

FIGURE 3-3 Identify the landmarks: the suprasternal notch *(circle),* the clavicle *(dashed lines),* and the clavicular bend. The insertion site is 1 cm inferior and 1 cm lateral to the bend (marked with an *X*).

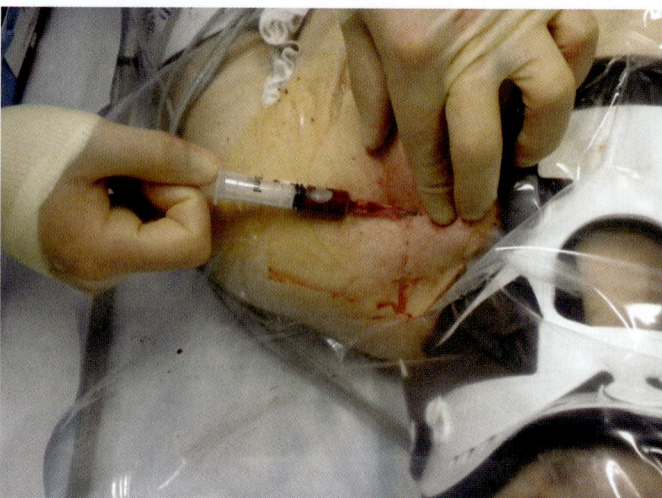

FIGURE 3-5 You should enter the subclavian vein as the needle passes under the inner third of the clavicle. Ensure blood aspirates freely and continuously.

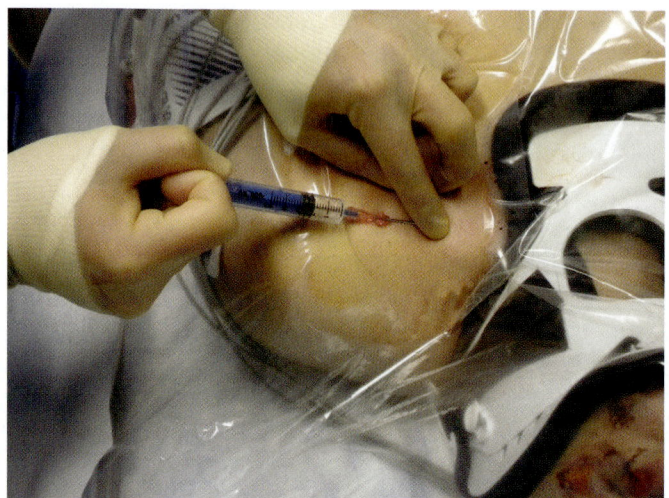

FIGURE 3-4 After appropriate local anesthesia, insert the needle directed toward the suprasternal notch, keeping the needle parallel to the ground and aspirating continuously. If you hit the clavicle push down on the needle with your free fingers to get below the bone.

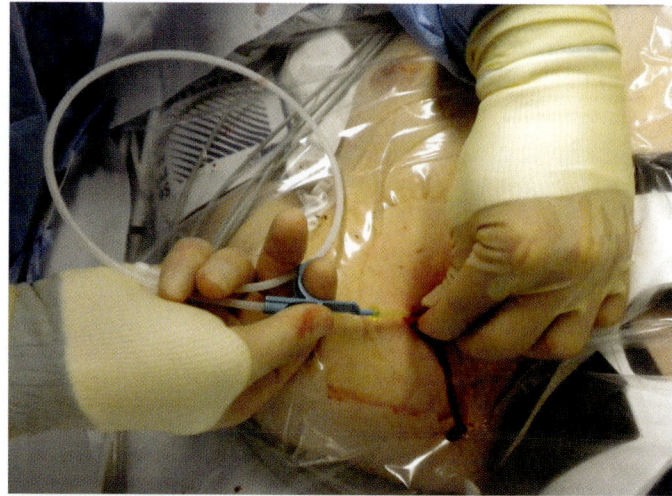

FIGURE 3-6 Thread the guidewire. Do not force it; if it does not thread smoothly, pull the wire out and recheck the needle for easy aspiration of blood. As you thread the guidewire point the J-curve caudally to prevent misdirection of the line into the contralateral IJ vein. Watch and listen for ectopy as you advance the guidewire. Once the guidewire is in, remove the needle leaving the guidewire in place.

Chapter 3 SUBCLAVIAN VEIN CATHETERIZATION

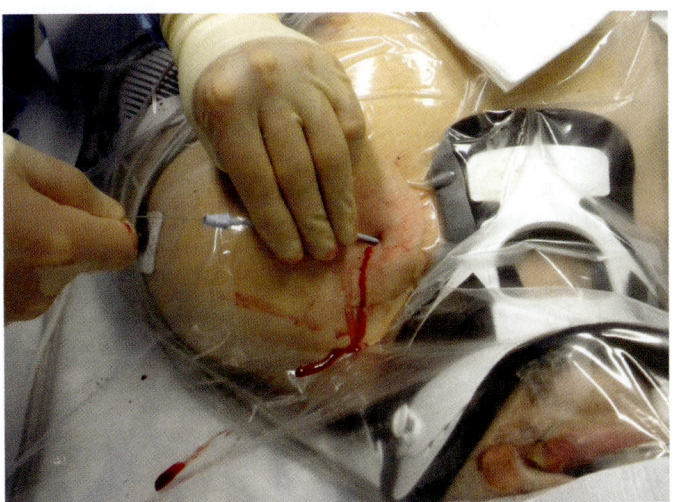

FIGURE 3-7 Make a skin incision along the guidewire and then advance the dilator over the guidewire. Holding the dilator close to the skin and using a gentle twisting motion will facilitate smooth placement. Remove the dilator, keeping the guidewire in place.

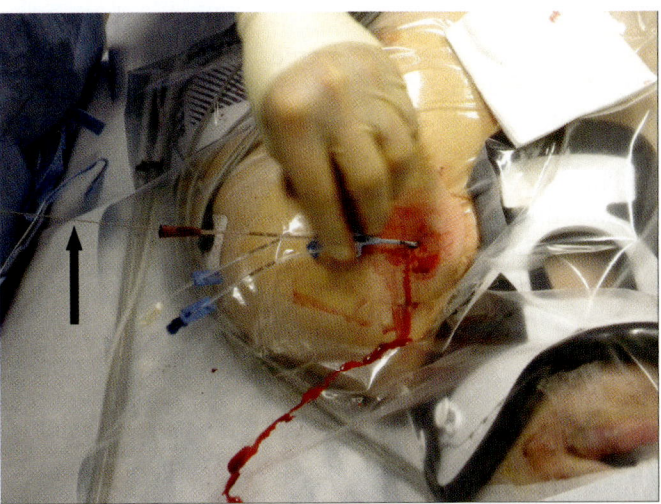

FIGURE 3-8 Advance the catheter over the guidewire, watching for the guidewire *(arrow)* to exit the distal port (which is usually brown). Once you have the guidewire gripped distally, continue advancing the catheter as you withdraw the guidewire until the catheter is inserted to the appropriate depth.

COMPLICATIONS

- Placement of catheter in IJ (up to 5%)
- Arterial puncture (3–5%): more common with IJ than subclavian
- Pneumothorax (1.5–3%) or hemothorax (0.5%): most common with subclavian
- Venous thrombosis (1–2%): least common with subclavian site
- Catheter-related bloodstream infection: least common with subclavian site
- Catheter or guidewire embolism

TROUBLESHOOTING

- You hit the artery. Damn! Well there's no real way to put pressure on it. Sometimes there's such a big hole it needs surgical repair, which is difficult given the position of the hole. The best treatment is always prevention. Don't go deep, and don't aim high. That's where the artery is. Keep the needle parallel to the ground as you advance toward the suprasternal notch, and push down on the needle with your free fingers to get the depth you need.

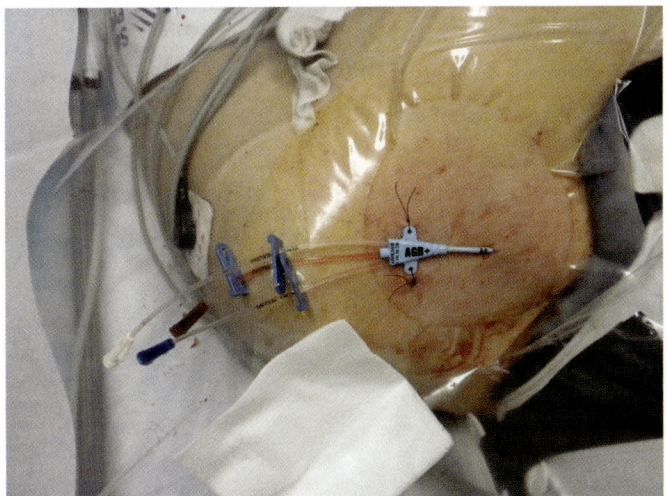

FIGURE 3-9 Confirm aspiration of blood from each port and then flush and clamp them. Suture in the catheter, clean up, apply a sterile dressing, and you're done. Confirm appropriate placement and the absence of a pneumothorax by chest x-ray. (Note: There is not a Bio-Patch® on this line. Some would argue you should have such an additional measure in place to reduce infection.)

- You dropped the lung. Damn! Stick a 14-gauge catheter in the second intercostal space in the midclavicular line to decompress the pneumothorax, and then get a surgeon to put a chest tube in for you.
- The guidewire and line went in seemingly smoothly, but on x-ray the catheter is pointing... up? Misplacement of a subclavian vein catheter tip in the ipsilateral IJ occurs in up to 5% of subclavian lines. It may also be detected when an abnormal waveform or CVP reading is obtained after transduction of the line. Misplacement in the IJ is associated with an increased risk of thrombosis, thrombophlebitis, and errors in transduced values. To ensure against IJ placement, point the J-curve of the guidewire caudally when inserting it through the needle. The "Ambesh maneuver" involves occluding the ipsilateral IJ while advancing the line. This can help to both prevent and detect IJ placement of the catheter. It may also be used as a salvage technique if you've found the line in the IJ, without having to take the whole line out.

CONCLUSION

Catheterization of the subclavian vein is usually a straightforward, fast approach to central vein cannulation. It is a skill worthy of attention and recalling at opportune times.

SUGGESTED READING

Ambesh SP, Pandey JC, Dubey PK. Internal jugular vein occlusion test for rapid diagnosis of misplaced subclavian vein catheter into the internal jugular vein. *Anesthesiology* 2001;95:1377–1379.

Describes the Ambesh maneuver to prevent or correct misplacement of a subclavian catheter into the IJ.

Czarnik T, Gawda R, Perkowski T, Weron R. Supraclavicular approach is an easy and safe method of subclavian vein catheterization even in mechanically ventilated patients: analysis of 370 attempts. *Anesthesiology* 2009;111:334–339.

A prospective cohort study analyzing the safety of using the supraclavicular approach for subclavian vein placement.

Fortune JB, Feustel P. Effect of patient position on size and location of the subclavian vein for percutaneous puncture. *Arch Surg* 2003;138:996–1000.

An ultrasonographic analysis of the effect of five different positions subclavian vein anatomy.

Kitigawa N, Oda M, Totoki T, et al. Proper shoulder position for subclavian venipuncture. *Anesthesiology* 2004;101(6):1306–1312.

A computed tomography radiographic study of the effect of three different shoulder positions on subclavian vein anatomy.

McGee DC, Gould M. Current concepts: preventing complications of central venous catheterization. *N Engl J Med* 2003;348:1123–1133.

A succinct review detailing the complications of central lines, contrasting different sites and outlining how to prevent these complications.

Thompson EC, Calver LE. Safe subclavian vein cannulation. *Am Surg* 2005;71(2):180–183.

A surgeons perspective on subclavian lines.

CHAPTER 4
CENTRAL VENOUS ACCESS IN THE PEDIATRIC PATIENT

LYDIA M. JORGE
AMANDA SAAB
RICHARD ELF

INTRODUCTION

Gaining central venous access in the pediatric patient can be a panic-inducing event, especially for those practitioners who require this skill on rare occasion. Unfortunately, it is those rare occasions where central venous access is imperative that can strike terror in the heart of the most experienced anesthesiologist. An update of the Pediatric Perioperative Cardiac Arrest (POCA) Registry, which evaluated anesthesia-related cardiac arrests in children (1994–2004), noted that a common anesthesia-related factor was underestimation of blood loss, insufficient peripheral IV access, and the absence of central venous catheter placement or monitoring. There also was a small percentage of catheter-related arrests, which included injuries associated with needle, guidewire, or catheter insertion.

"WOW! THAT'S A SMALL BABY!"

Haven't put an IV, let alone a central line, in something this tiny? Time to call for backup! You can always call your pediatric anesthesia attending, pediatric surgeon, or pediatric intensivist for help or guidance. Although inexperience is nerve racking, it is not an excuse to avoid adequate peripheral or central line placements in patients when they require it. This chapter guides you through the basics of gaining central venous access in the pediatric patient population. Of note, the best lines for resuscitation are large-bore peripheral IVs.

CENTRAL VENOUS ACCESS

Indications
- Infusion of vasoactive medications (e.g., epinephrine, norepinephrine)
- Bolus delivery of cardiac drugs with very short half-lives (e.g., adenosine)
- Providing a means to infuse medications that can be damaging if given in peripheral veins (e.g., hyperalimentation, vasopressors, antibiotics)
- Central venous pressure monitoring
- Pulmonary artery catheterization (PAC)
- Transvenous cardiac pacing
- Aspiration of air emboli (e.g., during intracranial procedures in the sitting position)
- Providing access for blood sampling

Contraindications
- Occlusion of the vessel from multiple previous lines at the site (as seen on ultrasound or catheterization)
- Severe trauma of the neck
- Outflow obstruction
- Infection at the site

General Complications of Central Venous Access
- Thrombosis
- Malposition/perforation
- Infection
- Hemothorax
- Pneumothorax

- Arrhythmias
- Systemic air emboli

Other Considerations

- If planning to place a pulmonary artery catheter (PAC) or pacing wires, consider the right internal jugular (IJ) (straight shot to heart) or the left subclavian vein (SC) (gentler angle to the heart).
  - However, in infants <1 year of age, the SC makes a much sharper angle into the heart than in older patients.[1]
- Infection risk? Subclavian lines often remain cleaner than either IJ or femoral lines.
- Coagulopathic? The subclavian artery cannot be compressed regardless of how hard you mash down on the clavicle. Consider the IJ or femoral lines where pressure can easily be applied by your assistant.
- Don't trust lines from the floor!
  - This can't be emphasized enough: lines can come down unsutured (are they even still in the vein?), clotted (check ports for blood return/flushing), interarterial (they put the fluids on an infusion pump for a reason), and with the guidewire STILL in place (why is the patient having ectopy?).

What Line Can I Place?

- Care should be taken when placing superior vena cava (SVC) catheters in patients smaller than 4 kg because of the risk of thrombosis (Table 4-1).
- A large study of central venous catheter (CVC) placements in infants and children developed a formula to approximate the correct insertion depth based on height and weight that would predict placement of the tip of the catheter above the right atrium in the SVC 97.5% of the time. Using this equation would approximate the catheter tip to be at 1 cm above the SVC-RA junction. This equation can be used for both IJ and subclavian catheter placement.[2]
  - Patient height <100 cm:

(Height in cm/10) − 1 cm = catheter insertion distance

  - Patient height ≥100 cm:

(Height in cm/10) − 2 cm = catheter distance

THE INTERNAL JUGULAR

The Anatomy of the Internal Jugular

- Along its entire length in the neck, the internal jugular vein runs in close proximity to the carotid artery and vagus nerve within the carotid sheath.

TABLE 4-1 Recommended Central Line Catheter Sizes and Length

Patient Weight	Internal Jugular/ Subclavian Vein	Femoral Vein
<10 kg	4F, 2 lumen, 8 cm	4F, 2 lumen, 12 cm
10–30 kg	4F, 2 lumen, 12 cm	4F, 2 lumen, 12–15 cm
31–50 kg	5F, 2 lumen, 12–15 cm	5F, 2 lumen, 15 cm
51–70 kg	7F, 2 lumen, 15 cm	7F, 2 lumen, 20 cm
>70 kg	8F, 2 lumen, 16 cm	8F, 2 lumen, 20 cm

F, French.
Data from Andropoulos DB. Vascular access and monitoring. In: Andropoulos DB. *Anesthesia for congenital heart disease.* Hoboken, NJ: Blackwell; 2010, pp 99–107.

- It is initially posterior to, then lateral to, and then anterolateral to the carotid artery during its descent in the neck.
- On the left side of the neck, the internal jugular vein is anterior to the thoracic duct, and therefore cannulation is usually avoided if possible to avoid injury to the thoracic duct.
- Appropriate exposure can be difficult in infants due to the large occiput and relatively short neck, making it nearly impossible to obtain the shallow angle of approach necessary to gain access.

Advantages

- A right internal jugular vein provides a direct route to the right atrium, making it the ideal line for floating pulmonary artery catheters.
- The location of the line in the patient's neck makes it more easily accessible intraoperatively (unless of course, the head of the bed is turned away from you).
- This is the line anesthesiologists have the most practice performing.

Disadvantages

- It is not very comfortable for the awake patient.
- Positioning, especially in the infant, can be nearly impossible.
- Tip migration can occur with head movement.

Procedure and Approach

- After induction, and securing of the airway, a shoulder roll should be placed under the infant, who is presumably in the supine position.
  - This functions to elevate the thorax and extend the head and neck slightly. Don't be overzealous, or you will distort the anatomy. Recheck the endotracheal tube position. Even minute adjustments to the head position of an infant can alter the position of the tube, leading to inadvertent endobronchial intubation (with head flexion) or (Eek!) extubation (with rotation or extension)!
- The head should be turned no more than 45 degrees to the left, as greater rotation will cause the internal jugular vein and carotid artery to overlap more. Recheck the endotracheal tube position and ensure the end-tidal carbon dioxide concentration (E_TCO_2) is still present; 45 degrees can mean an extubated baby! (Figure 4-1)
- Once the tube is in position, the landmarks should be palpated because identification may not be possible under the sterile drape (Figure 4-2).
- Strict aseptic technique with wide sterile prep and drape is required following Centers for Disease Control and Prevention (CDC) guidelines to reduce the risk of catheter-related infections.
  - Wash hands with sterile scrub or aseptic solution.
  - Apply sterile gown and gloves (assuming you are in the OR, you are already donning a scrub cap, and a mask with a shield).
  - Prep the skin in a circular motion, making sure not to overlap the area already cleaned, from the intended puncture site up to the earlobe and down to the clavicle and sternal notch.
  - Open the sterile drape and completely cover the patient and any areas that may cause you to contaminate yourself (Figures 4-3 and 4-4).
- Place the patient in the Trendelenburg position.
  - Ensure the E_TCO_2 and no change in tidal volumes and peak inspiratory pressures. (Do you see a pattern forming here?)
- Remove the catheter kit from the packaging, maintaining sterility. Open the kit on a sterile flat surface such as a Mayo stand covered in sterile towels. This should be placed on the side of your dominant hand; style points for not having to reach over your own body to pick up the next item in the sequence.
- Flush each of the ports with normal saline, and then clamp all but the distal port (since this is where the wire will emerge from).
- Palpate the carotid impulse using your nondominant hand.
- Using your dominant hand and a 22-gauge (G) needle loaded onto a 3-cc syringe, enter the skin at a 15- to 30-degree angle to the skin at the medial border of the sternocleidomastoid between the two heads of the muscle aiming toward the ipsilateral nipple.
- As you advance, constant gentle negative pressure should be applied. The vessel will be found less than 3 cm from the surface of the skin.
- Once you've entered the vessel, dark red blood will return into the syringe.
- Holding the catheter firmly in place, disconnect the syringe and allow backflow of blood. A slow ooze of dark red blood is promising. Pulsatile flow means you have entered the carotid—close, but no cigar.
- Transduce your line via connection to the central venous pressure (CVP) monitor with short extension tubing, which provides confirmation that this is truly venous flow.
- Now, still firmly fixing the catheter in place, disconnect the extension tubing and advance the wire into the catheter, taking care not to lose the wire.
  - If an arrhythmia develops, stop and back up a few millimeters; you are tickling the baby's ventricle.
  - If at any point you encounter resistance, STOP! It does not take much force to push through a vessel wall into the lung or, even worse, the right ventricle.
- Remove the 22-G catheter, taking care to maintain control of the wire at all times.
- Using a small scalpel in the dominant hand, sharp side pointing AWAY from the carotid artery, slightly extend the size of the puncture site by riding down the wire and making a small skin nick to facilitate placement of the larger catheter (Figure 4-5).
- Holding pressure and the wire (Figure 4-6), advance the dilator over the wire making sure that you have control of the wire at the distal tip before letting go of the proximal end (Figure 4-7).
  - This may require your backing up the wire slightly until it is accessible distally.
  - Use the dilator to dilate the skin and soft tissue further.
- Remove the dilator. Bleeding from the site is normal, so do not be alarmed, but if you have the manual dexterity, hold the wire AND pressure over the site.
- Carefully thread the central venous catheter over the wire, maintaining control of the wire throughout the procedure (Figure 4-8).

- Draw back from both ports, ensuring blood return, and then flush the lines with normal saline, confirming easy injection.
- Suture the catheter in place, taking care not to hit the external jugular in your suture path.
- Clean the area of any blood and fluid, and then secure with a antimicrobial patch or ointment and a clear occlusive dressing (Figure 4-9).
- Order the chest x-ray.
- Check the chest x-ray.

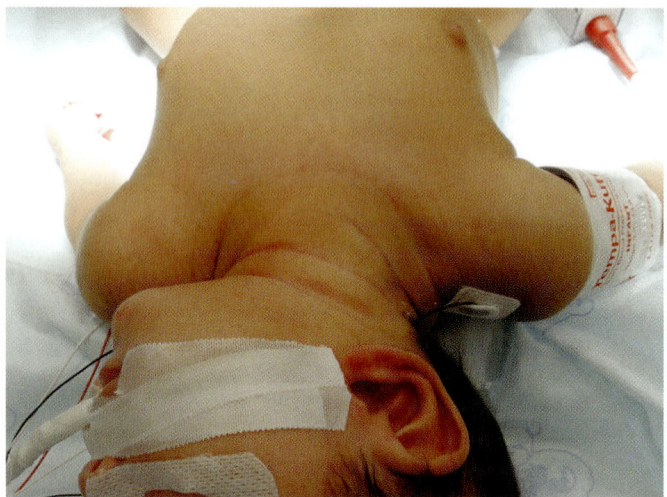

FIGURE 4-1 Positioning the patient.

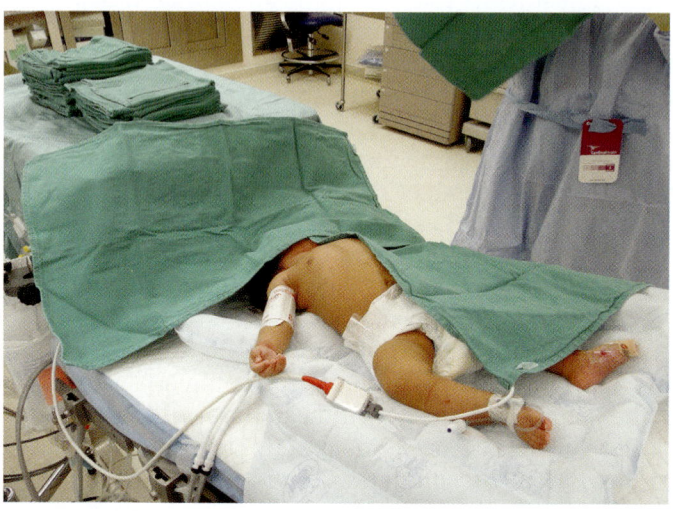

FIGURE 4-3 Use sterile drapes.

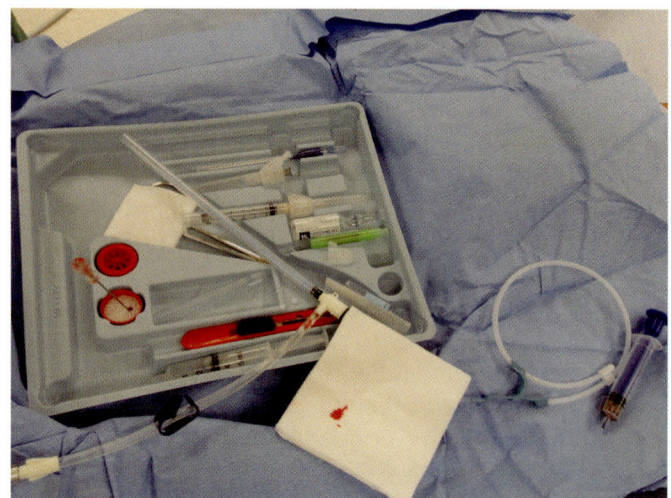

FIGURE 4-2 Have all your IJ equipment ready.

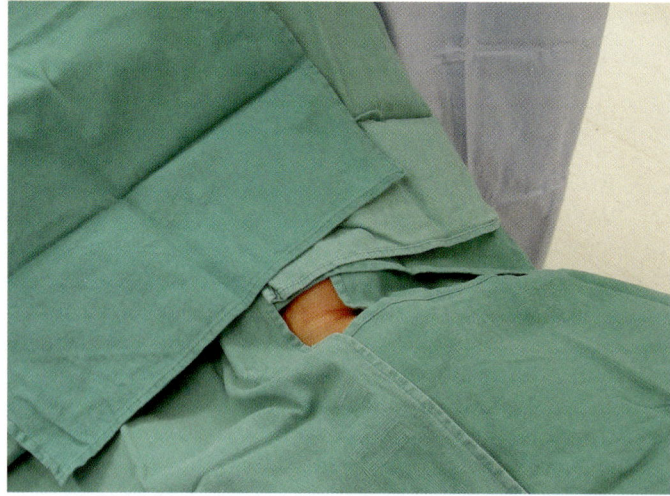

FIGURE 4-4 Place sterile drapes, well, duh, sterilely!

Chapter 4 CENTRAL VENOUS ACCESS IN THE PEDIATRIC PATIENT

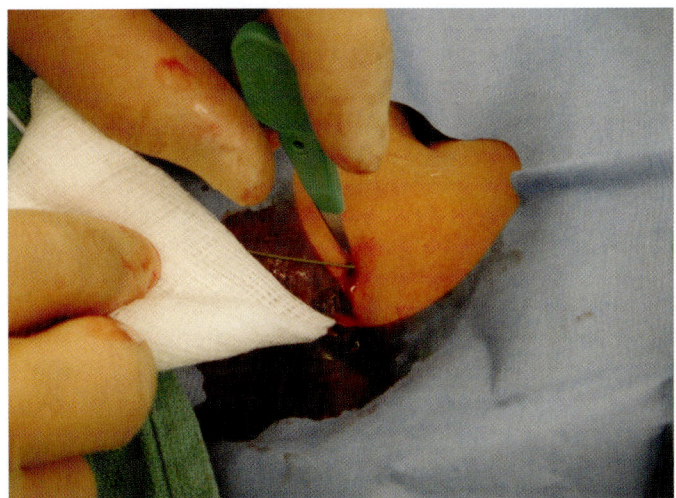

FIGURE 4-5 Nicking the skin.

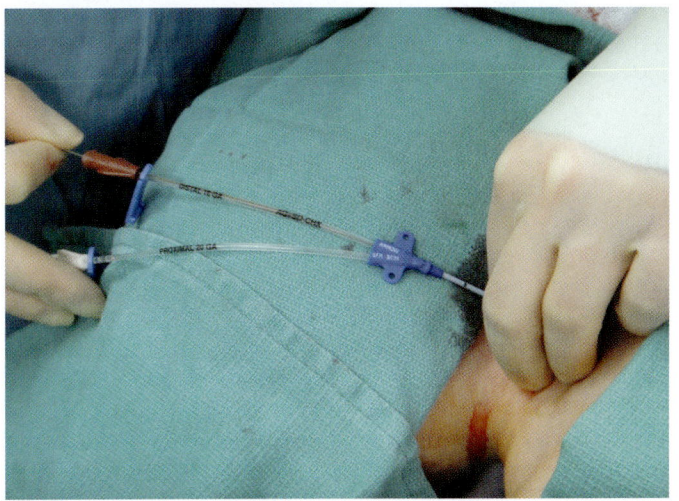

FIGURE 4-6 Holding the wire.

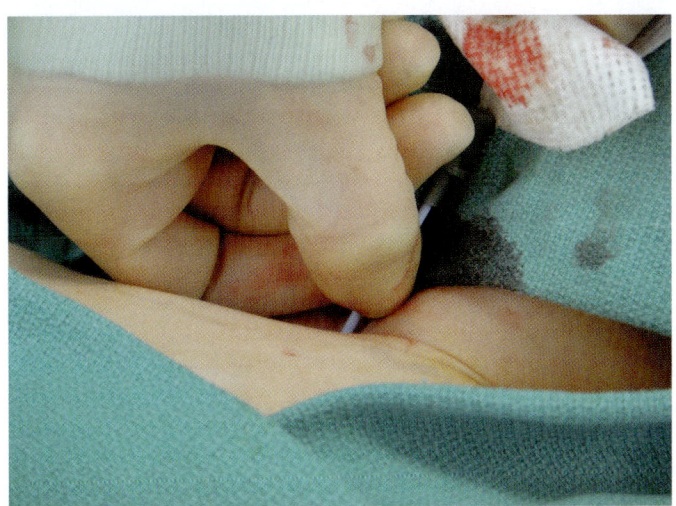

FIGURE 4-7 Placing dilator.

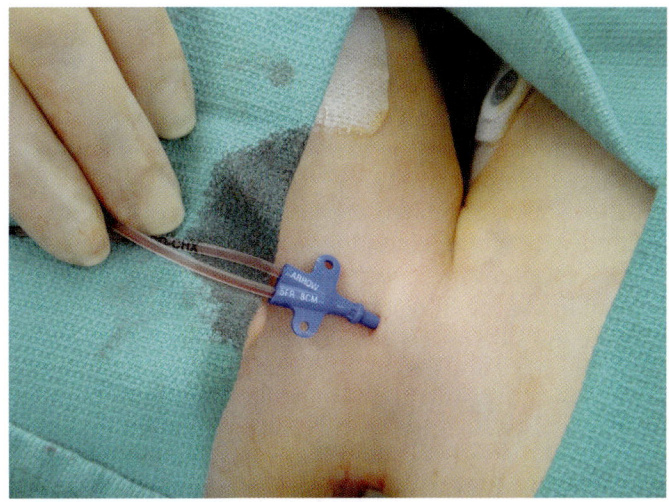

FIGURE 4-8 Insert to the proper depth.

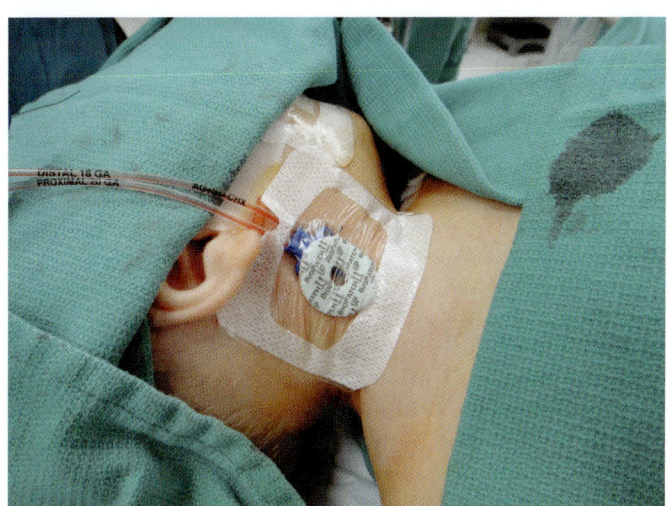

FIGURE 4-9 Apply sterile dressing.

Ultrasound Guidance

- The ultrasound can be a very useful tool in locating the internal jugular vein, especially when positioning is difficult (Figure 4-10).
- To use the ultrasound during your procedure, you will need a sterile ultrasound probe cover and the sterile probe goo that comes in the package that your facility carries.
- After donning a sterile gown and gloves, apply some goo into the sterile cover and have your assistant pull the cover over the probe.
- Apply a dime-sized dollop of goo to the neck.
- With the probe in your nondominant hand, place the probe perpendicular to the surface of the neck and begin to scan slowly for the vessels. Vessels will appear as circular to elliptical structures that are relatively well defined (Figure 4-11).

- Once you have encountered a pair of vessels, center them on the screen. Apply gentle downward pressure with the probe. *The vein will collapse under the probe, while the carotid artery will continue to appear round and pulsatile* (Figures 4-12 and 4-13).
- Once you've identified the structures, hold the probe still with the nondominant hand and pick up your 22-G needle loaded onto the 3-cc syringe.
- Looking at the ultrasound screen (not the patient), poke the skin gently with the needle, to determine the location of the needle in relationship to the probe. Ideally, both the image and your needle should be centered.
- Now puncture the skin and proceed with continuous negative aspiration on the syringe.
- You will see your needle enter the vessel and feel blood return into the syringe. Put the probe down, and proceed as indicated in the sections above (Figures 4-14 and 4-15).
- Once you have passed the wire, some practitioners advise utilizing the probe and visualizing the wire within the lumen of the internal jugular vein (Figures 4-16, 4-17 and 4-18).
- Now that the wire is in, proceed with placing the line as described earlier.

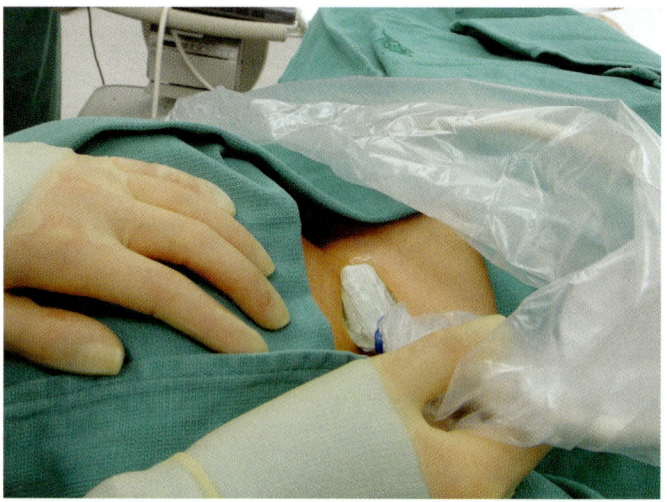

FIGURE 4-10 Ultrasound use is most righteously useful in kiddies.

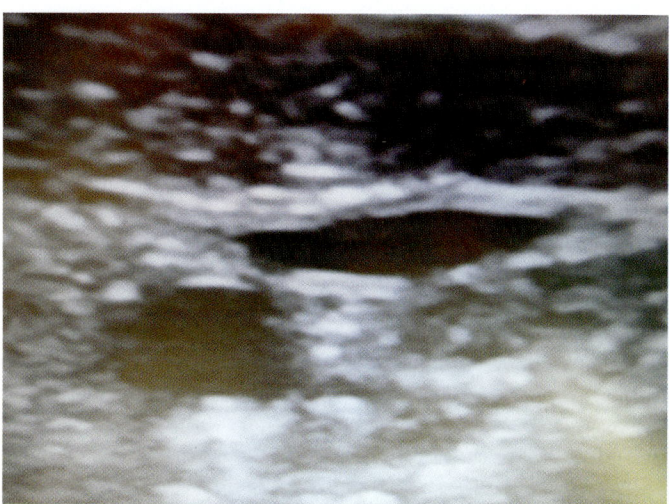

FIGURE 4-12 Note the IJ is squishable.

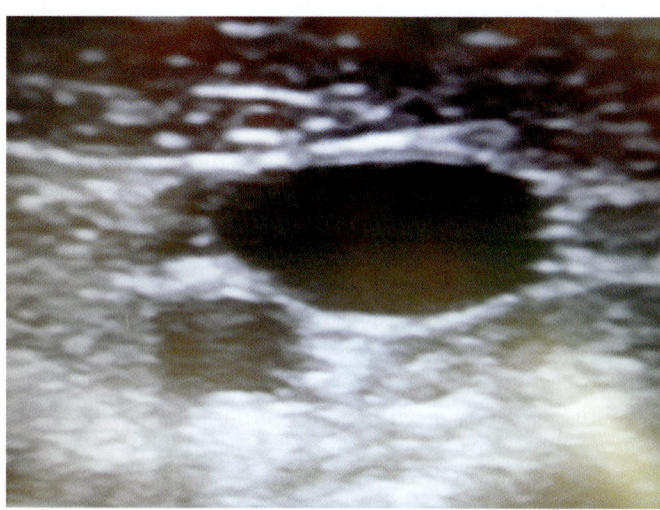

FIGURE 4-11 Ultrasound image of the vessels.

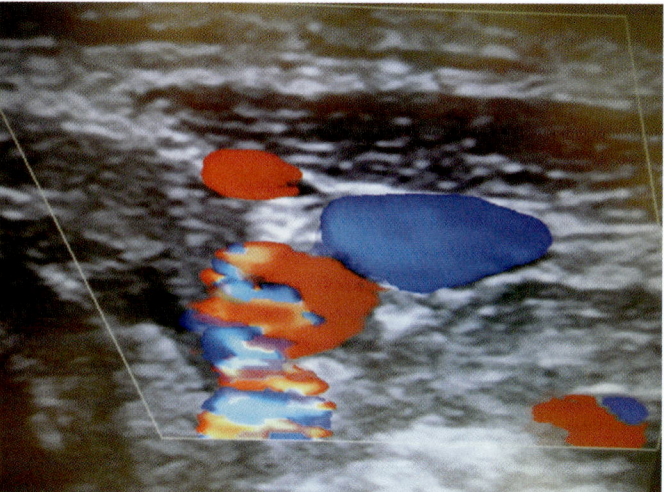

FIGURE 4-13 You can also use colorflow to identify the vein. Red means blood flows towards the probe and blue flows away.

Chapter 4 CENTRAL VENOUS ACCESS IN THE PEDIATRIC PATIENT

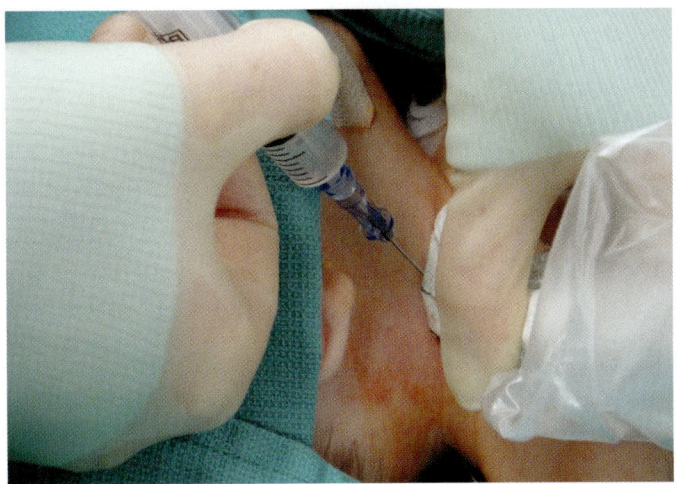

FIGURE 4-14 Watching the needle. Holding the ultrasound probe with your non-dominant hand and syringe/needle with your dominant hand can improve visualization.

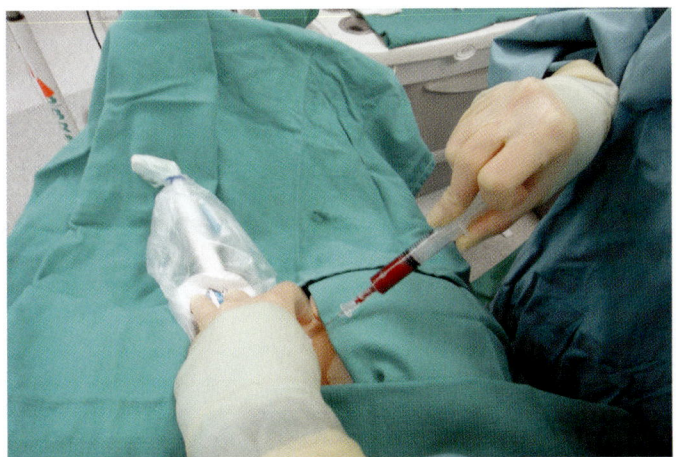

FIGURE 4-15 Still watching the needle. Remember to aspirate gently as you advance.

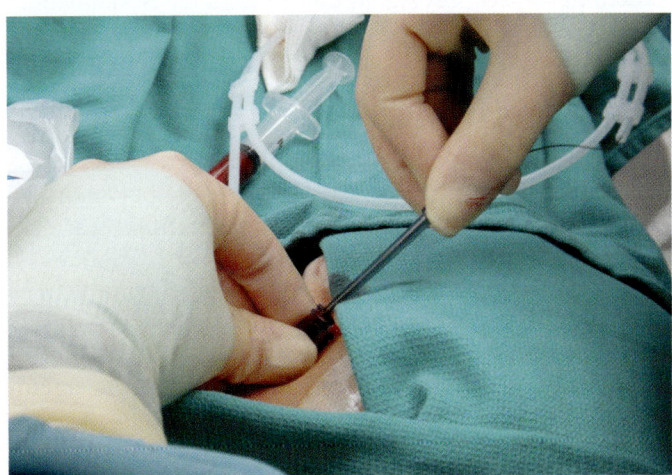

FIGURE 4-16 Watching the wire.

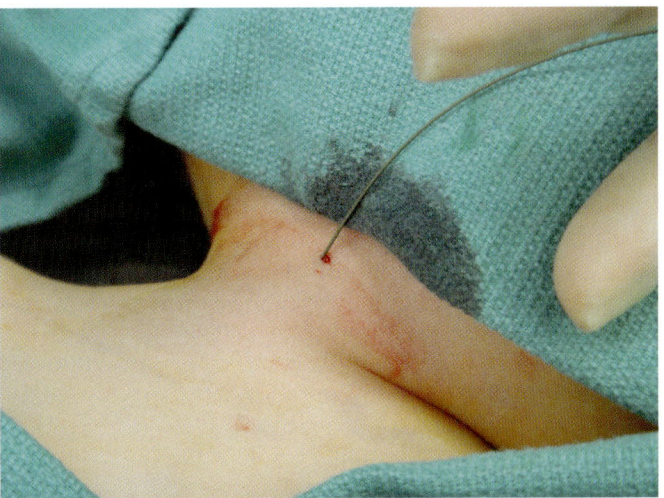

FIGURE 4-17 Still watching the wire!

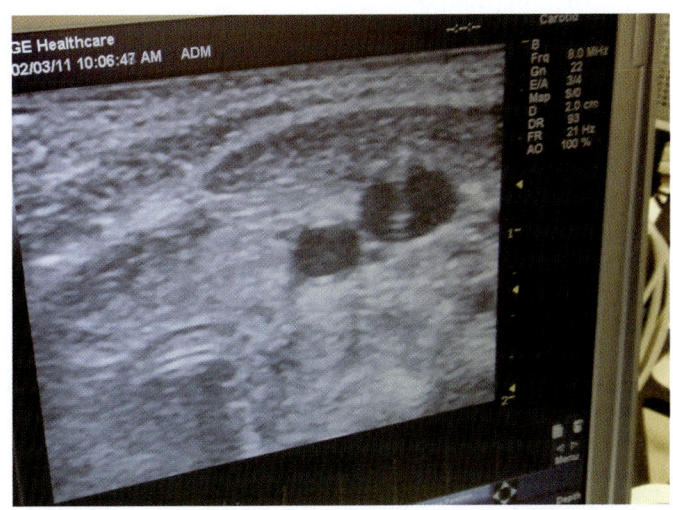

FIGURE 4-18 I can't get enough of this wire.

ISSUES AND TROUBLESHOOTING

- Children and babies will not hold still for even 30 seconds, much less than 10 to 15 minutes it takes to prep, place, and secure the line. Perhaps go for another site, if preinduction central venous access is necessary.
- Note that tip migration can be significant with rotation of the infant's head.
- "Uh-oh, I have torrential pulsatile flow"—you've hit the carotid.
  - The good news is that this artery is compressible and you used a small-caliber needle, so a tincture of time and continuous firm pressure will usually fix the problem.
  - However, after the bleeding is under control, you will need to find a new puncture site.

- "Hey, wait, I see my needle through the OTHER SIDE OF THE VESSEL on ultrasound but I still have no blood return. Now what?!"
  - Don't despair. It is possible that you tented the vessel wall as you were approaching it. Slowly pull back aspirating on the syringe. This pulls the superficial wall away from the deeper wall, widening the lumen. The key is to go slowly, so as not to pull all the way out of the tiny vessel. If there is no blood return, try a new stick.

Complications
- Carotid artery puncture
- Vertebral artery puncture
- Pneumothorax
- Venous air embolism
- Arrhythmias
- Tracheal perforation
- Venous thrombosis

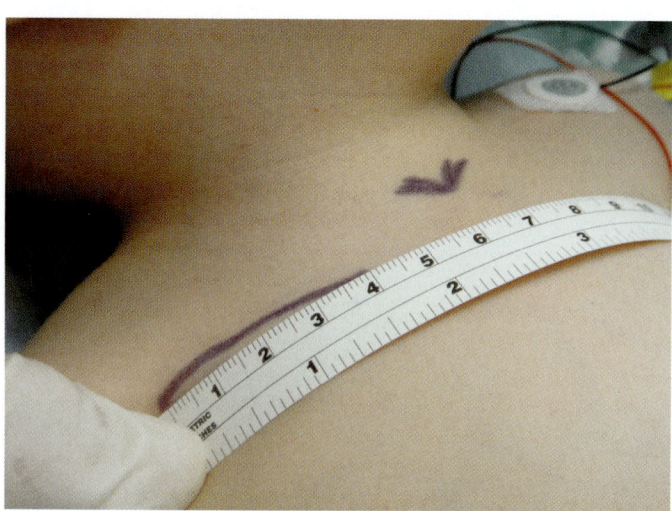

FIGURE 4-19 The clavicle is the linear marking. Suprasternal notch is marked with a "V".

THE SUBCLAVIAN

Anatomy of the Subclavian
- Recall that the subclavian vein is immediately posterior to the medial third of the clavicle (hence, "sub," meaning below, and "clavian," meaning relating to the clavicle). The artery lies superior and posterior to the vein. The dome of the pleura may extend above the first rib on the left, but rarely does on the right.

Advantages
- Its position in relation to surface landmarks is relatively constant among all age groups.
- Tip migration is less likely.
- It is tolerated better by the awake patient.

Disadvantages
- Higher incidence of pneumothorax
- The opportunity to place this line is often deferred by the anesthesiologist for fear of dropping the lung. Less practice means less confidence.
- Entry to the ipsilateral internal jugular vein or contralateral brachiocephalic vein
- Inability to compress the artery in the case of inadvertent puncture
- Inability to dilate the space between the clavicle and the first rib

Landmarks
- Clavicle
- Suprasternal notch (Figures 4-19 and 4-20)

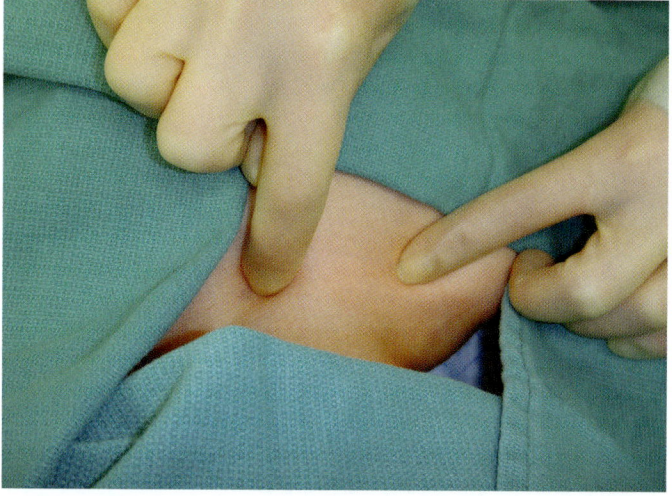

FIGURE 4-20 Yet Again Landmarks for Subclavian.

Procedure and Approach
- After induction, and securing of the airway, a shoulder roll should be placed vertically between the scapulae of the supine infant. The infant's arms should be neutral at his sides.
  - This position helps to move the subclavian vein anteriorly just under the posterior aspect of the clavicle.
  - Recheck the endotracheal tube position. As stated before, the slightest adjustments to the head position of an infant can alter the position of the tube, leading to inadvertent endobronchial intubation or extubation!

- The head should be turned TOWARD the side of the puncture (i.e., to the left for a left sided subclavian puncture).
  - This helps to collapse the ipsilateral internal jugular and prevents the guidewire from entering into it.
  - Recheck the endotracheal tube position and ensure the E_TCO_2 is still present. A rotated head and neck can mean an extubated baby!
- Once the tube is in position, palpate the landmarks. If a pulsatile structure is noted in the area of intended puncture, consider another site. Aberrant arterial anatomy can lead to an accidental subclavian artery puncture, an event that can ruin your day and buy the patient a surgery to gain control of the bleeding.
- Strict aseptic technique with wide sterile prep and drape is required following CDC guidelines to reduce the risk of catheter related infections.
  - Wash hands with sterile scrub or aseptic solution.
  - Apply sterile gown and gloves (assuming you are in the OR, you are already donning a scrub cap, and a mask with a shield).
  - Prep the skin in a circular motion, making sure not to overlap the area already cleaned, from the intended puncture site up to the earlobe and down to the nipple line and sternal notch.
  - Open the sterile drape and completely cover the patient and any areas that may cause you to contaminate yourself.
- Local anesthetic if in an awake/lightly sedated patient
- Check your equipment.
- Flush the ports and clamp all but the distal port (for the guidewire).
- Ensure free guidewire movement in its sheath.
- With the first finger of your nondominant hand, locate the sternal notch under the drapes. Keeping your finger there, use your thumb to locate the lateral third of the clavicle (which happens to be approximately where the clavicle takes a bend posteriorly).
- Holding the needle loaded onto a 3-cc syringe, and MAINTAINING THE NEEDLE PARALLEL TO THE GROUND, enter the skin approximately 1 cm medial to your thumb and aim for the sternal notch. You are trying to hit the clavicle! (Figure 4-21)
- Once you've hit it, SLOWLY and METHODICALLY walk off the clavicle until you drop just under it. Avoid the temptation to change your angle of entry drastically as THIS IS HOW YOU WILL DROP THE LUNG!
- Advance slowly, continuously aspirating in a SHALLOW course until blood is returned.
- As with the internal jugular, if you don't hit the vessel on advancement, pull back slowly, still aspirating, as up to 50% of infant subclavian veins are cannulated during withdrawal of the needle.
- Once you have blood return, disconnect the syringe and ensure NONPULSATILE FLOW! Connect the extension tubing to be extra sure it is not the subclavian artery you are about to cannulate.
- Confirm the blood you've got is actually venous. If you remove the syringe, does blood shoot across the room? As it turns out, color is a terrible indicator. Three good ways to do it:
  - Transduce the needle and hope you don't see an arterial waveform.
  - Connect a length of tubing, let it fill back with blood, and then elevate the tubing. If the blood drains back down, it's most likely venous. If it remains elevated (or is pulsatile), you're probably in the wrong place.
  - Send it to the lab for a blood gas analysis (slightly slower, may not be useful in patients with severe cardiopulmonary disease).
- Once venous flow is established, advance the wire. It should glide easily with NO RESISTANCE. Look for a few PACs as an indication that you are within the heart.
  - Kudos, but now pull the guidewire back a touch.
- Make a small skin nick to accommodate the dilator.
  - You want the guidewire to be included in the hole you just made. Remember, as opposed to the IJ, where you need to get through the platysma muscle, with this nick you're just making enough room for the dilator and catheter to pass through the skin.
- Advance the dilator over the guidewire. Never lose control of the guidewire. Sometimes the dilator has a little difficulty getting underneath the clavicle. Try lowering the angle on the dilator and twisting a little. You don't need to go deep with the dilator, just enough to get into the vein. Ensure free movement of the guidewire.
- Remove the dilator without losing control of the guidewire, and be ready with some gauze to sop up the blood. This is normal. You just made a big hole in the vein.
- Thread the catheter over the guidewire without losing control of the guidewire. The guidewire should come out of the distal port (often the brown, though not always). As with the dilator, sometimes threading the catheter can be tricky. The same tricks apply: lowering the angle and a gentle twisting motion. Holding the catheter close to the skin can also aid with advancing (Figure 4-22).

- Ensure good blood return on each port and flush with saline. Avoid causing an air embolism (even with the Trendelenburg position, up to 30% of all patients can have a patent foramen ovale [PFO], and small volumes of air are more significant in the pediatric population).
- Thread the catheter to the premeasured length and secure with suture. Try to secure tightly while avoiding strangulating the skin.
- Secure the line with suture.
- Clean and dry the area, and then apply the anti-germ patch your facility uses and a clear occlusive dressing (Figure 4-23).
- Order the chest x-ray.
- Check the chest x-ray.
- Happy dance!

Issues and Troubleshooting

- "My patient has a weird-looking clavicle."
  - Perhaps it has been broken, or maybe a congenital malformation. My best advice, avoid it. Look for another site.
- "Uh-oh. I have torrential pulsatile flow." You've hit the subclavian artery.
  - Ideally you have used a small-caliber needle and the patient is not coagulopathic. Monitor the patient closely and make the surgeons aware of the situation. The patient may need surgical repair of the hole.
- "I got a gush of air in the needle." You've hit trachea. Call the surgeons.
- "I felt a pop, and no blood return, and now my peak inspiratory pressures (PIPs) are sky high." You've dropped the lung.
  - Call the surgeons. Ideally, the surgery dictates the need for a chest tube on that side (e.g., a thoracotomy), and therefore the patient just got a chest tube a little early.
  - Remember, you can needle decompress using a 16-G angiocath at the second intercostal space, midclavicular line.
  - To avoid this, insert the needle PARALLEL to the ground. Don't go diving into the chest.

Complications

- Arterial puncture (3–5%)
  - Ideally, only with your needle, not your dilator. If you do happen to dilate the artery, call vascular surgery STAT.
- Pneumothorax (1.5–3%)
  - Choose patients wisely. Although not as common in pediatrics, try to avoid those with chronic obstructive pulmonary disease (COPD) and large

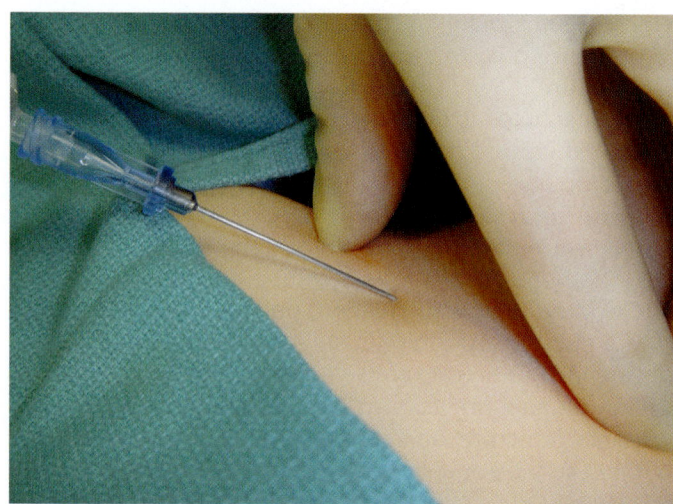

FIGURE 4-21 Needle placement.

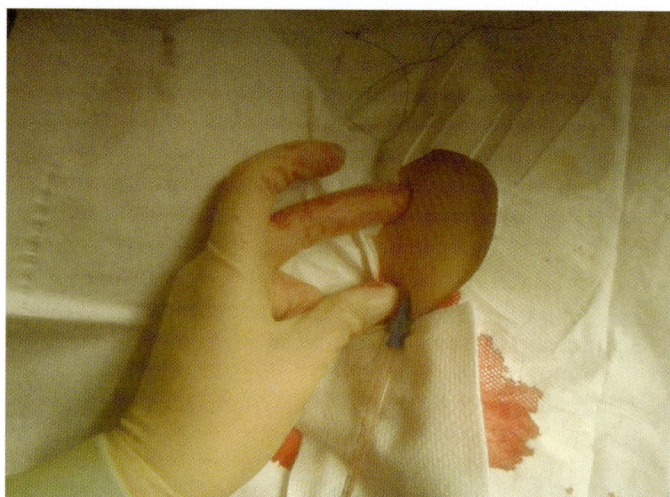

FIGURE 4-22 Subclavian Placement Extraordinaire.

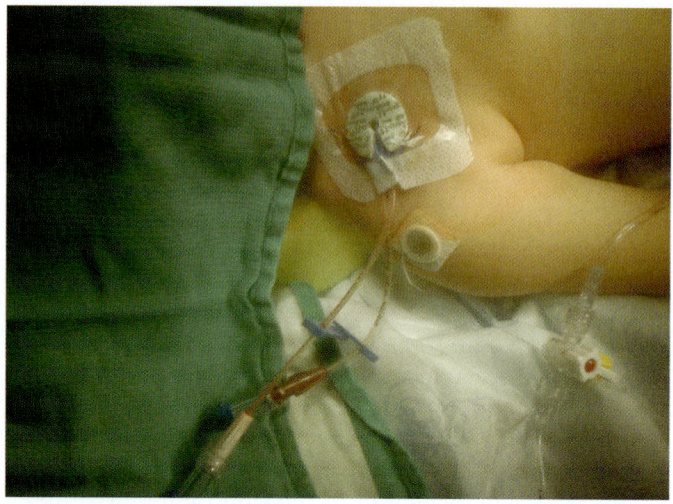

FIGURE 4-23 Dressing on Subclavian Line.

lung volumes. Select patients who are going to be getting a chest tube on that side anyway.
- If you need to decompress in a hurry, a large catheter in the second intercostal space at the midclavicular line works wonders. This is just a temporizing measure, though; get a surgeon to place a chest tube.
- Hemothorax (0.5%)
  - Try to avoid in patients with known coagulopathies. Remember, you can't compress the subclavian vessels.
- Catheter or guidewire embolism
- Tracheal perforation
- Arrhythmias
- Malposition of catheter

THE FEMORAL

The Anatomy of the Femoral

- The femoral vein travels out of the pelvis under the inguinal ligament in the sheath, along with its friends the femoral artery and femoral nerve.
- Recalling from anatomy, the nerve is the most lateral, the vein is the most medial, and the artery lies somewhere in between.
- In small infants the distance between the vein and the artery is minuscule. Therefore experience will help you to gauge the location of the vein after palpation of the arterial pulse.

Advantages

- The femoral is more easily accessible than either the IJ or the subclavian if the surgeons are working on the chest or head and intend to turn the head of the patient away from you.
- There is a lower risk of thrombosis, especially in children younger than 6 months of age.
- An arterial puncture, while not ideal, is more easily controlled and unlikely to have catastrophic consequences, unless of course you pass under the inguinal ligament; we will get to that shortly.

Disadvantages

- May not be ideal for long-term postoperative use if the patient is going to be moving around and flexing his hips.
- Proximity to the groin may make it more difficult to keep clean and dry.

Procedure and Approach

- After induction, and securing of the airway, a small roll should be placed horizontally under the hips of the supine infant to provide MODERATE hip extension. (This step does not apply to children over the age of 2 years.) This will aid in moving the child's legs out of the way and stretching any adipose tissue that might be obscuring your landmarks (Figure 4-24).
- Recheck the endotracheal tube position and ensure the E_TCO_2 is still present.
- Once in position, palpate the landmarks. Find the anterior superior iliac spine and pubic tubercle. The imaginary line drawn between these two structures demarcates the intraabdominal vs. extraabdominal areas. A puncture under and passed the inguinal ligament can lead to an unrecognized retroperitoneal bleed. Another way to ruin your day.
- Strict aseptic technique with wide sterile prep and drape is required following CDC guidelines to reduce the risk of catheter related infections.
  - Wash hands with sterile scrub or aseptic solution.
  - Apply sterile gown and gloves (assuming you are in the OR, you are already donning a scrub cap, and a mask with a shield).
  - Prep the skin in a circular motion, making sure not to overlap the area already cleaned, from the intended puncture site up to the umbilicus and more than halfway down the thighs.
  - Open the sterile drape and completely cover the patient and any areas that may cause you to contaminate yourself.
- Locate the femoral pulse using the first and second fingers of your nondominant hand.
- Puncture the skin.
  - For children under 2 years we use the following technique: With your fingers still on the pulse, puncture the skin using a 22-G needle 1 to 2 cm inferior to the inguinal ligament and approximately 0.5 to 1 cm medial to the femoral impulse aiming toward the umbilicus.
  - For children older than 2 years we use the small needle loaded onto the 3-cc syringe and proceed just as with the internal jugular or subclavian.
  - For children between 2 and 3 years, use either technique.
  - Ultrasound guidance may be useful to ensure success in the first pass.
- Return of blood may not be noted in the hub of the needle. Disengage the needle and pull back slowly and hope for venous flow (Figure 4-25).
- As soon as venous blood return is noted, pass a sterile guidewire through the catheter. It should pass smoothly with no resistance.
- Remove the catheter and leave the wire.

- Proceed to make a skin nick along the wire away from the artery.
- Dilate the subcutaneous tissue.
- Advance the catheter over the wire while maintaining control of the wire.
- Remove the guidewire.
- Aspirate blood from all ports and then flush each of them with normal saline.
- Secure the line with suture.
- Clean and dry the area, and then apply the germ repellant patch your facility uses and a clear occlusive dressing (Figure 4-26).
- Order the chest x-ray.
- Check the chest x-ray.

Issues and Troubleshooting

- "Uh-oh. I have torrential pulsatile flow." You've hit the artery.
  - Thankfully, it was a small needle well below the inguinal ligament in an easily compressible area.
  - Hold pressure and monitor the site.
  - Consider a new puncture site.
- "My patient is going to get up and walk tomorrow." Try another site. This is uncomfortable for ambulatory or excessively wiggly patients.
- "My patient was a little coagulopathic, and now after the line, his hemoglobin and hematocrit (H/H) is dropping for no reason." You likely have a retroperitoneal bleed.
  - Determining the rate of blood loss and the ability to control it or replace it and avoiding surgery are key.
  - Call the surgeons, though, just in case.

Complications

- Arterial puncture
- Retroperitoneal hematoma
- Bladder perforation
- Bowel perforation
- Creation of arterial venous fistula

CONCLUSION

Central venous access in pediatric patients can be a daunting task, but with a little planning and a heaping dose of care and vigilance, it can become a worthy weapon in your anesthetic armamentarium. Pediatric internal jugular, subclavian, and femoral veins can be cannulated in very similar ways to their adult counterparts, albeit on a smaller scale. Concerns about the sterility, sizes of catheters, and the depths of insertion are extremely important in pediatric patients. In those

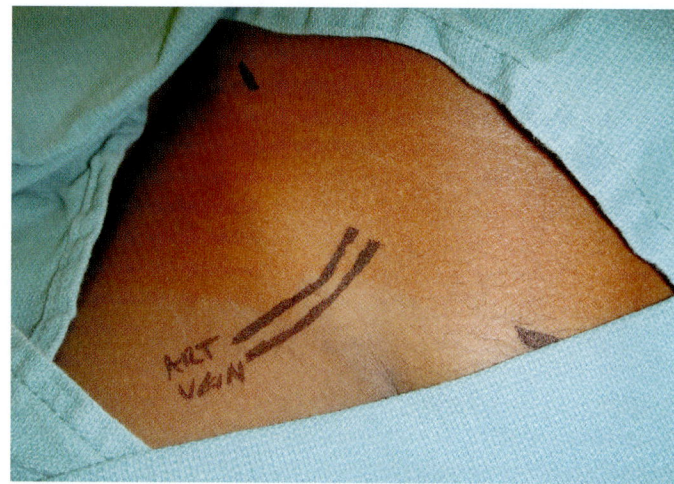

FIGURE 4-24 Femoral Landmarks.

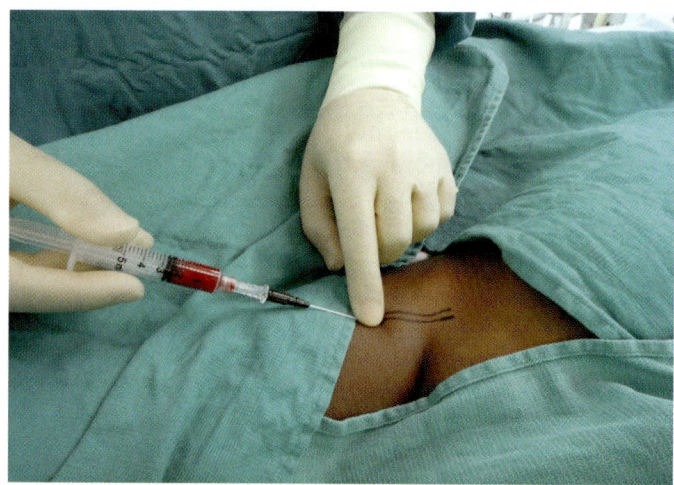

FIGURE 4-25 Placing the Femoral Line.

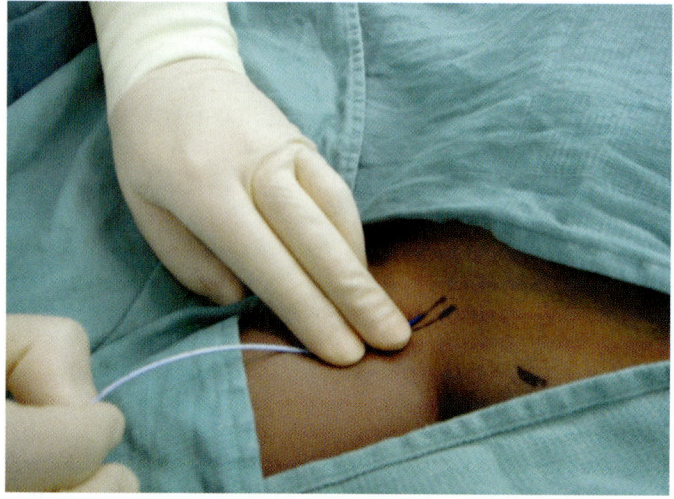

FIGURE 4-26 Another Magnificent Femoral Line Placement!

patients for whom a preinduction line is necessary, consider a peripheral IV or a peripherally inserted central catheter (PICC) line placed by persons specializing in PICC access (and, in some cases, you may even need to consider surgical assistance), followed by a postintubation central line. As with any procedure, indications, risks, benefits, and alternatives must always be considered when dealing with a patient requiring central access. Possible complications should be known, but more importantly, the anesthesiologist should know how to handle those complications should they arise.

REFERENCES

1. Cobb LM, Vinocur CD, Wagner CW, Weintraub WH. The central venous anatomy in infants. *Surg Gynecol Obstet* 1987;165(3):230–234.
2. Andropoulos DB, Bent ST, Skjonsby B, Stayer SA. The optimal length of insertion of central venous catheters for pediatric patients. *Anesth Analg* 2001;93:883–886.

SUGGESTED READING

Wald SH, Cote CJ. Procedures for vascular access. In: Cote CJ, Lerman J, Todres ID, eds. *A practice of anesthesia for infants and children,* 4th ed. Philadelphia: Saunders Elsevier; 2009, pp 1051–1057.

CHAPTER 5

FEMORAL VENOUS ACCESS—THE THUNDER DOWN UNDER: THE FEMORAL VEIN

ROSE ALLOTEH
ARLENE LAMBA

Accept the challenges, so that you may feel the exhilaration of victory.

General George S. Patton

INTRODUCTION

The femoral line has always been labeled as a dirty competitor in the tournaments of lines. Like an unrelenting bad rumor, the femoral line has never been able to ditch its image of being a dirty line, even though this thunder down under has come through as a savior on many occasions. Maybe we are afraid of something a bit unknown to our daily practice. The fact is, we just don't place femoral lines as much, but once we do its thunder just may shock us (no pun intended)! Let's get to know the femoral line a little better; maybe we will be pleasantly surprised and just maybe befriend it. After all, you can't judge a book by its cover or, in this case, by its location!

The center of the bad rap the femoral line gets is the prevailing myth that it's a line that lurks close to infections. But the truth of the matter is that femoral lines do not get infected any more than other central lines.[1] Femoral lines can be done emergently with anatomical landmarks or even under ultrasound guidance.

What gives these lines the real thunder down under besides their location? Femoral lines are great "just in case" lines. Put them in at the start of a case and that makes you say "yikes!," but if at the end your worst fears didn't materialize, just take the femoral line out.

Many times this line is the savior when those you depended on just didn't come through, like when you try to poke your old friends the subclavian or jugular but you hit the artery by mistake. Now in the neck this can lead to many sticky situations. Hey, you may have just hit the carotid, which could mean you may now have a cerebrovascular problem, which could mean you have a hematoma, or a bleeding problem or even an airway problem.[2] But in the femoral region the arterial stick is not that catastrophic. It'll be easy to get to, easy to fix, and, at best, you won't lose the airway.

You get the drift? Not bad for a mislabeled dirty line.

However, there in a new Sheriff in town: The ultrasound. Ultrasound-guided femoral vein stick ensures a 100% success rate.[3]

INDICATIONS

- Volume access[4] (emergent or otherwise)
- Inotropic access/central venous pressure (CVP) monitoring. You can even float a Swan catheter from a femoral introducer, but be aware that you won't be able to adjust the Swan during surgery

since you'll be near the head of the patient and not the groin!
- Hypertonic fluids (total parenteral nutrition [TPN], for example)

CONTRAINDICATIONS

- Infection at the site, but remember all lines can get infected!
- Penetrating abdominal trauma (your femoral infusion will spill into the abdomen)
- Occlusion of the inferior vena cava from tumor (consider this the "lower" variant of superior vena cava syndrome)
- Prior groin surgery is a relative contraindication (e.g., an arterial graft placement).

EQUIPMENT

- Keep it clean and simple: sterile prep, drape, and gloves (lights, camera, and action!)
- Central line kit
- Helper, aka an elf or a medical student will do, in helping pull the abdomen out of the way, should the patient require help in exposing the anatomy.
- Ultrasound machine for venipuncture, if available

If the femoral lines are hanging out on the floor:
- Don't be nervous. When someone comes with a femoral line, it's usually from the cardiac cath lab. So most likely someone put it in who actually loves and relies on these lines. Someone who respects what they stand for and what they can do for us.
- When the cath lab calls and are going to send someone down, I always tell them, "Don't pull your groin lines!"

THE PHILOSOPHY OF FEMORAL LINES

- Doing a neuro case? Need good access? Want to be able to get at and troubleshoot a central line? Hey, a femoral line works just right. You don't cut off venous drainage from the head, you won't have to crawl up and under the drapes, bumping the patient and infuriating the "looking through the microscope" neurosurgeons.
- Surgeons working high in the chest? Hey, the "northern route" into the heart might get cut off. How will you resuscitate? Try the "southern route" via the femoral approach.
- If you really sit down and THINK about how you'll get stuff into the patient's heart, you may be surprised at how often a femoral line makes sense.

FEMORAL LINE HISTORY AND PHYSICAL

- Location, location, location! Look at the groin. See it? Great! Now, check for the usual stuff (infection, hematoma). Nada? OK, look for the unusual stuff (inguinal lymphadenopathy compressing and distorting the anatomy). All good? March onward!
- Be wary. If the inferior vena cava (IVC) is likely to be interrupted (renal cell cancer, for example, blocking passage), then don't use the femoral approach.

Imagine driving a van from the inner to the outer lane: VEIN → ARTERY → NERVE.

TECHNIQUE

- Prep it, drape it, and light it[5] (good lighting that is) (Figure 5-1).
- If the patient's abdomen protrudes, have a helper pull the pannus back and give you a straight shot.
- The landmarks, from lateral to medial, are, using the mnemonic NAVEL, nerve, artery, vein, empty space, lymphatics.
- For the irreverent, the landmarks, from lateral to medial, are, using the mnemonic, NAVY, nerve, artery, vein, Yahoo! The yahoo implies some degree of happiness affiliated with the pudendal region, and has nothing to do with the Internet search engine.
- Localize the area with lidocaine, just enough to make a nice wheal. Don't be shy with the numbing; the patient will thank you for it! (Figure 5-2)
- Light sedation may be necessary if your patient is awake. Remember, you might need his or her cooperation. ("Hold still, sir/ma'am, this will only take a minute.")
- Numb → Numb'er → Numb'est
- This hurts and is more than a little scary, so if you can do this when the patient is under general anesthesia, then do that.
- Feel the pulse, go medial, and advance at a 45-degree angle to the skin. No need for a finder here.
- Use the long needle; the catheter will get kinked and scrunched.
- Aspirate while advancing.
- Once you get blood flow, disconnect the needle and watch for arterial spurting (if it spurts, hold pressure).
- Alternatively, if you do not have ultrasound, you could leave the needle in for a moment and stick another one medial to it. Take the first needle out when you get a venipuncture.
- If both arterial and venipuncture are required, then presto! You have both!

- However, bear in mind that the complication of an arteriovenous (AV) fistula may develop.
- If you're in the vein, advance the wire (Figure 5-3).
- Once the wire's in, lay the dull edge of your blade against the wire and guide it to make a nice clean nick in the skin. Remove the needle.
- Introduce the dilator over the wire, but not too much (a few centimeters) to avoid tearing a gaping hole in the vein.
- Advance the line.
- Aspirate and flush.
- Sew in place.
- Hook up to your infusion.
- It's just like knitting, left then right, but careful no poking yourself! (Figure 5-4)

Stabilize your needle and thread wire. No kinks, just glide it in nice and easy and under control.

Things that make you go Hmm:[2]

- The femoral is deep. In larger patients, it's real deep, and it can be a source of genuine frustration to find the femoral vein. So don't get frustrated!
- Whoops, somehow with your fine needle work you dropped a lung by this approach! If you do drop a lung with the femoral approach, you may want to call Ripley's Believe It or Not!
- If the patient is going to ambulate soon after the case, a femoral line is clumsy and probably not a good idea in general. Try ambulating with that in you. Yes, our thoughts exactly: bed rest is best.
- If you're going femoral, don't put a dinky short line in. The thing will pull out. Remember its nickname is thunder down under!
- If you're right handed, go for the right femoral; the mechanics are just easier.
- If you are having a terrible time of it, consider an ultrasound to help you "find" the vessel.[3] There's no shame in using the ultrasound; if you have it, then use it!

Things that make you go Mmmmmmmm and Grrrrrr and Mmmmmm all at once:

Imagine yourself in the midst of a pediatric femoral central line placement, and instead of aspirating blood, you aspirate a clear, yellow fluid. Or maybe you detect some feculent material in your syringe. Bowel and bladder are just a peritoneal reflection away from the groin, so be careful, especially in the pediatric population.[4]

Next, imagine a patient who is a tad on the coagulopathic side, so you go the femoral route to avoid a potential bleeding problem in a more clinically important region. That femoral stick can ooze (or trickle or gush) its way into a retroperitoneal hematoma.[2] So if your patient is becoming unstable for no other apparent reason, think of this and do serial hematocrits.

Finally, imagine your patient already has a femoral arterial line and needs a venous line (or vice versa). If you place the complementary catheter on the same side as the existing line, it is possible for an AV fistula to develop.

OK, don't get so dramatic! We had to let it be known but now that it is, move forward with the confidence that you may have possibly befriended this line whose thunder will now be your strength. Go forward, learn it, practice it, use it, and own it!

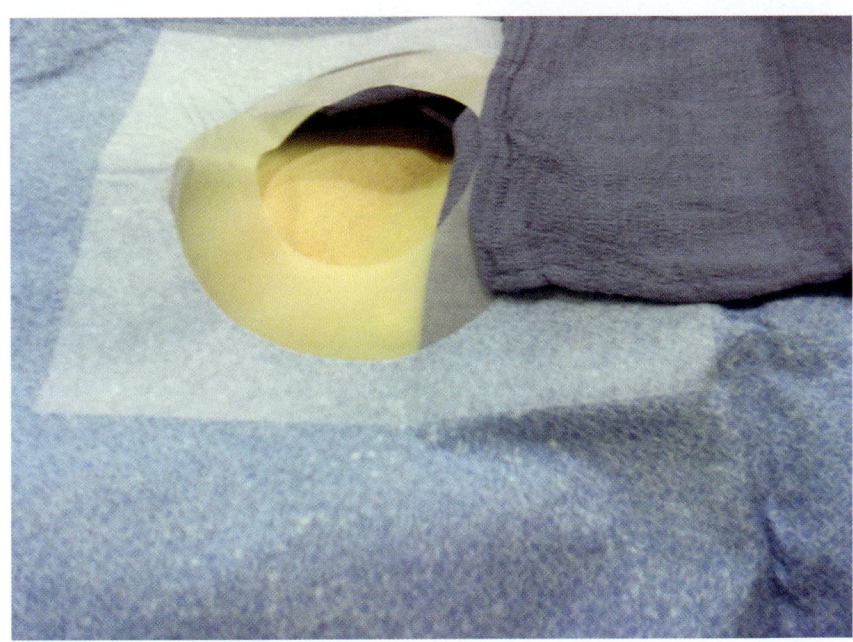

FIGURE 5-1 Sterile, prepared, and draped groin.

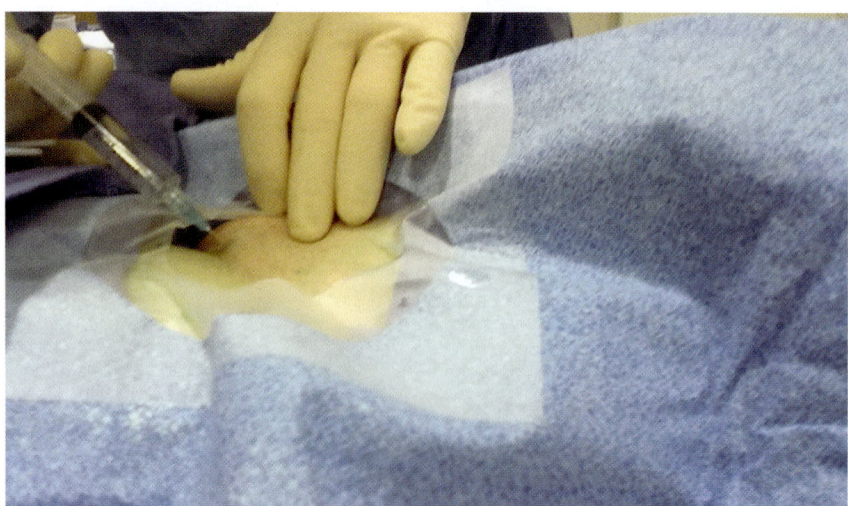

FIGURE 5-2 Numb and number.

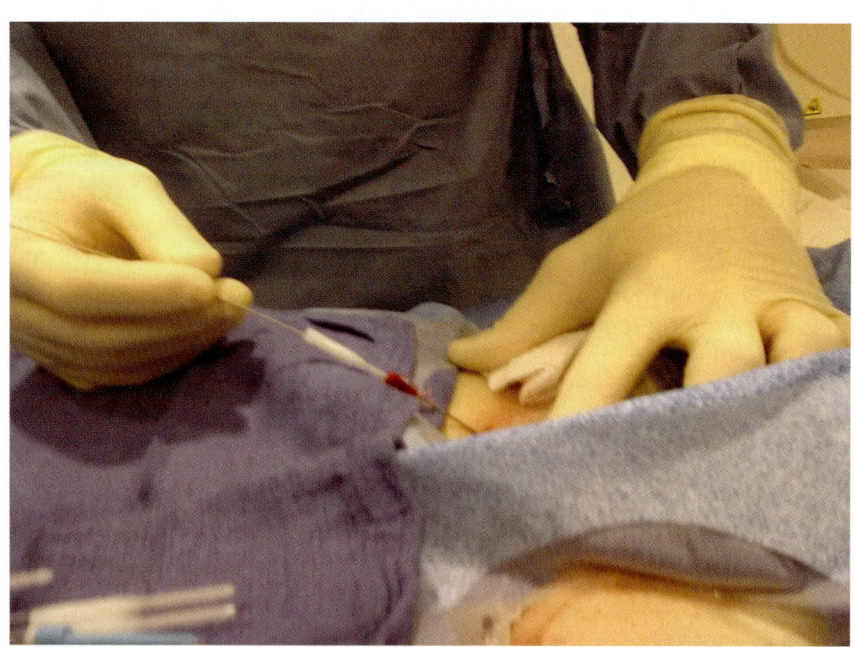

FIGURE 5-3 Advancing wire.

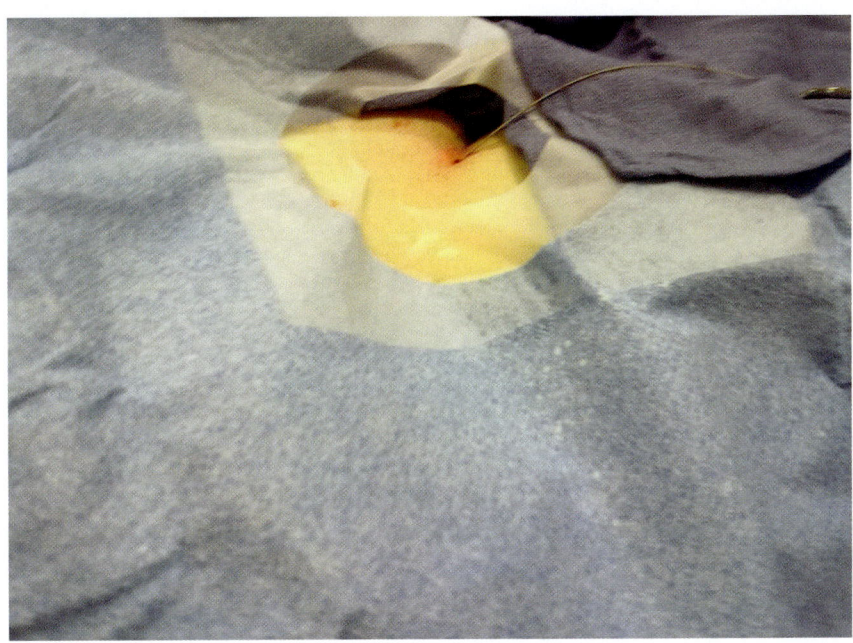

FIGURE 5-4 Guidewire in femoral vein.

REFERENCES

1. Williams JF, Seneff MG, Friedman BC, et al. Use of femoral venous catheters in critically ill adults: Prospective study. *Crit Care Med* 1991;19:550–553.
   This study pre-dates the Deshpande group study and also concludes that the rate of major infectious complications associated with femoral venous catheters in the ICU setting is acceptably low.
2. Eisen LA, Narasimhan M, Berger JS, et al. Mechanical complications of central venous catheters. *J Intensive Care Med* 2006;21(1):40–46.
   The study analyzed 385 consecutive central venous catheter (CVC) attempts over a 6-month period. Complications included failure to place the CVC, arterial puncture, improper position, pneumothorax, hematoma, hemothorax, and asystolic cardiac arrest of unknown etiology. The subclavian approach had a higher complication rate than the internal jugular or the femoral approach.
3. Abboud PA, Kendall JL. Ultrasound guidance for vascular access. *Emerg Med Clin North Am* 2004;22(3):749–773.
   Research focuses on ultrasound (US) guidance to achieve vascular access, which in turn increases the safety and efficiency of venous access procedures. Support the use of US guidance over the traditional landmark approach for venous access.
4. Marino PL, Sutin KM. Establishing venous access. In: Marino PL, ed. *The ICU book,* Vol 1, 3rd ed. New York: RR Donnelley; 2007, pp 108–128/6.
5. Tsui JY, Collins AB, White DW, Lai J, Tabas JA. Placement of a femoral venous catheter. *N Engl J Med* 2008;358:e30.
   Video that shows the placement and important uses for femoral line catheters.

SUGGESTED READING

Durbec O, Viviand X, Potie F, Vialet R, Albanese J, Martin C. A prospective evaluation of the use of femoral venous catheters in critically ill adults. *Crit Care Med* 1997;25(12): 1986–1989.

Study consisted of 80 consecutive patients admitted to the ICU who underwent right femoral venous catheterization over a 13-month period. Conclusion was that femoral vein catheterization with a polyurethane catheter is associated with an 8.5% frequency rate of femoral vein thrombosis. Femoral venous catheterization is an alternate site of insertion to the jugular and subclavian veins for central venous access in the critically ill.

CHAPTER 6

PICC LINES—JUST REALLY, REALLY LONG IVS

JUSTIN HAMRICK
DEBORAH SCHWENGEL

"Dr. Catheter, this just came for you."
"Ah, splendid. This must be my malaria."
Dr. Catheter, Gremlins, The New Batch (1990)

INDICATIONS

- Poor peripheral access
- Long-term medication administration (usually 3 weeks to 1 year)
  - Chemotherapy
  - Total parenteral nutrition (TPN), hyperalimentation, hyperosmolar solutions
  - Blood products
- Repeated venous sampling—limits venipunctures
- Measurement of central venous pressure (CVP)

RELATIVE CONTRAINDICATIONS

- Massive anasarca/edema—not a true contraindication, but may be more difficult to obtain
- Burns—might also be a relative contraindication; a central line might also be a necessity in some cases
- Renal failure or impending renal failure—may need to use upper extremity vein for graft or fistula formula (may not be a problem in pediatrics)
- Sclerosis
- Thrombosis—have to weigh risk/benefit ratio; if patient has history and if vein already thrombotic, the line just will not go
- Phlebitis

- Extremities on ipsilateral side of radical mastectomy or arteriovenous (AV) fistula
- Cellulitis
- Veins that drain the neck in the setting of increased intracranial pressure (ICP)—not ideal but sometimes a judgment call

EQUIPMENT

- Peripherally inserted central catheter (PICC) kit
  - Polyurethane or silicone catheter of appropriate size (usually 2-, 3-, 4-, or 5-French catheters)
  - Single or double lumen
  - Ultrasound and gel
  - Sterile drapes, gown, and gloves

PERTINENT HISTORY AND PHYSICAL EXAMINATION

- History of difficult IV access
- Need for ongoing medication administration
- Patency of vessels, history of thrombosis?
- Vascular procedures?
- Contraindications to alternative access
- Usually no preprocedural blood work needed (unless the patient is severely coagulopathic or unstable); even so, it is probably a safer line than neck or subclavian; sticking a vein in the arm doesn't mess with hemodynamics, and coagulopathy is not very risky for peripheral sticks.

VEIN SELECTION[1]

- ≤3 months
  - Superficial temporal, posterior auricular, saphenous, median cubital, cephalic, basilic, scalp
- 4 months to 12 months (or until ambulation)
  - Saphenous, cephalic, basilic, and median cubital
- >12 months (or after ambulating)
  - Cephalic, basilic, brachial, and median cubital

TECHNIQUE

- Full assessment of the patient's veins will increase your likelihood of success. The road less traveled may be the one to go down. Thanks, Frost.
- Full sterile prep and drape.
- Identify the vessel with small 22- or 24-gauge Angiocath (usually with ultrasound guidance using a small-size linear array probe). Look on BOTH sides for best site BEFORE draping and cleaning.
  - Basilic vein preferred about 3 cm above elbow
  - Cephalic vein has more acute angle at the junction to axillary vein, making catheter advancement difficult.
- Cannulate the vessel with introducer needle, like starting an IV or use Seldinger technique.
- Place guidewire into appropriate vessel (may observe under ultrasound or fluoroscopy) (Figure 6-1).
- Dilate to proper size (Figure 6-2).
- Insert peel-away sheath (Figure 6-3).
- Cut catheter to length.
- Insert PICC line to appropriate depth via peel-away sheath (or needle in large vein) (Figure 6-4).
- Cuff (if present) is advanced into the soft tissue.
- At exit site catheter is secured with Steri-Strips or a device like a Stat Lock® (these are usually not sutured because of the risk of silicone catheters breaking off at the suture and then proximal catheter embolizing) (Figure 6-5).
- Confirm placement with x-ray.
  - Ideal central placement is at the superior vena cava/right atrium (SVC/RA) junction.
    - Central placement decreases fibrin sheath and thrombus formation.
  - Position will vary with arm position.
- Secure and apply dressing.

KIDS, JUST SMALL ADULTS?

- Need to explain it twice (once to child and once to parents!)
- May need sedation (not just local)
  - May use Sweet-Ease® in the neonate
  - Older children may need local versus sedation versus general anesthesia.
- May use numbing cream (30 to 60 minutes PRIOR to procedure). Patient may not be talked into holding still for lidocaine injection.
- Various sites not routinely used in adults (saphenous, etc.). Some patients may not be walking.
- Better securing. Kids try to pull things out!
- May need ultrasound more often.
- One size DOESN'T fit all! Need to measure length and adjust size to patient.

COMPLICATIONS

- Noncentral catheters have a higher complication rate than central catheters (28.8% vs. 3.8%).[2]
- Overall complications (especially infection) directly proportional to catheter duration.[1-3]
- Hematoma
- Catheter occlusion (1.7–6.5%)
- Infection (1–3%, similar to tunneled central venous catheter [CVC])[4]
  - Related to catheter duration[3]
    - Risk increases by 14% every day until about day 20.
    - Risk increases by 33% every day after day 35.
    - May consider changing PICC after 30 days.
- Arterial puncture
- Thrombosis (1–4%)
  - Adults have a 6.6 risk ratio versus a peripheral catheter[5]
- Vascular injury/tip perforation
- Chronic venous insufficiency
- Pulmonary embolization
- Fracture of line with embolization
- Cardiac tamponade
- Nerve injury
- Phlebitis (1–10%)
- Leaking catheter (0.1–11.2%)
  - Sutured catheters leak less than does standard taping. Sutureless securement devices and staples aren't different from sutured catheters.[6]

COMMENTS

- PICC success
  - Parents and patients seem to be genuinely satisfied with therapy when the PICC line works correctly. Studies have shown that patients report a higher satisfaction with medication administration in PICC lines versus peripheral catheters.[7] You hear less screaming during blood draws and you aren't getting called all night to figure out how to administer 13 drugs that all have to run over 4 hours through a single shoddy 24-gauge peripheral intravenous (PIV) line. The lack of headaches may be worth it.

Chapter 6 PICC LINES—JUST REALLY, REALLY LONG IVS

Table 6-1 PICC Line Flushing Recommendations[8,9]

Patient Weight (kg)	Locking Solution (Patency)	Minimum Flush Volume (0.9% NaCl)
>50	Heparin 100 units/mL	• 10 mL pre- and postmedication administration • Draw 10 mL waste before blood sampling (20 mL if PT/PTT/INR), and flush postsampling with 20 mL
5–50	Heparin 100 units/mL	• 3–5 mL pre- and postmedication administration • Draw 1.5 mL of waste before blood sampling and flush postsampling with 3 mL
<5	Heparin 50 units/mL	• 3 mL (1.5 mL if patient is fluid restricted) • Draw 1.5 mL waste before blood sampling and flush with 3 mL postsampling

PT/PTT/INR, prothrombin time/partial thromboplastin time/international normalized ratio.

- Less IV restarts and sticks for blood draws. It is not uncommon for medications, labs, or other treatments to be delayed in pediatric patients due to lack of access.
- Cost compared to maintenance and replacement of peripheral catheters can be similar.[7]
- PICC failures/limitations
  - Access to placement. It is not uncommon for a PICC service to exist in a hospital. Due to the nonemergent nature of a PICC line, it may be quite difficult to get a PICC line placed before 8 am, after 4 pm, or on a weekend. Don't be above begging to get it done, though. A skilled PICC service can be your best friend.
  - Patients with no peripheral veins are harder and take longer to place, but you can use ultrasound to place/find a vein that you can't see or palpate.
  - Vasospasm can make it harder to place.
  - It is possible to accidentally place into an artery; you don't want to cannulate "Big Red."
- Line maintenance
  - PICCs need to be maintained with a constant fluid infusion or heparin flush if the line is locked between uses.
  - Heparin flush is recommended (Table 6-1).

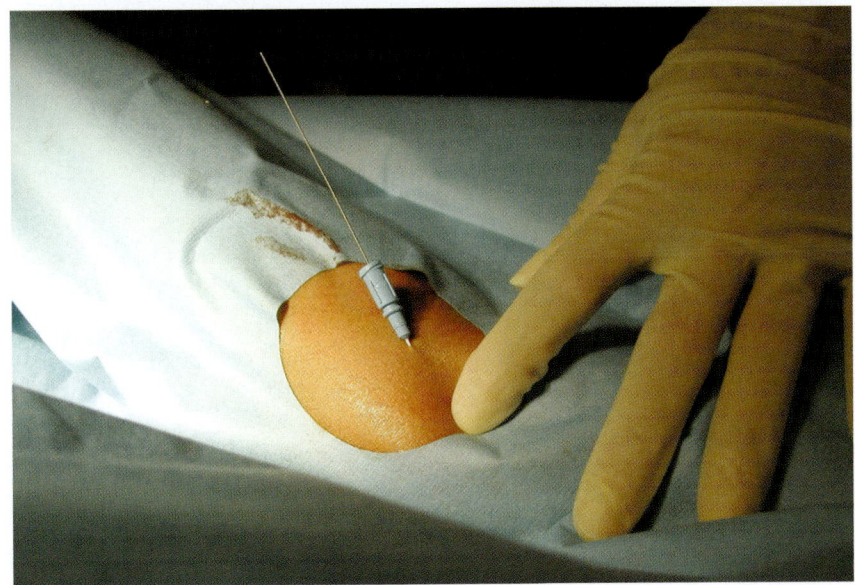

FIGURE 6-1 After cannulation of the vein, a wire is inserted through the catheter.

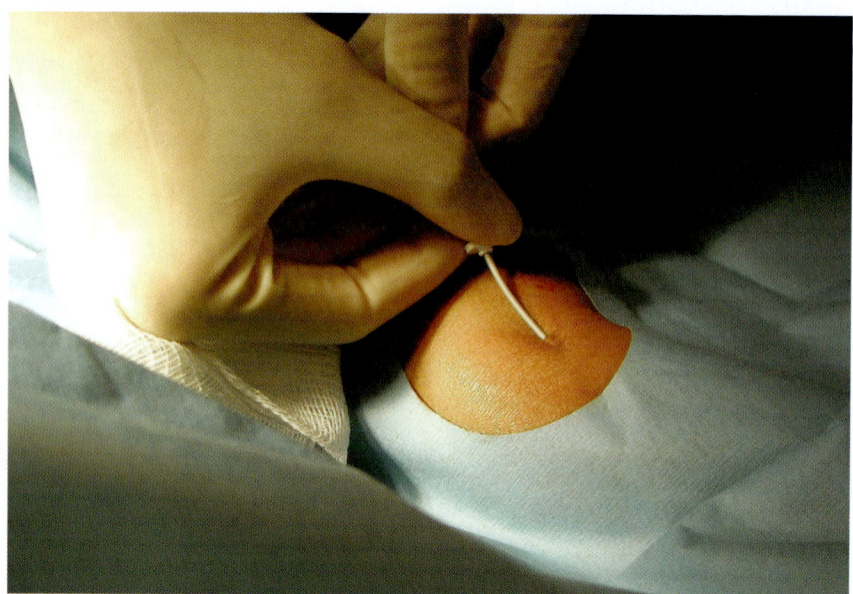

FIGURE 6-2 The IV catheter is removed and a dilator is passed over the wire to dilate in preparation for the sheath.

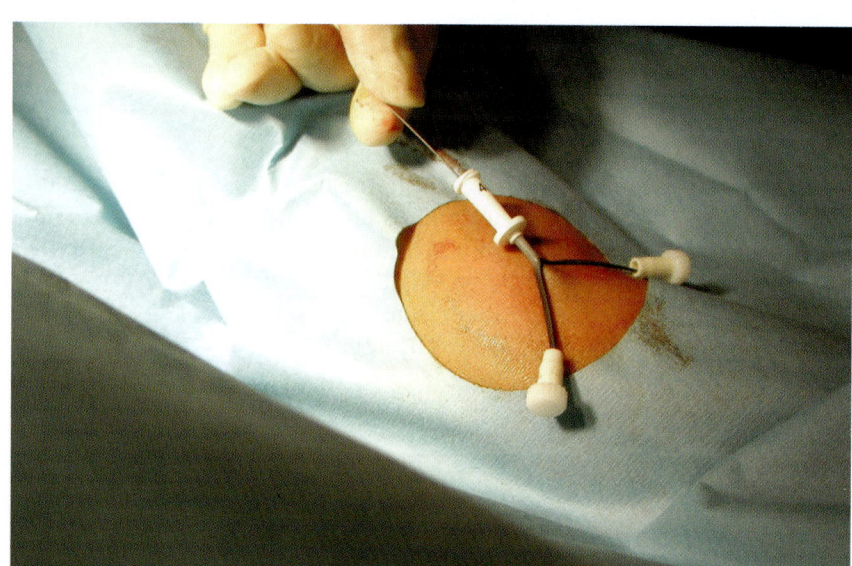

FIGURE 6-3 The peel-away sheath with a dilator is passed over the wire into the vein.

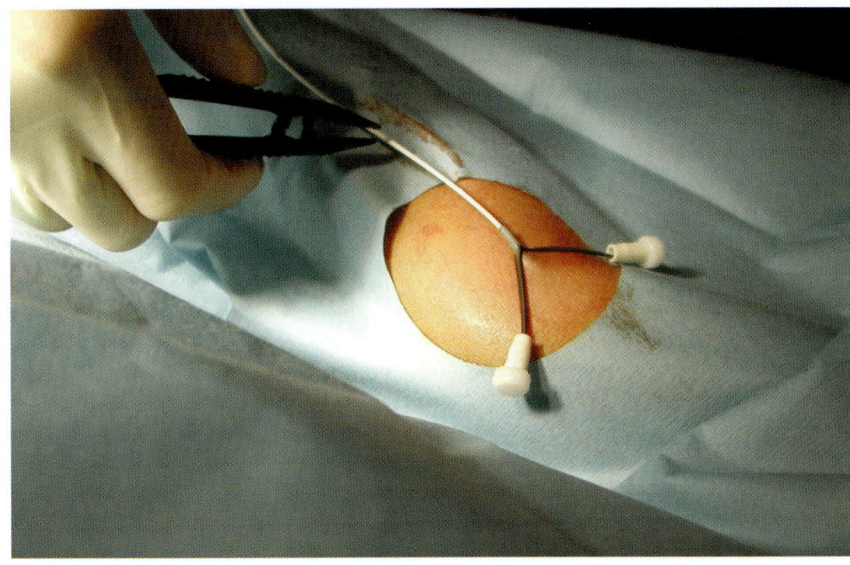

FIGURE 6-4 After removing the wire and dilator, the PICC is inserted into the peel-away sheath and advanced until in place.

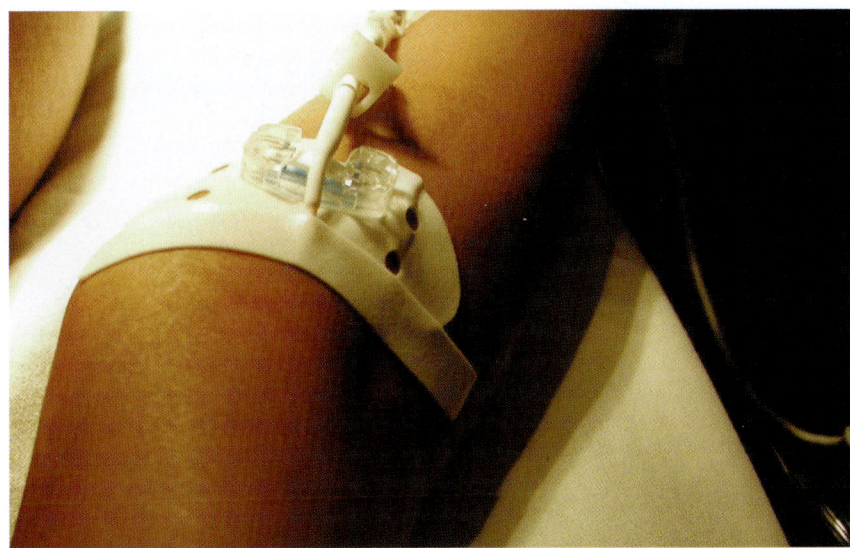

FIGURE 6-5 After confirming PICC placement by x-ray, the sheath is removed and the PICC is secured with a device like a Stat Lock®.

REFERENCES

1. Mickler PA. Neonatal and pediatric perspectives in PICC placement. *J Infus Nurs* 2008;31(5):282–285.
2. Racadio JM, Doellman DA, Johnson ND, et al. Pediatric peripherally inserted central catheters: complication rates related to catheter tip location. *Pediatrics* 2001;107(2):E28.
3. Sengupta A, Lehman C, Diener-West M, et al. Catheter duration and risk of CLA-BSI in neonates with PICCs. *Pediatrics* 2010;125(4):648–653.
4. Al Raiy B, Fakih MG, Bryan-Nomides N, et al. Peripherally inserted central venous catheters in the acute care setting: a safe alternative to high-risk short-term central venous catheters. *Am J Infect Control* 2010;38(2):149–153.
5. Periard D, Monney P, Waeber G, et al. Randomized controlled trial of peripherally inserted central catheters vs. peripheral catheters for middle duration in-hospital intravenous therapy. *J Thromb Haemost* 2008;6(8):1281–1288.
6. Graf JM, Newman CD, McPherson ML. Sutured securement of peripherally inserted central catheters yields fewer complications in pediatric patients. *JPEN J Parenter Enteral Nutr* 2006;30(6):532–535.
7. Schwengel DA, Periard D, Monney P, Waeber G, et al. Peripherally inserted central catheters: a randomized, controlled, prospective trial in pediatric surgical patients. *Anesth Analg* 2004;99(4):1038–1043.
8. Rocca N. PICC Line-Technical Skills Program. Queen's University, 2010.
9. Fry B. Intermittent heparin flushing protocols. A standardization issue. *J Intraven Nurs* 1992;15(3):160–163.

PART II
ARTERIAL ACCESS

CHAPTER 7

THE RADIAL A-LINE: A VERSATILE AND ESSENTIAL TOOL

JULIAN B. KERTSMAN
VINCENT DEANGELIS

A man is as old as his arteries.
Thomas Sydenham (1600s)

INTRODUCTION

If there is one thing that makes an anesthesiologist breathe easy when taking over a big case, it is knowing you have "great access," and at the top of the list is the access to an arterial line. An A-line is extremely useful because it provides beat-to-beat blood pressure monitoring as well as several other uses described in this chapter. The radial artery is the most commonly utilized and convenient site for A-line placement.

INDICATIONS: WHY PLACE AN A-LINE?

- Beat-to-beat blood pressure monitoring: If doing a big case with severe blood loss or dosing medications in a hemodynamically compromised patient, having real-time blood pressure monitoring can be lifesaving! The noninvasive blood pressure cuff may be fine in routine surgeries for healthy patients, but waiting for it to cycle in an unstable patient is suboptimal. Having an A-line prior to induction is extremely helpful in minimizing the hypotension of induction and the hypertensive response to intubation by allowing instantaneous diagnosis and treatment.
- You never regret having an A-line; you often regret NOT having one!
- Access for frequent blood sampling: Frequent blood sampling, such as blood gases or activated coagulation time (ACT) monitoring is easily facilitated by having an A-line. Blood sampling from an A-line is usually technically simple, as it is with a central line. Attempting to draw back blood from a peripheral IV or having to stick a patient is inconvenient and inefficient when compared to sampling from an A-line. In addition, sampling from an A-line is less prone to dilution when compared to a line used to administer fluids.
- (Joke)And if the above didn't convince you to place an A-line yet, most vascular surgeons will ask you to place an A-line anyway.
- It is the best option for long-term monitoring, such as in the ICU. Have a patient who is bound for an extended ICU stay? A radial A-line is the best option in this case because along with its utility intraoperatively, it may be used for long-term blood pressure monitoring and blood sampling.
- Low rate of complications: Although complications (listed below) exist, they are fairly rare.

RISKS/COMPLICATIONS

Radial A-lines are routinely used in most institutions with minimal reported complications.
- Limb ischemia: Absent pulses, dampened waveform, mottled/blanched skin, delayed capillary refill, and finger pain or weakness are all signs of limb

ischemia. Although no consensus on treatment exists, early recognition is the key to reducing likelihood of permanent injury.[1] The Allen test (described below) can be used prior to placement of an A-line as a tool to predict hand ischemia from a radial A-line.
- Infection: Infection at the site of cannulation may occur if sterile technique (see below) is not observed. Most infections resolve with removal of the catheter and a course of IV antibiotics.[2]
- Pseudoaneurysm/thrombosis: Radial artery pseudoaneurysms present as a palpable pulsatile mass over the artery with possible overlying tissue necrosis. Diagnosis is confirmed by Doppler sonography showing thrombosis and turbulence.[2]
- Nerve damage: Damage to the median or radial nerve is possible as they both course in close proximity to the radial artery. Knowledge of the anatomy (see below) is key in avoiding possible nerve damage.
- Hematoma formation/compartment syndrome: Hematoma formation may occur with multiple punctures of the artery. Patients particularly at risk are those who are anticoagulated or those with clotting disorders. Direct pressure on the site decreases the chance of hematoma formation and compartment syndrome occurrence.

ANATOMY

- Anatomy of the radial artery: The radial artery arises from the bifurcation of the brachial artery in the cubital fossa and runs on the anterior aspect of the lateral forearm and winds laterally around the wrist through the anatomical snuff box, where it anastomoses with the ulnar artery in forming the palmar arches.[1]
- Anatomy of ulnar artery: The ulnar artery also arises from the bifurcation of the brachial artery but courses the medial forearm into the hand where it forms the deep palmar arch and joins with the radial artery in formation of palmar arches.[1]
- Radial versus ulnar artery cannulation: Although the diameter of the ulnar artery is larger at the level of the cubital fossa, the diameter of radial artery is equal or larger than that of the ulnar artery at the level of the wrist. Although both of these arteries may be cannulated, the consistent anatomical location of the radial artery compared to the tortuous course of the ulnar artery makes the radial artery a better choice for cannulation.

THE MODIFIED ALLEN'S TEST

- How it is performed:
  - The patient is asked to elevate the hand and clench his/her fist several times for approximately 30 seconds until the skin is blanched.
  - Direct pressure is held over the ulnar and radial arteries at the level of expected artery cannulation.
  - The patient is instructed to open his/her hand (which should appear blanched).
  - Pressure on the ulnar artery is released and the time for return of color to the hand is monitored.
  - In the inverse modified Allen's test, the pressure on the radial artery is released.
  - In a normal exam, color should return to the hand within 7 to 10 seconds.
- Although the modified Allen's test is a widely accepted test to monitor collateral blood flow to the hand, its clinical use is controversial. Slogoff et al. performed the modified Allen's test of 411 patients and found a greater than 15-second reperfusion time in 16 patients (3.9%). Despite this, radial artery cannulation was performed on each of these patients without any ischemic complications. The literature suggests that although a normal modified Allen's test is reassuring, a negative test has not been proven to predict hand ischemia with radial artery cannulation.

METHODS FOR INSERTION

Direct Cannulation

Tools: Arrow kit, wrist support, chlorhexidine pads, gauze, 1% lidocaine in a syringe with a 25-gauge needle, sterile gloves.

Step-by-step guide to A-line success:
- Perform the Allen test to gain reassurance of sufficient collateral circulation.
- Palpate for an area with an appreciable radial pulse.
- Place wrist support onto patient's wrist with adequate extension to open up the "landing zone" to eliminate the thenar eminence as an obstacle. In addition, abducting the thumb and attaching it to the work area with a piece of tape may augment wrist extension. Make certain to avoid overextension to prevent median nerve injury and overtightening of wrist guard straps because that may compress the radial artery and make the pulse difficult to palpate.
- Clean the "landing zone" with a chlorhexidine. Sterile drapes are not necessary; however, sterile gloves and sterile prep are recommended (Figure 7-1).

- Inject sufficient lidocaine subcutaneously to numb the skin (1–3 cc is usually sufficient) (Figure 7-2).
- With sterile gloves and wrist extended, palpate for the pulse with the nondominant hand while slowly advancing arrow at a shallow angle (Figure 7-3).
- When a flash is seen in the chamber, advance the catheter another millimeter. This is the key to ensure successful cannulation (Figures 7-4 and 7-5).
- Lower the arrow kit parallel to the forearm and slowly advance the guidewire to the black line on the clear chamber, signifying that the wire has been advanced adequately. As with most techniques in anesthesia (and usually in life), DO NOT FORCE IT! The wire should slide relatively easily and smoothly.
- Slide the catheter over the wire until the hub is at the skin (again, the catheter should slide relatively smoothly) (Figure 7-6).
- Compress the artery proximally while removing the wire to keep the work area clean while attaching the catheter to A-line tubing (Figures 7-7 and 7-8).
- You may choose to protect your A-line from being pulled out by creating a loop with the tubing around the patient's thumb (Figure 7-9).

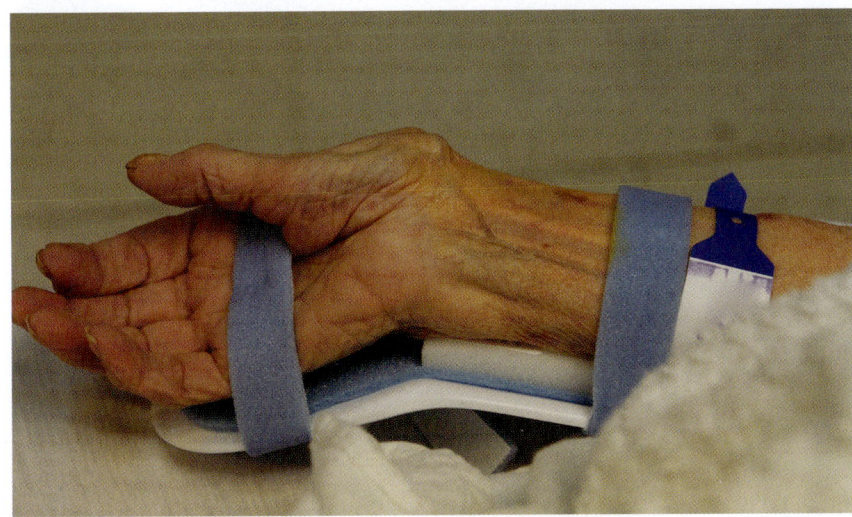

FIGURE 7-1 Clean the "landing zone" with chlorhexidine. Sterile drapes are not necessary; however, sterile gloves and sterile prep are recommended.

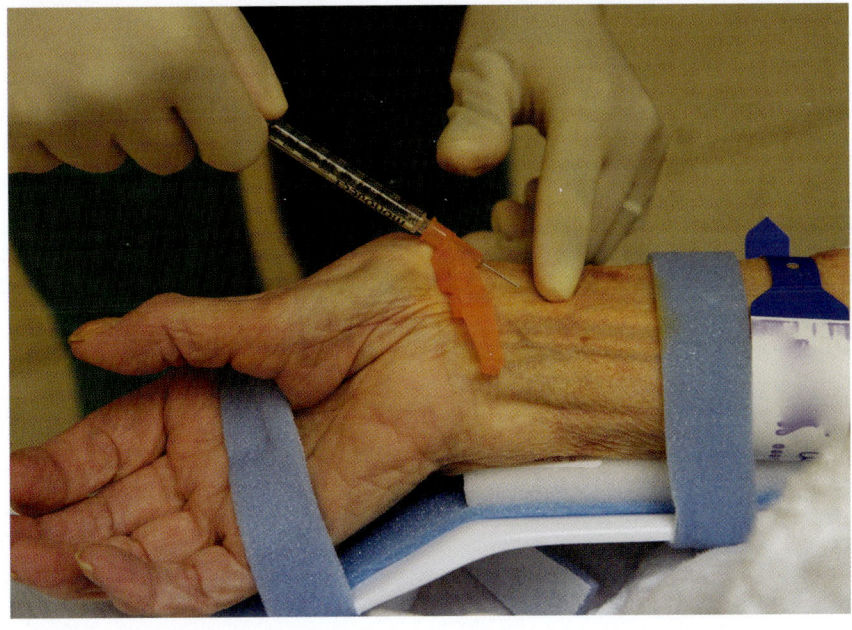

FIGURE 7-2 Inject sufficient lidocaine subcutaneously to numb the skin (1-3 cc is usually sufficient).

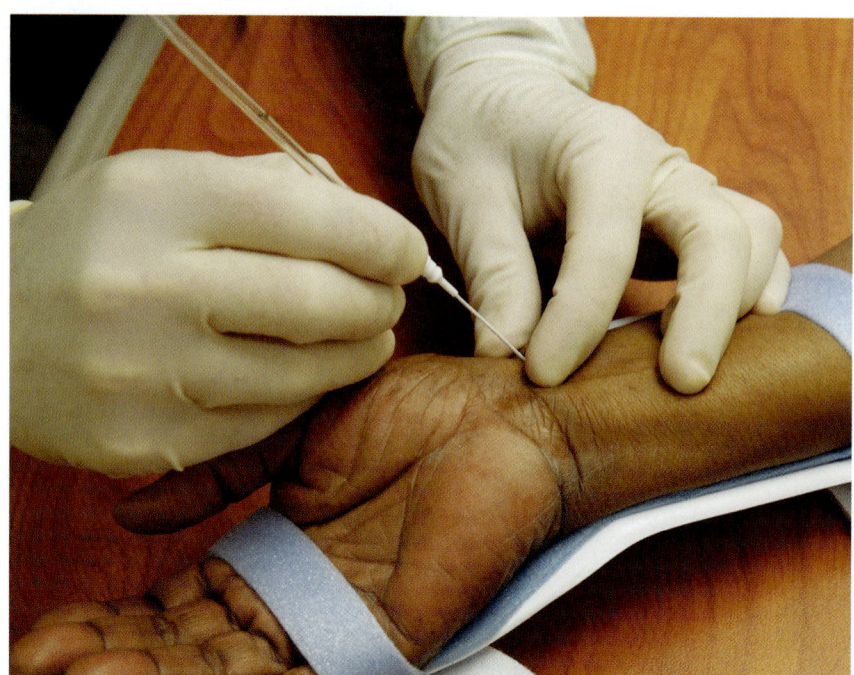

FIGURE 7-3 With sterile gloves and wrist extended, palpate for the pulse with the nondominant hand while slowly advancing the 20-gauge IV catheter at a shallow angle.

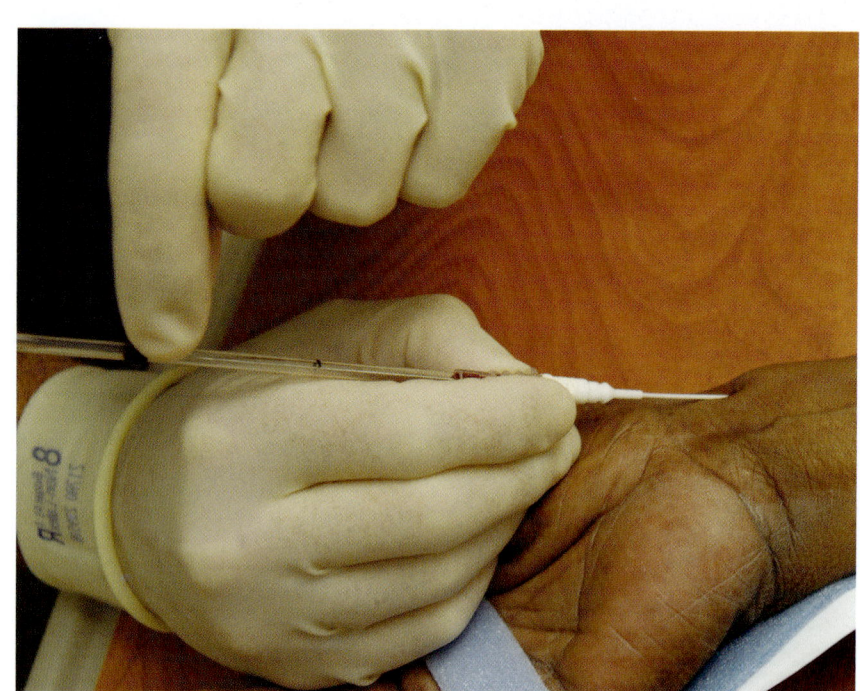

FIGURE 7-4 When a flash is seen in the chamber, …

Chapter 7 THE RADIAL A-LINE: A VERSATILE AND ESSENTIAL TOOL

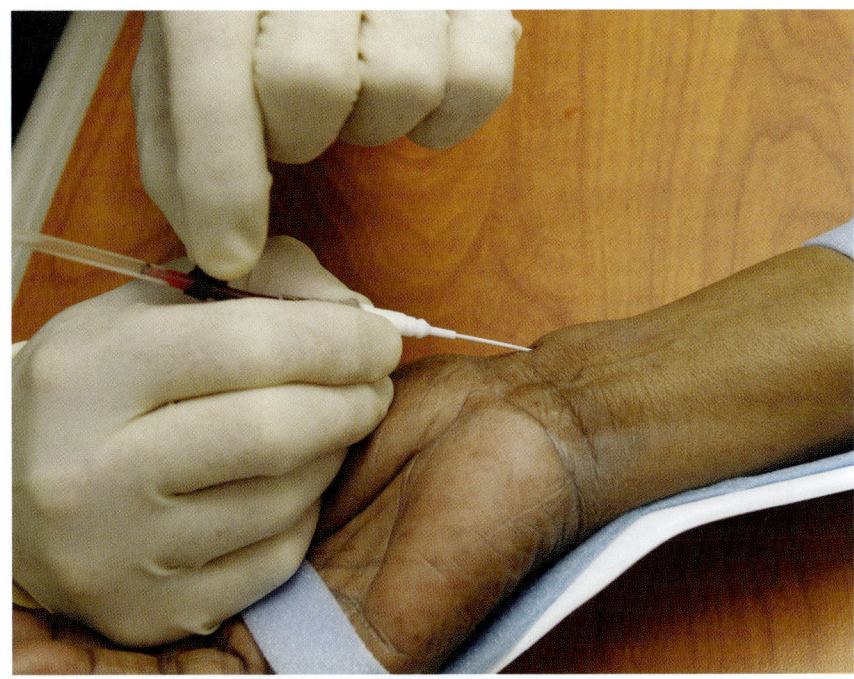

FIGURE 7-5 …advance the needle (not the catheter) further 1 to 2 cm.

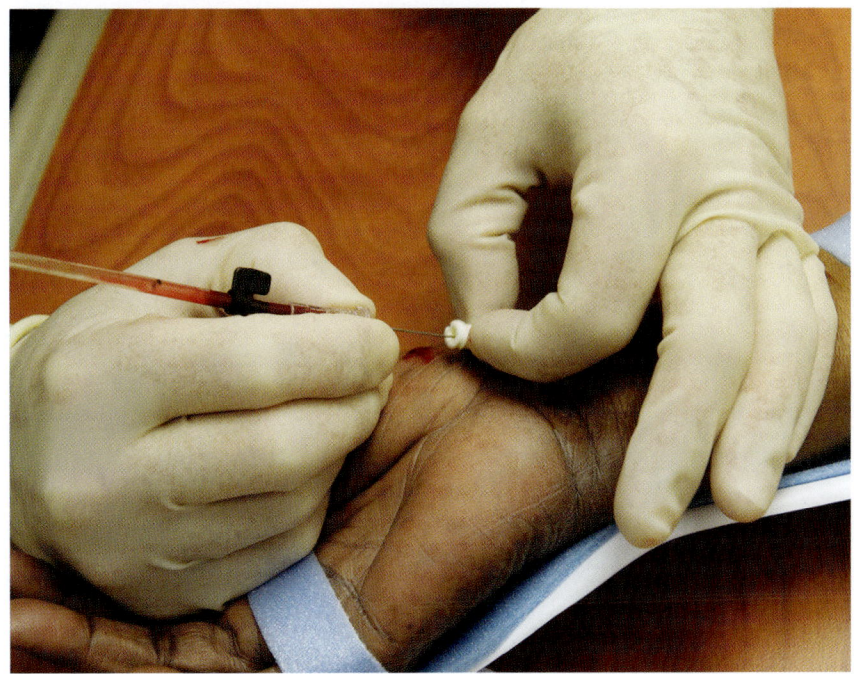

FIGURE 7-6 Slide the catheter over the wire until the hub is at the skin (again, the catheter should slide relatively smoothly).

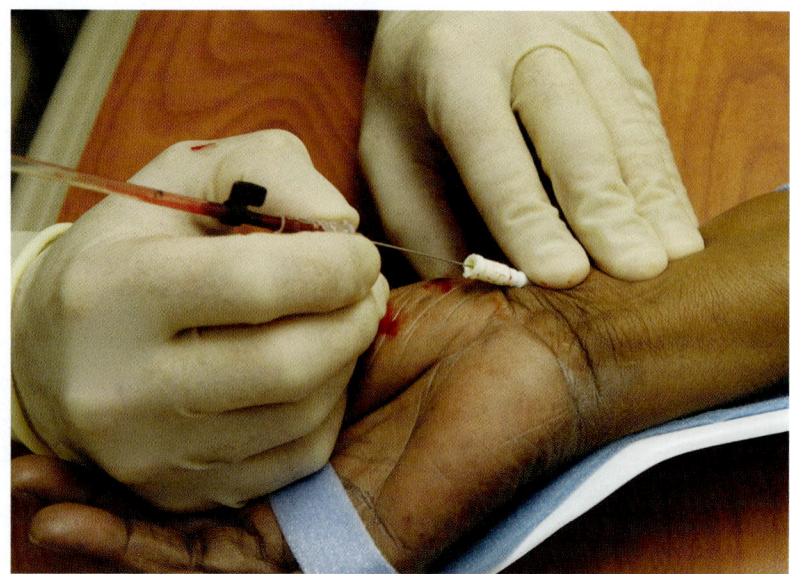

FIGURE 7-7 Compress the artery proximally while removing the wire to keep the work area clean...

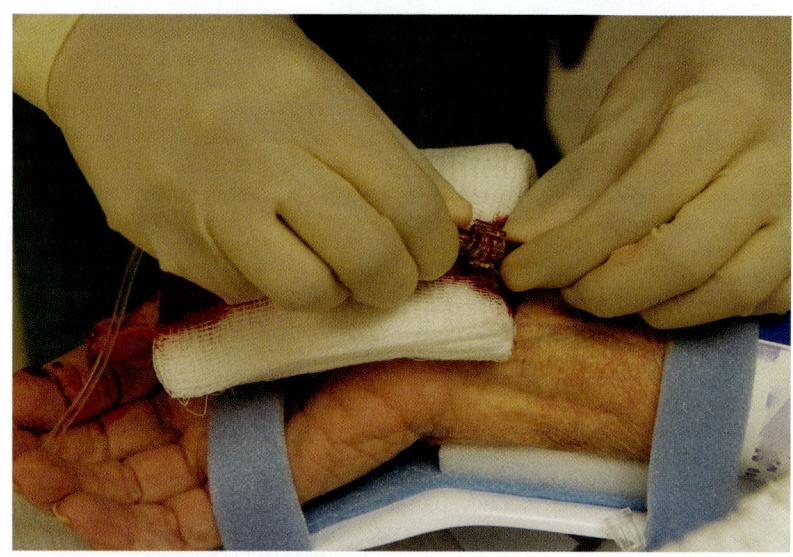

FIGURE 7-8 ...while attaching the catheter to A-line tubing.

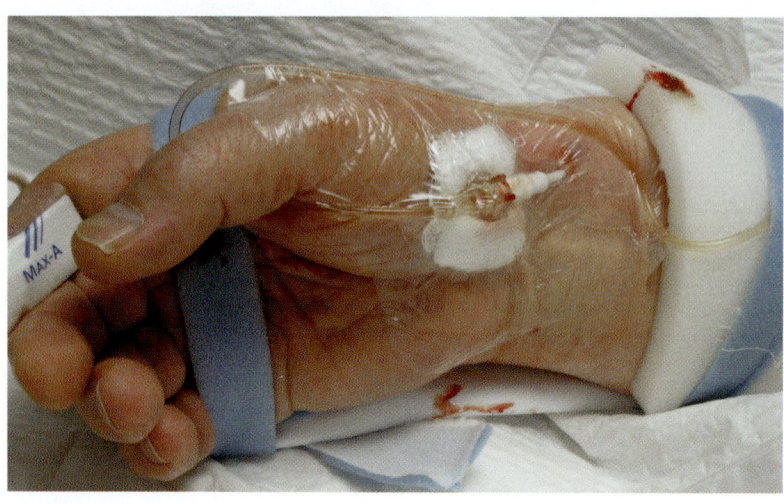

FIGURE 7-9 Arterial line secured.

Chapter 7 THE RADIAL A-LINE: A VERSATILE AND ESSENTIAL TOOL

Through-and-Through Technique

Tools: 20-gauge IV catheter, guidewire, wrist support, alcohol pads, gauze, 1% lidocaine in a syringe with a 25-gauge needle, sterile gloves.

Step-by-step guide to A-line success:
- Perform the Allen test to gain reassurance of sufficient collateral circulation.
- Palpate for an area with an appreciable radial pulse.
- Place wrist support onto the patient's wrist with adequate extension to open up the "landing zone" to eliminate the thenar eminence as an obstacle. In addition, abducting the thumb and attaching it to the work area with a piece of tape may augment wrist extension. Make certain to avoid overextension to prevent median nerve injury and overtightening of wrist guard straps because that may compress the radial artery and make the pulse difficult to palpate (Figures 7-10 to 7-14).

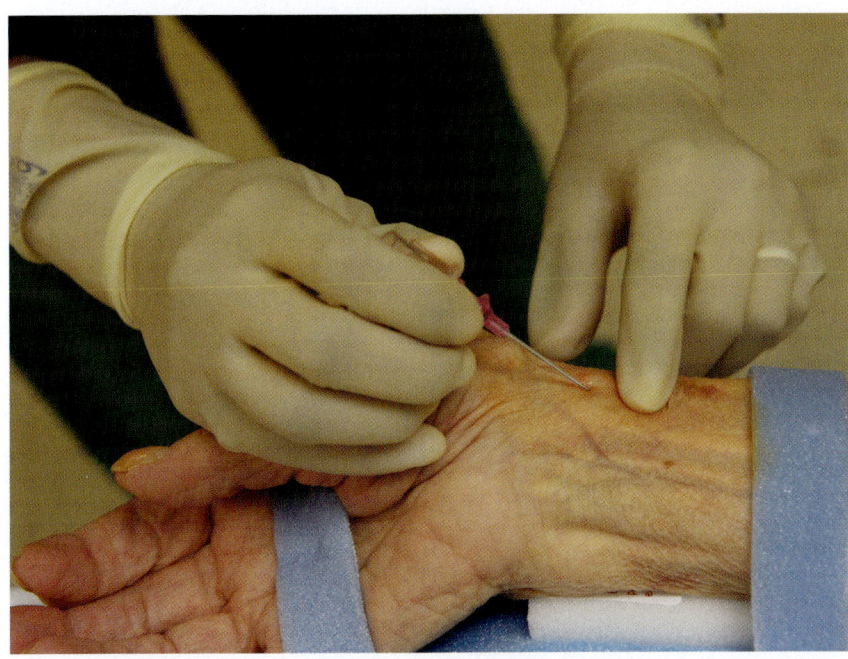

FIGURES 7-10 to 7-14 Through-and-through technique for arterial line insertion.

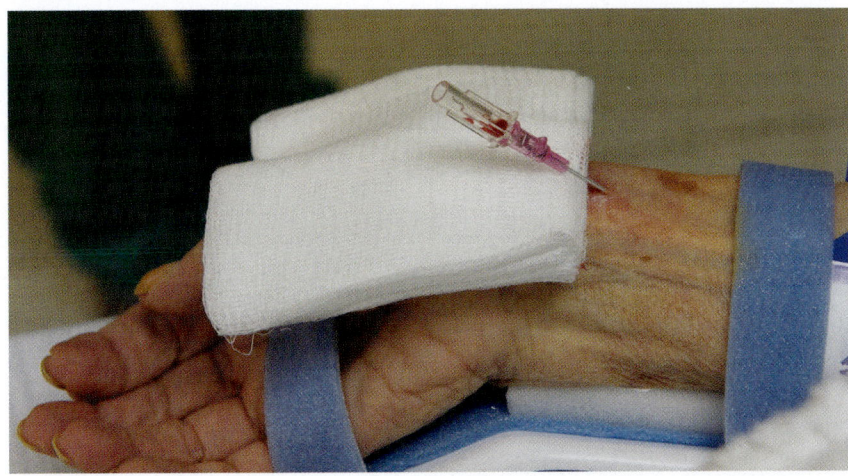

FIGURE 7-11

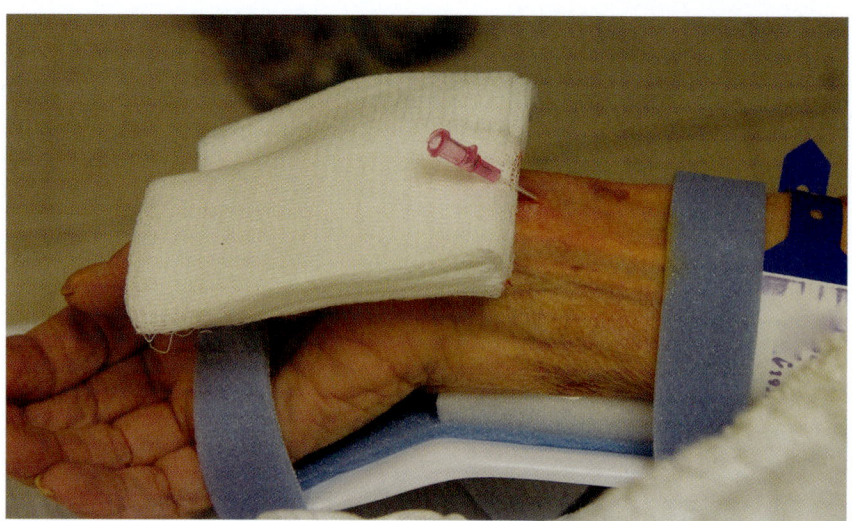

FIGURE 7-12

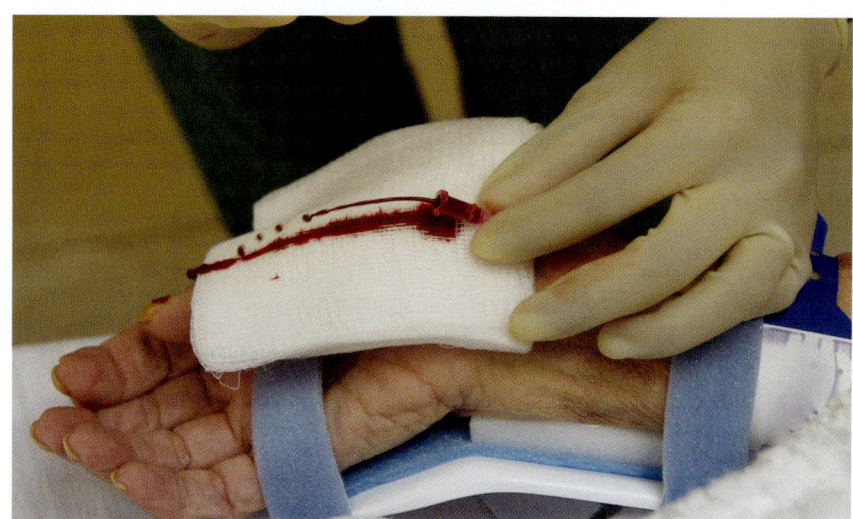

FIGURE 7-13

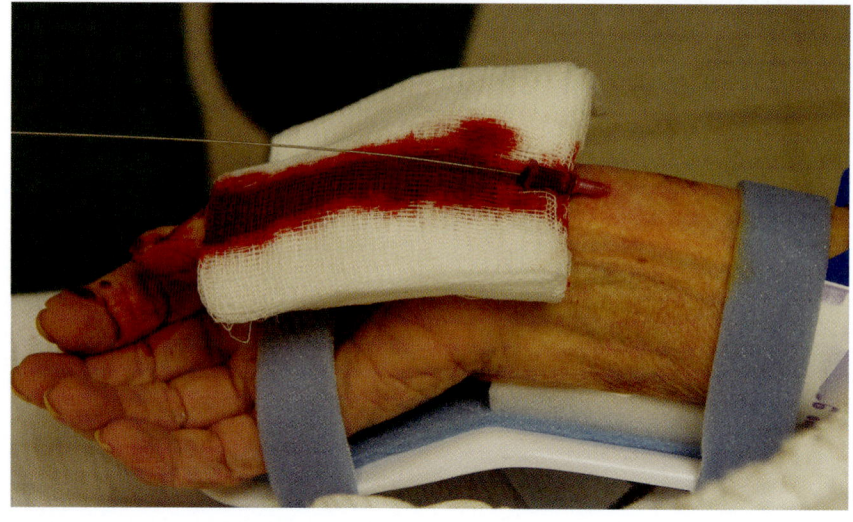

FIGURE 7-14

US-Guided Technique as a Rescue

Repeated unsuccessful attempts may make subsequent cannulation difficult due to vasospasm, hematoma formation, or intimal dissection. The radial artery runs deep to the brachioradialis muscle proximally, and although difficult to palpate, it can be easily visualized using ultrasound. Ultrasound guidance can be used for both direct cannulation and the through-and-through technique.[3]

Ultrasound-guided cannulation in infants in particular is key because it has been shown to improve the success of cannulation. A study performed in small children of ages 40 ± 33 months resulted in 100% cannulation using the ultrasound technique versus 80% success rate using the traditional palpation method.[4]

What to Do Once Your A-Line Is Secure

- Attach tubing via a three-way stopcock to pressure transducer attached to pressure bag
- Normal saline (NS) or NS with 2 units per cc of heparin solution may be used. Heparin solution has not been proven to keep the vessel open; however, it may play a role in heparin-sensitive patients. Proceed cautiously!
- The transducer should be secured and zeroed at the level of the right atrium. Placing the transducer above or below the level of the right atrium will cause artificially lower or higher respectively.
- Look at our transducer holder/circuit holder: All in one (University of Medicine and Dentistry of New Jersey, patent pending) (Figure 7-15).

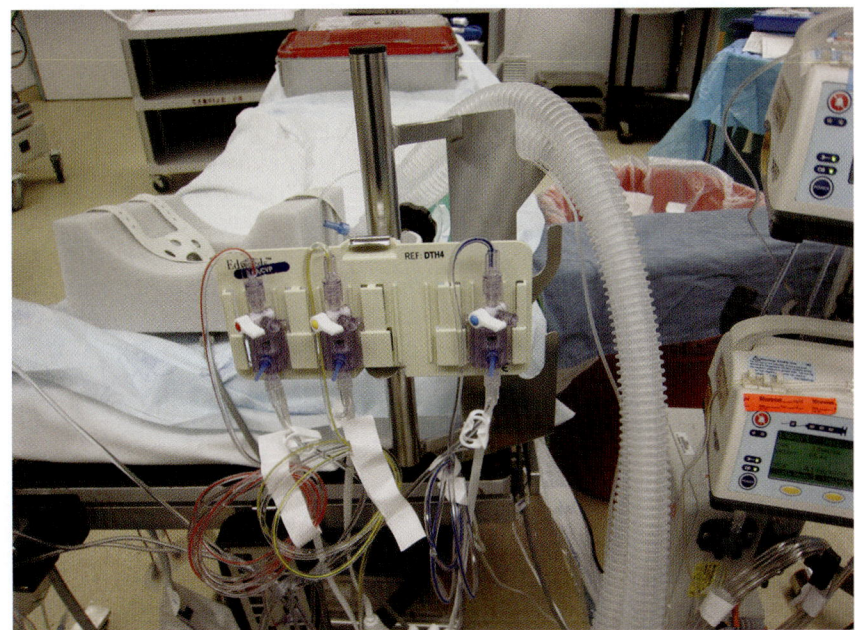

FIGURE 7-15 Transducer holder, patent pending.

Interesting Techniques

- Topical localization with EMLA cream: Studies show that application of EMLA cream 2 hours prior to A-line placement can increase success rate, decrease pain score of the patient during cannulation, and decrease time of cannulation.[5]
- Subcutaneous nitroglycerine: Subcutaneous administration of nitroglycerine has been shown to decrease spasm of the artery after unsuccessful cannulation. Relief of vasospasm allows return of palpable pulse and increases success rate of cannulation.[6]
- Anterograde artery cannulation: Although anterograde cannulation does not have any significant advantage when compared with retrograde cannulation, it may be used effectively when anterograde cannulation is unsuccessful.[7]
- Techniques for neonates: Neonates' radial artery cannulation is challenging due to perivascular interstitial fluid. Direct pressure may cause displacement of perivascular fluid and ease radial artery cannulation.

REFERENCES

1. Brzezinski M, Luisetti T, London MJ. Radial Artery cannulation: a comprehensive review of recent anatomic and physiologic investigations. *Int Anesth Res Soc* 2009;109:1763–1781.
   A comprehensive review of uses of radial A-line, Allen test, techniques of placement and possible complications of placement.
2. Kang GC. Simultaneous infected pseudoaneurysm and suppurative tenosynovitis resulting from radial artery cannulation. *Surg Infect* 2008;9:489–492.
   Case report of pseudoaneurysm of radial artery and suppurative tenosynovitis following radial A-line insertion.
3. Sandhu NS, Patel B. Use of ultrasonography as a rescue technique for failed radial artery cannulation. *J Clin Anesth* 2006;18:138–141.
   Article illustrating the utility of ultrasonography as a method of placing radial A-line in patients with difficult anatomy or after several unsuccessful attempts with the traditional methods.
4. Schwemmer U, Arzet HA, Trautner H, Roewer N, Greim CA. Ultrasound-guided arterial cannulation in infants improves success rate. *Eur J Anaesth* 2006;23:476–480.
   Article describing the use of ultrasound for placement of A-lines in infants.
5. Joly LM, Spaulding C, Monchi M, Ali OS, Weber S, Benhamou D. Topical lidocaine-prilocaine cream (EMLA) versus local infiltration of anesthesia for radial artery cannulation. *Anesth Analg* 1998;87:403–406.
   Comparison of EMLA cream versus subcutaneous local anesthetic prior to placement of radial A-line.
6. Pancholy SB, Copola J, Patel T. Subcutaneous administration of nitroglycerine to facilitate radial artery cannulation. *Cathet Cardiovasc Intervent* 2006;68:389–391.
   Description of advantages of subcutaneous nitroglycerine in radial A-line placement.
7. Karacalar S, Meltem C, Bayrak IK, Yegin S, Sarihasan B, Keceligil HT. Feasibility and safety of anterograde radial artery cannulation. *Eur Soc Anesthes* 2009;26:207–212.
   Description of safe/effective placement of an anterograde radial A-line.

CHAPTER 8
THE BRACHIAL A-LINE

EDGAR PIERRE
JORDAN TAYLOR

I am always doing that which I cannot do, in order that I may learn how to do it.

Pablo Picasso

INTRODUCTION

Yes, the radial artery is the most common place to get your arterial line, and yes, the safety of radial lines has been well documented in multiple studies. If you want to ruffle some feathers, however, then the brachial A-line is for you. The brachial arterial line remains a point of much controversy; it has the bad reputation of being an end artery and lacking the benefit of collateral circulation. Historically, many have avoided the site for fear of forearm and hand ischemic complications. Some smaller studies showed increased frequency of complications after brachial artery cannulation; in contrast, Bazaral et al.[1] described over 3000 brachial cannulations in which only a single patient required a postoperative thrombectomy. So before you completely blackball the brachial A-line, peruse the literature and then decide for yourself. So you botched the job on your radial and the femoral is a no go; it is now time to take a long look at that brachial.

INDICATIONS

- Major surgery where fluid shifts and large swings in blood pressure are expected
- When there is a need for rigorous control of blood pressure
- When there is a need for frequent arterial blood gas analysis
- Possibly more reliable than radial arterial blood pressure measurement in the postcardiopulmonary bypass period

CONTRAINDICATIONS

- Vascular insufficiency
- Arteriovenous fistula
- Infection at brachial site

EQUIPMENT

- Use a femoral arterial kit (20-gauge, 12 cm) (Figure 8-1).
- A short catheter like those used for radial lines could easily come out and cause a compartment syndrome.
- Transducer and pressure tubing (Figure 8-2).

PHILOSOPHY

- If you have no other options, brachial will work; it is done all the time.
- The brachial artery is larger and thus often easier to hit.
- If you poked and struggled to get the radial line, it probably will fail later in the case; it might be wise to just move up and place a fresh brachial line.

TECHNIQUE

- First explain the procedure and obtain informed consent from patient.
- Then start by positioning the arm out nice and flat.
- Palpate the brachial artery, which is found just medial to the midline in the antecubital fossa overlying the lateral border of the brachial muscle (Figure 8-3).

- Prep and drape in the usual sterile fashion (Figure 8-4).
- Place local anesthesia if the patient is awake.
- Use Seldinger technique to get flow (Figure 8-5 and 8-6).
- Pass a guidewire.
- Remove the needle (Figure 8-7).
- Slide the catheter over the wire, taking care not to lose sight of wire (Figure 8-8).
- Once you are ready to hook up the line, pull the wire and then attach the arterial line (Figure 8-9).
- Confirm the A-line trace (Figure 8-10).
- If the catheter will be in for a long period of time, suture the catheter.
- Place a dressing.

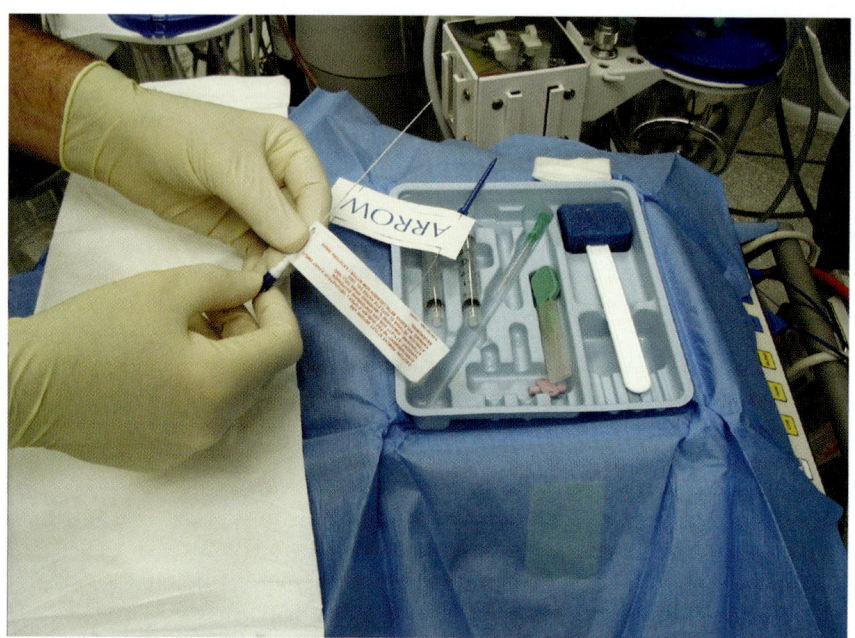

FIGURE 8-1 Typical femoral arterial line kit (20-gauge, 12 cm).

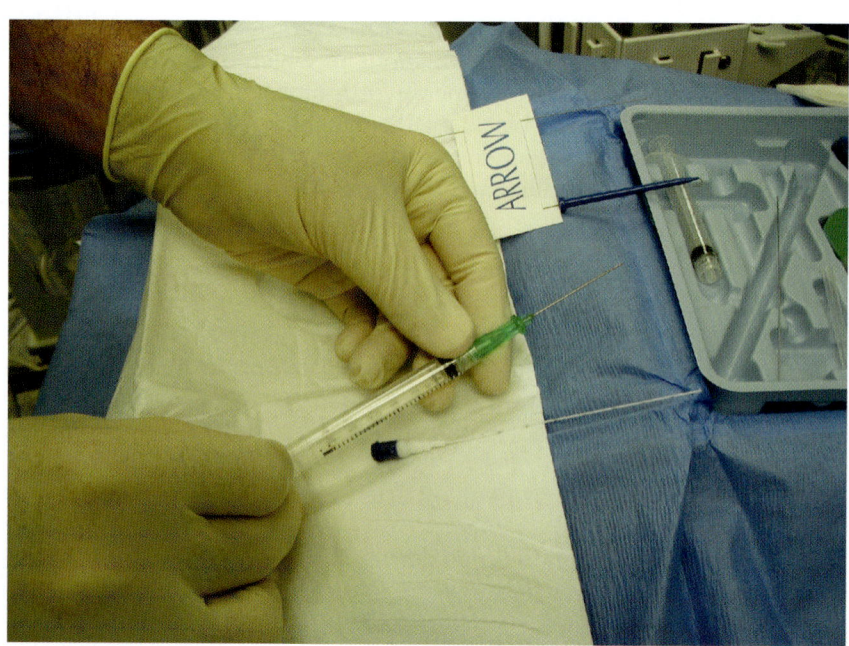

FIGURE 8-2 Use an Angiocath and syringe to find the vessel.

Chapter 8 THE BRACHIAL A-LINE

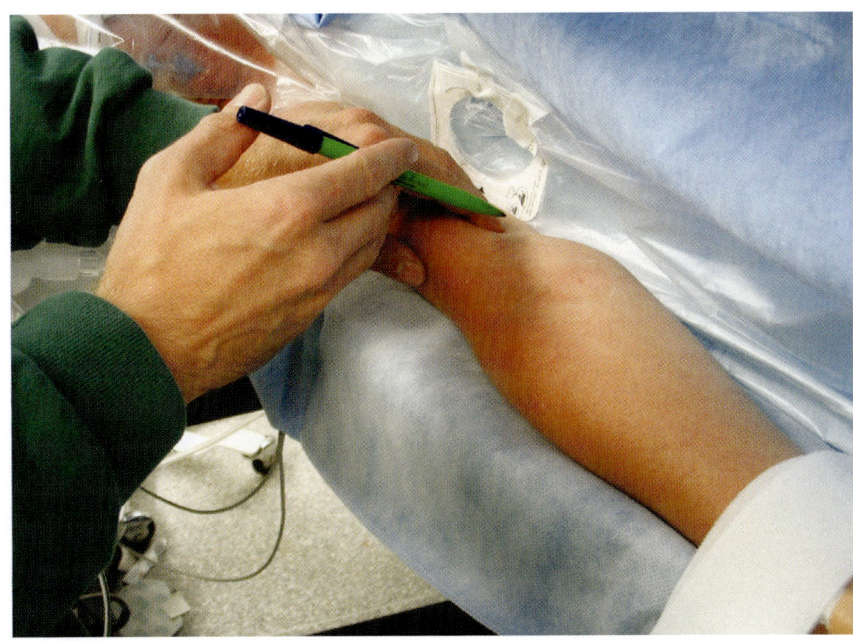

FIGURE 8-3 Palpate the brachial artery, just medial to the midline antecubital fossa.

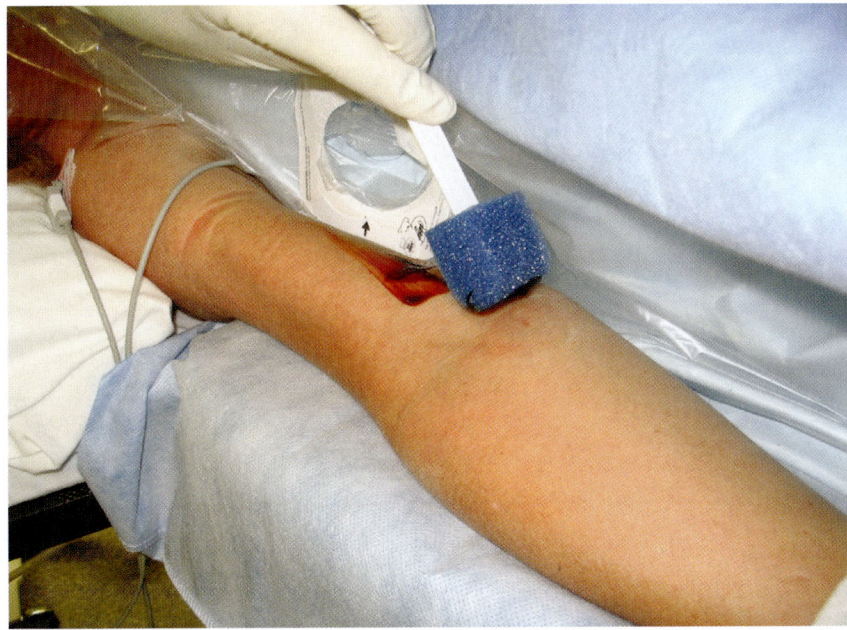

FIGURE 8-4 Prep and drape in usual sterile fashion.

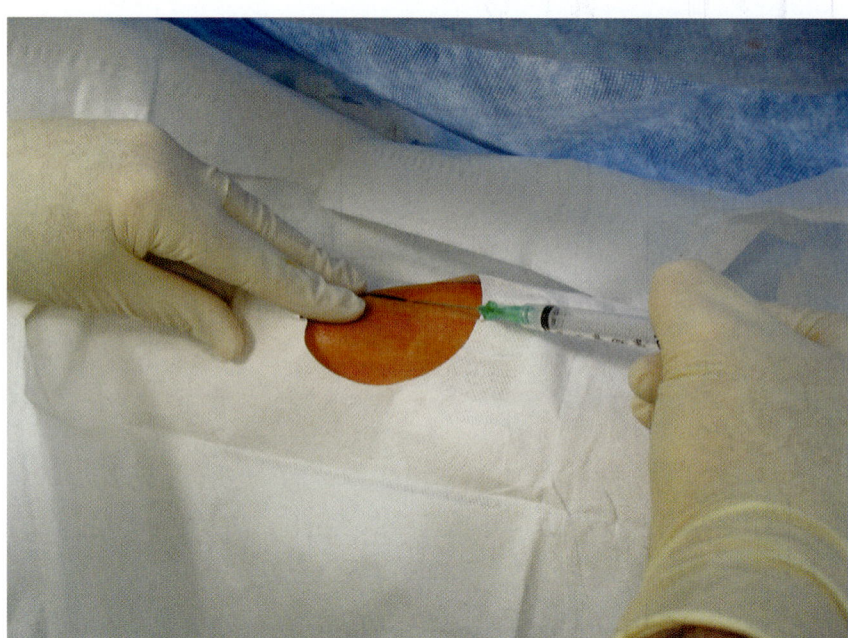

FIGURE 8-5 Stabilize the vessel and use Seldinger technique to get flow.

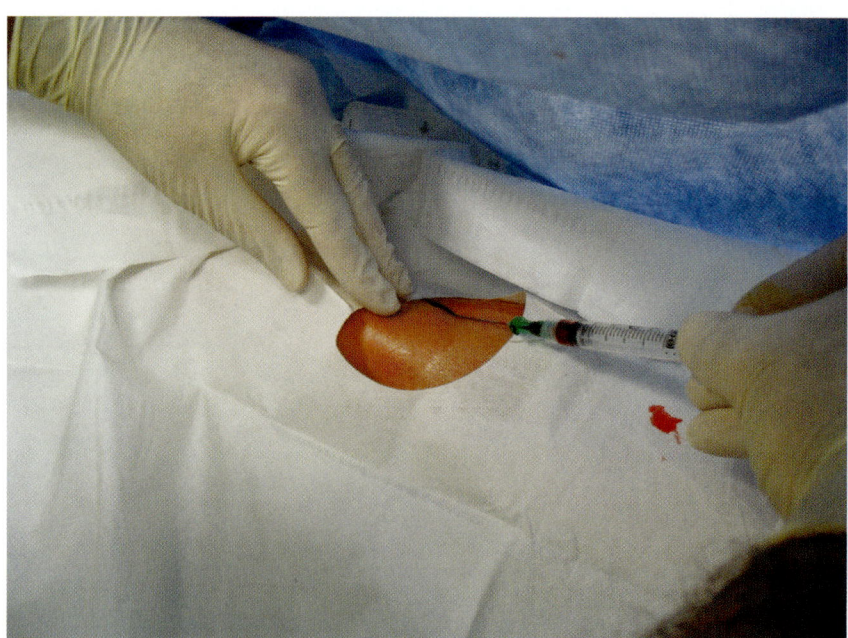

FIGURE 8-6 You should get bright red pulsatile blood flow.

Chapter 8 THE BRACHIAL A-LINE

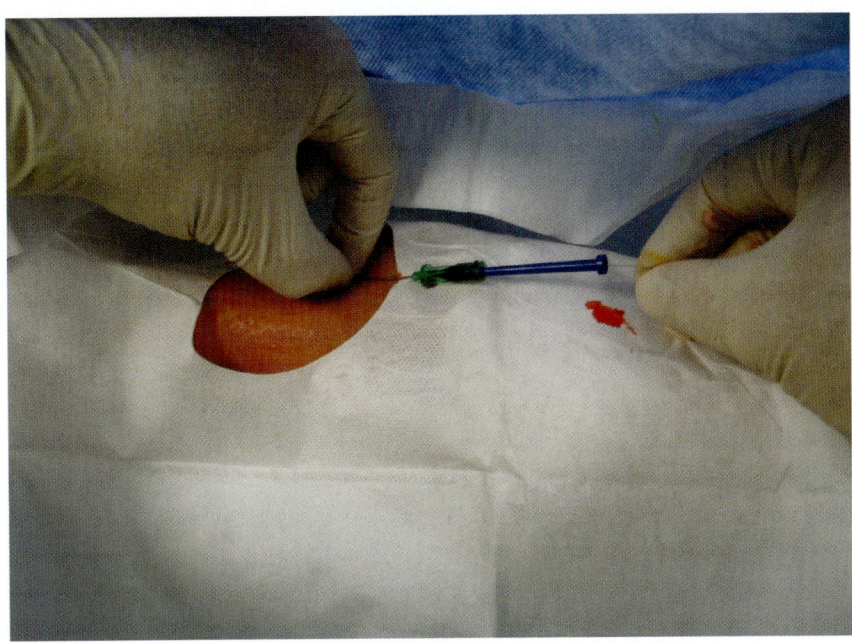

FIGURE 8-7 Thread the wire and remove Angiocath.

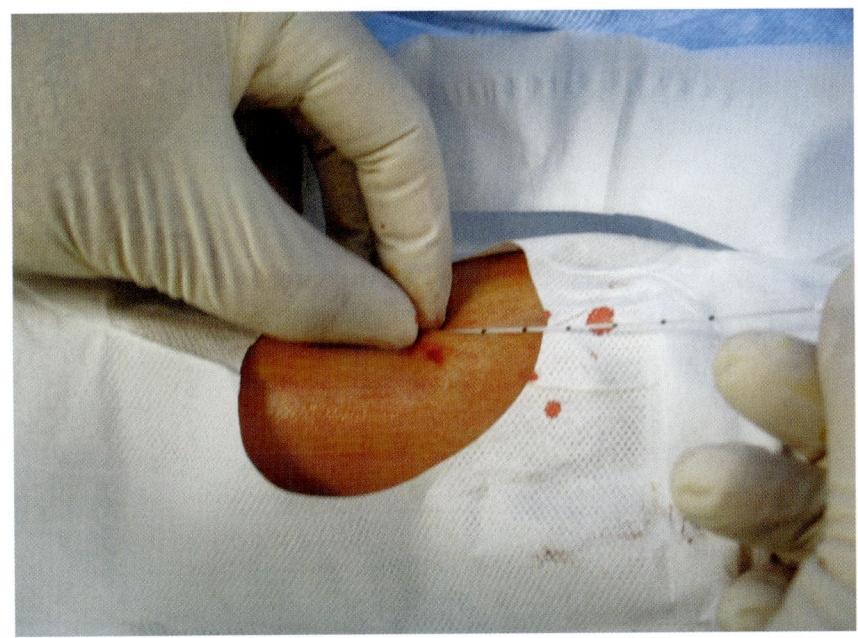

FIGURE 8-8 Maintain visual of the wire at all times when sliding the long catheter.

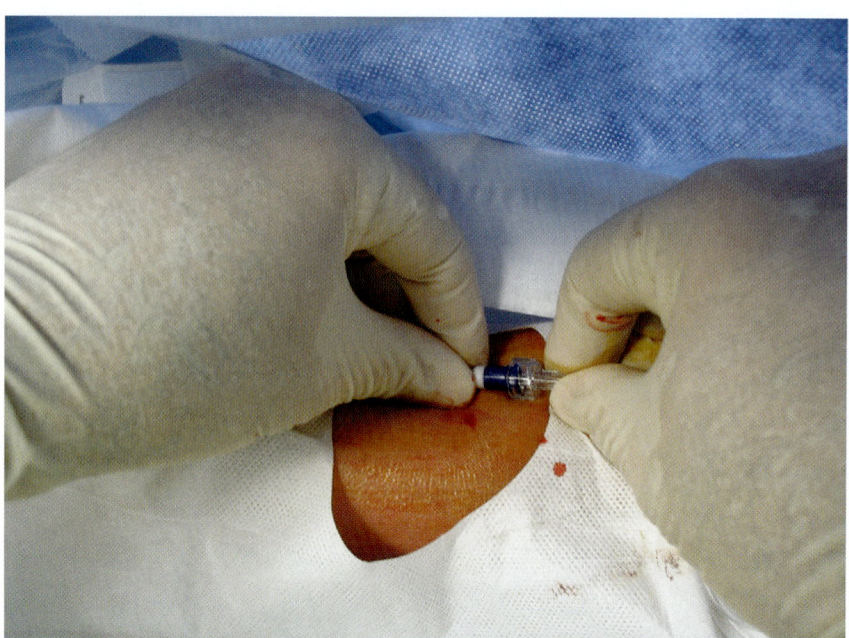

FIGURE 8-9 Attach the tubing and transducer.

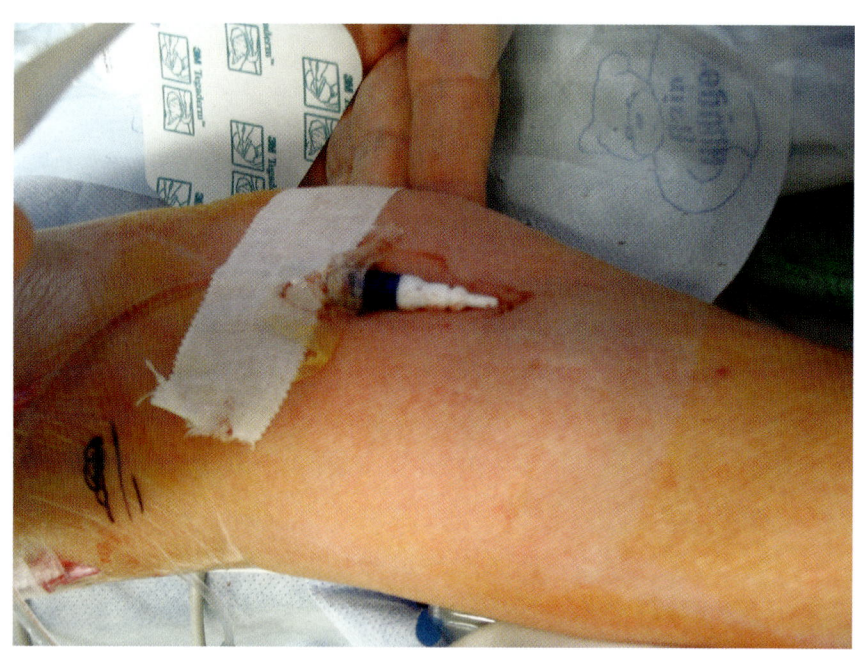

FIGURE 8-10 Once an arterial tracing is confirmed, secure the A-line well.

COMPLICATIONS

- Thrombosis
  - The most frequently reported major complication from arterial puncture is thrombosis at the site of entry with distal ischemia. Factors significantly increasing the risk of ischemic complications include female gender, history of hypertension, arthritis or vascular disease, catheter size, duration of cannulation, and use of pressors.
- Neuronal or adjacent structure injury
  - A 0.2% to 1.4% incidence of median nerve injury after brachial cannulation has been described, with ischemia, compression, and direct nerve trauma resulting in appreciable long-term disability.
- Hemorrhage
- Infection
- Vascular insufficiency
- Ischemia
- Embolization

CONCLUSION

An arterial line of any kind can provide us with data that are often invaluable for management in the operating room and ICU. Arterial lines allow the continuous display of hemodynamic measures and pulse contour. Lines placed at any site are not without risk, and thus we must always weigh the risk-to-benefit ratio before proceeding. Your clinical skill, the patient's positioning, the potential for neuronal injury, and pathophysiologic attributes all should be considered before selecting a site. That being said, if the need for a brachial line presents itself, crack your knuckles and get down to business.

REFERENCE

1. Bazaral MG, Welch M, Golding LA, Badhwar K. Comparison of brachial and radial arterial pressure monitoring in patients undergoing coronary artery bypass surgery. *Anesthesiology* 1990;73:38–45.
   This study compares radial and brachial arterial cannulation in patients receiving cardiopulmonary bypass. Results showed that brachial artery cannulation in adult patients is safe, practical, and may even provide more accurate information than radial A-lines in certain circumstances; 3,057 brachial A-lines were placed, with only one known patient requiring postoperative thrombectomy.

SUGGESTED READING

Kennedy AM, Grocott M, Schwartz MS, Modarres H, Scott M, Schon E. Median nerve injury: an underrecognised complication of brachial artery catheterization? *J Neurol Neurosurg Psychiatry* 1997;63:542–546.
Discusses the role of median nerve injury following brachial A-line placement. Describes a 0.2% to 1.4% incidence of median nerve injury after brachial cannulation with resulting appreciable long-term disability.

Khoury M, Batra S, Berg R, Kumara R. Influence of arterial access sites and interventional procedures on vascular complications after cardiac catheterizations. *Am J Surg* 1992; 164:205–209.
Discusses the various complications specific to each cannulation site and describes an increased rate of complications following brachial artery cannulation.

Lazarides MK, Tsoupanos SS, Georgopoulous SE, et al. Incidence and patterns of iatrogenic arterial injuries; a decade's experience. *J Cardiovasc Surg* 1998;39:281–285.
Discusses the various complications of arterial cannulation and their multifaceted impact; also describes a rising incidence of iatrogenic arterial injuries.

Moran KT, Halpin DP, Zide RS, Oberfield RA, Jewell ER. Long term brachial artery catheterization: ischemic complications. *J Vasc Surg* 1988;8:76–78.
Small retrospective study of patients with transbrachial catheters that showed a high frequency of radial pulse diminution following cannulation.

Van Beck JO, White RD, Abenstein JP, Mullany CJ, Orszulak TA. Comparison of axillary artery or brachial artery pressure with aortic pressure after cardiopulmonary bypass using a long radial artery catheter. *J Cardiothorac Vasc Anesth* 1993;7:312–315.
Study describing the inadequacies of radial aline in post–cardiopulmonary bypass (CPB) patients. Showed frequent aortic to radial disparity post-CPB with systolic gradients >10 mmHg in 52% to 77% of patients, and 15% of patients with gradients >20 mmHg.

CHAPTER 9

STAND BY ME: THE FEMORAL ARTERIAL LINE

SYLVIANA BARSOUM

It is possible to fail in many ways, while to succeed is possible in only one way.

Aristotle

INTRODUCTION

So you need an arterial line. Maybe in spite of your better judgment, you let the residents try both radials without success. Here is a famous quotation of residents: "It just wouldn't thread." Interpretation: it is the artery's fault or the kit's fault. Just like my kids tell me "the vase just fell off the shelf." Interpretation: the vase sprouted legs and jumped off the shelf. Or perhaps, your patient has had radial artery harvesting for coronary artery bypass graft (CABG); or perhaps you anticipate the need for an intraaortic balloon pump (IABP). Nothing will stand by you like the femoral arterial line. Our cardiology buddies utilize this site more than any other (it is large bore and easily compressible). And we shouldn't forget it when the need arises. No need to have the surgeons breathing down your neck while you make repeated attempts at the radials.

ANATOMY

A little refresher for those of us to whom anatomy was more than just yesterday[1] (all my troubles seemed so far away).
- The common femoral artery (CFA) is a continuation of the external iliac artery as it passes under the inguinal ligament (Figure 9-1).
- It lays midway between the anterior superior iliac spine (ASIS) and the symphysis pubis.
- It branches into the superficial and deep femoral arteries about 4.5 cm distal to the inguinal ligament.
- A couple of memory aids: (1) the VAN (vein-artery-nerve) pulls away from the driveway (medial = driveway, lateral = away). Or if you prefer, (2) NAVEL (nerve-artery-vein-empty space-lymphatics) toward the navel (umbilicus). Or recall the famous NAVY mnemonic from Chapter 5.

INDICATIONS

- Beat-to-beat blood pressure measurements
- Frequent arterial blood gas (ABG) measurements or blood sampling throughout the procedure
- Anticipated need for IABP (although once you have the IABP, the parameters of interest to you will be proximal to the balloon and you won't be able to use that line for blood sampling)
- An occasional case where it may be important to know the arterial blood pressure (BP) distal to the aortic cross-clamp, since femoral arterial pressure will also reflect perfusion pressure to the kidneys and a large portion of the spinal cord via the artery of Adamkiewicz
- Previous harvesting of radial artery for CABG
- More reliable reflection of aortic BP post–cardiopulmonary bypass (CPB) than radial arterial pressure (secondary to transient changes induced by CPB). Why the radial artery tracing craps out postbypass is OOTMOL (one of the mysteries of life).

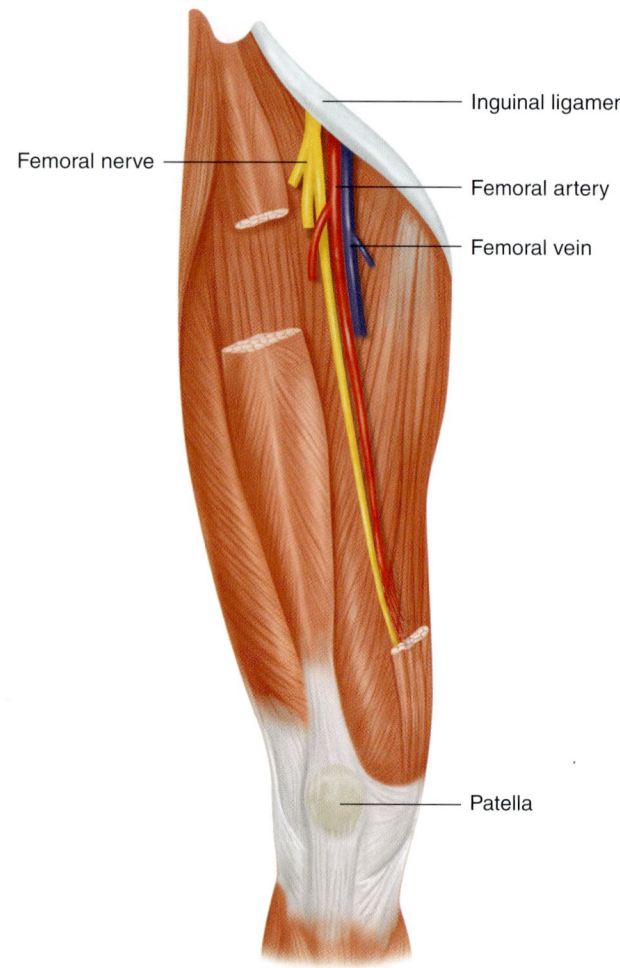

FIGURE 9-1 Common femoral artery anatomy.

CONTRAINDICATIONS

- Femoral bypass surgery, either currently—you will be in the field (duh)—or a history thereof. You don't want to be poking holes in the graft.
- A venous catheter in the same location (increased risk of arteriovenous [AV] fistula formation). Although when the cath lab becomes the crash lab, they usually come down with both on the same side without any concern.
- Peripheral arterial disease (PAD): the accuracy of your readings will be questionable (narrowing of the arteries), and there is a possibility of increasing limb ischemia.
- Aortic surgery/compression may interfere with the readings.
- Infection at the site

COMPLICATIONS

The rate is less than 1% for all whether the CFA is accessed for diagnostic or interventional use.[2,3]
- Limb ischemia, although if you are an avatar, blue toes may be quite becoming
- Pseudo-aneurysm
- AV fistula formation
- Hematoma
- Bleeding
- Vessel laceration
- Acute vessel closure
- Venous thrombus
- Pericatheter clot
- Infection

Most complications result from puncturing the vessel too proximal or too distal. Remember, it is a continuation of the external iliac artery. So if you puncture too proximal, you actually have an external iliac arterial line with the attendant risk of life-threatening retroperitoneal hemorrhage. The retroperitoneal space can accommodate a massive amount of blood, and this may not be apparent until you have hemodynamic collapse. The problem continues once your line is removed; you can't compress the external iliac artery no matter how much you try. If you puncture too distal, you could be in the superficial and/or deep femoral artery instead of the CFA. This will increase your chances of the above-noted complications.

Regarding infectious complications, the incidence of local site infections for femoral arterial catheters was 0.78% (vs. 0.72% for radial arterial catheters). Catheter-related sepsis was found to occur in 0.44% of patients with femoral arterial catheters (vs. 0.13% with radial arterial catheters).[2]

So here, as in Chapter 5, the idea that the femoral is an inherently dirty line is disproven.

TECHNIQUE

Just as there's more than one way to skin a cat, there's more than one way to sink your needle into that CFA.[3]
- Traditional palpatory methods: The problems with any of these methods are that they can be altered secondary to obesity, prior hematomas, scarring, and severely reduced BP or shock.
  - Using the inguinal crease: This is based on the belief that the inguinal crease overlies the inguinal ligament (remember separating the external iliac artery from the CFA). Be aware that there is a significant variation in the distance between the crease and the ligament, anywhere from 0 to 11 cm (average 6.5 cm). This can be worse in women.

- Using the strongest femoral pulse: This seems to be the more reliable method. The point of strongest femoral artery pulsation is projected over the CFA in about 93% of patients. This may be difficult to feel in vasculopaths.
- Using bony landmarks: If your patient is thin enough, you may be able to feel the femoral head. Even on most obese patients, you should be able to feel the ASIS and the symphysis pubis (Figure 9-2).

• Fluoroscopy: Interventional radiologists, vascular surgeons and cardiologists use fluoroscopy routinely. A recent prospective trial comparing fluoroscopy with traditional landmark methods suggests their equality. So I don't think the surgeons will look kindly on you dragging in the C-arm to place your A-line.
• Ultrasound Guided[4]: One group recently demonstrated that ultrasound (US) guidance decreased the number of attempts and time to puncture only in obese patients or patients with poor to absent femoral pulses. They also found that if the patient has a good pulse, then the use of US actually prolonged the time to access the CFA. There was no difference in complications. Color Doppler can show the patency of a vessel and help differentiate artery from vein in patients with weak pulses. Likewise, color Doppler can allow puncture of a partially thrombosed vessel (but would you want to?!).

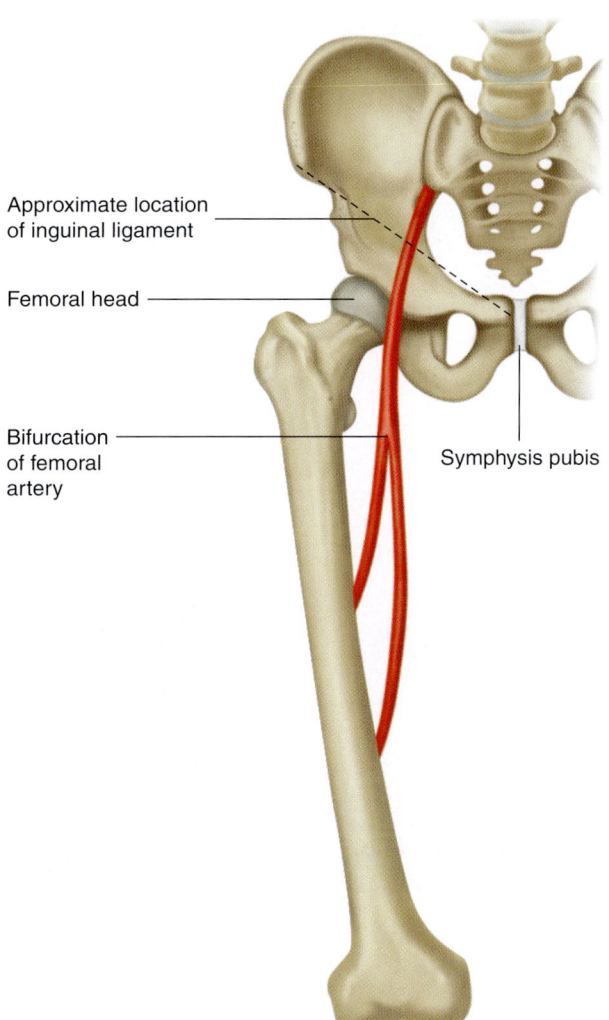

FIGURE 9-2 Bony landmarks in relation to the femoral artery.

EQUIPMENT

Learn to be self-reliant. Have everything ready to go before you start. When you keep asking for things, the nurses notice and label you "needy." You don't want that label.

- Either a short catheter (7.5 cm) placed directly or a longer catheter (15 cm) placed over a wire. Some people even use a single-lumen central venous pressure (CVP) kit. Familiarize yourself with the kits used in your hospital (Figures 9-3 and 9-4).
- Pressurized transducer system—heparinized (to a final concentration of 1 unit/1 cc normal saline (NS)) or not (no difference).[5] Others say 2 units/1 cc NS or not at all. In this age of heparin-induced thrombocytopenia (HIT), it is probably better to avoid it if you can.
- Have the transducer set up and zeroed before you start.
- Make sure all Luer lock connections are tight. Check this yourself even if you are lucky enough to have someone else set it up for you. Most often, when you take over a case and the line keeps damping, it's a loose connection somewhere.
- Use the usual sterile prep and drape.
- You may need an extra hand to hold a pendulant abdomen out of the way or consider taping out of the way.

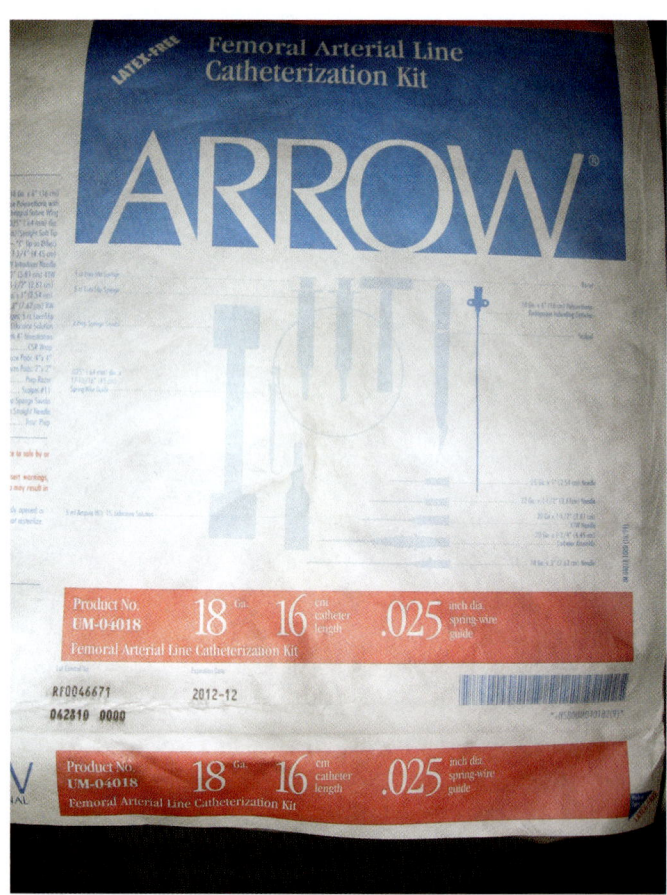

FIGURE 9-3 Arrow™ Femoral Arterial Line Catheterization Kit. (This kit is used in the author's hospital.)

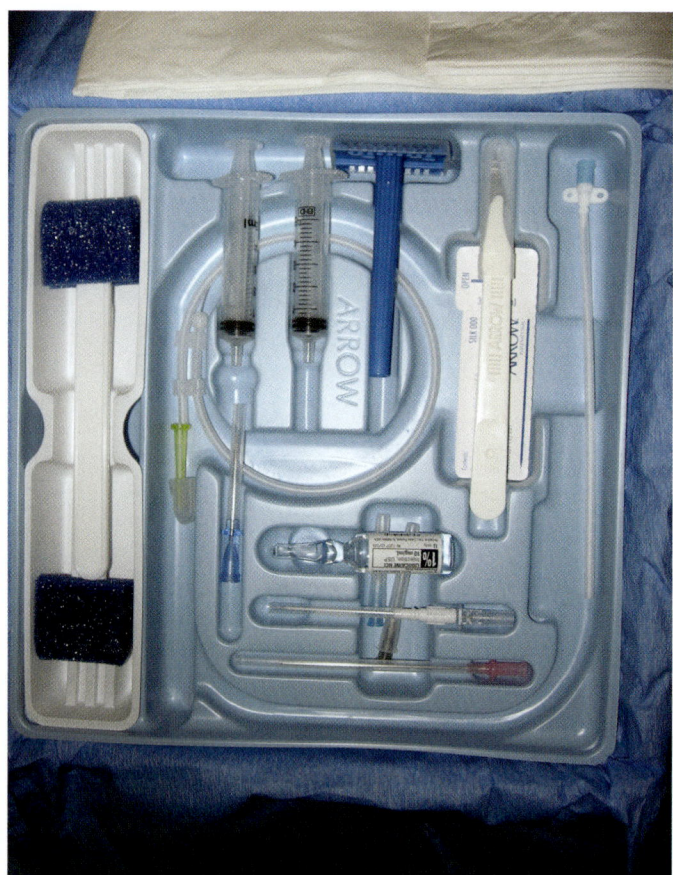

FIGURE 9-4 Arrow™ Femoral Arterial Line Catheterization Kit contents.

Chapter 9 STAND BY ME: THE FEMORAL ARTERIAL LINE

PROCEDURE

- Go on the same side as your handedness.
- For the sterile prep and drape, chlorhexidine solution is more effective than povidone-iodine solution.[2]
- If the patient is awake, remember to sedate and anesthetize the area (Figure 9-5).
- Use the needle straight (no finder, no catheter) (Figure 9-6).
- Use any or all combinations of techniques described earlier.
- If these don't work or you just can't feel the pulse, use the US.
- Once you get pulsatile flow of bright red blood, thread your wire into the artery. It should slide easily and smoothly with no resistance. NEVER force a wire. You will bend the wire (get another kit), lacerate the artery (increased risk of the complications discussed above), and dislodge plaques (resulting in possible blue toes) (Figure 9-7).
- Adjust the angle of your needle. Sometimes laying your needle a little flatter makes it easier to thread the wire (be sure that you still have pulsatile flow).
- Once the wire passes easily, remove your needle. NEVER let go of the wire.
- Make a small nick in the skin only. There is no need to stab the artery itself. Find another outlet for your anger.
- Thread and advance your catheter over the wire.
- Remove your wire. Now you can let go of the wire.
- Attach transducer (Luer lock tightly). Aspirate (should be easy). Flush (make sure there are no bubbles). Look at your tracing (which should have already been zeroed and ready to go).
- Now suture in place.
- Make sure transducer tubing has gentle loop back toward you (no kinks).
- Make sure the stopcock is not digging into the patient's side.
- Make sure all connections are TIGHT. Unrecognized disconnections can lead to exsanguinations. And you would be surprised at how much blood the drapes can hide before it starts dripping on the floor (by the way, that's where your patient's blood pressure will be—on the floor).

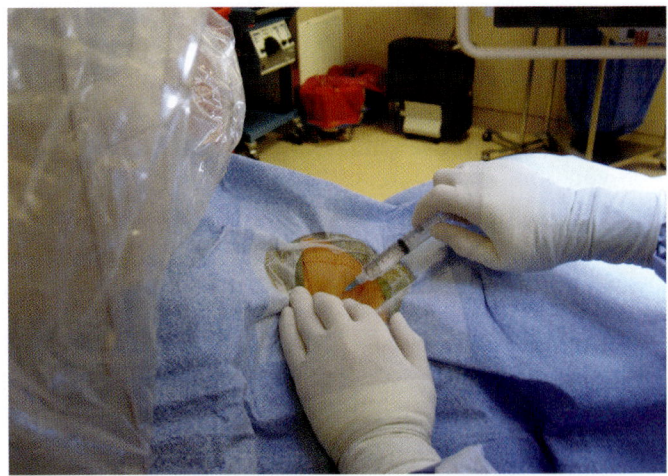

FIGURE 9-5 Don't forget to anesthetize the area if the patient is awake.

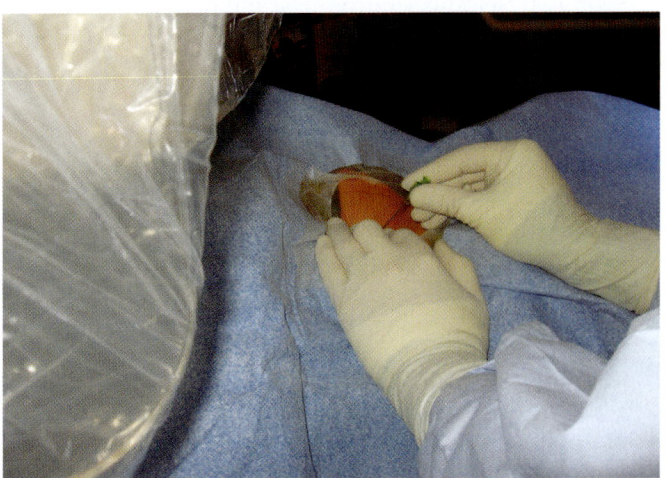

FIGURE 9-6 Locate the artery, and puncture the vessel.

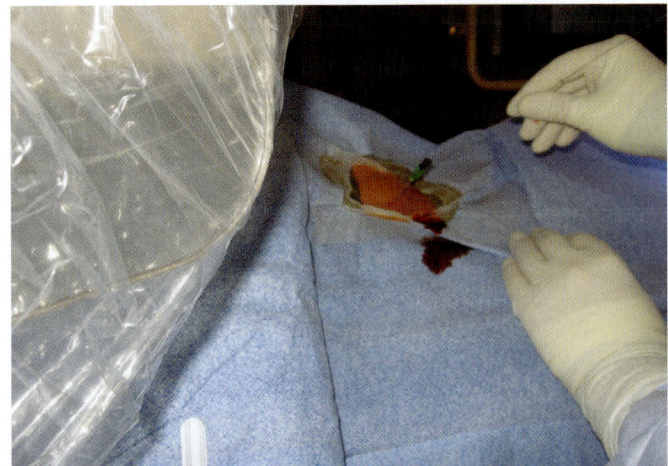

FIGURE 9-7 Once you have confirmed pulsatile flow, insert the wire. It should have no resistance.

TROUBLESHOOTING

- Make sure you still have a tracing once the patient is positioned but before the drapes go up. It's no fun poking around under there later.
- If you don't have a tracing and/or you can't aspirate, then check your line. Make sure there are no kinks or closed-off stopcocks. Also check for kinks at the insertion site itself.
- If you can't fix it, get another line. Don't start the case with a handicap and pray for a quick case or a miracle.
- If the trace looks damped: (1) check the pressure bag (probably not enough pressure), and (2) check your line (is there something partially disconnected or loose?).

SOME TRIVIA (THAT'S NOT SO TRIVIAL)

- Sven Ivar Seldinger introduced the percutaneous vascular access technique that bears his name about half a century ago.
- Do not inject medications into any arterial line. The classic scenario of the line switch is the cath lab disaster that comes flying into the room and you have ZERO time. Someone injected etomidate and sux into a femoral artery that way. No complications, but you will worry for days.
- The CFA is the most commonly used artery for percutaneous coronary interventions (PCI) (although cardiologists also use the radial and brachial).
- It is considered ideal because of its large size and because of its course over bone (making compression easier).
- Several large multicenter registries—the Coronary Artery Surgery Study (CASS); the Society for Cardiovascular Angiography and Intervention (SCA-I); the acute catheterization and urgent intervention triage strategy (ACUITY) trial—found similar complication rates for the femoral, brachial, and radial.
- The cath lab patient (or for that matter the ICU patient with multiple line spaghetti) usually has femoral arterial and venous lines. Hook up your transducers to be sure which is which. Don't rely on the color coding or the labeling alone. In the rush to transfer, things could be wrongly labeled. Better to check now than after the drapes are up.
- Pulse pressure undergoes a natural amplification as it traverses the arterial tree. This distortion results in an exaggerated systolic blood pressure (SBP) and pulse pressure (PP). Normally, radial SBP > aortic SBP, radial diastolic blood pressure (DBP) < aortic DBP, and radial PP > aortic PP. This is the sort of question that appears on the written boards.
- Post-CPB: Secondary to transient changes induced by CPB (decreased vascular resistance with warming), radial SBP < aortic SBP, and radial mean arterial pressure (MAP) < aortic SBP.
- Vasodilating drugs can accentuate the discrepancy between central and distal arterial blood pressure measurements.
- Patients with severe PAD may also have discrepancies between central and distal measurement sites.
- It is a good idea to take the noninvasive blood pressure measurements periodically for correlation and to aid in troubleshooting. Overall, automated oscillometric noninvasive measurements of blood pressure correlate well with invasive measurements of mean and diastolic blood pressures but may underestimate systolic blood pressures.[6]
- Never forget: when you lose the arterial tracing, you may have just lost the patient. When this happens in conjunction with perhaps no end-tidal carbon dioxide concentration (E_TCO_2), no electrocardiogram, and no pulse oximeter tracing, someone is trying to tell you something.

REFERENCES

1. Gray H. *Anatomy of the human body*, 20th ed. Philadelphia: Lea & Febiger; 1918.
   Good old standard anatomy, now available on the Internet.
2. Scheer BV, Perel A, Pfeiffer UJ. Clinical review: complications and risk factors of peripheral arterial catheters used for haemodynamic monitoring in anaesthesia and intensive care medicine. *Crit Care* 2002;6:199–204.
   Detailed review of complications.
3. Irani F, Kumar S, Colyer WR. Common femoral artery access techniques: a review. *J Cardiovasc Med* 2009;10:517–522.
   Goes over every possible way to access the femoral artery and also complications.
4. Dudeck O, Teichgraeber U, Podrabsky P, Lopez Haenninen E, Soerensen R, Ricke J. A randomized trial assessing the value of ultrasound-guided puncture of the femoral artery for interventional investigations. *Int J Cardiovasc Imaging* 2004;20:363–368.
   There is some limited benefit to ultrasound-guided femoral artery access.
5. Randolph AG, Cook DJ, Gonzales A, Andrew M. Benefit of heparin in peripheral venous and arterial catheters: systemic review and meta-analysis of randomised controlled trials. *BMJ* 1998;316:969–975.
   Beneficial for those of us who remember always adding heparin to the transducer system.
6. Riachy M, Azar M. [Interest of the noninvasive techniques for the measurement of the blood pressure in critical care] [French]. *Lebanese Med J* 2006;54(1):17–21.
   Confirms good correlation between invasive and oscillometric blood pressure measurements.

CHAPTER 10

THE BEAT-TO-BEAT FAUCET DOWN YONDER: THE PEDAL A-LINE

ARTEMUS FLAGG
DEBORAH SCHWENGEL

Step on it!

*Bonnie Parker to Clyde Barrow
in the movie Bonnie and Clyde
(screenplay by David Newman
and Robert Benton)*

INDICATIONS

- The same as any other arterial catheter
- Cannulation of other arteries has failed or placement in the upper extremities is not advised due to infection, burns, contractures, amputation, etc. Let's face it, you have your good and bad days and sometimes you screw up placement in the radial artery.
- Advantages: low risk of complications, collateral flow is excellent, and cannulation is fairly easy to perform. The posterior tibial (PT) artery is larger than the radial, and the dorsalis pedis (DP) artery is superficial with bone behind it.

CONTRAINDICATIONS

Absolute Contraindications
- Infection at the site of insertion
- Traumatic injury proximal to the site of insertion

Relative Contraindications
- Failure to demonstrate collateral flow
- Arterial insufficiency in the distribution of the artery to be cannulated
- Disadvantages: surgical positioning (prone cases) may lead to a dampened tracing, not much help if the aorta is to be clamped (liver transplant, cardiac surgery), might get in the way of compression stockings and devices for deep venous thrombosis prophylaxis, and provides significant patient inconvenience in terms of patient ambulation (but how many patients with arterial lines are ambulating?).

EQUIPMENT

- Something to hold the foot in position (no, not ropes and chains, but good old tape will do and an arm board)
- Local (if the patient is not sedated)
- Arterial line kit or a cannula (a 20-gauge for an adult, a 22- or 24-gauge for the little ones)
- A wire
- Transducer and pressure tubing

ANATOMY

- The arterial supply of the foot involves a three-artery distributing system with extensive anastomoses (good for collateral circulation!).
- The DP artery, a continuation of the anterior tibial artery, passes along the medial side of the dorsum

of the foot to the first intermetatarsal space where it divides to form the first dorsal metatarsal and the deep plantar arteries.
- The PT artery, the larger terminal branch of the popliteal artery, courses down and medially through the lower leg. It ends midway between the medial malleolus and the most prominent part of the heel.

TECHNIQUE

- Ensure that all preprocedure steps and preparation are used just like other arterial cannulations (see Chapter 6).
- DP cannulation
  - Place the patient's foot in plantar-flexion, prep, drape, and then approach the artery, keeping the anatomy in mind. The extensor hallucis longus tendon is an excellent landmark for the dorsalis pedis artery. If you are having trouble feeling the pulse, have the patient flex the big toe, and you can see or feel the course of the tendon. The artery should be right next to it (Figure 10-1).
  - This artery has the advantage of being very superficial and has bone behind it, but it can roll. So adopt a flat, shallow approach while palpating the artery with your nondominant hand.
  - Cannulate the artery as you would any other artery by direct cannulation or transfixion (the through-and-through technique). Each person seems to prefer one technique or the other.
- PT cannulation
  - Place the foot on the lateral side down and the medial malleolus pointing up. In infants, it is helpful to tape the foot to a splint or arm board to hold it in position. Prep and drape like you usually do.
  - Palpate the pulse posterior to the medial malleolus. Notice that this artery will be a little deeper than the DP, but it is less likely to roll because it lies within a neurovascular sheath and is bounded by tendons.

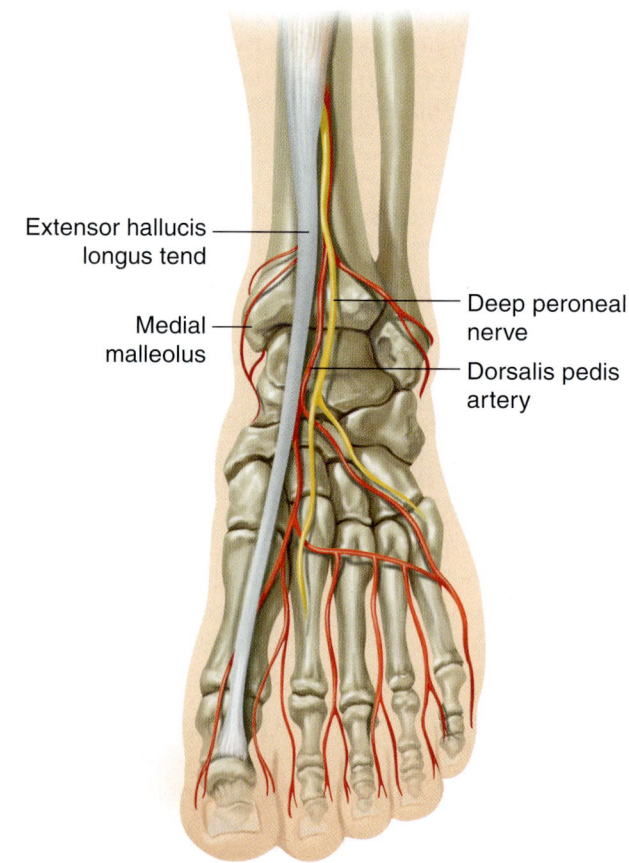

FIGURE 10-1 Anatomy of the foot showing the proximity of the dorsalis pedis artery to the flexor hallucis longus tendon. (Drawn by Tim Phelps.)

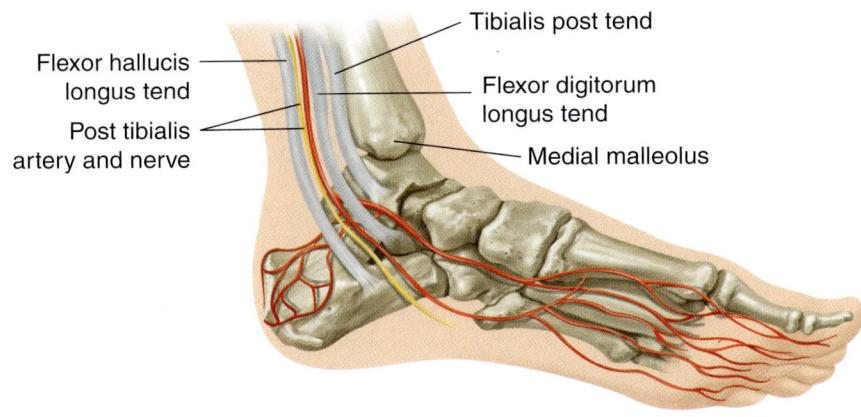

FIGURE 10-2 Anatomy of the posterior tibialis artery and its relationship to tendons, medial malleolus, and the posterior tibialis nerve. (Drawn by Tim Phelps.)

- Approach the artery at the point where it is posterior to the malleolus. It takes a straight trajectory at that point. If you go more caudad, it curves (Figure 10-2).

COMPLICATIONS

- Hematoma
- Infection
- Embolization
- Overall, like the radial art line, the pedal A-line is a pretty safe procedure.

HELPFUL HINTS

- Many provider types like to penetrate the back wall of the artery with the needle and then slowly pull the needle back until the tip is in the lumen of the artery, but this doesn't work if the artery is in spasm, and unfortunately arterial spasm is fairly common. Who wouldn't spasm when being chased by a needle?!
- Keep in mind that the artery is typically not very deep.
- You can attempt to use the fingers of your other hand to keep the artery from rolling while performing the stick.

- Tread lightly! Most rookies push down harder when the pulse is weak or difficult to palpate. This actually occludes the artery (duh!) and you won't feel the pulse at all. Instead, lessen the amount of pressure on the artery and the pulse is usually easier to feel. (The artery and the patient will say "aaahhh"!).
- When cannulating baby arteries, don't be disappointed if you miss. Even seasoned veterans miss. If you have ever seen how small these vessels are during a cut-down, you won't believe that anyone can ever hit them percutaneously!

SUGGESTED READING

Franklin CM. The technique of dorsalis pedis cannulation. An overlooked option when the radial artery cannot be used. *J Crit Illn* 1995;10(7):493–498.

Gordon LH, Brown M, Brown W, Brown EM. Alternative sites for continous arterial monitoring. *South Med J* 1984; 27:1498–1500.

Naguib M, Hassan M, Farag H. Cannulation of the radial and dorsalis pedis arteries. *Br J Anaesth* 1987;59(4):482–488.

Spoerel WE, Deimling P, Aitken R. Direct arterial pressure monitoring from the dorsalis pedis artery. *Can Anaesth Soc J* 1975;22(1):91–99.

PART III

AIRWAY

CHAPTER 11

MASK VENTILATION: THE MASK OF ZORRO

KIMBERLY SCHINNERER COVER
LAUREN BERKOW

"Why do you wear a mask? Were you burned by acid or something?"

"Oh no. It's just they're terribly comfortable. I think everyone will be wearing them in the future."
The Princess Bride
(screenplay by William Goldman)

INTRODUCTION

Mask ventilation is one of the most important skills you can learn as an anesthesia provider. Intubation gets all the press. Each edition of *Anesthesiology News* has a dozen ads for whiz-bang intubation gizmos. But don't forget the basics!

You need to *walk* before you *run*, and you need to *mask ventilate* before you *intubate*.

If you mask ventilate well, you will prevent yourself from getting into disasters, *and* if you mask ventilate well, you can extricate yourself from disasters.

This is a craft worth learning.

INDICATION

- Ventilatory support
- Not only is this important for routine induction, but it is also of utmost importance when intubation fails. It is better to ventilate than to mess around with a difficult intubation when your patient begins to desaturate.
- With mask ventilation you are at least providing for gas exchange. Not as elegant as intubating, but your patient is alive!

CONTRAINDICATION

- Full stomach or risk of aspiration
- That being said, you can mask ventilate through cricoid pressure in an effort to prevent aspiration if you must mask ventilate (for example, if you are unable to intubate).
- It is important to note here that the topic of cricoid pressure is controversial. While many use cricoid pressure in standard practice in an effort to decrease the risk of aspiration (and improve visualization of the vocal cords), studies have shown that cricoid pressure may in fact cause the esophagus to be displaced laterally and may reduce lower esophageal sphincter tone, thus increasing the risk of aspiration.[1]

EQUIPMENT

- In the operating room, an anesthetic circuit with supplied oxygen
- On the floor, an Ambu-bag with supplied oxygen (for pediatrics, a Mapleson circuit will also work) (Figure 11-1)

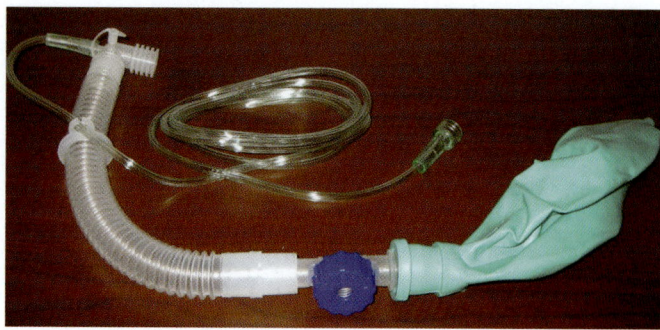

FIGURE 11-1 Mapleson circuit.

- A properly fitting mask
- Suction nearby in case of airway secretions, vomiting, or blood. (Make sure it's on and that you can reach it!)
- Optional: A black strap to hold the mask on and free up your hands. This can be extremely helpful to preoxygenate the patient while you place monitors or IVs. Note: this may not go over well with your claustrophobic, mask-fearing patients, and you may have to hold off on using this handy device.

PHILOSOPHY OF MASK VENTILATION

- In a code or near-code situation on the floor, mask ventilate the patient while the intubation stuff is being opened and readied.
- Get the patient's saturation as high as you can before intubating. You never know who might give you trouble.
- Develop a smooth mask ventilation style that keeps you at ease. You are "setting up the intubation" while you're mask ventilating.
- Do a good job with the mask, and you will have all the time in the world when the intubation approaches.
- Do a bad job with the mask, and you'll be listening to the saturation drop while you're intubating, you'll get panicky, and you will be more likely to make a mistake.
- You also want to develop a style of mask ventilation where you are able to relax your upper body and especially your hand. If you clench your hand into the "claw of death," it will quickly tire.
- If you are comfortable, you can mask ventilate all day. And one day, you just might have to!
- And if you get good at it, your attending might ask you to mask ventilate the case and do the charting simultaneously!

MASK HISTORY AND PHYSICAL

- Read old records to see if the patient was hard to mask ventilate or to intubate.
- Take a good look at the face and see if the patient will be tough to mask.
- Beard? Big mustache? These will make a mask seal hard to obtain.
- Obese? Masking may be hard; plus, obese people are at greater risk for aspiration.
- Obstructive sleep apnea (OSA)? Not only does OSA make masking more challenging, but some patients with OSA will not tolerate lying flat while awake. Be sure to find out how severe the patient's obstructive symptoms are BEFORE induction. You may need to deviate from your usual preoxygenation and mask routine.
- Is the patient lying on an a weird bed? Those orthopedic jungle gyms can make access tough and masking even more difficult.
- Unstable neck from injury or arthritis? While masking, the tendency is to pull the chin up toward the head of the bed, thus extending the neck. This could be catastrophic when the cervical spine is at risk.
- No teeth? Yeah, easy intubation, but guess what—expect a difficulty mask seal. Oral airways can be very helpful in this situation.

TECHNIQUE

- To keep your hands free, put a black face strap on the mask. No kidding, this makes your life a lot easier.
- Make sure the oxygen is on. (Don't laugh, it happens.)
- Hold the mask with your left hand.
- Use your right hand to squeeze the bag.
- With your thumb and index finger form a "C" on the surface of the mask and hold it on the patient's face (Figure 11-2).
- Use your middle, ring, and pinky finger to support the mandible and lift the face up to the mask.
- Important: Don't squish the mask into the patient's eyes and injure them. They will need those when they wake up!
- Speaking of eyes, make sure your ID badge, pens, stethoscope, lucky amulets, and "Go Bulldogs" pins are not hanging down in the patient's eyes. Tape the eyes as soon as the patient is asleep to avoid corneal abrasions.
- When you squeeze the bag, finesse the air into the lungs. Don't use huge volumes or you'll just pump

air into the stomach. A good rule of thumb: keep your eye on the pressure gauge and make sure it stays under 20 cm of H_2O.
- Make sure you have a good seal. For small-handed folks, air can sometimes escape out the right side of the mask. A helping hand (or even finger) to push down the mask on that side is sometimes all that you need. (Figure 11-3)
- If air doesn't go in (chest doesn't rise, no CO_2 on trace, embarrassing flatulent sounds are produced), then try a lifting the chin toward you and tilting the head back (assuming no neck pathology).
- Be sure you are pulling up on the bone of the chin, not the soft tissue (because compressing the soft tissue may cause you to obstruct the airway).
- Next on the list of maneuvers: The jaw thrust. Place your pinky behind the angle of the mandible, pull the entire jaw toward the ceiling (i.e., make the patient have an underbite for the moment).
- If all that doesn't work, try this trick: turn the patient's head to the side a little. You'll be amazed, this really does open up the airway a lot of times.
- Still no air? If the patient can tolerate it, place an oral airway. (Figures 11-4, 11-5)
- To place the oral airway, start by flipping the oral airway upside-down and put it in the patient's mouth (so that tip of it is running across the patient's palate and the curve is pushing the tongue down). Once it is halfway into the mouth, flip it over and place it the rest of the way in (making sure it actually opens up the airway and doesn't just jam the tongue back into the pharynx).
- Alternatively, you can use a tongue depressor; depress the tongue and push the oral airway in right-side up.
- Important: Make sure you are using the right sized oral airway. With the flange at the center of the lips, the tip should reach the angle of the mandible. If it is too small, it will act more like a bite block than an airway adjunct; if it is too big, it can reach back far enough to close the glottis.
- If you're still having trouble, consider a nasal airway. As with the oral airway, make sure you have the right size (measured from the nares to the thyroid notch).
- Caution: the nasal airway can help you, but it can also stir up bleeding and hurt you!
- If you place the nasal airway, goop it up well with lubricant and place it gently. Don't force it or you'll cause bleeding.
- To make ventilation easier, especially in obese patients, put the table in the reverse Trendelenburg position. This takes weight off the diaphragm and makes your life much easier.
- If you're having a tough go of it, use two hands to give a head tilt, chin lift, jaw thrust (the whole shebang), and have a second person squeeze the bag. (Figure 11-6) If you don't have extra help, use the black mask strap to help you hold the mask in place.
- One extra trick to keep up your sleeve: use a shoulder roll as a way to open up the airway in difficult to mask patients (this can be especially helpful in obese patients).
- In an anesthetic induction, ventilation will often be tough until the "relaxant hits." This creates a Catch-22. "Hmm, he's hard to ventilate, should I now give him a relaxant (making it easier to ventilate), or if I give him relaxant will I burn my bridges and find that he's STILL hard to ventilate, and now we're driving toward Disaster Junction?" The answer to this question is definitely provider dependent, but it is smart to consider using a short-acting relaxant if you do bite the bullet and give one.

MASK INDUCTION

- This is a common form of induction in pediatrics.
- You can do it in adults, though this is much less common.
- A wild, thrashing, hold-on-for-dear-life mask induction is always a possibility, but why make your life miserable? Sedate the patient ahead of time (midazolam PO with or without ketamine, IM midazolam, ketamine, and atropine, for example) and everybody wins.
- Another tip: Use a scented Chap Stick to line the inside of the mask. Not only will it help to distract the child from the noxious smell of inhaled anesthetics, but kids really enjoying picking their own flavor and painting it onto the mask. You can also let them carry the mask into the OR. Some will even think of it as a toy!
- Keep the kid comfortable. You can, for example, put the kid in your lap, or even better on Mom's or Dad's lap! A previously cooperative patient may turn into a biting, kicking "strongman," and help will be needed to prevent injury to the patient, parent, and staff members. Beware: a well-placed kick could incapacitate certain team members!
- Place the mask on the child and turn on a non-pungent vapor such as nitrous oxide plus oxygen.
- Next add a potent anesthetic agent, increasing it incrementally every 5 to 10 seconds.

- If the child becomes restless the minute he enters the OR, don't waste time giving him nitrous oxide and slowly adding in the other volatile agent. Put all your cards on the table and turn up the hurry-up-and-fall-asleep-flurane as high as it will go and get that mask sealed. A crying child will take in enough agent in the first 10 seconds to put him to sleep in no time.
- Children will often get a little wild in phase II. Keep your eye on the prize and do not lose your grip on the mask. It often helps if you use your right hand to support the back of the child's head while your left hand is on the mask (that way you have a Kung Fu grip if the child tries to move).
- Once the child is asleep and breathing easily, then place your IV.

MASK GLITCHES

- Taking masking lightly. "We can always intubate, after all." Guess what, that is NOT a given!
- Not doing a real assessment of how hard it might be to mask ventilate. This is especially common on orthopedic beds where, all of a sudden, you just can't get at the patient.
- Beards. Big ones are big problems!
- Want a trick when a Santa Claus beard comes along? Once the patient is induced, place a large Tegaderm over his chin and mouth, smash it down, flatten all the facial hair, poke a hole in the mouth, and voila! Perfect seal for a mask!
- Hair pieces. With this new fashion statement, large attached hair pieces at the crown of the head will push the patient's head in a flexed position, making it hard to achieve good positioning for mask ventilation. Turning the patient's head to the side and then trying to extend the neck may help.
- Obesity. For obese patients, you may consider intubating them awake, because it can be very difficult or even impossible to mask ventilate them.
- Vomiting. Put the patient's head down, turn it to the side, and suction like mad.
- Have a supraglottic airway available at all times (and for an anticipated difficult mask and/or airway you will want to have it open and ready to go). While you shouldn't use these as a way to escape from the challenging mask, they can really save your you-know-what in a pinch!

MASK VENTILATION PICTORIAL

See Figures 11-2 to 11-6.

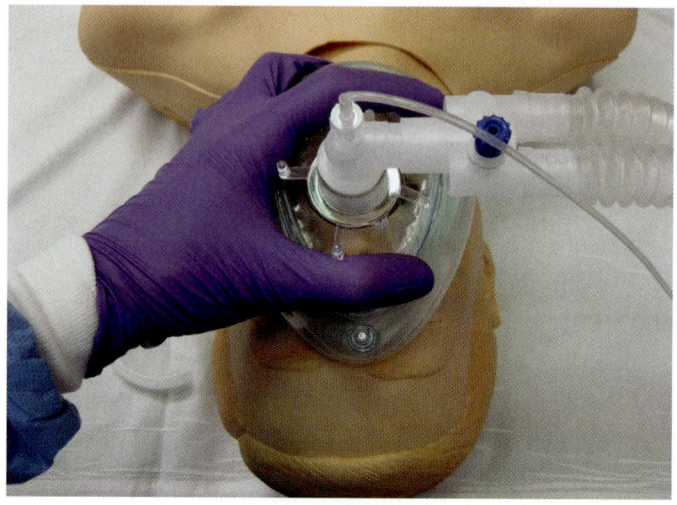

FIGURE 11-2 As an anesthesia provider, you should always be ready for the routine induction that turns into an unexpected failed intubation. You'll see how important good mask ventilation is when things go sour! Here, the procedure starts, and mask ventilation proceeds. Your left hand creates a C-shaped seal on the mask with your thumb and index finger, and your other three fingers support the mandible.

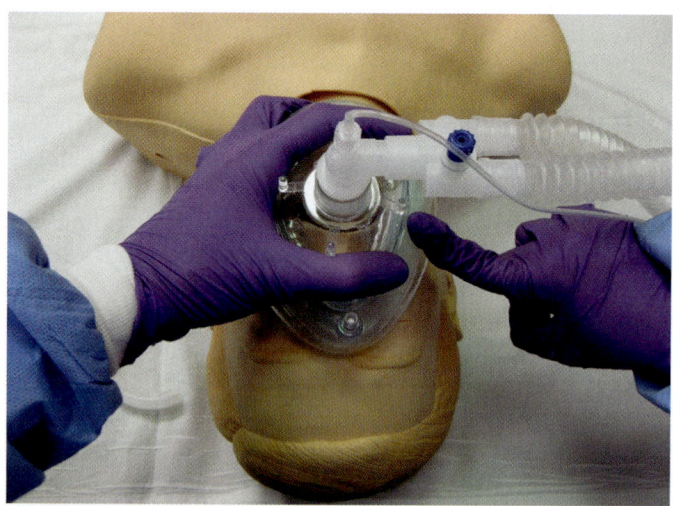

FIGURE 11-3 Note on the right side, where ventilation can "escape." A helping hand (here, a finger), presses down on the right to help "seal the deal." Even with this assistance the patient is still difficult to ventilate.

Chapter 11   MASK VENTILATION: THE MASK OF ZORRO

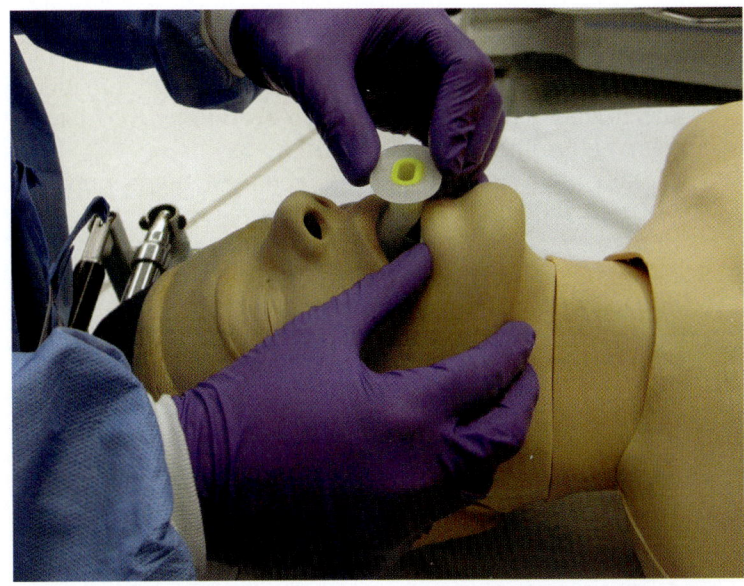

FIGURE 11-4 In goes the oral airway (which is usually helpful).

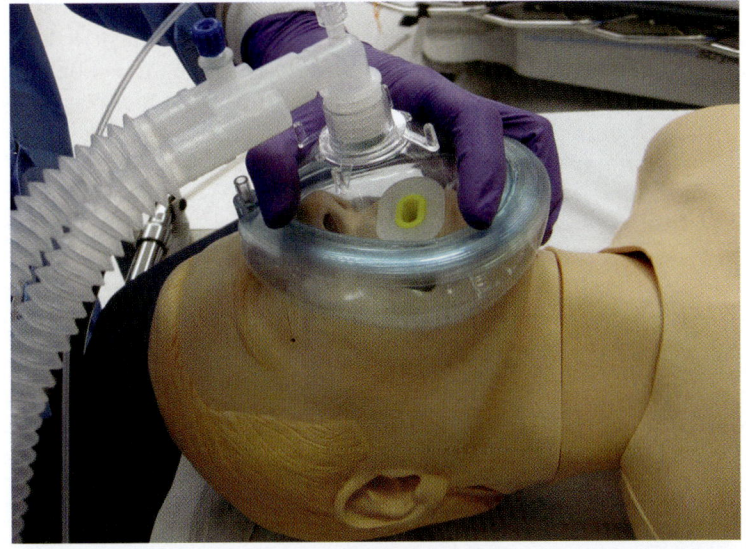

FIGURE 11-5 Still no ventilation.

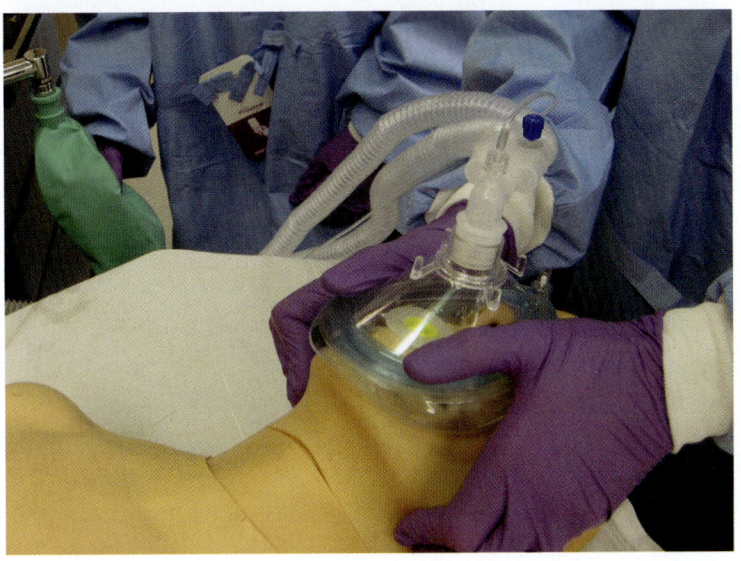

FIGURE 11-6 Next, you can move onto two-handed mask ventilation, where the more skilled person holds the mask, and the helper squeezes the bag. All efforts are focused on masking, and finally air sneaks in! In a situation where attempts at intubation fail, rather than "pursue failure," you should focus on the all-important ventilation. You never HAVE to intubate, but you always HAVE to ventilate.

VENTILATION PEARLS

The Good Ol' Face Strap

To keep your hands free, preoxygenate by holding the mask in place with a face strap. This will allow you to preoxygenate while you do other preparations—put on monitors, strap down the patient's arms, look over your stuff one last time (suction, vital signs, equipment). It also allows you to push your own drugs for induction. An efficient "take-off" is much appreciated by one and all! Just be mindful not to use the face strap for prolonged periods of time, as excessive pressure from the face mask can lead to motor and sensory nerve damage.

But wait, is it that big of a deal to preoxygenate?

Yes, yes, a thousand times yes. Consider every case a scuba dive into the unknown. Before any scuba dive, you fill up your tanks with air. Similarly, before every anesthetic induction, you "fill the tanks with oxygen." Those tanks are the patient's lungs. Furthermore, if you preoxygenate for a full 3 or 4 minutes, you saturate the patient's functional residual capacity (FRC) with oxygen, giving you "little reserve oxygen tanks" to draw on. That complete preoxygenation can provide valuable time (we're talking minutes!) before desaturation during periods of apnea.

How valuable is extra time in a catastrophic airway Armageddon? Priceless! That extra time can allow you to call for help, try something new, get in a supraglottic airway, even cut the neck if you absolutely have to!

People do not come down with tattoos on their forehead that say, "I will be the surprise you never wanted to see, a perfectly normal person who turns out to be impossible to ventilate and impossible to intubate."

Go on the assumption that anyone and everyone can be the big bad surprise, and preoxygenate them completely. You will never regret preoxygenating. You may well regret NOT preoxygenating.

The Claustrophobic Patient

If you really have to preoxygenate, what do you do when someone absolutely cannot tolerate the mask? Do you just say, "The heck with it, I'll not preoxygenate and hope nothing goes wrong?"

Holy desaturation Batman!

Instead, take the mask off and have patients put the elbow of the circuit in their mouth and breathe in oxygen like a straw. No one is claustrophobic of a straw. Then you induce, and as soon as the patient is unconscious, you put the mask on the circuit and away you go. This is useful for both children and adults.

A Little Bit of Reverse Trendelenburg Makes the Medicine Go Down

Look at people who in any way are having trouble breathing: they sit upright. Whether its epiglottitis, congestive heart failure, asthma, mediastinal mass, obesity, pregnancy—you name it, there is one universal behavior that patients seek to improve their breathing mechanics. They sit up. They do everything they can to get weight off their diaphragm.

Take their cue! Tilt patients about 30 degrees upright prior to induction. You will take weight off their diaphragm, making them easier to ventilate, and just a tad bit less likely to desaturate.

That little tip up may make all the difference!

The Oxyhemoglobin Curve Revisited

It's worth taking a look at the oxyhemoglobin dissociation curve at this time. We always think of that curve in its "scary" direction—once the oxygen saturation goes below 90%, it plunges like a roller coaster. But keep in mind that that same curve works for you as well as against you.

If a patient desaturates badly, and you readjust things and get just a little more oxygen in (for example, just a few little puffs of air after readjusting the mask), then that saturation will jump up pretty fast, too. You'll be hip deep in you-know-what; then you finesse a few breaths, and you at least get up into the high 80s on the pulse oximeter (Figure 11-7).

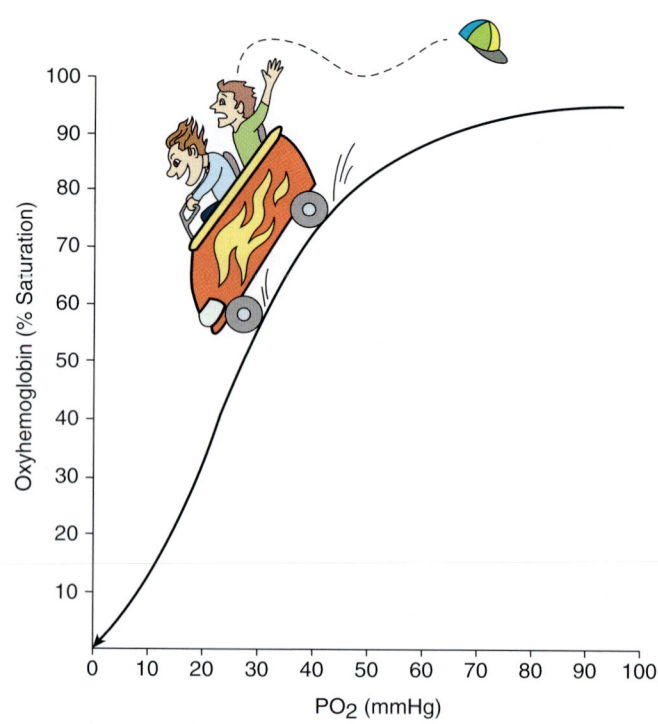

FIGURE 11-7 Oxyhemoglobin dissociation curve. (Drawn by Kelly Brenan-Rothschild.)

The Hardest Sometimes Are the Easiest

One interesting fact about mask ventilation: sometimes the hardest people to mask are the easiest to intubate. Look at edentulous patients. Their face falls away from their mouth, and it can be difficult to "gather" enough face into the mask to get a good seal. Fortunately, their lack of teeth can make them quite easy to intubate, so when you're getting frustrated as heck trying to mask them, consider trying to place the tube. The same concept is also true of a healthy, thin man with a full beard.

Don't Mess With Perfection

An important patient population to consider before masking away: patients after rhinoplasty (or other procedures involving the nose).

After you extubate, you can get into airway trouble and have to mask ventilate. If some plastic surgeon just finished carving the perfect nose, and you smash the mask down on this aesthetic creation, you may undo the beauty (and make enemies with the surgeon).

To keep the mask off the nose, yet still ventilate, just turn the mask around 180 degrees and seal it over the mouth and nose (with the narrow part near the chin, and the wider part near the nose). Yes indeed, you can ventilate this way and spare the nose from your brutality.

Thus you can serve the cause of oxygenation and beautification at the same time! (Figure 11-8).

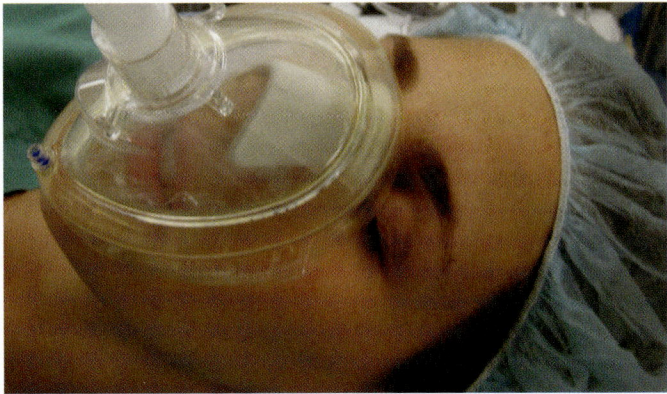

FIGURE 11-8 Mask turned 180 degrees for a rhinoplasty patient.

Beware of CPAP on the Floor

Mask continuous positive airway pressure (CPAP) at home is one thing. Mask CPAP in the hospital is quite another. If you are called to assess a patient on the ward, and his or her oxygenation status is so tenuous that only a tightly applied mask with a high level of continuous pressure will keep the patient going (e.g., CPAP of 20), think strongly about intubating the patient or moving him or her to the ICU for CPAP or bi-level positive airway pressure (BiPAP) therapy.

Breaking Laryngospasm, the Ultimate Test of Mask Ventilation

Most of the focus on mask ventilation is at the beginning of the procedure. The patient gets induced, you "take over," and mask ventilation happens. At the end of the procedure, the patient is breathing on his or her own, you pull out the tube, go to the postanesthesia care unit (PACU), fill out grossly overweighted paperwork, and head to the yacht club.

Piece of cake.

Only one zinger in this deal: sometimes when you pull the tube out, the patient goes into laryngospasm and your yacht sinks! Now you have to mask ventilate *with attitude*. The patient is desaturating, and the chest is moving up and down, generating negative pressure pulmonary edema, and you are in a world of hurt.

As with everything else in medicine, an ounce of prevention is worth a pound of personal injury lawyer subpoenas. Do your best to extubate the patient when laryngospasm won't happen. That means either a deep extubation or an awake extubation. By awake, I mean this: the patient's *brain* is awake as well as the *airway*. If just your airway is awake, then you cough, buck, and flail around. Remember, your *airway alone* has only one way to protect itself—slam the vocal cords shut. When your *brain* is awake (enabling you to respond to commands such as "open your eyes"), you have more ways to protect your airway.

So you blew it and the patient is in laryngospasm. Now what?

Apply the mask and get "the mother of all seals"; you need to ventilate this patient pronto. Don't be shy about asking for help; laryngospasm is scary as heck and can get ugly fast. It often helps to have both hands on the mask and have someone else handle the bag. Drive your fingers behind the ramus of the mandible and pull toward the ceiling like there is no tomorrow (i.e., perform a mean jaw thrust). Apply CPAP with the bag. Some clinicians suggest putting pressure at the "laryngospasm notch" (located between the mastoid process and the ear lobule) as a way to break the process. If this doesn't work, try deepening anesthesia by giving a small dose of propofol. Still no love from the closed vocal cords? Show them a lesson and give a small dose of succinylcholine. This can be given IV, or on the off chance that you have no IV access (oh my!), have no fear: you can give it IM[2]!

CONCLUSION

By now you appreciate why mask ventilation is one of the most important skills you can learn as an anesthesia provider. Knowing how to mask ventilate, and how to do it well, not only can buy you time in a disaster, but it can mean the difference between life and death for your patient. So pick up that mask, get a good seal, and ventilate away!

REFERENCES

1. Smith KJ, Dobranowski J, Yip G, et al. Cricoid pressure displaces the esophagus. An observational study using magnetic resonance imaging. *Anesthesiology* 2003; 99:60.
2. Al-alami AA, Zestos MM, Baraka AS. Pediatric laryngospasm: prevention and treatment. *Curr Opin Anaesthesiol* 2009;22(3):388–395.

SUGGESTED READING

Benumof JL. Obstructive sleep apnea in the adult obese patient: implications for airway management. *Anesthesiol Clin North Am* 2002;20(4):789–811.

Berkow LC. Strategies for airway management. *Best Pract Res Clin Anaesthesiol* 2004;18(4):531–548.

Review of the American Association of Anesthesiologists guidelines for management of the difficult airway, including specifics on airway evaluation and mask ventilation.

El-Orbany M, Woehlck HJ. Difficult mask ventilation. *Anesth Analg* 2009;109(6):1870–1880.

Reviews the definition, pathophysiology, and management of difficult mask ventilation.

Greenberg RS. Facemask, nasal and oral airway devices. *Anesthesiol Clin North Am* 2002;20:833–861.

Detailed review of the fundamentals of airway management.

McGowan P, Skinner A. Preoxygenation—the importance of a good face mask seal. *Br J Anaesth* 1995;75:777–778.

Shows that air dilution occurs with failure to obtain a tight mask seal during spontaneous respiration.

CHAPTER 12

"GOODNIGHT, SLEEP TIGHT": SETUP AND MASK INDUCTION FOR PEDIATRIC PATIENTS

PEGGY SEIDMAN
KATHLEEN DUBROW

ROOM SETUP

- First things first: crank up the heat in the operating room. Pediatric patients, in particular neonates and infants, are more susceptible to heat loss, and their only mechanism of heat production, nonshivering thermogenesis, is limited at best. Turn up the thermostat, turn on the fluid warmer and the warming Bair Hugger© on the OR table.
- Choose your endotracheal tube. A rough estimate of tube selection can be calculated as follows: (age/4) + 4. Have an endotracheal tube (ETT) a half size above and half size below what you calculate you need (Figure 12-1). Stay "green," though; no need to open every size ETT and keep it on your anesthesia cart. Then, hug a tree.
- Uncuffed tubes are recommended for patients under the age of 6. This decreases the risk of postintubation croup and minimizes the risk of barotrauma. Since the early 1990s, cuffed tubes for younger and younger patients are being used, but this remains an area of controversy.
- How about an emergency backup airway device? A laryngeal mask airway (LMA) perhaps? Have an appropriate-size LMA out and ready for use if necessary.
- Which blade will you use? The pediatric airway differs from the adult in several ways (see Table 12-2). Traditionally, the straight blade is a good choice, but there are many straight blades to use; personal preference may rule (Figure 12-2).
- Time to enter the "crazy box." Set up your fluid line and knock out all the bubbles! Bubbles like to hide in all the stopcocks, ports, and connectors. Everybody knows that kids LOVE bubbles, but let's not give them these bubbles. Entrained air in the IV tubing could lead to an air embolism. Small amounts of air are usually filtered out through the venous circulation in the lungs, but pediatric patients may have a patent foramen ovale or intracardiac shunt that would allow the air into the arterial circulation.
- Put together an IV kit so it's ready to grab and an IV can be quickly popped into those tiny veins. Your IV kit should have the IV needle/catheter, a flushed saline lock, tourniquet, alcohol swabs, and gauze (Figure 12-3). Depending on the size of the patient and type of case, a 24-, 22-, or 20-gauge (G) IV will be appropriate.

- DRUGS! What do you absolutely need? This is about pediatric mask induction, so please make sure that the sevoflurane has been topped off and is ready to go. What bad things can happen to the kiddies? That's right—laryngospasm and bradycardia! The rescue drugs necessary for pediatric patients include succinylcholine and atropine with a 22-G needle for intramuscular (IM) delivery of the drug if necessary (Figure 12-4). Correct dosing for succinylcholine is 1.5 to 2 mg/kg IV, 5 mg/kg IM, and for atropine is 0.01 mg/kg IV, 0.02 mg/kg IM.

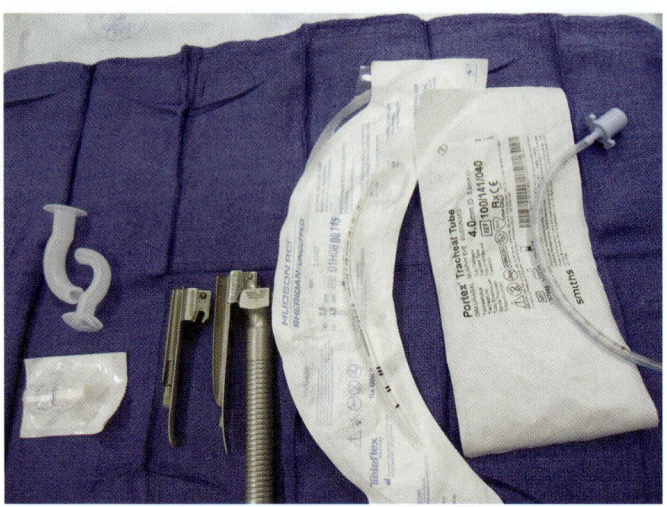

FIGURE 12-1 Airway setup.

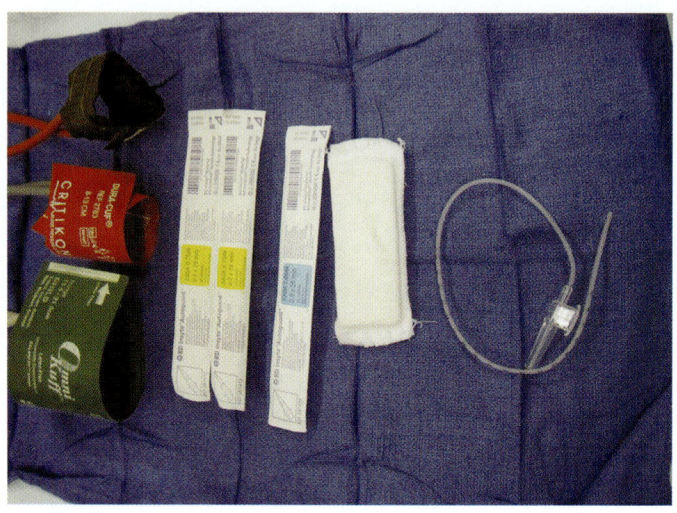

FIGURE 12-3 IV setup.

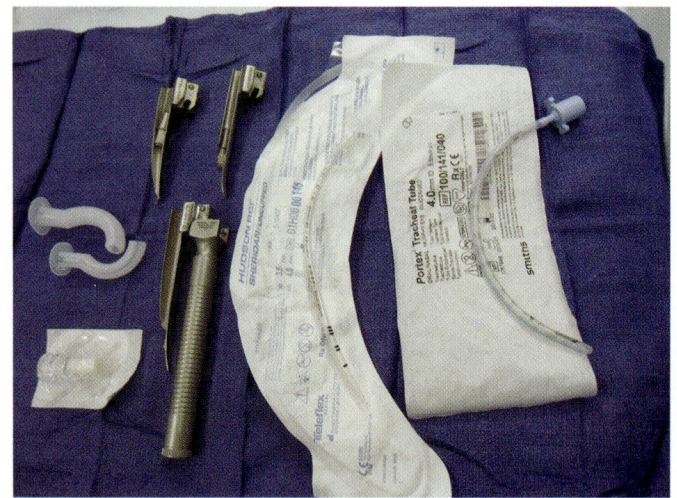

FIGURE 12-2 Note the straight blades of this airway setup.

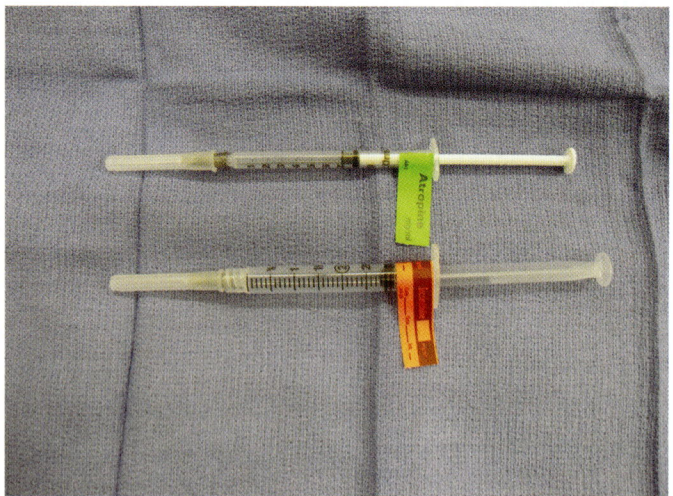

FIGURE 12-4 Emergency drugs.

PREOPERATIVE ASSESSMENT AND PREMEDICATION

- What are the patient's allergies? How much does the patient weigh? This information is crucial.
- How about a history and physical examination? At what gestational age, in weeks, was the child born? Did the patient need to spend any time in the neonatal intensive care unit (NICU)? Once a preemie, always a preemie. Premature gestational age (PGA) is important until 6 months of age, and prematurity problems are for life. Any other medical problems? Has the patient had anesthesia before? Problems? Any recent upper respiratory infections (URIs)? Cough? Fever? Snotty nose? Are the lungs clear? Can you do an airway exam? Any loose teeth to be aware of?
- When did the patient last have anything to eat? The NPO status is also crucial for every single patient (Table 12-1).
- When is it appropriate to premedicate the patient? When is it best to bring in a parent? Can you premedicate the parents?
- Pediatric patients who show signs of separation anxiety, usually at about age 10 months old, are good candidates for premedication. Of all the choices for premedication, midazolam 0.5 mg/kg given orally 30 minutes prior to induction has been shown to ease the anxiety and lead to a calmer and smoother mask induction and the least amount of postoperative negative behaviors. Some may say that midazolam has delayed discharge, but this has NOT been proven.

TABLE 12-1 NPO Guidelines

Substance	Minimum Hours of Fasting
Solids	8
Formula	6
Cow's milk	6
Citrus juice	6
Breast milk	4
Clear liquids	2

- To bring in the parent or not to bring in the parent? Studies have shown that parents believe that they are helpful during induction. Anesthesiologists feel that they are NOT helpful during induction. The anxiety of both the parent and child may be detrimental, but a prepared and calm parent's presence could be beneficial. The controversy battles on.

THE PATIENT ARRIVES

- When the pediatric patient arrives, everyone in the operating room tends to ooh and ahh and fawn over the patient. When is the last time anyone tried to cuddle with a vasculopath undergoing a fem-pop bypass? Never. So it shouldn't be done for a pediatric patient either.
- Pediatric patients have a smoother induction with a quiet room, no harsh lighting, and only one person speaking to them. This person should be the anesthesiologist. This may be difficult with a parent in the room, but the overall goal should be to limit the noise.
- Good luck strapping on all the standard American Society of Anesthesiologists (ASA) monitors on a squirming 2-year-old. What is important is quickly putting on the pulse oximeter and beginning the induction of anesthesia (Figure 12-5).
- Start with a 30:70 mixture of O_2 and N_2O; once the patient has taken several breaths, crank up the sevoflurane to 8% (Figure 12-6). The patient will be down for the count in a few short breaths. Having the circuit primed with this mixture has been shown to induce patients more quickly compared to incremental increases of sevoflurane. Sevoflurane has also been shown to have good hemodynamic stability as an induction agent and is less noxious compared to the other volatiles. Sevoflurane is the volatile agent of choice for a mask induction.
- Begin to assist the patient in breathing to drive all that sevoflurane to distal most alveoli. Always keep an eye on the patient; watch the chest rise and fall. The expired sevoflurane level should be at least 4.68% to ensure depth of anesthesia necessary for the patient will tolerate laryngoscopy and ETT placement.
- Now that your patient is being much more cooperative, connect the rest of the monitors! (Figure 12-7)

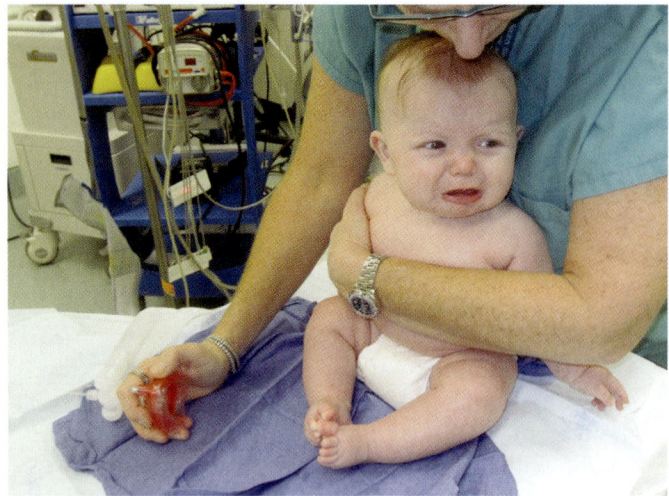

FIGURE 12-5 Hug the kiddie to hold safely.

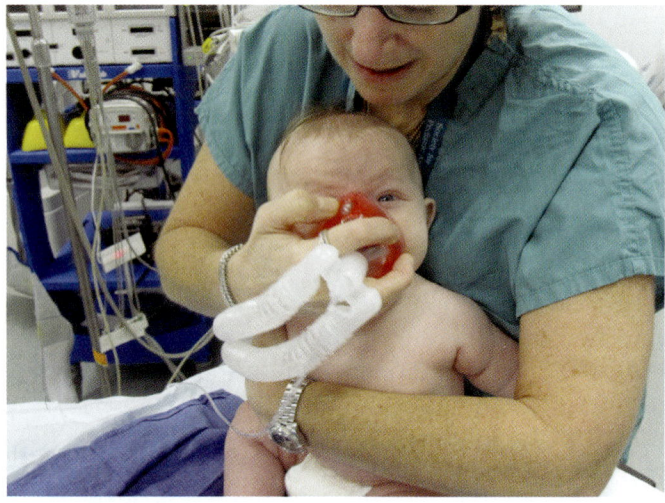

FIGURE 12-6 Holding the mask on the baby.

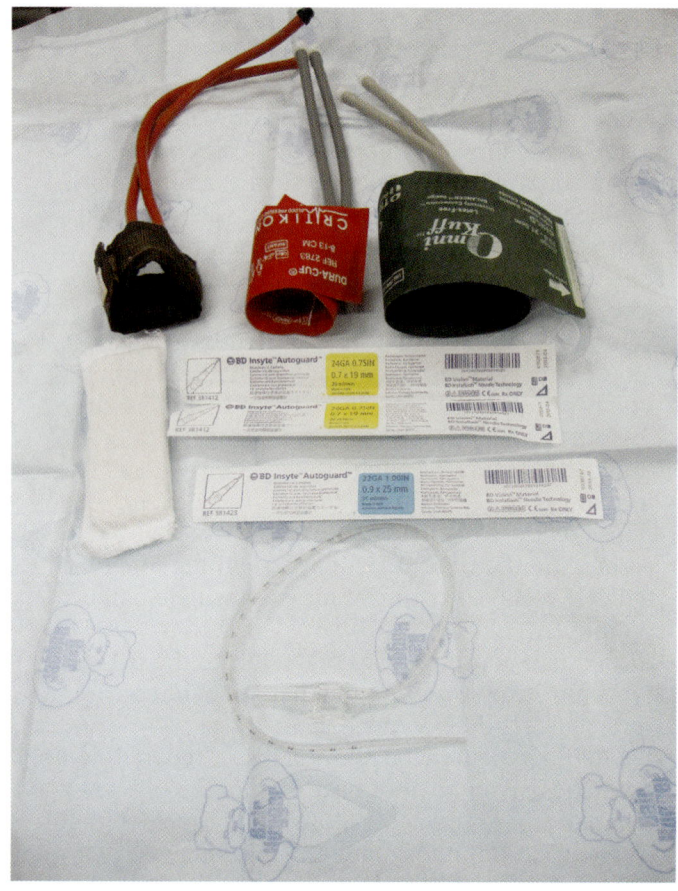

FIGURE 12-7 Different size blood pressure cuffs.

PLACEMENT

- Do babies actually have visible veins? Is this an impossible task? Where is the best place to aim for?
- Once the patient has been properly anesthetized, someone trained in advance airway management needs to continue to monitor the airway, while you go for that IV!
- Take your handy-dandy pre-made IV kit and go for it! Strap the tourniquet above the wrist to find dorsal veins of the hand or above the ankle for that elusive, but great, saphenous vein. Try to avoid the antecubital space, as those IVs are more difficult to place and secure and are much more problematic for the child when he or she awakens.

ENDOTRACHEAL TUBE TIME! (DON'T BE SCARED)

- First off, placing an ETT should be smooth, quick, and atraumatic. There is no need to jam this large foreign body down a poor innocent baby's throat.

TABLE 12-2 Comparison of Pediatric and Adult Airways

	Pediatric Airway	Adult Airway
Larynx	C3-4	C4-5
Most narrow	Cricoid cartilage	Glottic rim
	• Tongue larger in size in proportion to mouth • Large, stiff epiglottis • Small nares	

- Before attempting direct laryngoscopy, there are some important differences that should be emphasized about the pediatric airway compared to the adult airway (Table 12-2).
- Straight blades are narrower, which is advantageous in successful intubations of pediatric patients, given their anatomy. Pediatric patients have a large epiglottis, which typically obstructs the view of the vocal cords if a curved blade is used. The straight blade will lift the epiglottis and bring the vocal cords into view.
- Using your straight blade of choice, enter the mouth from the right, and sweep the tongue to the left. Make sure that the tip of the blade has covered the epiglottis. Lifting gently up with the blade should bring the vocal cords into view. With your right hand, gripping the tube near the top with your thumb and forefinger, carefully put the tube in between the vocal cords.
- The best method for tube depth placement is to place the ETT endobronchial and pull the ETT slowly back until bilateral breath sounds are heard. The anesthesiologist always needs to confirm proper tube placement by auscultation of the lungs to ensure bilateral breath sounds.
- Once the tube is in the correct position, take note of the number depth the tube is, and then properly secure the tube to the patient.

EXCUSE ME, DOCTOR, BUT WHAT IS THAT SQUEAKING NOISE?...LARYNGOSPASM!!!

- Laryngospasm is nothing to be afraid of as a trained advance airway specialist like yourself, but it should always be anticipated and the anesthesiologist needs to be ready to quickly diagnose and treat the laryngospasm. If not treated in a timely manner, then laryngospasm may lead to desaturation, bradycardia, cardiac collapse, and even death.
- Laryngospasm is glottic closure from reflex constriction of the intrinsic laryngeal muscles. Laryngospasm is more likely to occur in children than in adults.
- Laryngospasm is brought on from an irritation to the larynx, such as from secretions or blood. Laryngospasm is a protective mechanism from these irritants. It is most likely to occur during induction or emergence.
- Laryngospasm can be treated in several ways. For an incomplete obstruction, attempts to remove the irritant should be made, deepening the anesthesia, and applying continuous positive pressure with a tightly sealed mask.
- For a complete obstruction, a strong jaw thrust should be done in addition to continuous positive pressure. If this move is not successful, then the use of a muscle relaxant, succinylcholine, becomes the next option. By this time, the patient is likely bradycardic from the hypoxia, so atropine should be given prior to or concurrently with the succinylcholine.
- Prevention and anticipation with each case is the key. Identifying patients who are at high risk of laryngospasm, using non-noxious volatiles for inhalation induction, suctioning thoroughly prior to extubation, and providing positive pressure while extubating will help aid in the fight against laryngospasm.

SUGGESTED READING

Cassey JG, King RA, Armstrong P. Is there thermal benefit from preoperative warming in children? *Paediatr Anaesth* 2010;20(1):63–71.

Dullenkopf A, Gerber A, Weiss M. Fluid leakage past tracheal tube cuffs: evaluation of the new Microcuff endotracheal tube. *Intensive Care Med* 2003;29(10):1849–1853. Epub 2003 Aug 16.

Epstein RH, Stein AL, Marr AT, Lessin JB. High concentration versus incremental induction of anesthesia with sevoflurane in children: a comparison of induction times, vital signs, and complications. *J Clin Anesth* 1998;10(1):415.

Inomata S, Nishikawa T. Determination of end-tidal sevoflurane concentration for tracheal intubation in children with the rapid method. *Can J Anaesth* 1996;43(8):806–811.

Kain ZN, Mayes LC, Wang S-M, Caramico LA, Hofstadter MB. Clinical investigations of parental presence during induction of anesthesia versus sedative premedication: which intervention is more effective? *Anesthesiology* 1998;89(5):1147–1156.

Mariano ER, Ramamoorthy C, Chu LF, et al. A comparison of three methods for estimating appropriate tracheal tube depth in children. *Pediatr Anesth* 2005;15(10):846–851.

CHAPTER 13

LARYNGEAL MASK AIRWAY AND OTHER SUPRAGLOTTIC AIRWAY DEVICES

MELTEM YILMAZ
RENA BECKERLY

"What are two off-label explanations of what LMA stands for?"

"Lose My Airway and Let 'em aspirate."

Overheard in the locker room

INTRODUCTION

How many times have we heard surgeons say, "An LMA should be fine; we'll be done in no time"? Supraglottic airways (SGAs) have become such a staple in our practice that even our surgical colleagues can recognize their utility over endotracheal tubes. However, like every other device that promises eternal bliss, the SGA's role in our practice needs to be carefully considered. When selected for the right patient and appropriate procedure, the SGA can offer a safe, smooth, and seemingly effortless airway management technique.

The laryngeal mask airway (LMA), the first SGA device, was introduced by a British anesthesiologist, Dr. Archie Brain, in 1981, and finally made its way to the United States in 1989. It was designed to serve as an intermediary between the face mask and endotracheal tube (ETT). Anesthesiologists had a new toy to play with that freed their hands from mask ventilation and allowed them to avoid the more invasive ETT. The LMA has become a core instrument in managing airways for over 30,000,000 patients in the U.S. and U.K. It has even become one of the first supraglottic device to be recommended by the American Society of Anesthesiologists' (ASA) difficult airway algorithm for the "cannot intubate—cannot ventilate" scenario.

The LMA is archetypical of all supraglottic devices. Due to its success, new-generation supraglottic devices with advanced features such as intubating and gastric suctioning capabilities, better seal pressures, and improved anatomical design have been developed. These newer SGA devices have also been integrated to the ASA's difficult airway algorithm for the "cannot intubate—cannot ventilate" scenario (Figure 13-1).

TYPES OF SGAs

There is multitude of different designs of SGAs. Although there have been some attempts to classify these devices, it is easier to distinguish them by focusing on their functional design (Figures 13-1 to 13-5).

The SGAs can simply be categorized as follows:
- *SGA only*, e.g., LMA, Cobra perilaryngeal airway (Cobra PLA), King Laryngeal tube disposable (King LTD), Streamlined Sealer of the Pharynx Airway (SLIPA)
- *SGA with gastric suctioning capability*, e.g., Proseal LMA/LMA Supreme, newer generation AirQ, King Laryngeal Tube-Suction (LTS), I-Gel, Combitube/Easytube
- *SGA with intubating capability*, e.g., Intubating LMA (ILMA), AirQ, Ambu Aura

Some of these devices can serve multiple purposes. When necessary, with the aid of a fiberoptic bronchoscope and some extra effort, intubation can be achieved with any SGA in experienced hands.

Next-generation supraglottic airways (SGA) include:
- LMA: 4G iPad
- SGA: Bluetooth
- AirZ: Facebook

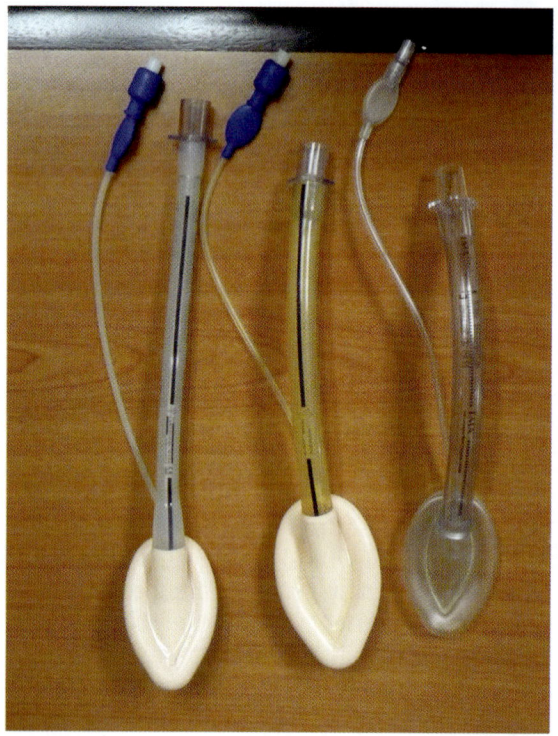

FIGURE 13-1 Classic LMAs: flexible, classic, and unique.

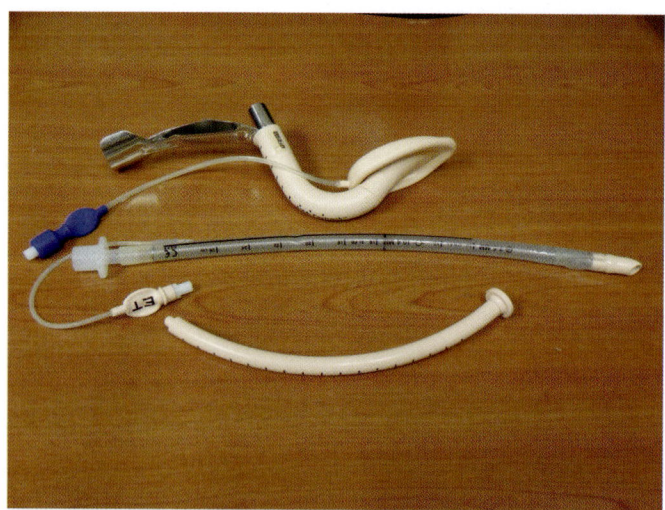

FIGURE 13-2 Intubating LMA (Fastrack LMA).

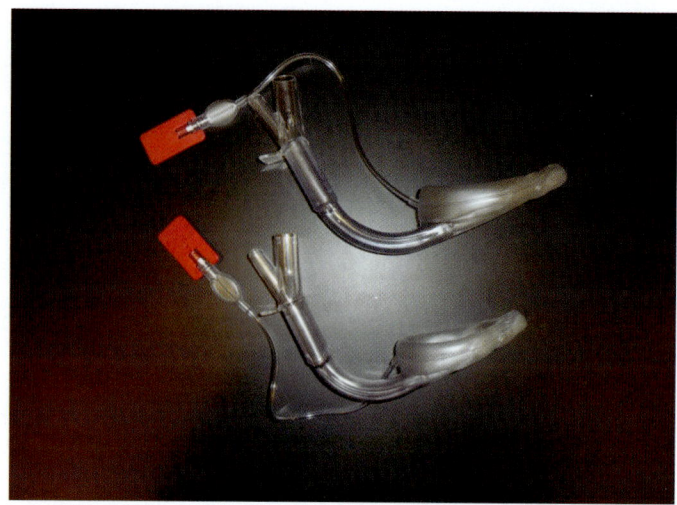

FIGURE 13-3 LMA Supreme (disposable Proseal).

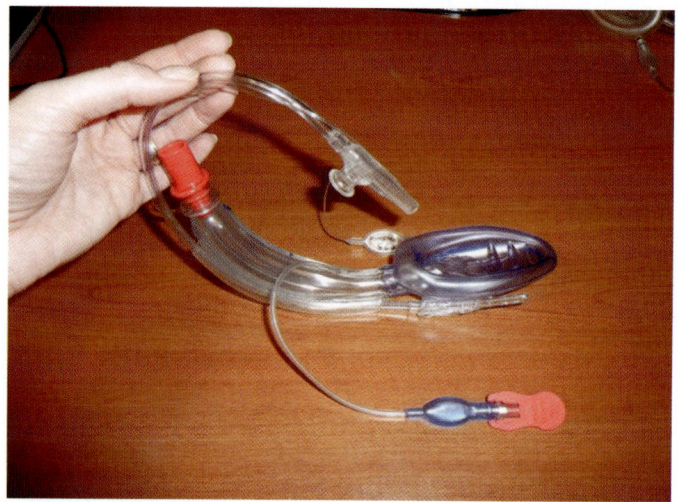

FIGURE 13-4 AirQ.

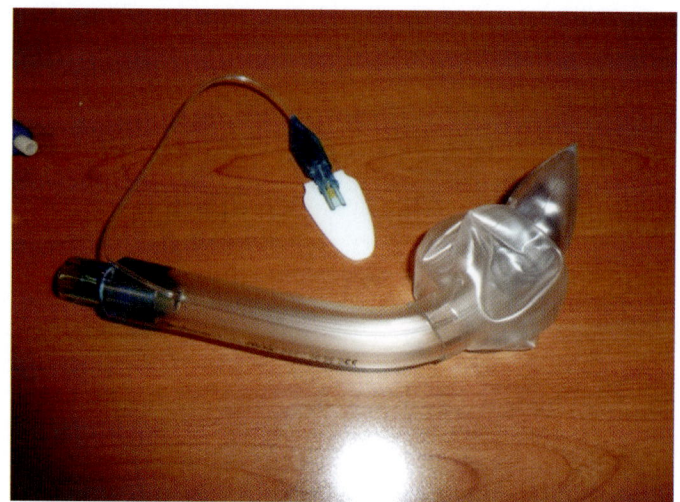

FIGURE 13-5 Cobra PLA.

Chapter 13 LARYNGEAL MASK AIRWAY AND OTHER SUPRAGLOTTIC AIRWAY DEVICES

INDICATIONS

Who is a good candidate for an SGA device, and which procedure allows for its successful use? The indications for SGA placement seem to be growing quickly. In Britain, anesthesiologists are even using SGAs for pregnant women requiring C-sections. Routinely, cases are handed off with the patients with SGAs in the lateral position or even prone position. YIKES!

- The good news is that there are newer SGAs with better sealing capabilities that allow for positive pressure ventilation, provide a gastric suction port to assist in drainage of gastric contents, and are designed to perform as a bridge to intubation.
- Everyone respects the SGA for its critical role in managing a difficult airway where mask ventilation and intubation are impossible.
- SGAs without a gastric suction port are safe for routine general anesthetics that require airway support where the patient is not considered to have a full stomach or to be at increased aspiration risk.
- SGAs are considered easier to place, less stimulating than direct laryngoscopy with intubation, and offer smoother emergence than with an ETT. This often makes them ideal for a myriad of surgeries that does not require muscle paralysis, including cystoscopies and surgeries of the extremities in both adults and children.

CONTRAINDICATIONS

With all these advantages, how can you get yourself into trouble?

- The main disadvantage of the SGA is the lack of a secure airway that protects against regurgitated gastric contents, thus further increasing the patient's aspiration risk.
- We all know not to put SGAs without intubating capability and/or gastric suction port in patients with morbid obesity/pregnancy/ascites, obstructive sleep apnea (OSA), large tonsils, bloody airways, oral/pharyngeal masses, or significant facial trauma.
- We also know that SGAs are contraindicated for laparoscopic surgeries or surgeries that require paralysis. Hmm... or is it possible? (Newer generation SGA's with better seal pressures allow positive pressure ventilation) Additionally, the SGA might not work in everyone and the patient may require intubation. Even if the SGA sits right, you might struggle with adequate ventilation, especially in patients with decreased lung compliance.

EXAMPLES OF PATIENTS

Let's consider the following patients, who you may struggle with if you manage the airway with an SGA.

Patient 1

A 60-year-old woman presents with long-standing diabetes (HbA_{1c} of 12), hypertension, and coronary artery disease scheduled for a transurethral resection of a bladder tumor (TURBT).

You weigh the risks and benefits of ETT versus an SGA. You ultimately convince yourself to go with the SGA. After all, there will be less hemodynamic changes during induction, less airway stimulation (less coughing, gagging, breath holding, bronchospasm), and the procedure is relatively simple and short. Soon after you induce anesthesia with propofol/fentanyl, you notice what looks like last night's dinner in the patient's oropharynx. OOPS! You quickly suction the oral cavity, push succinylcholine, and intubate the patient. What went wrong?

- This patient was not a good candidate for an LMA since she has long-standing and poorly controlled diabetes (as evidenced by the HbA_{1c} of 12). While she denied any symptoms of reflux, she suffers from diabetic gastroparesis with delayed gastric emptying/motility. This automatically increases her risk for aspiration.
- Every patient undergoing anesthesia is at aspiration risk. Endotracheal intubation offers a secure airway once the tube is in place and the cuff is inflated. However, patients are still at aspiration risk during induction and after extubation.
- Similar rates of aspiration have been reported in patients at low risk for aspiration with an LMA or an ETT.
- In this patient with an aspiration risk, such as gastroparesis, consider other supraglottic devices that have the capability to be intubated through (such as an intubating LMA or AirQ) or devices with a good laryngopharyngeal seal that provide a much better seal around the glottic opening with a gastric suction port, such as the Proseal LMA, LMA Supreme, Ambu aura or AirQ.

Patient 2

A 55-year-old woman, weighing 150 pounds, and 66 inches tall, with a thick neck and a large tongue, presents for a skin mass excision.

You decide on an LMA since the patient denied gastroesophageal reflux disease (GERD) and obstructive sleep apnea (OSA), and because the procedure would be relatively short. You induce general anesthesia with propofol and fentanyl, place a size 4 LMA, inflate the cuff with 20 cc of air, and hand ventilate. You notice a leak and put another 20 cc of air into the cuff. Still you hear a leak and inject another 10 cc of air. You then notice the whole LMA pop out. You switch to a size 5 LMA and still can't get a good seal. You attempt to mask ventilate the patient, but it is unsuccessful, and her oxygen saturation is now 75%. You quickly grab your Miller blade and intubate the patient. How did this happen?

- Everyone swears by a technique that never fails them for LMA placement. Dr. Brain initially meant for the LMA to be positioned with the nondominant hand on the occiput, to extend the neck and to open the mouth, and the LMA in the dominant hand (positioned as an extension of the index finger, at the junction of the tube and the mask). The LMA is advanced against the hard palate and behind the tongue until you feel the resistance of the upper esophageal sphincter.
  - BE CAREFUL to make sure that the tip of the LMA has not bent on itself. There have been case reports of significant mucosal tears caused by aggressive LMA placement with a bent LMA tip, resulting in pharyngeal and mediastinal abscesses. The cuff should be inflated until an effective seal is established.
- How much air can you safely inject to obtain an adequate seal? The manufacturers of the LMA recommend inflation pressure of up to a maximum of 60 cm H_2O. This is the pressure that is recommended, the maximum amount of air is usually marked on the LMA itself and it is different for each size (Table 13-1).
  - The LMA is intended to be positioned so that the distal tip of the LMA mask sits in the esophageal inlet and rests against the upper esophageal sphincter in the hypopharynx. The sides of the cuff rest in the pyriform fossae (site of recurrent laryngeal nerve). The upper border rests against the base of the tongue.
  - It is understandable how longer procedures or high inflation pressures can put the patient at risk for tongue ischemia and nerve injury (lingual, recurrent, and hypoglossal). Manometry studies have shown that inflation pressures of less than 44 cm H_2O are associated with fewer complications and slightly less sore throats. REMEMBER, nitrous oxide can increase your pressures.
- Selecting the appropriate size LMA is based on the patient's weight (Table 13-1). Patients between 50 and 70 kg require a size 4 LMA. Patients heavier than 70 kg require a size 5 LMA. If I think I will need a size 5 for a patient in an elective procedure,

TABLE 13-1 Specific Recommendations for Each LMA Size (per Patient Weight, Max. Cuff Volume, Largest Diameter of ETT, and Fiberoptic Bronchoscope Size That Can Be Inserted)

LMA Size	Patient Weight (kg)	Maximum Cuff Volume (cc)	Largest ETT	Fiberoptic Scope Size (mm)
1	<5	4	3.5	2.7
1.5	5–10	7	4.0	2.7
2	10–20	10	4.5	3.5
2.5	20–30	14	5	4
3	30–50	20	6.0 cuffed	5
4	50–70	30	6.0 cuffed	5
5	>70	40	7.0 cuffed	6

I start to reconsider my decision to use an LMA. Is this patient really a good candidate for an LMA, or should I just secure the airway with an ETT or switch to another supraglottic device with a better pharyngolaryngeal seal and a gastric suction port, such as a Proseal LMA/LMA Supreme (the disposable version), I-Gel, or an AirQ?

Patient 3

A 45-year-old man with ischemic cardiomyopathy, asthma, and pulmonary hypertension presents for a knee arthroscopy.

You decide on an LMA to minimize the hemodynamic stress of intubation and hope to better manage his asthma. You induce with propofol/fentanyl and place the LMA without complication. You continue to support his ventilation manually as he is breathing irregularly with small tidal volumes (expired CO_2 of 65 mm Hg). Also, you are continuously giving boluses of phenylephrine to support his blood pressure. Eventually, you are forced to titrate down your volatile agent to maintain hemodynamic stability, as he does not respond to fluid challenge. Upon incision, he gags and becomes stridorous. You quickly give him a propofol bolus to deepen the level of anesthesia (chase it with phenylephrine) and continue to give positive pressure ventilation to try and break the laryngospasm. The laryngospasm doesn't break, and so you administer succinylcholine. He is now paralyzed and you decide to put him on the ventilator. Luckily, your surgeon is finished and it is time to wake the patient. This is a disaster! You thought you were decreasing this man's anesthetic risk, but now you see that this was the wrong choice for airway management in such a complicated patient. Let's review this closely.

- SGAs are great for asthmatics in that they do not instrument the trachea. However, this patient needed very tight management of his ventilation as he already had pulmonary hypertension, which is worsened by hypercarbia.
- Additionally, hypotension in this patient would reduce perfusion to his compromised heart. He did not tolerate the vasodilation from the volatile agents, and you appropriately titrated down the agent.
  - This is DANGEROUS in a patient with an SGA, as light anesthesia can trigger the gag reflex and coughing. Secretions around the SGA can drip on the vocal cords or the tip of the SGA can irritate the vocal cords, resulting in laryngospasm/bronchospasm. So you are stuck. You need the agent at an appropriate depth to tolerate the SGA, but his blood pressure and myocardium were at risk.
- It is appropriate to give succinylcholine for laryngospasm that does not break with positive pressure ventilation. Many anesthesiologists will put the patient on a ventilator as long as airway pressures are kept under 20 cm H_2O. Reports have shown that this technique can increase the patient's aspiration risk, as it continuously forces air into the stomach.

Patient 4

A 35-year-old woman brings a letter confirming past difficult intubation when she presents for a lumpectomy.

You take over this case from a colleague; the patient has an SGA and everything is going smoothly. As your colleague rushes out the door, he tells you: "Oh, she has a history of a difficult intubation but you should be fine." No sooner than when you sign the chart, the patient bucks and vomits. You quickly suction out the airway, call for help and a fiberoptic bronchoscope.

- Should you ALWAYS secure a difficult airway or try to "get away with it"? Once this scenario happens to you, you might think twice about dodging this bullet. You have to secure the airway after a patient aspirates with an SGA. How this is done depends on the clinician. Some may argue that you already have an established airway through which you can ventilate, so keep the SGA in place until a fiberoptic bronchoscope is available. Others may suggest removing the SGA and try intubating the patient with direct laryngoscopy.
  - Many institutions use intubating SGAs so that the patient can readily be intubated with the help of a fiberoptic bronchoscope. Newer SGA devices such as the I-Gel, AirQ, AMBU Aura, and AMBU Once, among others, have become popular options as bridging devices to intubation. An Aintree catheter can also be used over a fiberoptic bronchoscope through any of the above devices until a more appropriate-sized ETT can be inserted over it. This catheter decreases the diameter difference between a pediatric bronchoscope and a larger size ETT.
  - REMEMBER, airway always comes first. You need to deliver oxygen to the patient regardless of what the patient is aspirating. If patients are spontaneously breathing, then they probably already aspirated what you have just noticed in their oral cavity.
- Intubating LMAs are excellent instruments for blind tracheal intubation with either an intubating tracheal stylet or a fiberoptic bronchoscope. Blind tracheal intubation with an LMA and cricoid pressure has a reported 45% to 60% success rate. Fiberoptic intubation through the LMA is reported to have close to 100% success. The lumen of the LMA usually leads you directly to the vocal cords and the trachea. There are three critical points of caution while using this technique:
  - Ensure the ETT you are going to pass will fit through the lumen of the LMA.
  - Make sure the ETT is long enough so that it can pass below the vocal cords and still pass through the LMA without losing the airway.
  - Carefully remove the LMA over the ETT without losing the airway.

TIPS AND TRICKS

Standard and Disposable LMA

- Successful placement of all supraglottic airways relies on good insertion technique. The most successful technique (and there are many different ways) of insertion of an LMA requires one to extend maximally the head of the patient, which pulls the tissues away from the posterior pharynx and opens up room for the LMA to slide into place. The other point is to have an approximately 90-degree bend in the wrist that is inserting the LMA and to start positioning with the tip of the LMA behind the incisors and to continue to push cranially with the index finger toward the hard palate as the LMA is advanced further into the mouth and pharynx. The objective of these two key steps is to keep the dorsal surface of the LMA in constant contact with the hard palate and the soft palate to prevent the tip from folding over on itself toward the nasopharynx (Figure 13-6).

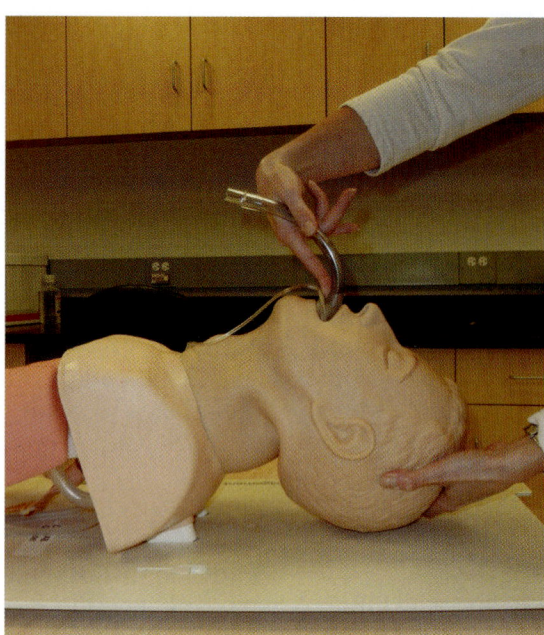

FIGURE 13-6 LMA insertion technique.

- Another insertion technique for advanced users is to do the insertion from across the patient, rather than standing at the head, with the thumb instead of the index finger in the groove between the cuff and the shaft of the LMA.
- When removing the LMA to remove secretions simultaneously, the LMA cuff can be kept partially inflated.
- Use a smaller size SGA for obese patients and a larger size for older and edentulous. Beware, edentulous patients can be challenging to place SGAs!

INTUBATING LMA (ILMA)

Insertion Technique

- A fully deflated and lubricated ILMA is held in the dominant hand.
- With the patient's head in neutral position, the handle of the ILMA is held parallel to the chest as the tip of the cuff is placed behind the incisors.
- Insertion continues with pressure being applied in the cranioposterior direction to maintain contact with the hard palate. As the soft palate is reached, the hand directing the ILMA should follow the direction of the curve of the shaft.
- Once the ILMA is inserted, the teeth should be at the 1- to 2-cm mark on the shaft.
- The cuff is then inflated and the ILMA is connected to the circuit, ventilation is begun (Figure 13-7).

Intubation Technique

- Intubation should begin only after finding the most optimal ILMA position for ventilation, with the least amount of resistance.
- "Chandy's maneuver" has been shown to help in finding the optimal position. This consists of moving the ILMA on a sagittal plane while ventilating to find the optimal position while slightly lifting the ILMA without tilting to provide a good seal against the glottic opening.
- Before we continue, some information regarding the designated tube of the ILMA: There are two lines on the tube to be aware of that are used during intubation and for troubleshooting. First is a longitudinal line seen along its length; second is a horizontal line at around the 16-cm mark.
  - The tube should be inserted with the longitudinal line placed facing cranially to allow the conical bevel to be positioned to the right side of the patient.
  - The horizontal line is a depth marker and points to the depth at which the tube starts to exit the ILMA bowl, pushing the epiglottic elevating bar along with the epiglottis away as the tube is advanced into the trachea.
- As the tube is advanced through the ILMA with the vertical line positioned cranially, at the 16-cm mark the practitioner will feel some resistance but then a release as the tube pushes the epiglottic elevating bar and continues without further resistance (Figure 13-8).
- The endotracheal tube cuff is inflated 5 to 10 cc and the ETT connected to the circuit and ventilation started.

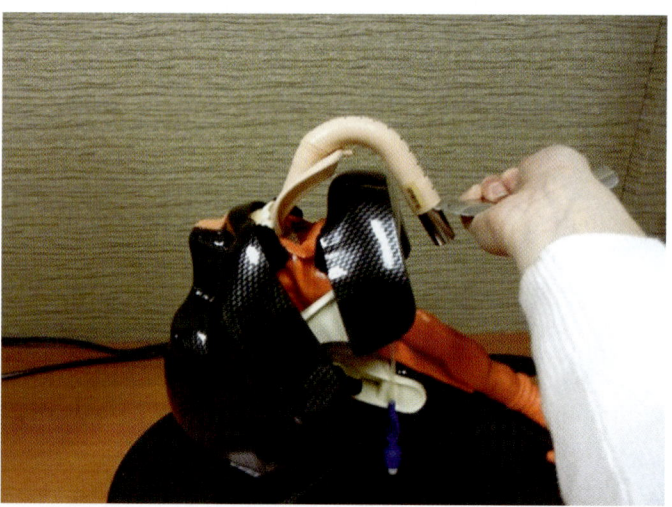

FIGURE 13-7 Insertion of ILMA.

Chapter 13 LARYNGEAL MASK AIRWAY AND OTHER SUPRAGLOTTIC AIRWAY DEVICES

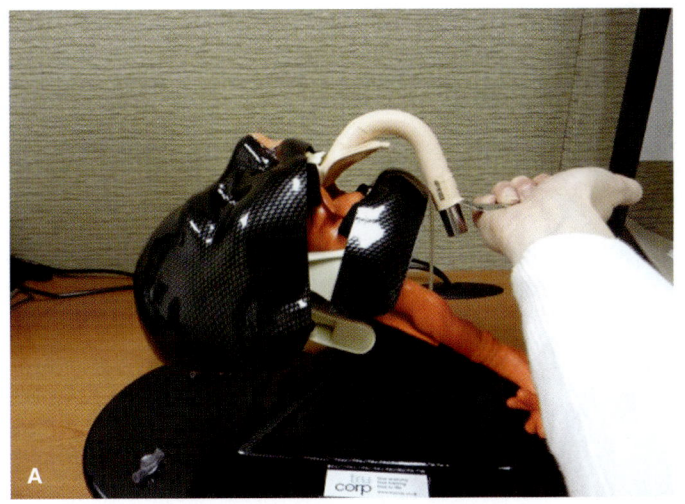
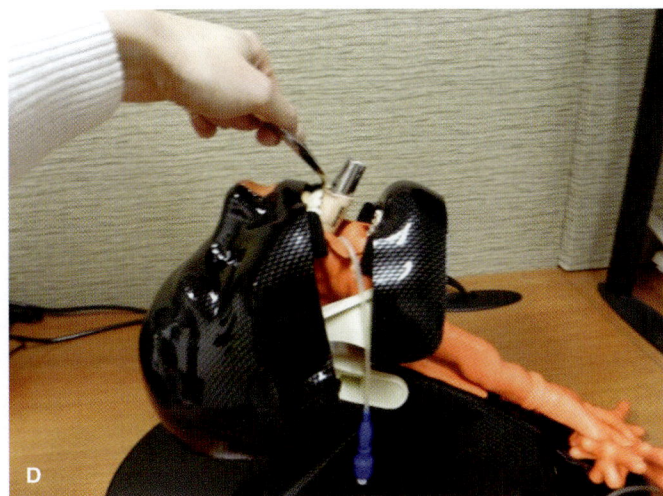
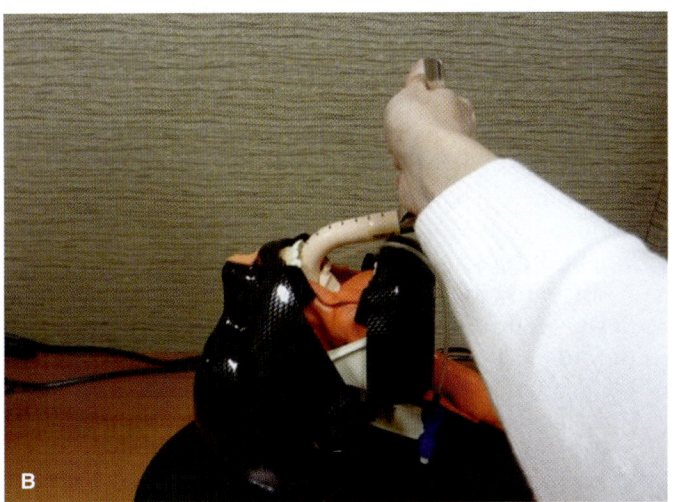
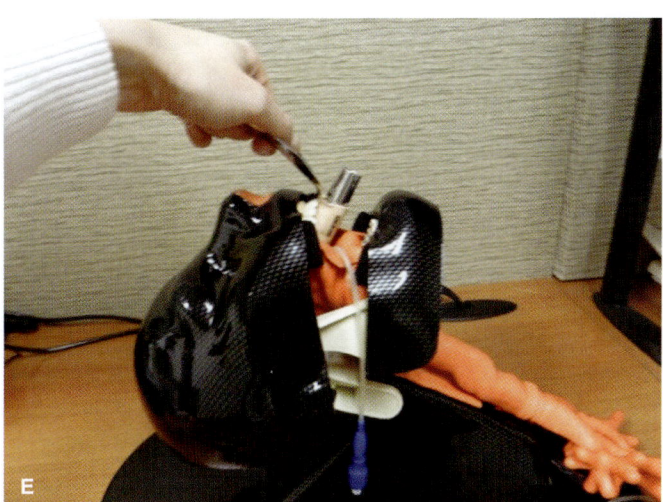
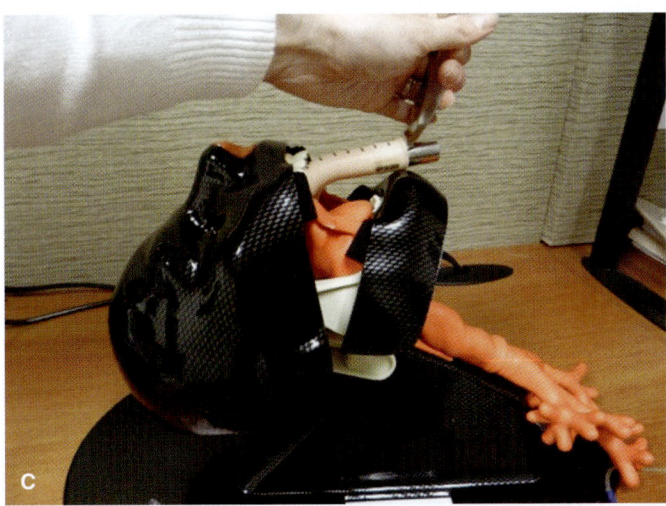
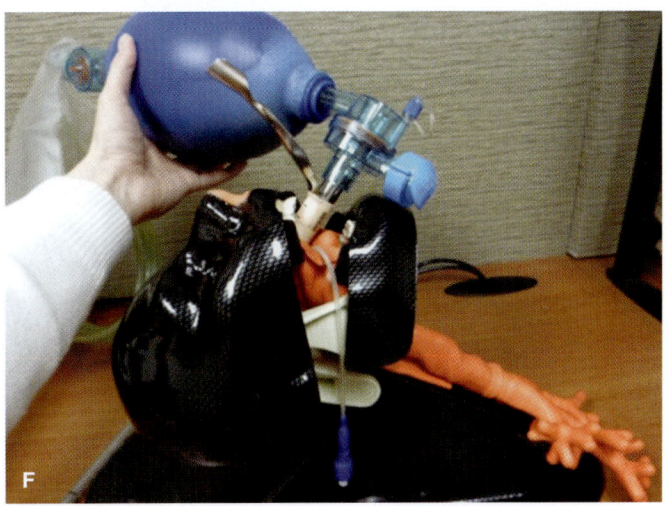

FIGURE 13-7 *(continued)* (A) Start placement like this. (B) Note how the handle goes to the vertical position as you advance. (C) Making the corner can be a little tricky. This is where a lot of hang-ups occur. (D) Now the handle is flat and you're in position. (E) Doing the Chandy maneuver. (F) Hook up Ambu and get some oxygen in there!

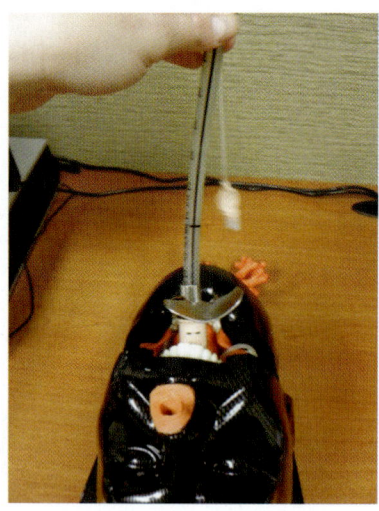
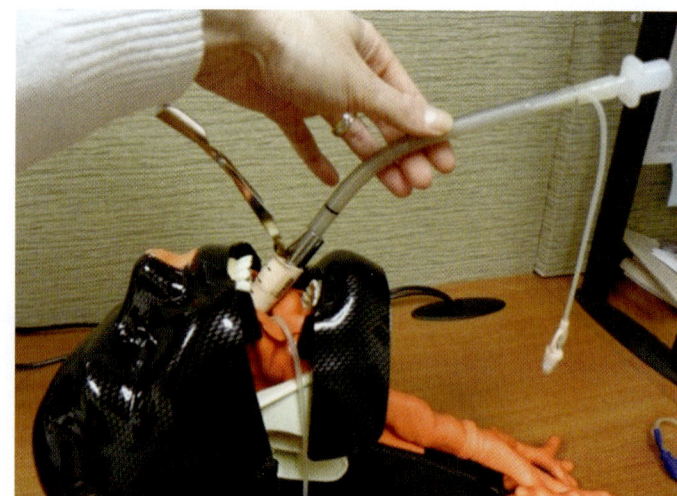

FIGURE 13-8 Intubation via ILMA with the designated ETT.

Removal of the ILMA

- Once correct placement is confirmed by end-tidal CO_2, the ILMA can be removed after removing the ETT connector, using the stabilizing rod.
- It is important to pull the stabilizing rod out of the ILMA shaft once the ETT is securely held inside the bowl of the ILMA. The reason is that the pilot balloon of the ETT will not slide through the shaft with the rod in place as the ILMA is being pulled out of the mouth, and if pulled too quickly the ETT may inadvertently be removed with it (Figure 13-9).
- The ILMA should not be left in place for long periods to prevent any injury to laryngopharyngeal tissues due to its metal shaft.
- The designated tube of the ILMA has a high-pressure, low-volume cuff and should not be used for long procedures. A tube exchanger should be used to remove the ILMA and replace it with a regular ETT whenever possible.
- A soft bite block should be placed next to the designated tube so that the patient will not bite the tube. This could result in the devastating consequence of the wire-reinforced designated tube losing its round shape, narrowing the orifice, and increasing the resistance to the flow of air and even occluding the lumen making ventilation impossible.

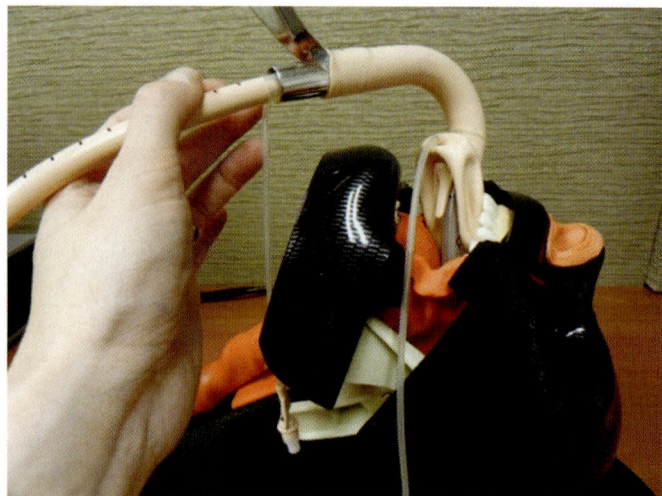
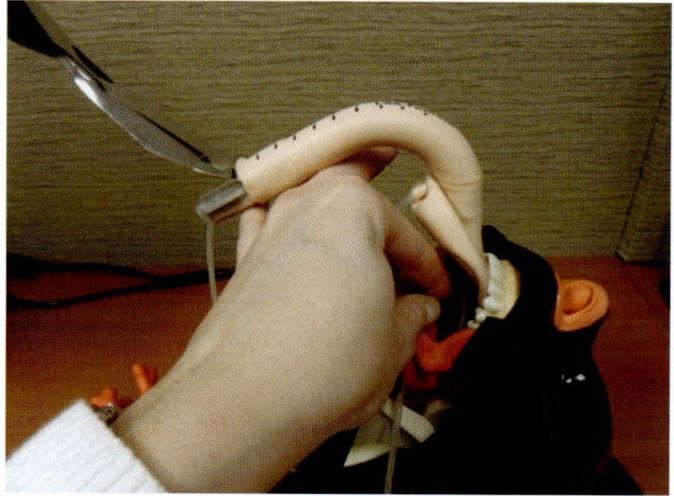

FIGURE 13-9 Removal of ILMA over the designated tube using the stabilizing rod.

Chapter 13 LARYNGEAL MASK AIRWAY AND OTHER SUPRAGLOTTIC AIRWAY DEVICES

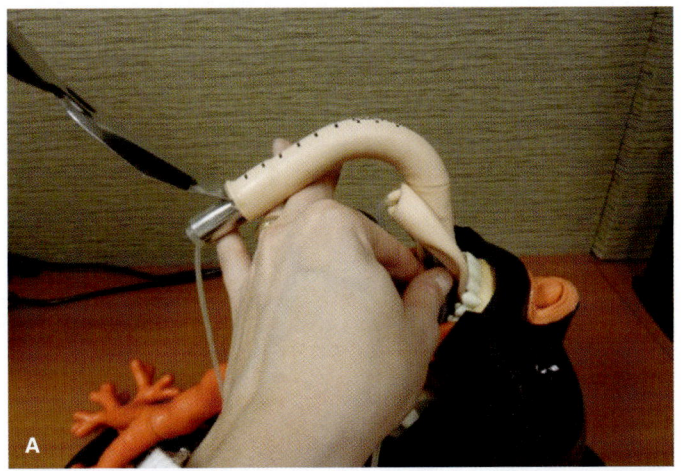

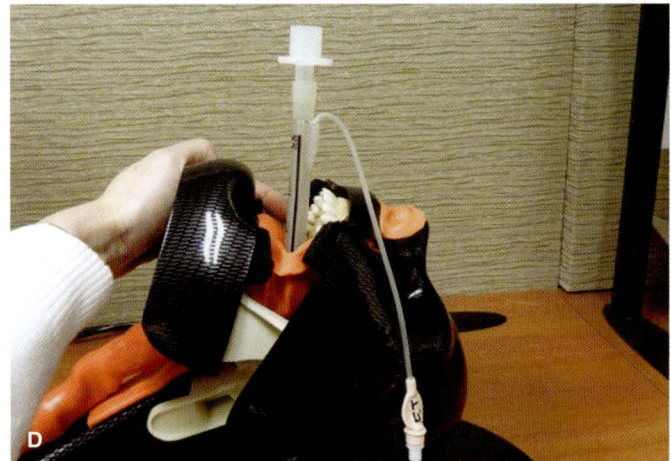

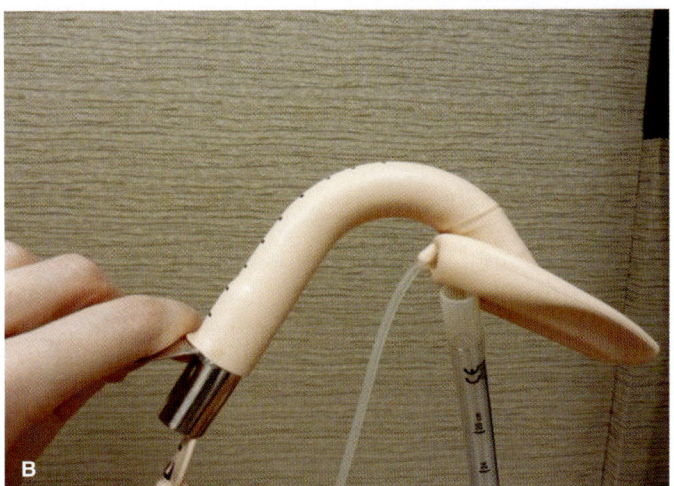

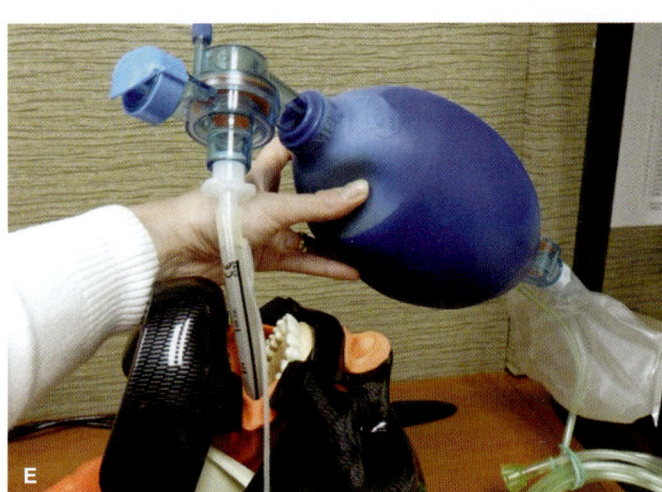

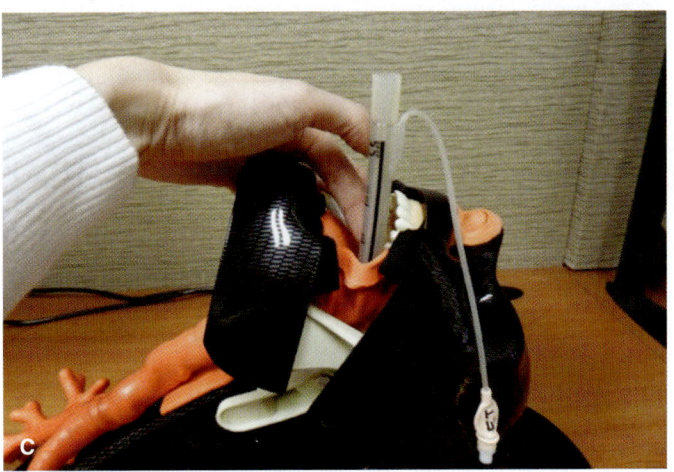

FIGURE 13-9 *(continued)* (A) Grab that endotracheal tube. (B) Sliding the ILMA out is NOT trivial. (C) Now the ILMA is gone (whew!). (D) Make sure you're still in! (E) Don't forget to oxygenate after all your hard work (Humans are not facultative anaerobes.)

Factors Affecting the Blind Intubation Success Rate

- Factors that increase success rate:
  - Using a conical rather than a straight bevel ETT, such as the designated tube of the ILMA or Parker tube
  - Using a regular ETT for intubation and reversing the angle of the ETT
  - Pulling the handle of the ILMA cranially
- Factors that decrease the success rate:
  - Using size 3 rather than size 4 or 5 ILMA
  - Lifting the handle of the ILMA
  - Cricoid pressure
  - Use of a collar
  - Lack of experience

Troubleshooting

- Once the ILMA is inserted, the cuff is inflated and connected to the circuit. If there is no CO_2 return with ventilation, the epiglottis is downfolded.
  - *Solution*: The ILMA is withdrawn 6 cm, which can be measured by the markers on the ILMA shaft and reinserted with the cuff inflated. This is called the "up-down" maneuver.
- Correct sizing of ILMA allows for better ventilation, but, more importantly, successful intubation is the key. Troubleshooting when the intubation is not successful by looking at the depth of tube insertion beyond the depth marker will clue the operator:
  1. When the ETT is inserted via the ILMA, if there is resistance felt immediately with the depth marker still showing, the ILMA size is most likely too large for the patient. The epiglottic elevating bar is stuck posterior to the arytenoids, not allowing the tube to be inserted. This is most likely a patient with a thin neck.
     - *Solution*: Change to a smaller ILMA.
  2. Upon insertion of the ETT, if resistance is felt at 4 to 5 cm beyond the depth marker, the ILMA size is again too large. This is most likely a patient with a wide, short neck.
     - *Solution:* Change to a smaller ILMA.
  3. If resistance is felt at 2 to 4 cm beyond the depth marker, the ILMA is too small.
     - *Solution*: Change to a bigger ILMA.

Observing the bowls of different SGAs reminds us that the epiglottic elevating bar of the ILMA needs to lift for the fiberoptic bronchoscope or ETT to pass. The classic LMA has aperture bars that may make intubation challenging. Remember that the only size of ETT that can pass through a size 3 LMA is a 6-mm ETT. An adult bronchoscope will not fit through a 6-mm ETT; therefore, a pediatric bronchoscope needs to be available (Figure 13-10).

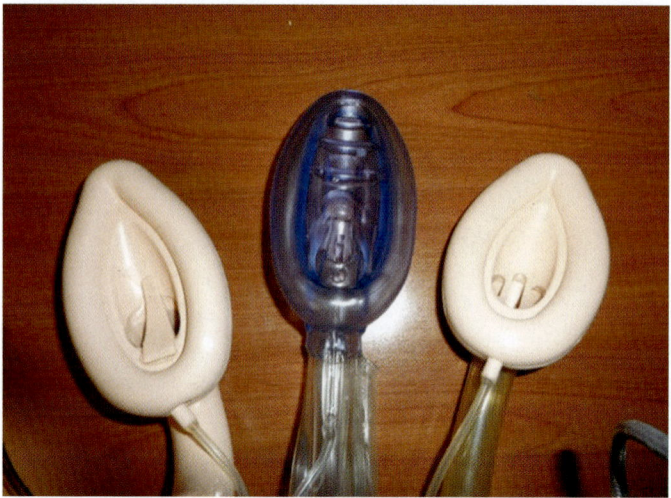

FIGURE 13-10 Bowls of different SGAs (intubating LMA, AirQ, and Classic LMA).

CONCLUSION

Overall, the utility of the SGA devices are rising, and anesthesiologists are relying on them more heavily in elective and emergency situations. When they work, they are excellent. When they fail, we all age! It is important to remember that patient selection and positioning of the supraglottic device within the airway are the most important factors for a successful anesthetic with these devices. Patients must receive full doses of induction agents when using SGAs without muscle relaxants, so as to avoid laryngospasm/bronchospasm on induction of anesthesia.

Underdosing the induction agent, so that the patient resumes spontaneous ventilation faster, is unacceptable and dangerous. Additionally, an adequate depth of anesthesia must be maintained so that the patient tolerates the SGA in their oral cavity. If you find yourself struggling with an SGA, despite confirming proper positioning, consider calling for an extra pair of hands and changing it to an ETT under the drapes. Furthermore, always have a supraglottic device of your choice in each of your practice areas available to use when you are in an emergency situation or are struggling with a difficult intubation. It pulls through, most of the time.

SUGGESTED READING

Barash PG, Cullen BF, Stoeling RK, eds. *Clinical anesthesia*, 6th ed. Philadelphia: Lippincott Williams & Wilkins; 2009, pp 751–789.
Nice review of supraglottic devices and LMAs.

Brimacombe JR, Berry A. The incidence of aspiration associated with the laryngeal mask airway: a meta-analysis of published literature. *J Clin Anesth* 1995;7:297.

One of the authors is such a proponent of LMA that he has placed an LMA Proseal in his mouth and has sat in a swimming pool under water and drank wine through its orogastric port. The article has nice pearls for the use of LMA.

Domino KB, Posner KL, Caplan RA, et al. Airway injury during anesthesia a closed claims analysis. *Anesthesiology* 1999;91:1703.

It is important to know the closed claims analysis in anesthesia, to learn from our mistakes and improve upon them.

Hagberg CA. *Benumof's airway management: principles and practice*, 2nd ed. Philadelphia: Mosby Elsevier; 2006.

Nice overview of the LMA by the inventor Dr. Archie Brain himself and Dr. David Ferson in Chapter 21. Great review of other supraglottic devices from experts in the field in other chapters, with a beautiful three-dimensional radiologic reconstruction of the human airway with an LMA in situ.

Practice guidelines for the management of the difficult airway: an updated report by the American Society of Anesthesiologists Task Force on Management of the Difficult Airway. *Anesthesiology* 2003;98:1269.

The ASA difficult airway guidelines include, for the first time, the use of LMA in the "cannot ventilate—cannot intubate" scenario. This difficult airway algorithm is always on the board exam. These were updated in 2007. Interestingly, the Glidescope® is not to be found in the difficult airway algorithm!

Verghese C, Brimacombe J. Survey of laryngeal mask airway usage in 11,910 patients: safety and efficacy for conventional and nonconventional usage. *Anesth Analg* 1996;82:129.

This article describes the conventional and unconventional uses of LMAs for the adventurous anesthesiologist.

CHAPTER 14
LARYNGOSCOPY

FOUAD SOUKI
MICHAEL C. LEWIS

"This is a perfect example of esophageal intubation."
Spoken by the professor,
ironically, after our first laryngoscopy

INTRODUCTION

Direct laryngoscopy is the act of visualizing the larynx and vocal cords using a handheld scope. It is the most simple and commonly used method for tracheal intubation. Laryngoscopy is the first thing you must learn if you ever need to put a breathing tube down a patient's throat.

INDICATIONS

- Provide a patent airway (surgical procedures, care of critically ill, advanced cardiac life support)
- Protect the airway against aspiration of gastric contents
- Ventilation or oxygenation

EQUIPMENT

All essential equipment should have a readily available backup in case of unexpected failure. Preparatory efforts enhance success and minimize risk to the patient (Figure 14-1).
- Oxygen source
- Ventilation bag
- Appropriately sized face mask
- Appropriately sized oral airway, in case mask ventilation proves to be difficult
- Tongue blade and soft bite block
- A properly checked anesthesia machine, ventilator, and breathing circuit
- Endotracheal tubes (ETTs) of appropriate sizes, generally have half a size smaller and larger than the one you intend to use
- Stylet that helps to stiffen and shape the tube
- A gum elastic boogie (never leave home without it)
- Syringe to inflate the ETT cuff, 10 mL
- Laryngoscope handle and blades, usually two sizes of a curved (Macintosh) and straight (Miller) blade, with confirmation that the light works and the blade attaches to the handle appropriately
- Suction apparatus for oral secretions and potential regurgitation
- Drugs: intravenous anesthetics, muscle relaxants, vasopressors (ready to administer)
- Monitors: pulse oximeter, electrocardiogram (ECG), noninvasive blood pressure, end-tidal CO_2 monitor (quantitative or qualitative)
- Stethoscope
- Tape or tie to secure the endotracheal tube

Many hands make light work. An experienced aide can provide items and apply cricoid or laryngeal pressure if needed.

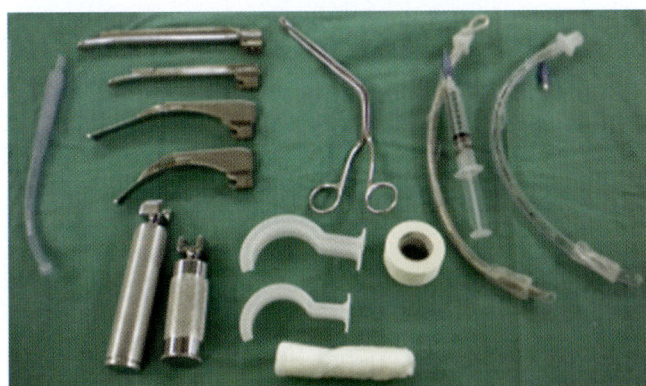

FIGURE 14-1 Equipment.

HISTORY AND PHYSICAL EXAMINATION

Securing the airway could get really nasty. Direct laryngoscopy requires neck flexibility, a wide mouth opening, and no excessive pharyngeal tissue or large tongue that gets in the way. A combination of clinical tests can help in assessing the beast you're up against. No single test is sufficiently predictive on its own. The best predictor of difficult airway management is the old anesthetic record.

- Mouth opening: inter-incisor distance should exceed 4 cm in an adult
- Thyromental distance (>6.5 cm): shorter distances suggest an anterior larynx, which would be difficult to visualize by laryngoscopy (Figure 14-2)
- Mallampati classification: Investigate the posterior pharynx by having the sitting patient fully extend his neck, maximally open his mouth, and stick out his tongue with or without phonation (Figures 14-3 and 14-4)
- Determine the patient's ability to bite the upper lip
- Evaluate neck mobility: full extension through full flexion should exceed 80 degrees
- Evaluate neck circumference: more than 40 cm (17 inches) implies increased difficulty
- Record loose teeth, missing teeth, and removable dentures

Some patients require extra care when performing direct laryngoscopy:

- Patients with cervical spine pathology (rheumatoid arthritis, Down syndrome, stenosis)
- Patients with questionable or confirmed trauma to cervical spine
- Patients with a history of difficult intubation
- Patients with airway pathology (vocal cord tumor, neck radiation scar, congenital malformation, tracheal stenosis, tracheostomy scars)
- Patients with a history of snoring, sleep apnea, or morbid obesity
- Congenital conditions (Pierre Robin syndrome, Treacher Collins syndrome, Down syndrome, etc.)
- Acquired conditions (epiglottitis, Ludwig angina's, arthritis, tumors, acromegaly)

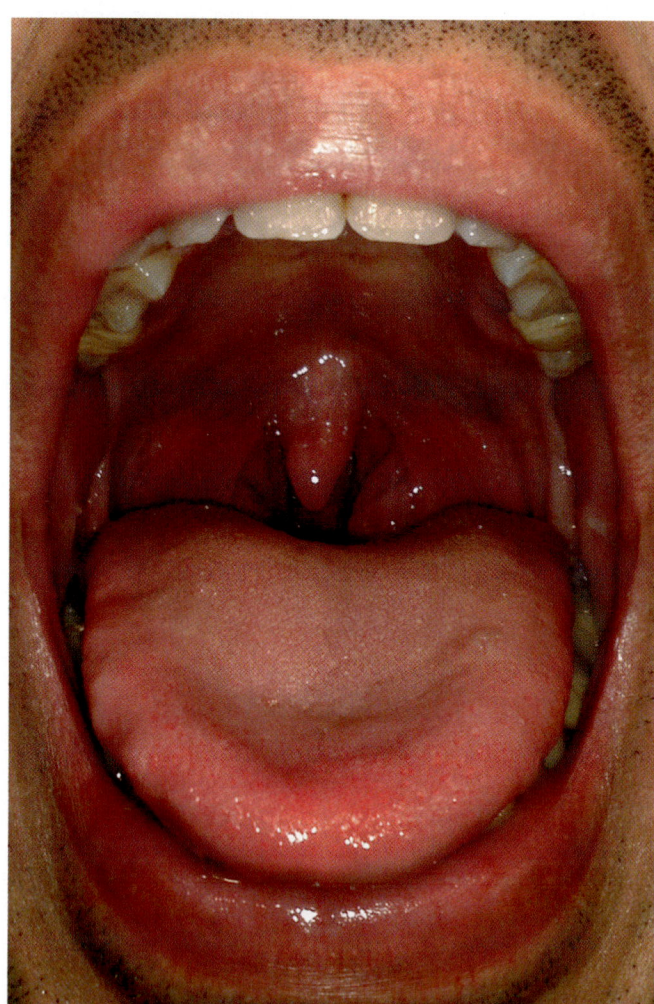

FIGURE 14-3 Mallampati I.

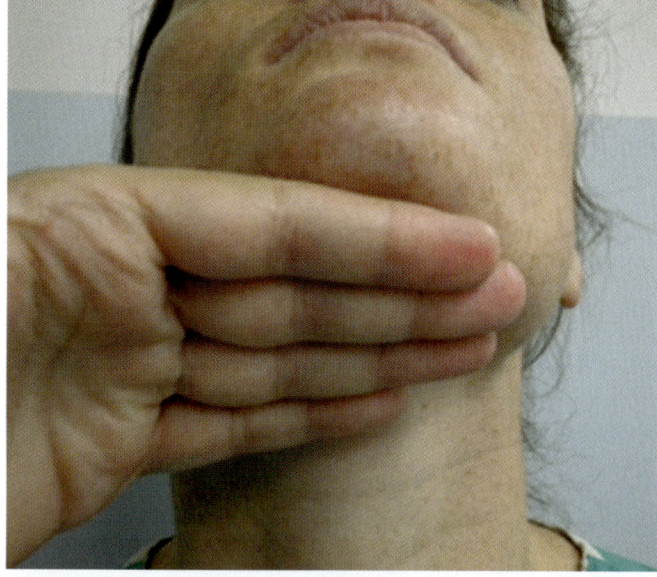

FIGURE 14-2 Thyromental distance: more than three fingers breadth.

Chapter 14 LARYNGOSCOPY

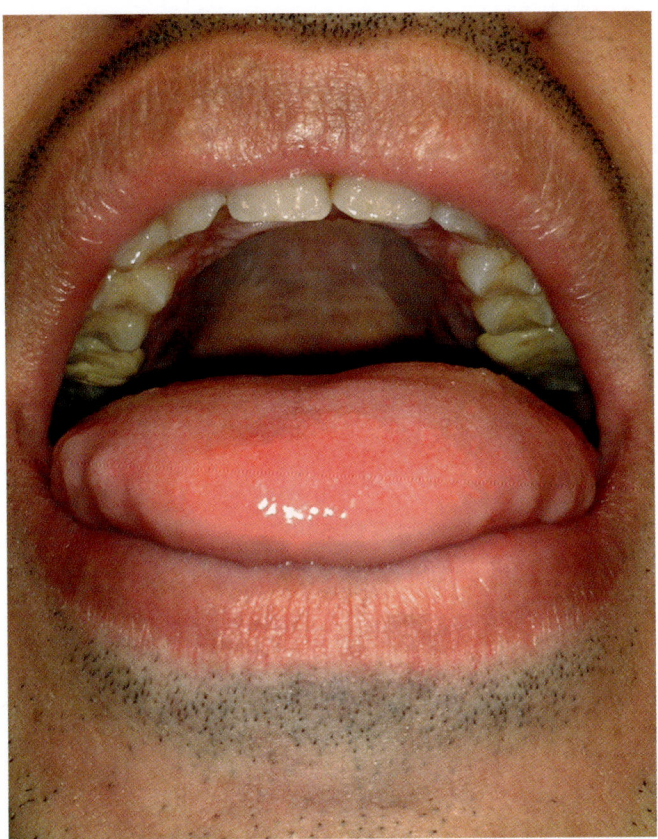

FIGURE 14-4 Mallampati IV.

LARYNGOSCOPIC METHODS

Laryngoscopy could be performed orally or nasally. Visualizing the larynx can be done by a laryngoscope, fiberoptic scope, or the recent video laryngoscopes.

DIRECT LARYNGOSCOPIC OROTRACHEAL INTUBATION

Access and Positioning

Endotracheal intubation may be emergent, urgent, or elective. The most challenging is to intubate someone on the ward, or in a regular hospital bed squeezed against the wall and surrounded with furniture. No matter what, you have to make the odds in your favor.

- Create adequate access to the head of the bed or table. Ensure that the bed/table is locked in position and the patient's head is at the edge. The height of the surface should be adjusted to the level of your chest or xiphoid (if you're going to do this for the rest of your life, you might as well protect your back).
- Proper positioning of the patient is the key to easier laryngoscopy. The three-axis theory has proposed that the oral, pharyngeal, and laryngeal axes should be brought into approximate alignment in order to best facilitate orotracheal visualization and intubation. The "sniffing" position involves flexion at the neck and extension at the head. This is accomplished by supporting the head on a firm pillow. However, neck extension may sometimes prove useful. Don't be committed to one technique (Figure 14-5).
- Occasionally, in obese patients it is necessary to place blankets under the scapula, shoulders, and nape of the neck, as well as the head; this is known as "stacking." Take a look from the lateral side of the patient to ensure appropriate positioning; you should be able to draw a line parallel to the floor between the patient's ear and sternum.

Technique

The smooth placement of an endotracheal tube requires skill and practice.

- There are two basic types of laryngoscope blades: the curved blade (Macintosh) and the straight blade (Miller). Take the laryngoscope in your left hand; the right hand is responsible for everything else (those medical television series and movies still don't get it).
- When you put that blade in, avoid the patient's teeth (you break them, you fix them). If teeth are loose, a mouth guard may help.
- To open the mouth and facilitate the introduction of the blade, perform a scissor-like maneuver with the right thumb and index finger to open the patient's jaw (Figure 14-6).
- Advance the laryngoscope down the right side of the mouth to the base of the tongue while avoiding entrapment of the lower lip. Sweep the tongue to the left as you bring the laryngoscope to the midline (Figure 14-7).
- The straight blade tip should extend just behind or beneath the laryngeal surface of the epiglottis. The curved blade is placed at the base of the epiglottis, i.e., the vallecula. With both blades, forward and upward movement (in the direction of the laryngoscope handle) exposes the glottic opening. Do not pry or crank with the laryngoscope! Teeth might be broken. Straight blades are preferred in infants, pediatric patients, and patients with an anterior larynx. Large patients with long thyromental distance will require the longest blades (Mac 4 and Miller 3).
- The glottis is located in the midline, has a triangular shape, and contains the prominent knobs of the arytenoids posteriorly and the pale white true vocal

cords bilaterally. The esophageal opening is round and puckered, with no structures around it.
- Occasionally, you may need to apply external laryngeal pressure with your right hand to improve laryngoscopic view. Optimal external laryngeal pressure is usually back up right pressure (BURP) on the thyroid cartilage. Find the appropriate view and get a third hand to hold pressure in that position while you grasp the tube for intubation.
- Hold the endotracheal tube like a pencil and advance the tip, under direct vision, into the trachea just until the cuff disappears completely beyond the vocal cords. The ETT should be introduced into the far right corner of the mouth and passed along an axis that intersects the line of the laryngoscope blade at the glottis. In this manner, the tube does not interrupt the view of the vocal cords down the channel of the blade.
- The use of a stylet may be valuable in controlling the direction of passage of an ETT. A stylet should not extend beyond the tip of the tube. A curved, styleted ETT may impinge on the anterior tracheal wall; hence, after the ETT tip is through the vocal cords, the stylet should be withdrawn to permit further passage distally.
- Inflate the cuff only to the point of no air leakage.
- Confirm adequate tube position (time to use that stethoscope you've been holding onto).
- Fix the tube to the skin of the maxilla and tape the eyes (again a missed step in TV shows and movies).
- A bite block, rolled gauze, or an oral airway should be placed between the teeth to prevent the patient from biting down and occluding the lumen of an oral tube.

Things that complicate laryngoscopy:
- Inserting the blade too deep
- Tongue protrusion over the flange of the blade toward the right side of the mouth, thus obstructing a clear path through which the vocal cords must be visualized
- Displacement of the blade tip to the right of the midline. This position obscures the view of the epiglottis and may precipitate trauma and bleeding from friable tissue in the tonsillar bed.
- Barrel-chested, obese, or large-breasted patients. Obstruction to movement of the handle of the laryngoscope by the chest wall may occur. In these patients, further initial neck extension or a rotation of the laryngoscope handle to the right permits easier introduction of the blade of the laryngoscope into the mouth. Alternatively, a short laryngoscope handle may be used.

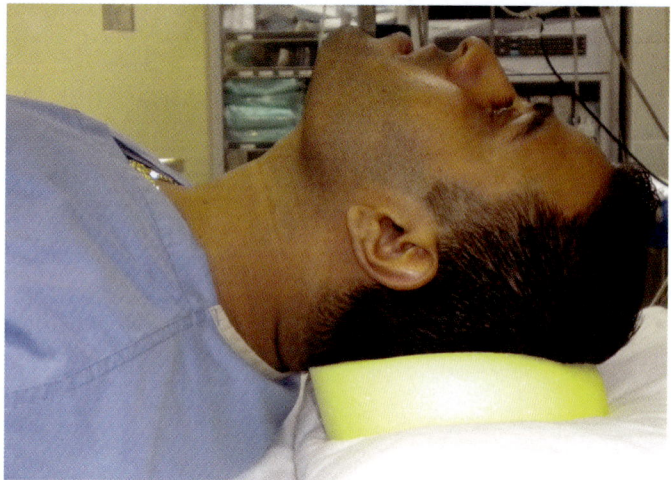

FIGURE 14-5 Sniffing position: neck flexion/head extension.

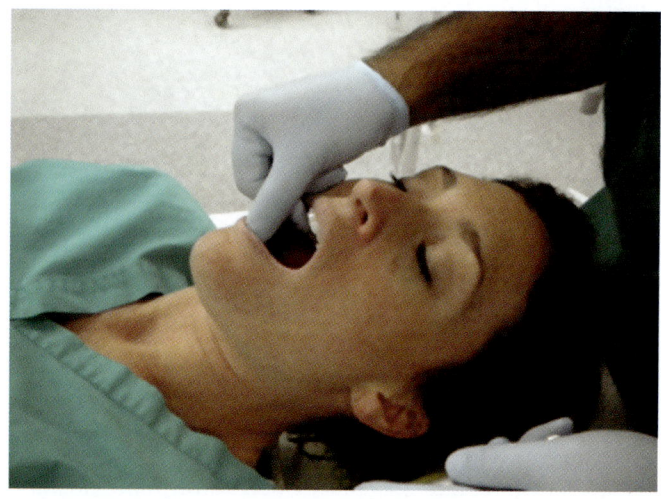

FIGURE 14-6 Scissor-like maneuver.

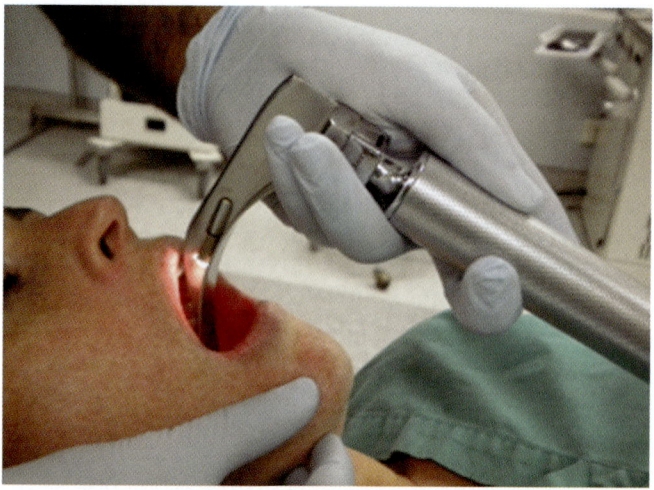

FIGURE 14-7 Laryngoscope insertion.

Verification of Tube Position

- The only absolutely reliable methods of definitively determining tracheal intubation are direct observation of the ETT going through the vocal cords (laryngoscopy) and the use of a fiberoptic bronchoscope (impractical as a clinical routine).
- Confirmation of exhaled CO_2 is the gold standard, quantitative capnography as in the operating room, or colorimetric sensors.
- Palpation of the ETT cuff in the suprasternal notch (notable by the bounce felt while squeezing the pilot balloon)
- Condensation in the clear plastic ETT during exhalation
- Breath sounds, while not definitive for tracheal placement, should be present across the chest and absent over the stomach. Rule out endobronchial intubation when good breath sounds are heard bilaterally.
- Chest movement should be symmetric.
- A chest radiograph, both posteroanterior (PA) and lateral, confirming location in the trachea would also work, but is similarly impractical for OR applications. Ideally, the tip of the tube should be 2 to 4 cm above the carina.

NASOTRACHEAL LARYNGOSCOPY

- Intubation by the nasal route is a cool technique that you must master somewhere down the line in your career. Generally, it's a more complex procedure than oral intubation.
- Nasotracheal intubation is currently confined to surgical procedures involving the oropharynx. It can also be used for blind and fiberoptic intubation.
- Prior to insertion of the nasotracheal tube, the nasal mucosa should be sprayed with a vasoconstrictor drug and the tube softened by soaking it in a warm saline solution (a little lubrication doesn't hurt either). This decreases the incidence of mucosal damage and bleeding.
- Select the more patent naris and gently insert the tracheal tube. Once the tube has reached the oropharynx, it can be guided into the glottis under conventional direct laryngoscopic vision, or it can be grasped by a Magill forceps and thus directed into the glottis.
- The nasal route limits the size of tube to 7.5 mm or less.

VIDEO LARYNGOSCOPY

- Video laryngoscopes are new intubation devices. They consist of a miniature video camera attached to the laryngoscope, allowing an indirect view of the upper airway. In difficult airway management, they improve the Cormack–Lehane grade and achieve the same or a higher intubation success rate compared with direct laryngoscopy.
- Limitations include difficulty inserting the blade, difficulty in getting the tube through the vocal cords, and injury to the soft palate.
- Each particular device has advantages or disadvantages. Some have a standard Macintosh blade, while others have an angulated blade or anatomically shaped blade. The visualization screen may be connected directly to the laryngoscope or separate. A special J-shaped stylet aids in maneuvering the tube in position.
- The collection includes Storz, V-Mac and C-Mac, Glidescope, McGrath, Pentax-Airway Scope, Airtraq, and Bullard (Figure 14-8).
- Overall, they are used as backup devices in cases of difficult or questionable airway examination.

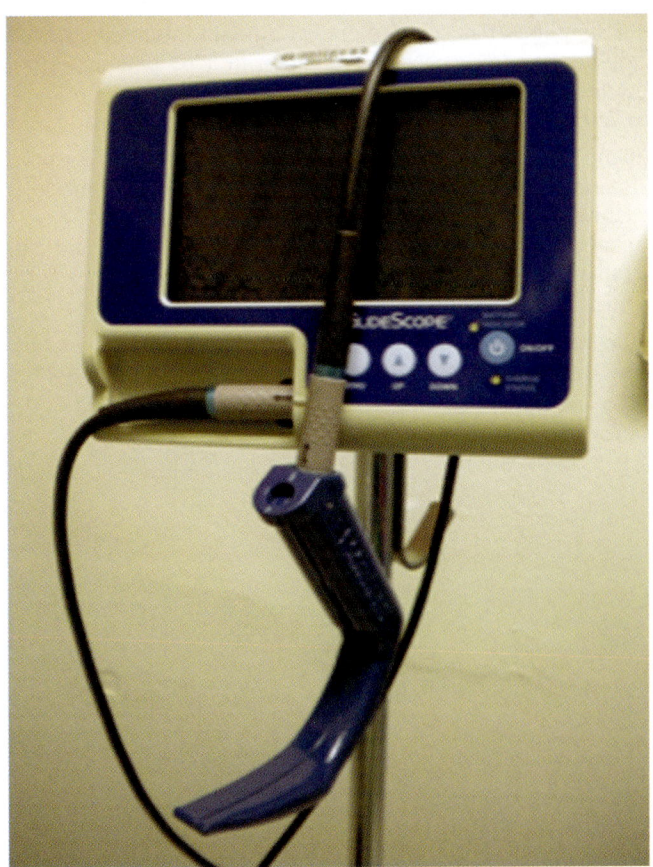

FIGURE 14-8 Glidescope.

CONCLUSION

Laryngoscopic intubation is a continually evolving branch with a wide choice of devices and techniques. The fastest and simplest means of achieving tracheal intubation is direct laryngoscopy. Adequate airway evaluation, preparation, and proper patient positioning are required to ensure that the first attempt at laryngoscopy is the best attempt. Experience is paramount. Practice makes perfect.

SUGGESTED READING

Ayoub CM, Kanazi GE, Al Alami A, Rameh C, El-Khatib MF. Tracheal intubation following training with the GlideScope compared to direct laryngoscopy. *Anaesthesia* 2010;65(7):674–678. Epub 2010 May 17.
Videolaryngoscopy is so easy that a med student can do it.

Baker PA, Depuydt A, Thompson JM. Thyromental distance measurement—fingers don't rule. *Anaesthesia* 2009;64(8):878–882.
Three finger breadths are not accurate enough in assessing thyromental distance.

Barash PG, Cullen BF, Stoelting RK, ed. *Airway management. Clinical anesthesia*, 5th ed. Philadelphia: Lippincott, Williams and Wilkins; 2006, pp 595–642.

Eberhart LH, Arndt C, Aust HJ, Kranke P, Zoremba M, Morin A. A simplified risk score to predict difficult intubation: development and prospective evaluation in 3763 patients. *Eur J Anaesthesiol* 2010;27(11):935–940.
The latest in airway difficulty prediction.

Euliano TY, Gravenstein JS. *Airway management. Essential anesthesia: from science to practice.* New York: Cambridge University Press; 2004, pp 24–37.

Hagberg CA, ed. *Benumof's airway management*, 2nd ed. Philadelphia: Mosby-Elsevier; 2007.
A must read for every anesthetist.

Lundstrøm LH, Møller AM, Rosenstock C, Astrup G, Gätke MR, Wetterslev J; Danish Anaesthesia Database. A documented previous difficult tracheal intubation as a prognostic test for a subsequent difficult tracheal intubation in adults. *Anaesthesia* 2009;64(10):1081–1088.
Good history taking helps in identifying subsequent difficult tracheal intubation.

Manoach S, Paladino L. Manual in-line stabilization for acute airway management of suspected cervical spine injury: historical review and current questions. *Ann Emerg Med* 2007;50(3):236–245. Epub 2007 Mar 6.
What you need to know about cervical spines and laryngoscopy.

Myneni N, O'Leary AM, Sandison M, Roberts K. Evaluation of the upper lip bite test in predicting difficult laryngoscopy. *J Clin Anesth* 2010;22(3):174–178.
This test is a poor predictor of difficult laryngoscopy when used as the single bedside screening test.

Niforopoulou P, Pantazopoulos I, Demestiha T, Koudouna E, Xanthos T. Video-laryngoscopes in the adult airway management: a topical review of the literature. *Acta Anaesthesiol Scand* 2010;54(9):1050–1061. Epub 2010 Jul 28.
It is a review!

Rudraraju P, Eisen LA. Confirmation of endotracheal tube position: a narrative review. *J Intensive Care Med* 2009;24(5):283–292. Epub 2009 Aug 3.
Strengths and weaknesses of particular methods are highlighted.

Serocki G, Bein B, Scholz J, Dörges V. Management of the predicted difficult airway: a comparison of conventional blade laryngoscopy with video-assisted blade laryngoscopy and the GlideScope. *Eur J Anaesthesiol* 2010;27(1):24–30.
Video laryngoscopy is a useful instrument in the management of the predicted difficult airway.

Shiga T, Wajima Z, Inoue T, Sakamoto A. Predicting difficult intubation in apparently normal patients: a meta-analysis of bedside screening test performance. *Anesthesiology* 2005;103(2):429–437.
Combination of the Mallampati classification and thyromental distance are the most useful for predicting difficult intubation but remain limited.

CHAPTER 15

AWAKE INTUBATION

SARAH LASALLE
GEZA K. KISS
JOHN DENNY

Ah, Pray, make no mistake, we are not shy; We're very wide awake, the moon and I.

Sir William Gilbert, Patience, 1881

THIS CHAPTER IS LONG FOR A REASON

Better tuck yourselves in for a long read, for this chapter is a little more "detail friendly" in describing one of the most important procedures that we do as anesthesiologists. Securing an anticipated difficult airway for a surgical procedure requires a method that gives you a high success rate with the lowest mortality. To date, the awake fiberoptic intubation is the gold standard for an elective anticipated difficult airway intubation.

IF YOU'RE STILL NOT CONVINCED, HERE ARE SOME SCARY STATISTICS

"The ability to successfully manage very difficult airways has been responsible for as many as 30% of deaths totally attributable to anesthesia."[1] According to the American Society of Anesthesiologists' (ASA) closed data base, adverse respiratory events "form the largest single class of injury."[1]

DIFFICULT AIRWAY: WHAT IS IT?

A difficult airway is "the clinical situation in which a conventionally trained anesthesiologist experiences difficulty with mask ventilation, difficulty with endotracheal intubation or both."[2]
- The ASA algorithm begins with the difficult airway either being recognizable or unrecognizable. Let's start with a recognizable difficult airway: think Santa Claus with buck teeth and a bulging neck mass! And now a not quite so obvious unrecognizable difficult airway: a 6-foot-tall runway model comes in for elective surgery. Unfortunately, under direct laryngoscopy you discover that her vocal cords somehow ended up in the far-off land of deep and anterior.
- Other management options exist in the ASA difficult airway path; however, here we focus on awake intubations, which primarily include *recognizable* difficult airways. These are determined by (a) a previous history of difficult intubation; (b) physical examination assessment demonstrating prominent protruding teeth, small mouth opening (scleroderma, temporomandibular joint pathology, anatomic variant), narrow mandible, micrognathia, macroglossia, short muscular neck, very long neck, limited range of motion of the neck, congenital airway anomalies, obesity, pathology involving the airway (tracheomalacia), malignancy involving the airway, or upper airway obstruction; (c) trauma to the face, upper airway, or cervical spine; (d) anticipated difficult mask ventilation; (e) severe risk of aspiration; (f) respiratory failure; or (g) severe hemodynamic instability.[1]

The Good, the Bad, and the Ugly
- The good: the advantages of choosing the "awake" airway management pathway: the natural airway is preserved; spontaneous breathing is maintained; a patient who is awake and well topicalized is easier to intubate (airway patency maintained, larynx less anterior); the patient can still protect his or her airway from aspiration; and the patient is able to monitor his or her own neurologic symptoms.
- The bad: there are no absolute contraindications to an awake intubation (AI) other than the patient's

refusal, a patient who is unable to cooperate (e.g., a small child, a mentally challenged patient, and an intoxicated individual), or a patient with a documented true allergy to all local anesthetics.
- The ugly: the only true contraindication, according to some, is lack of time.

PREOPERATIVE VISIT

The ASA taskforce recommends that "review of history and prior records if available with time permitting may improve detection of difficult airway."[2]
- Review a patient's history, including old anesthesia/OR records and possible events that may have changed the airway since the last intubation. Key items to look for include the ability to ventilate, ease of laryngoscopy, number of attempts at intubation, maneuvers/outcomes, tolerance of drugs, evidence of reactions to local anesthetics, and apnea with minimal doses of narcotics.
- Look for scenarios that may have changed the airway since the patient was last intubated (e.g., weight gain, laryngeal stenosis from previous airway intervention, previous surgeries such as facial plastic surgery, radiation, burns, trauma, tumors, and infection).
- Other medical conditions that could influence the airway are osteoarthritis, rheumatoid arthritis, temporomandibular joint (TMJ) stiffness, cervical disk disease, morbid obesity, obstructive sleep apnea, enlarged epiglottis, scleroderma, narrowed glottis, diabetes mellitus (DM), acromegaly, and congenital anomalies.
- Physical examination should include an airway evaluation looking for the usual suspects (short chin, thick neck, previous tracheal scar, etc.).
- Adjuvant studies such as chest radiographs (tracheal deviations), cervical spine films (trauma, rheumatoid arthritis [RA]), and computed tomography (obstructing tumor, mass compression). Finally, consider the environment and establish plan A and plan B for ease and access to the patient.

THE PREOPERATIVE DIALOGUE

Compassion and empathy during the interview are a must for adequate communication, cooperation, and information gathering. The patient needs to be convinced that this is the optimal, safest route for intubation, and must be well informed of what to expect as well as possible complications. However, discretion over brutal honesty, and sound clinical judgment to finesse the situation, can never hurt. In general, complications include local anesthetic toxicity, awareness, discomfort, and recall.

After reviewing the situation your patient becomes a little testy, and refuses, saying, "Knock me out, Doc! I mean it!" A possible response would be, "This will be a little unpleasant, but I'll tell you everything that's going on, I will make you as comfortable and relaxed as possible, and we'll get through this OK."

Recruiting the primary care physician and surgeon could be another tactic.

ADVANCED PREPARATION

- Gaining familiarity with maneuvering the fiberoptic prior to "going live" is essential. There are fiberoptic simulators and training devices available. The Fiberoptic Training Jig is one such device (*Anaesthesia* 2007;62:190). The AccuTouch Virtual Reality Bronchoscopy fiberoptic simulator has been described by Kai Boldmann (*Journal of Clinical Anesthesia* 2006;18). Another invaluable and accessible technique would be to practice "asleep" fiberoptic intubations on healthy patients. You need the right attitude; it's too easy to not practice and let potential fiberoptic opportunities slip by. Don't let this happen to you. Find opportunities to use the fiberoptic.
- Aside from lack of experience with awake intubations, one of the biggest impediments to doing an AI is all the stuff and equipment that needs to be set up in advance as well as getting the appropriate trained help. This is particularly difficult in the middle of the night and on holidays.
- As mentioned previously, having the right attitude about AI is essential. Doing an AI is just another procedure like putting in an A-line or starting an IV. Your comfort level will flourish with practice. The best thing about an awake intubation is you haven't burned any bridges; the patient's still breathing, the airway's intact. It's not the end of the world if you take a few extra minutes (despite what the angry surgeon says). Another way to avoid disaster is having an educated (or well-bribed) ancillary staff and a preset customized advanced difficult airway cart in an accessible location.

STRATEGY

Always have a specific plan in mind as to how the intubation is going down. Are you going to be in the OR? Are you doing a bedside emergency intubation? Is the patient going to be on an inaccessible ortho bed? If the AI is going to be done with a fiberoptic bronchoscope that you then discover doesn't work, what are your other options? Nasal intubation? Intubating laryngeal mask airway (LMA)? Retrograde wire? Will you need to have a surgeon nearby to perform an emergency trach? Have everything you need as well as an extra pair of hands in the room. Insist that someone be there to assist, or, better yet, another anesthesiologist. It's easier to call across the room than across town for help.

EQUIPMENT

See Figure 15-1.

Flexible Fiberoptic Bronchoscope

- The flexible fiberoptic bronchoscope consists of fiberoptic light bundles that transmit light to the airway and an image back to the viewer. The bronchoscope also consists of a channel for suction and passage of other instruments such as brushes and forceps, a controller knob for ante- or retroflexing the instrument, and fine and gross adjustment foci.
- The outer diameter of the bronchoscope is of relevance to anesthesia. The outer diameter of the bronchoscope should be at least 2 mm narrower than the lumen of the endotracheal tube (ETT) to prevent excessive increases in airflow resistance and decreased tidal volume.
- The fiberoptic scope needs to be attached to the light source and camera. Make sure the bronchoscope fits easily inside the ETT (remember the 2 mm difference).
- Test the adjustment focus against the writing on the airway cart or camera.
- Practice maneuvering the scope, rotating it, and ante- and retroflexing before use. Make sure that you have the scope centered. Attach an appropriate ETT to the scope after removing the connector and place the connector in a known obvious place.

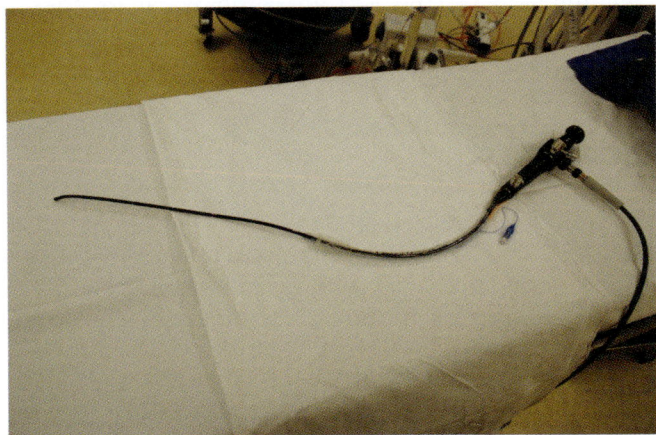

FIGURE 15-1 Flexible fiberoptic bronchoscope.

FURTHER PREPARATION

- Preassemble a difficult airway cart in an accessible and known location. Included in our general ancillary list would be nasal pledgets and trumpets, Williams or Ovassapian airways, topicalization devices (atomizer, nebulizers, sprayers, tongue depressors) or nerve block equipment (discussed later), source of oxygen, source of suction, cotton-tipped applicators, Ambu bag, supplemental oxygen supplies, monitors (pulse ox, capnograph, ECG, noninvasive BP monitor), lubricants, tape, premedications (e.g., antisialagogues, sedatives, hypnotics, aspiration prophylaxis, nasal mucosal vasoconstrictors, appropriate hemodynamic stabilizers).
- Adequate staff or another anesthesiologist present
- Surgeon trained in performing surgical airway with a tracheostomy-cricothyrotomy tray ready to be utilized

SECRETIONS BE GONE!

- If a potentially difficult airway presents itself, start drying the patient immediately. Glycopyrrolate, either IV or IM, takes at least 20 minutes to really set in well. Glycopyrrolate can also be given IM, so if a patient does not yet have an IV, you can get the ball rolling. Worst case: the patient has a dry mouth; best case: awesome drying time for prepared slick AI.
- Word on the street: glyco IM allows for more stable levels in the body. Topical anesthesia only works when it comes into contact and soaks into the mucous membranes you are trying to topicalize.
- Secretions are the enemy. As pointed out in the first edition of this book, trying to topicalize an airway full of secretions is like trying to paint your garage floor with two inches of water floating on top. Furthermore, lots of secretions will obscure your view.
- *Antisialagogues:* Drying agents to use include glycopyrrolate, atropine, scopolamine, or diphenhydramine. Briefly, atropine tends to cause more tachycardia and scopolamine does cross the blood–brain barrier (BBB) and can weird out your patient. Diphenhydramine can be beneficial, as it dries the patient out and causes some sedation.
- Without good topicalization/sedation, say hello to bucking and say goodbye to hemodynamic stability while you're on a train to nowhere fast with a disgusted surgeon as your conductor.

As Mentioned Earlier But Bears Repeating

- Start drying the patient immediately; administer glycopyrrolate the second a difficult airway (DA) walks through the door
- Talk to the patient. Good rapport is everything. Keep it simple; patients don't need to be bogged down

with details. The patient does not need to hear a detailed lecture on how the oropharynx is innervated by this nerve so we are going to use a sodium channel blocker called such and such. Just say, "We are going to numb up your airway and look in your mouth with a special light. You will be sleepy and numb but may experience a few seconds of slight discomfort. Once the tube is in place, you will be off to sleep." Answer all questions and emphasize that the patient's safety is your main concern.

ASPIRATION PROPHYLAXIS

Some patients are at higher risk than others for aspiration (e.g., full-stomach trauma victim, obese patient, etc.). There are multiple combinations of antiemetics out there with different ways of working.

Supplemental Oxygen

Supplemental oxygen should be administered during the entire procedure of any difficult airway management, including sedation, topicalization, nerve blocks, intubation, and extubation. O_2 is always job number one! There are also many ways to enhance FiO_2.

Sedation

As with any sedative, don't forget your audience. Think comorbidities and by all means keep the patient breathing! Many patients with compromised airways require conscious muscle tone to maintain airway patency, so be careful with these agents! Most importantly, don't convert your patient to an apneic mass of hypoxic protoplasm! Again, good rapport is the best way to start!

Sedation usually works best if it is started prior to topicalization or nerve blocks. Finally, keep in mind the patient needs to be coherent enough to follow commands.

- Benzodiazepines: Although there are others, midazolam is usually the benzo of choice due to the ease of titration, it's a good anxiolysis, and it provides anterograde amnesia. Midazolam can be administered IV, IM, or orally; onset is usually 1 to 5 minutes, and it has a shorter half-life than lorazepam and diazepam. Finally, benzos can be reversed; thank you, flumazenil.
- Opioids: There are many opioids available, and it can be a nice complement to local anesthetics because of their ability to suppress airway reflexes and help prevent coughing. Furthermore, they alter the respiratory pattern to a slower and deeper rhythm. Like benzos, they can be reversed. However, narcotics also can cause respiratory depression, muscle/chest wall rigidity, and decrease respiratory reserve. Of all the available opioids, fentanyl would be the most useful in regard to its benefit/risk ratio.

Intravenous Hypnotics

- Special K (ketamine) is a phencyclidine (PCP) drug that produces dissociative anesthesia for a nice analgesic effect. Pros: does not cause significant respiratory depression (except for large doses), upper airway muscle tone is maintained, and it is a good bronchodilator. Cons: emergence delirium (requiring midazolam), increases secretions (so must give glyco), and is a sympathetic stimulant (increasing BP, HR, heart O_2 consumption, and increased intracranial pressure [ICP]).
- Propofol: Pros: good amnesia, adequate anxiolysis, good antiemetic, rapid induction and emergence, and greatly attenuates airway response with induction doses. Cons: must titrate carefully to avoid overt apnea. It is not traditionally used.
- Dexmedetomidine: produces sedative analgesia and anesthetic-sparing effects that cause sedation without a change in ventilatory status. Unlike patients sedated with propofol, patients receiving dexmedetomidine are easily arousable and able to cooperate, and thus are able to take deep breaths and clear secretions during AI. Some clinicians swear that this is the Cadillac of AI sedation! Unfortunately, in the real world this "Cadillac" drug is not always accessible. Give a loading dose and then start a drip, preferably using an infusion pump so it doesn't get away from you! Dexmedetomidine takes about 20 minutes to work, which is about the same amount of time you need to topicalize.
- Inhalation anesthetics: Not typically used with adult AI; they do have a unique role in pediatric difficult airway situations. Also, with bronchoscopy and pregnancy: 50/50 doses of $N_2O:O_2$ to assist with conscious sedation along with bitty doses of midazolam.

Optional: place the ETT in warm water or stick it (while still in packaging) in the end of a Bair hugger so it will be nice and soft, which is less traumatic.

TECHNIQUE

As with all procedures, there is more than one way to skin a cat. This is a basic description of an AI technique (nasal or oral approach), with typical medications used. The important thing is timing, how to trouble shoot, the what and the why.

- Topicalization: VERY, VERY IMPORTANT. You must be thorough and give this time to work. Make sure the agent is going where it needs to go (i.e., deep breathing), and if you're not sure, test the patient beforehand! Typically, one would start with the nebulization process (if that is the form of topicalization you choose). Pending patient cooperation, the response to the gag test, the neck habitus, etc., will dictate forms of topicalization; clinical competence and flexibility with your airway tools is the key (Figure 15-2)!

Topicalization Devices

Regardless of what agent you use, it's always important to keep in mind the onset of action, the mechanism of action, the optimal concentration, and the maximum amount of drug that can be used safely. Also, some topical anesthetics can also cause methemoglobinemia (fatigue, weakness, headache, dizziness, and tachycardia). So keep your methylene blue close by. "Cocaine interferes with the reuptake of norepinephrine. It should therefore be used with caution in patients with known hypersensitivity, coronary artery disease, hypertension, pseudocholinesterase deficiency, preeclampsia, or hyperthyroidism, as well as in children, elderly patients, and patients receiving monoamine oxidase inhibitors."[1]

- Lidocaine lollipop: place 5% lidocaine ointment on the top of a gauze-wrapped tongue blade, kind of like an ice cream cone. This needs to be placed way back in the posterior pharynx where you would swab for a strep throat test. Have patients stick their tongue out and slowly advance this luscious lidocaine lollipop to the back of the tongue themselves. This is the ultimate gaga-licious spot, which is the hardest to numb and where you will get the most resistance, so it is the best place to start. You could also use the swish and swallow.
- Nasal versus oral: nasal is a more direct pathway to the larynx; oral may require increased patient cooperation and operator skill to perform; oral requires at least a minimal mouth opening. Nasal contraindications: coagulopathy, severe intranasal pathology, basilar skull fracture, and proposed involvement of nasal passages in surgery. Oral intubation is usually the preferred route; however, if nasal intubation it is, then we need to start vasoconstricting the mucosa to prevent a nose bleed.

Nasal Intubation

1. Start with a few squirts of 1% phenylephrine (or Afrin spray) up each nostril while telling the patient to breath way in. Then 4% lidocaine (as it is a dilator), using a mucosal atomization device, can be sprayed into each nostril. Cocaine, which causes local anesthesia as well as vasoconstriction, is commonly used in otolaryngologic procedures and could be entirely appropriate in this situation. Another good technique to really coat up those hard-to-reach places is to use a more viscous or goopy solution of 1% to 2% lidocaine jelly. Fill a 10 cc syringe and schmooze it up into each nostril. (OK, old horror movie fans, think of "the blob" infiltrating every nook and cranny of those nostrils.)
2. Allow at least 10 to 15 minutes for the vasoconstrictors and the local anesthetic to do its job.
3. Next, let's make sure the pathway is clear; use a small nasal airway and slip it gently on through.
4. The next step is to pass a lidocaine jelly-drenched tube into the nose. As the Miami Tag Team eloquently described, you will feel a pleasant "Whoomp! there it is" as the tube passes into the posterior pharynx ("can you dig it?"). Now this isn't the most pleasant for the patient, so you can distract them by saying something like "focus on breathing through your mouth" and then without ado go for it.

Regardless of Oral or Nasal Route: Topicalization Must Continue

- Nebulization: Except for small children and uncooperative patients, this technique is easy and safe. A standard nebulizer uses 5 mL of 4% lidocaine to be nebulized with O_2 with a flow rate between 6 and 8 L/min (usually gives optimal droplet size) for about 10 to 15 minutes (Figures 15-3 and 15-4).
- Atomization: Sprays and atomizers with long delivery systems are available to deliver local anesthesia to the larynx and trachea. You can use this in place of a nebulizer or in addition to a kind of spray-as-you-go technique. Again, keep in mind the amount and concentrations of local anesthetics being used. If atomization is your main topicalization, than make sure the patients are breathing deeply, panting to get the most in!
- Transtracheal anesthesia: A needle is passed through the cricothyroid membrane at a 45-degree angle, then, using a 20-gauge (G) angiocatheter with a 10 cc syringe, 4 to 5 mL of local anesthesia is injected in the caudad direction at the end of the patient's deep inspiration. Usually the patient will cough (which helps spread the local) and jump. Make sure he is stabilized and watch your needle.[3]
- "Spray as you go": In addition to the atomizer and nebulizer, this technique basically involves injecting local anesthetic through the injection port of the fiberoptic bronchoscope (FOB).[3]
- Nerve blocks: The lingual and glossopharyngeal nerve provide sensation to the posterior third of the tongue and oropharynx are blocked by bilateral injection of 2 mL of local anesthetic into the base of the palatoglossal arch with a 25-G spinal needle. For the airway below the epiglottis, you need bilateral superior laryngeal nerve blocks and a transtracheal

block. The superior laryngeal nerve requires some degree of neck extension. After negative aspiration of heme, inject 2 cc of 2% lidocaine to each side of the hyoid bone with the needle directed anterior to the greater cornu of the hyoid bone and inserted into the thyrohyoid membrane. To bring the bone to you, push on the opposite side that you are injecting. See above discussion of transtracheal block.[1]

- Oral intubation: If we're going in orally, then you can place a Williams or Ovassapian airway. Coat either with 5% lidocaine ointment; wherever it touches, it will become numb (Figure 15-5).

Quick Tips!

- Help with bucking: You can also test the gag reflex using a tongue depressor or oral airway just to be sure the patient is well topicalized before you head in.
- VERY IMPORTANT: Have an assistant perform a chin lift on the patient! This locks the airway between the teeth and aligns the vocal cords more toward the middle. The straighter the pathway, the better; otherwise, you're staring at a lot of PINK (Figure 15-6).
- Some like to load the ETT tube as close to the cords as possible; others prefer to place the ETT tube on the scope and lightly secure with a small piece of tape (Figure 15-7).
- For the final FOB scope touches: Remember, this is a very delicate and precious instrument. You have already learned to manipulate your view without too much force or twisting. Again, part of the preparation is the setup. Make sure you hook up your oxygen to the suction port of your FOB; this can help blow out secretions, provide supplemental oxygen, and reduce lens fogging during the intubation. Don't lose your connector, and make sure the ETT tube can fit through your pink airway (Figure 15-8).
- Hold your FOB straight and lower the OR bed as much as possible (for vertically challenged folks,

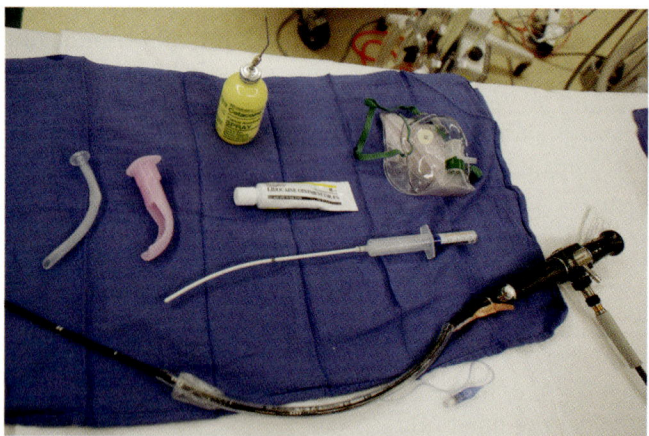

FIGURE 15-2 Topicalization devices.

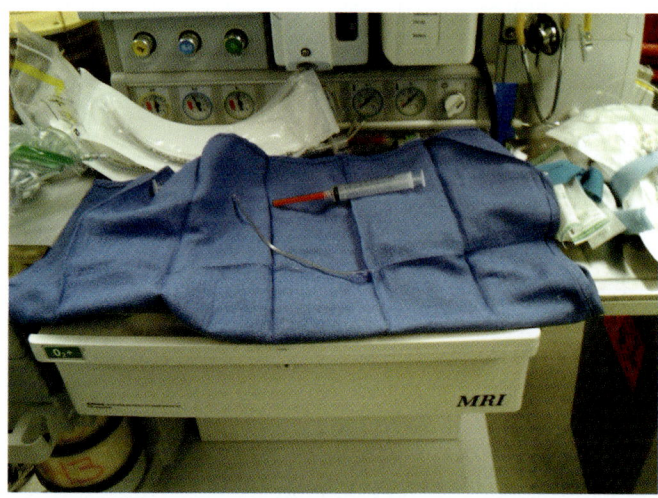

FIGURE 15-4 A lone atomizer.

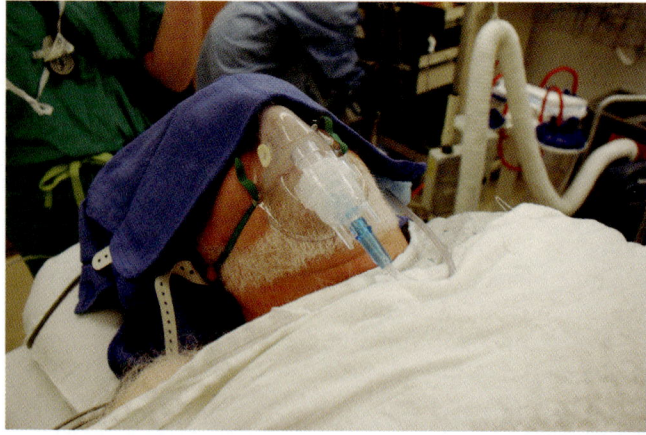

FIGURE 15-3 Nebulizing away! Patient is also ferociously panting!

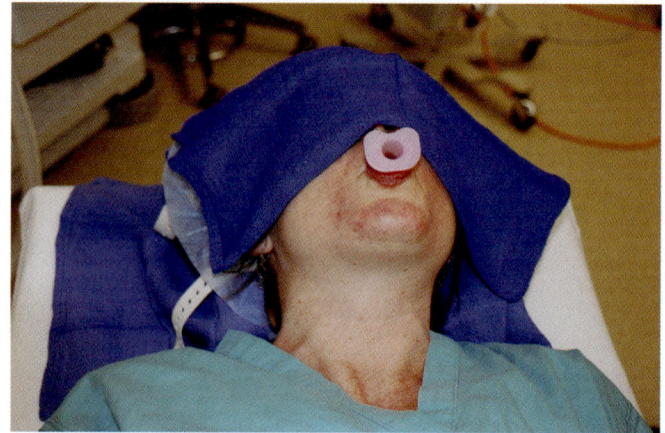

FIGURE 15-5 Williams airway from above; don't try this at home.

Chapter 15 AWAKE INTUBATION

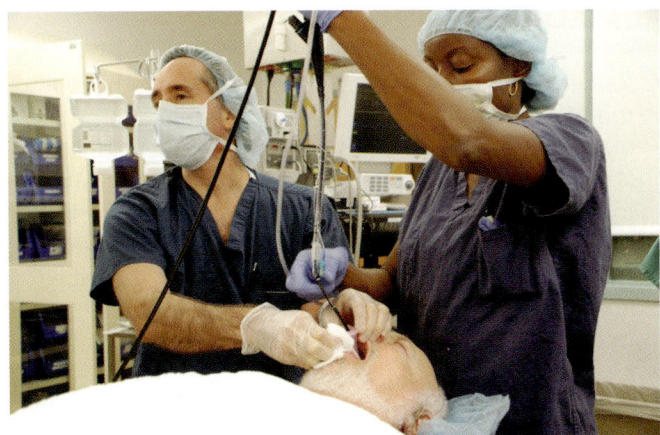

FIGURE 15-6 Not a chin lift exactly, but the assistant is manipulating the airway for a better view.

use stepping stools if necessary). Place and advance the tip through the Williams airway slowly; before you know it, you will enter an open cavern (aka the mouth) and see the epiglottis. Keep in mind to always use careful, minuscule movements; otherwise you will end up in "pinksville," the dreaded soft tissue hell. If that happens, then slowly back up, re-center your scope, and find that epiglottis (Figures 15-9 and 15-10).

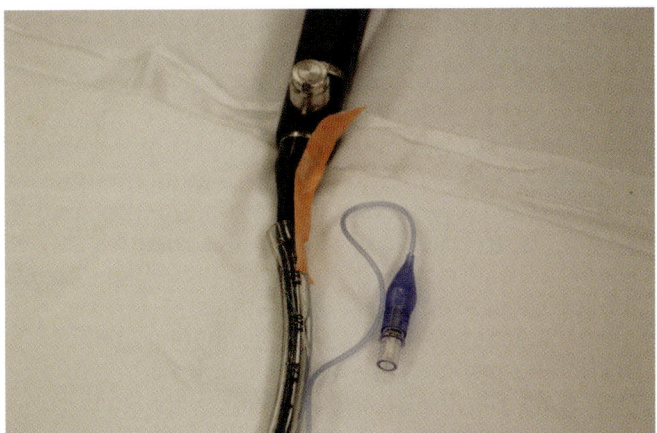

FIGURE 15-7 Fiberoptic with tape.

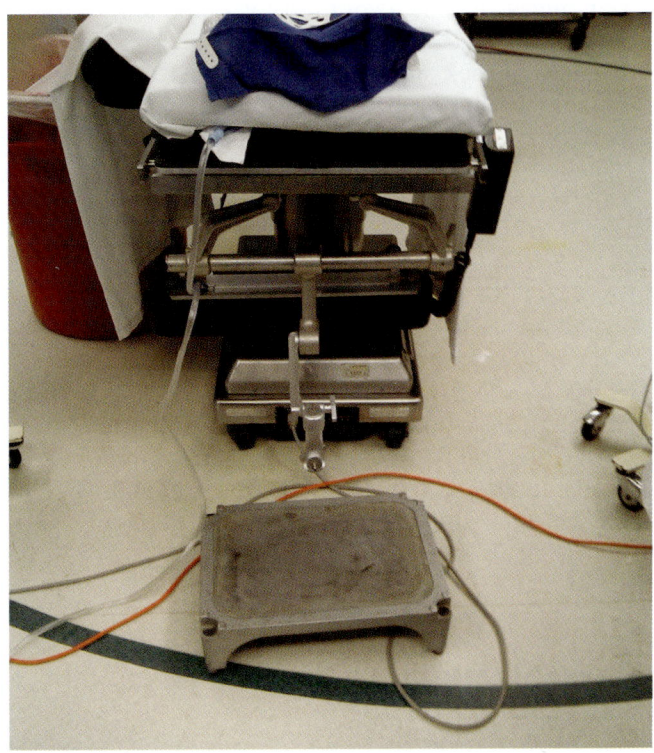

FIGURE 15-9 Lowered OR bed with step.

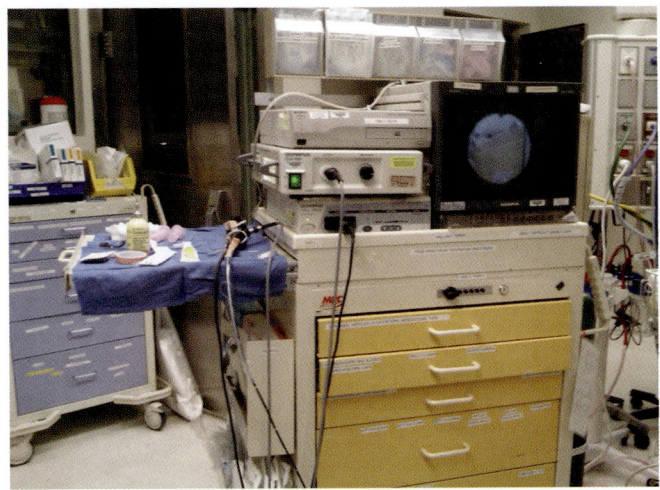

FIGURE 15-8 Difficult airway cart, with camera, scope, and topicalization supplies—ready to roll!

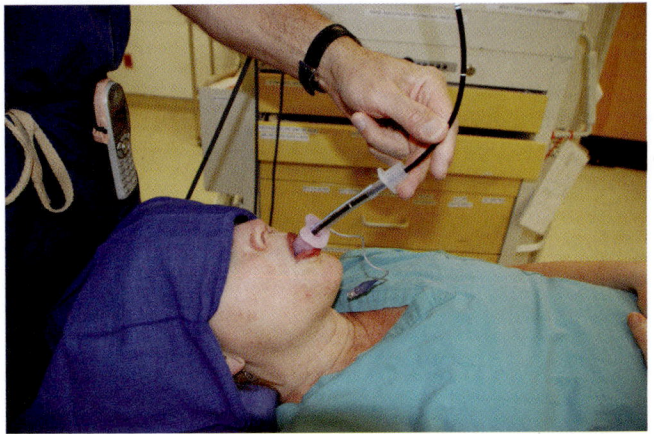

FIGURE 15-10 Again, don't try this at home: demonstration of a straight approach to advancing the fiberoptic.

TROUBLESHOOTING

- Make sure your assistant is performing an adequate chin lift on the patient. He or she can also perform some cricoid pressure, or move the neck around to try to find the right path; don't just keep going down the same road if the first is not working. You don't have to stay on this particular yellow brick road, Dorothy! Also, try repositioning the patient by turning the head left/right or whatever! Find out what works.
- Can always enhance your topicalization and "spray as you go" (see above).
- If you're a rock-star topicalizer, then you should be able to slip the ETT tube in without the patient even noticing! This can be particularly excellent if a neurologic postintubation check is in order!

ALMOST THERE!

- Now pull out the FOB, hook up your circuit, check for CO_2, and take out the oral airway.
- Voila! You are done. Once the tube is in, get the patient off to sleep; having some propofol ready could smooth this transition, depending on what the situation requires (e.g., frequent awake neuro checks? General anesthesia with paralytic?).

COMMON DIFFICULTIES AND REMEDIES

- Patient bucking: as discussed earlier, adequate preparation including time for drying and topicalization is everything; also careful sedation with a touch of fentanyl (suppress airway reflexes). If unsure, you can always test the gag reflex prior to starting.
- Difficulty inserting the tube over the fiberoptic bronchoscope: Anatomical considerations (such as bumps on the road to the vocal cords, so to speak), the arytenoids, a large tongue, long epiglottis, and airway deformity can all be factors. With nasal intubations, these roadblocks include deviated septum, inflamed turbinates, epiglottis, and or arytenoids.
- Other factors (both instrument and procedural): Murphy's eye of the ETT, cricoid pressure, airway intubator, and excessive jaw thrusting. A Parker tube is a bit longer and curved at the end. This design helps ease the tube through the vocal cords.

REMEDIES

- Remedy 1: "Mind the gap": reduce the gap between the fiberscope and the ETT. A possible technique to try would be to use a larger diameter fiberscope with a narrower ETT tube. Another gap reducer would be to fill the gap using a thinner and smaller tube inside of your ETT tube; thread both on the fiberscope (using judicious lubrication). Once all of the tubes are successfully in the cords, remove the inner (gap minimizer) and fiberoptic. These are suggestions, not laws.
- Remedy 2: Use an intubating LMA or LMA (see next section). This would not be a good technique to fall back on if you have never done it before.
- Remedy 3: Prewarming the ETT tube makes it softer and more malleable.
- Remedy 4: Load the ETT tube beforehand so the fiberoptic does not get stuck in the Murphy's eye; this might not be possible with nasal intubations.
- Remedy 5: Rotate the tube. Typically an unrotated tube tends to curve in such a way that the tip could impinge on the right arytenoids or vocal cord due to the bevel on the left. By rotating the tube counterclockwise about 90 degrees, the tip could avoid the arytenoids or subglottic structures as well as produce a posterior curvature, thereby reducing the possible esophageal intubation.
- Remedy 6: Similar to the troubleshooting tip in the technique section, ease up on the cricoid pressure, adjust the jaw thrust, use a laryngoscope to lift the tongue and epiglottis away from the fiberscope or use a glidescope for additional navigation (watch your fingers), and change or remove the airway intubator; find another path!
- Remedy 7: Esophageal intubation: If you feel resistance especially when advancing the ETT over the fiberoptic, you could be displacing the fiberoptic into the esophagus.

BRIEF LOOK AT OTHER WAYS OF PERFORMING AN AWAKE INTUBATION

- Intubating LMA/LMA: Advantage: intubation through an LMA is easier. First, the LMA positions you closer to the glottis and thereby bypasses a lot of soft tissue obstacles (remember "pinksville"?), which can be encountered in the oropharyngeal and epiglottal areas. It could also provide an easier path to the glottis for the fiberscope because the glottis is just below the grille of the mask. One disadvantage, however, is that some serious topicalization is going to be needed.

- Retrograde wire: This is an uncommon technique. Overall, the preparation in terms of topicalization and sedation are the same as with an AI. You penetrate the (already numbed) cricothyroid membrane with a wire and then work it up through the mouth or nose. Once the wire comes out on the other end, similar to the Seldinger technique for central lines, you advance the ETT tube over the wire. Complications include bleeding, subcutaneous emphysema, pneumomediastinum, breath-holding, catheter traveling caudad, trigeminal nerve trauma, advancing the tube over a flimsy wire, and pneumothorax.
- Awake Trach: This technique is usually reserved for patients who have some sort of massive elaborate tumor or structure in the oropharyngeal/epiglottal/subglottic space, where any manipulation of those areas could ruin the airway. Again, as with the AI technique, good rapport, sedation, and topicalization must be tailored to the individual patient. Once the airway is secured by the surgeon, general anesthesia can be initiated.

BRIEF LOOK AT PHYSIOLOGY

There are certain periods during bronchoscopy and intubation that the body finds particularly stressful physiologically.
- First to consider is the patient's anxiety about the procedure and surgery itself. Therein lies once again good rapport, sedation, and preparation!
- Now to the actual procedure: Maneuvering the fiberoptic through the vocal cords and suctioning are usually the most stressful. Basically any manipulation of the laryngeal area will induce stress in the form of hemodynamic changes, including blood pressure, heart rate, and mean arterial pressures. Cardiac dysrhythmia also tends to be the most prevalent during the "vocal cord violation." Basically the body is saying, "Houston, we have a problem."
- Pulmonary dynamics are also affected. Once the fiberoptic is inserted into the trachea, there is a decrease in the cross-sectional area and an increase in resistance, which will then lead to an increase in the work of breathing, decreased tidal volume, and the awful hypoxemia. Finally, suctioning can also cause problems. Suctioning in and of itself can be irritating and cause a reduction in a patient's functional residual capacity (FRC) by sucking out the remaining respiratory gases. Once again we are going down the road to hypoxemia—another reason why supplemental oxygen throughout the entire process is a MUST! Needless to say, nothing positive comes with hypoxia.

SURGICAL OPPOSITION

- Despite some of the obvious and profound reasons for an AI, some (not all) surgeons' interpretation of this technique is "delay of surgery," or "you'll give my patient a heart attack with your fiberoptic shenanigans!" It is incumbent upon us not only to educate and communicate, but also to be very cool, prepared, and slick with our AI. This is an excellent opportunity to remind others that us "gas passers" are capable of more than simple intubations and turning on a ventilator.
- Cole et al.[4] published a study detailing the instruction of novice residents in both fiberoptic intubation (FOI) and direct laryngoscopy (DL) during the first 4 months of their training. Subsequently, during a randomized study period, intubation times, hemodynamic changes, and complications were recorded for 71 FOI and 57 DL intubations. Mean intubation times were 56 seconds for FOI and 34 seconds for DL. There were no differences in hemodynamic indices or in sore throat between the two groups. No hypoxemia or hypercarbia was seen in either group.

EXTUBATION OF THE DIFFICULT AIRWAY

From ASA practice guidelines for the management of the difficult airway (2003): "The literature does not provide a sufficient basis for evaluating the benefits of an extubation strategy for the difficult airway. The Task Force regards the concept of the extubation strategy as a logical extension of the intubation strategy. Consultant opinion strongly supports the use of an extubation strategy."[2]

Basic ASA recommendations for an extubation strategy include:
- Awake versus unconscious extubation: consider factors that might impair ventilation postextubation.
- Have a preexisting airway management plan if a patient cannot maintain adequate ventilation post extubation.
- Finally, consider a short-term device that can serve as a guide for expedited reintubation, such as an airway exchange catheter (AEC), a nifty catheter that is placed through the existing ETT and stays in place after extubation.
- Mort[3] published a study of the effectiveness of the AEC; of 329 patients with difficult airways who were extubated over an AEC, 87 patients needed re-intubation; 51 still had an AEC in place, while 36 no longer had their AEC. To make a long story short, the rate of re-intubation was not reduced by a AEC. Rather, the AEC appeared to make difficult

re-intubations easier. In terms of "staged" extubation, the AEC has rockin' potential.

- AEC for "Dummies"
  1. It is important to premark your catheter so it can be inserted at the appropriate depth.
  2. Make sure your patient is well preoxygenated.
  3. Take an ETT (the same type you used to intubate) and hold it side by side with the AEC; mark where the tube starts (at the lip) and add an extra inch at the end. This should take you right to (not past) the carina.
  4. Insert the AEC through the tube that is still in the patient to the appropriate depth that you just marked. There is a connector that you can place at the tip of the AEC so you can ventilate the patient during this process.
  5. Next, slide the used tube over the AEC (keeping the AEC in the patient), and then you can slide the new tube over the AEC, which is firm enough to guide your new tube in the correct place.

Unfortunately, high-risk extubations tend to occur in settings under the care of physicians who are not familiar with these extubation guidelines.

REFERENCES

1. Sanchez A, Iyer R, Morrison D. Preparation of the patient for awake intubation. In: Hagberg CA, ed. *Benumof's airway management,* 2nd ed. Philadelphia: Mosby-Elsevier; 2007, pp 255–277.
2. Practice guidelines for management of the difficult airway. An updated report by the American Society of Anesthesiologists Task Force on Management of the Difficult Airway. *Anesthesiology* 2003;98:1269–1277.
3. Mort TC. Continuous airway access for the difficult extubation: the efficacy of the airway exchange catheter. *Anesthesia Analg* 2007;105:1357.
   An observational analysis from a difficult airway quality improvement database looking at AEC as part of an extubation strategy.
4. Cole AF, Mallon JS, Rolbin SH, Ananthanarayan C. Fiberoptic intubation using anesthetized, paralyzed, apneic patients. Results of a resident training program. *Anesthesiology* 1996;84:1101.
   A study to assess the effectiveness of a fiberoptic training program; the article also comment on the safety and efficacy of this training.

SUGGESTED READING

Goldman K, Steinfeldt T. Acquisition of basic fiberoptic intubations skills with a virtual reality airway simulator. *J Clin Anesth* 2006;18.
A study that concludes that the use of a virtual reality airway simulator enables residents to acquire basic FOI skills comparable to those of experienced anesthesiologists.

Rosenblatt W. The fiberoptic training jig. *Anaesthesia* 2007;62:201–202.
Explanation of what a fiberoptic training jig is and how it works, as well as comments on its effectiveness with resident training.

CHAPTER 16
WHIZ-BANG INTUBATION GIZMOS

KATHERINE S.L. GIL

I suppose it is tempting, if the only tool you have is a hammer, to treat everything as if it were a nail.

*Abraham Maslow,
Psychology of Science: A Renaissance (1966)*

INTRODUCTION

Difficult direct laryngoscopies (DLs) and intubations occur with a whopping frequency (1.5% to 8.5% of general anesthetics), while, horrors!, the failed intubation rate is 0.13% to 0.3%.[1]

Whenever you hear somebody say, "I can DL anybody," they're substituting intubation lingo into Maslow's maxim. In other words, they're claiming that laryngoscopes that have been around since World War II are as good as it gets! Gosh, even some young dogs can't seem to learn new tricks. They ignore three things:
- Studies reporting bad outcomes with repeated attempts at Macintosh/Miller direct laryngoscopy (MacDL/ MilDL)[2]
- Closed claims analysis noting high incidences of DL intubation difficulty
- New devices proven to have better success or better laryngeal views in comparison to DL.[3]

As much as we love our rigid laryngoscopes and flexible fiberoptic bronchoscopes, there's a whole new world out there: video laryngoscopes, optical laryngoscopes, optical stylets, and lighted stylets.

CUTTING-EDGE GADGET COMMONALITIES THAT WON'T BE DISCUSSED AGAIN

- Airway assessment: If you're going to drink the water, it's good to know who or what is upstream, so make sure the assessment is a good one.
- Elective intubation: Since the title of this chapter is "Whiz-Bang Intubation Gizmos," you can pretty much assume that indications for elective DL apply to all these gadgets.
- Cervical risk: They all cause less neck motion than DL, so patients can usually undergo their intubation journey in a neck-neutral position.
- Anesthetic: For these "gizmos," let's assume that airway management occurs with either perfect general anesthesia (asleep) or airway anesthesia (awake).
- Aids to intubation: Rigid DL tricks such as BURP (back, up, right neck pressure), tongue pull, or jaw thrust may help gizmo usage. (see Chapter 14, Laryngoscopy, for a review)
- Endotracheal tube placement: Let's also assume that correct endotracheal tube (ETT) placement is always adequately checked after each insertion.

VIDEO LARYNGOSCOPES

Video laryngoscopes (VLs) are high-definition, recordable, wide-angle, camera-assisted laryngoscopes for both indirect and direct visual ETT intubation.

Indications

- **Elective:** If the routine stuff is done everyday while thinking the exotic stuff will be tried tomorrow, often tomorrow never arrives. Become an airway champion! Periodically plan on blocks of 1 or 2 months for using exotics on a daily basis.
- Difficult airway patients, but not if an alternative airway technique is better
- Teaching: Yes![4]
- Diagnostic capability: Easier detection of vocal cord movement, abnormal airway anatomy, etc. Particularly advantageous are wide-angle VL devices with recording capacity.
- Direct visual placement of other devices such as:
  - For thyroid/parathyroid/neck surgery: Everyone can see the electrode-equipped ETT is correctly in contact with the vocal cords for electromyograph (EMG) monitoring.
  - For craniotomies: Everyone can see the electrode needles in the palate, tongue, or perilaryngeal areas for cranial nerve monitoring.
- Replacing ETT: Having to replace an ETT, especially in difficult circumstances, can be frightening. Under direct wide-angle vision VL, there's a much lower risk of airway loss.
- Combine with other airway devices to make the really tough intubations easier (e.g., VL use with flexible fiberoptic bronchoscope [FOB]).
- Removal of foreign body, from the upper airway down to the level of the larynx.

Contraindications

- Super-difficult airway, e.g., limited mouth opening, tons of loose teeth, extremely obscured soiled airway, upper airway blockage, very abnormal anatomy, etc., where another airway management device might be better.

Philosophy

Completely negative histories/physical examinations make you feel good about using any old intubation device, even DL, though almost no one knows what you're doing.

- How about VL? The next best thing to sliced bread; everyone in the OR loves seeing the views. The imaging is stunning and worth every dollar! Since it's a laryngoscope, the VL opens the airway and almost always finds the target.
- Ethics 101 (part A): A patient's history/physical examination indicated the potential for difficult intubation. We automatically fast forward to thinking about possible negative outcomes with a DL. Is it really ethical to use devices that are more likely to result in difficult and harmful intubations? So far, many practitioners might not consider this a problem because so many DL are still used. But, one day who knows? Would surgeons use older, though still commonly used techniques that are more likely to cause morbidity than newer ones? Hmmm.
- Ethics 101 (part B): And frankly, some requests from airway management practitioners just don't cut it. Have you heard this: "First look with DL, to 'evaluate' the degree of difficulty so that if the patient needs emergency intubation in the future, others will know how difficult it was." No, we want to use whatever is less difficult or harmful, even if the harm is as simple as a sore throat or broken tooth.
- Learning curve: Definitely! A great point is the much shorter learning curve with the VL compared to the DL.[3] In fact, newbies practicing on a mannequin with VL had more than three times higher success rates in using DL on patients than those practicing on the mannequin with DL before the live scenarios.[4] Also, instructors see what trainees see and can help them more. Plus, they aren't repeatedly asking, "What do you see?" when trainees suddenly fall into the dreaded "mute-trainee syndrome." Practice on mannequins first (in-services are great), and then select totally normal patients to get the technique down. Gradually work your way to increasingly complex airways. This goes for all "gizmos."
- Hemodynamic changes: Are usually less in comparison to DL.
- Multiple patient positions: With DL, supine positioning with the tongue to the left is important. With VL, any position is easier with its flexible midline approach.
- Environmental protection: For us? Really? Yes! With most VL devices your face doesn't have to be juxtaposed across from the patients' mouths as it is with DL. In other words, less chance that you'll get soiled.
- Cost (Part A): Yes. VL costs a lot. But if you start using VL on many patients, consider whether the VL over the course of 3 years will come out to be more cost-effective than cheaper gizmos mentioned later.
  - Higher Math: With frequent use, a VL costs less than $4 per patient if you do four cases a day, 5 days a week, 44 weeks a year for 3 years, even though you bought it for $10,000. What? It costs that much? Well, you pay for what you get! Besides, factor in money saved in time and emergency equipment not wasted on difficult intubations, more safety, less trauma, and fewer patient complaints. Plus, imagine your peace of mind!

- Lower or cheaper math: On the other hand, if expected VL use is less frequent, then the cheaper gadgets might be your ticket.
- Solution to cost (Part B): Try getting someone else to pay for the VL. That's always good! Research the literature. Hammer home the idea to your hospital/clinic/colleagues that VL devices are more successful and cause less morbidity, especially in difficult intubation patients where a ten-letter-word might disturb their peace: L-I-T-I-G-A-T-I-O-N. Even novices can make differences with proper data while using "patient safety" in every other sentence, during presentations to the "money controllers."

EXAMPLES OF VIDEO LARYNGOSCOPES (INDIRECT CAPABILITY DEVICES)

Examples of video laryngoscopes include the GlideScope® Video laryngoscope (GVL®)[3], Cobalt AVL®, Ranger®, and the GlideScope Direct (dual usage modes).

Good stuff (see Figure 16-1)

- Longest track record (since 2001)
- Intrinsic defogger and 60-degree blade
- Neonate to adult sizes
- Large video monitor
- Plastic disposable or nondisposable models; steel model for direct DL
- Use in the vallecula or to lift the epiglottis
- Mouth opening needs to be ≥1.4 to 1.8 cm

Indirect Technique

- Keep monitor by patient's abdomen in line of sight with airway, if possible.
- Slightly lowering the OR table, compared to DL height, helps.
- Turn power on ≥15 to 30 seconds for defogging.
- A big difference: Insert the VL midline under direct vision about 2 to 4 cm and lift.
- On video screen: palate, uvula, epiglottis, larynx; don't put VL too far in! (Figure 16-2)
- Important: Stop looking at the screen! Under direct vision, insert ETT about 3 to 4 cm.
- Return to the video screen and pass the ETT into the glottis (Figure 16-3).
- Strongly grip ETT and let someone pull the stylet out slowly.
- Pass the ETT down the trachea.

Direct Technique

The attachment, akin to a MacIntosh 3 blade is used similarly to a rigid laryngoscope, with the benefit of being able to monitor progress on the video screen.

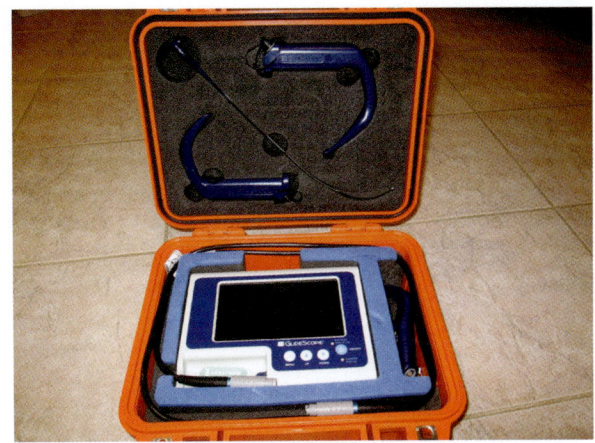

FIGURE 16-1 Portable GlideScope® Cobalt AVL®.

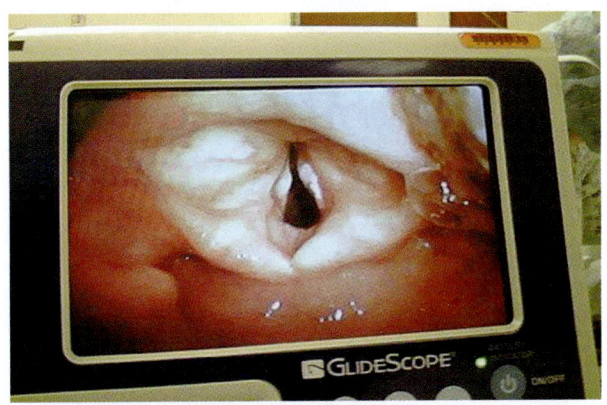

FIGURE 16-2 GVL® wide-angle anatomic larynx view.

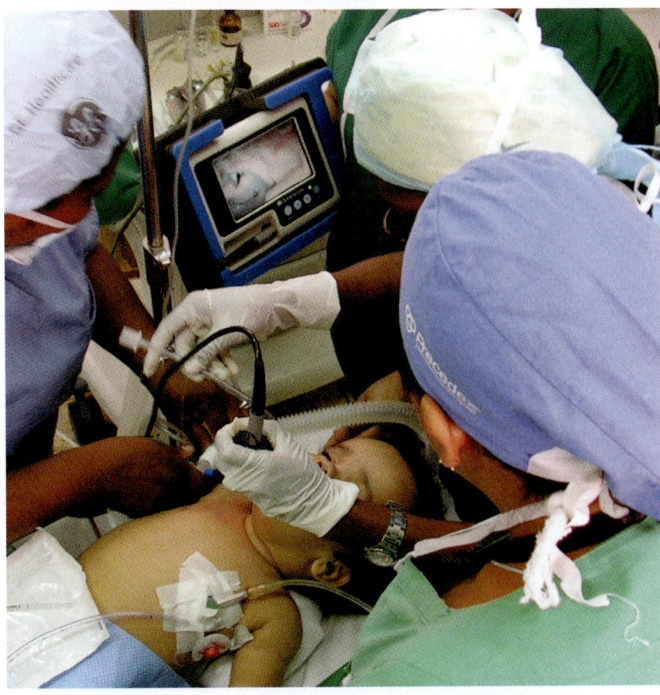

FIGURE 16-3 Pediatric intubation with GVL®.

McGRATH® VIDEO LARYNGOSCOPE

Good Stuff (see Figure 16-4)

- Introduced in 2006
- Angled CameraStick® within a thin disposable plastic blade
- Adjustable length, blade for small adults to Shaquille O'Neal–like patients (Figure 16-5)
- Super-portable, with a small screen mounted on the handle

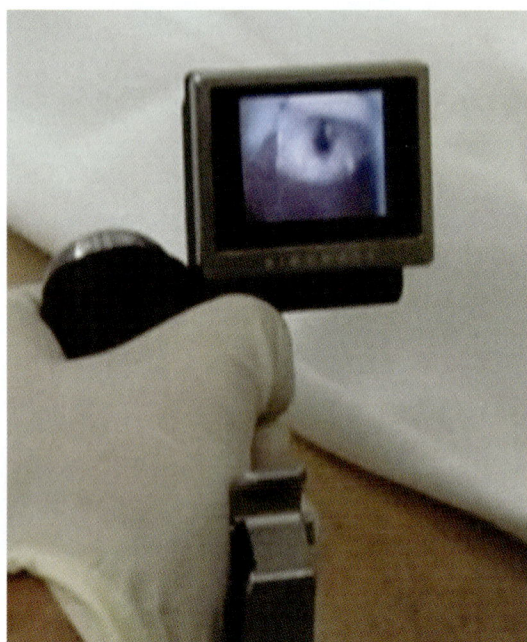

FIGURE 16-4 McGrath® VL view of larynx.

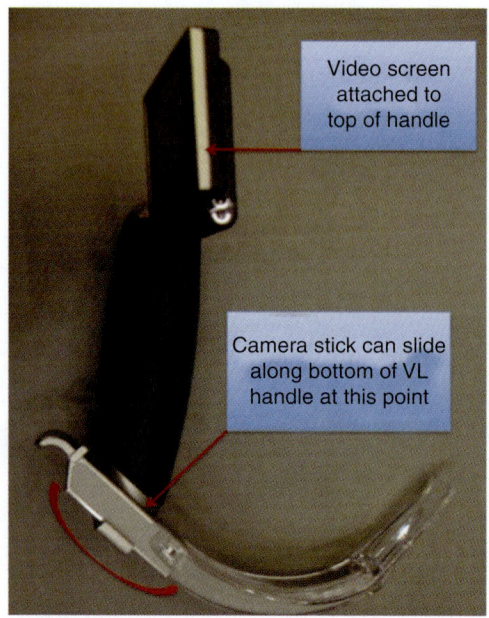

FIGURE 16-5 McGrath® VL adjustable length blade.

Tricky Stuff

- Definitely apply defogger.
- Must clean all contacts before use to avoid screaming as the screen turns staticky black.

Indirect Technique

Similar to that of other VL systems

McGRATH® MAC

Good Stuff (see Figure 16-6)

- Channeled and nonchanneled angled blades
- Much cheaper, plastic
- May be used with indirect or direct technique

Tricky Stuff

- Only one size, nonadjustable length
- No clinical studies; just came out (2010)

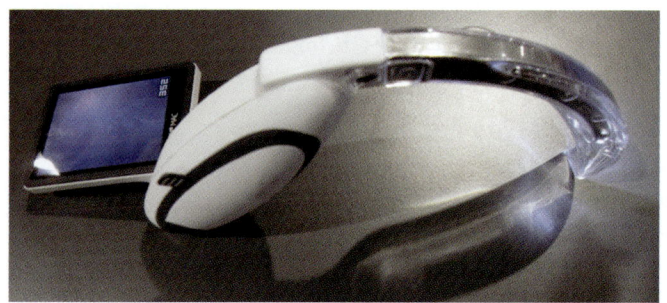

FIGURE 16-6 McGrath® Mac VL.

KING VISION™ VIDEO LARYNGOSCOPE

Good Stuff (see Figure 16-7)

- Also super-portable, small screen
- Channeled blade
- Much cheaper, plastic but estimated for only a 1-year life expectancy
- Disposable blades cost double other VLs since blade has the camera

Tricky Stuff

No clinical studies; just came out (2010).

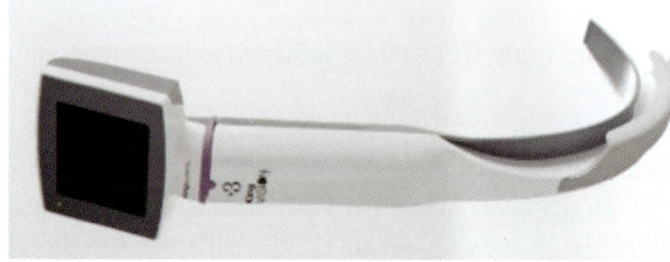

FIGURE 16-7 King Vision™ VL with channel for ETT.

PENTAX AWS® VIDEO LARYNGOSCOPE[5]

Good Stuff (see Figure 16-8)

- Introduced in 2006
- An ETT channel lies in an angled disposable plastic blade (Figure 16-9).
- Small screen mounted on the handle
- Screen has sighting crosshairs for glottic alignment (Figure 16-10).
- Suction conduit present

Tricky Stuff

- Apply defogger
- Very broad handle; those with tiny fingers will be straining
- Only one size
- Greater mouth opening needed (≥2.5 cm)
- To align the ETT with the glottis, you must lift the epiglottis.

Indirect Technique

Similar to VL except:

- Preload a well-lubricated ETT until its tip is barely seen on the video screen.

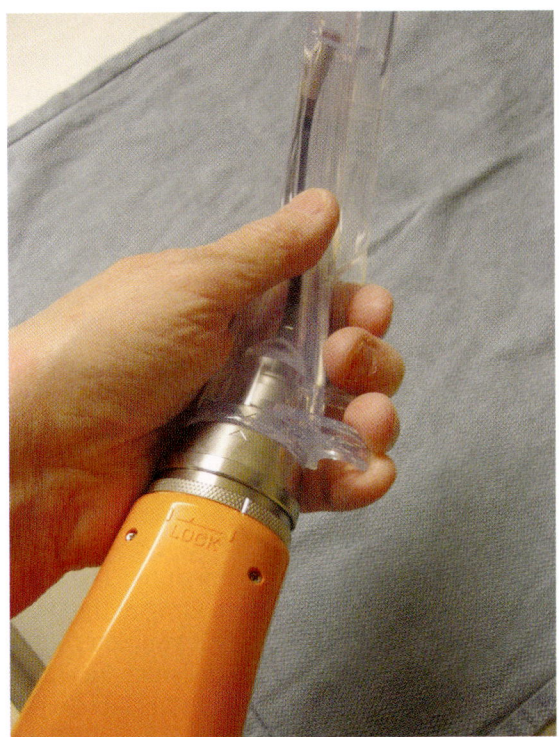

FIGURE 16-9 Pentax AWS®; putting on disposable blade.

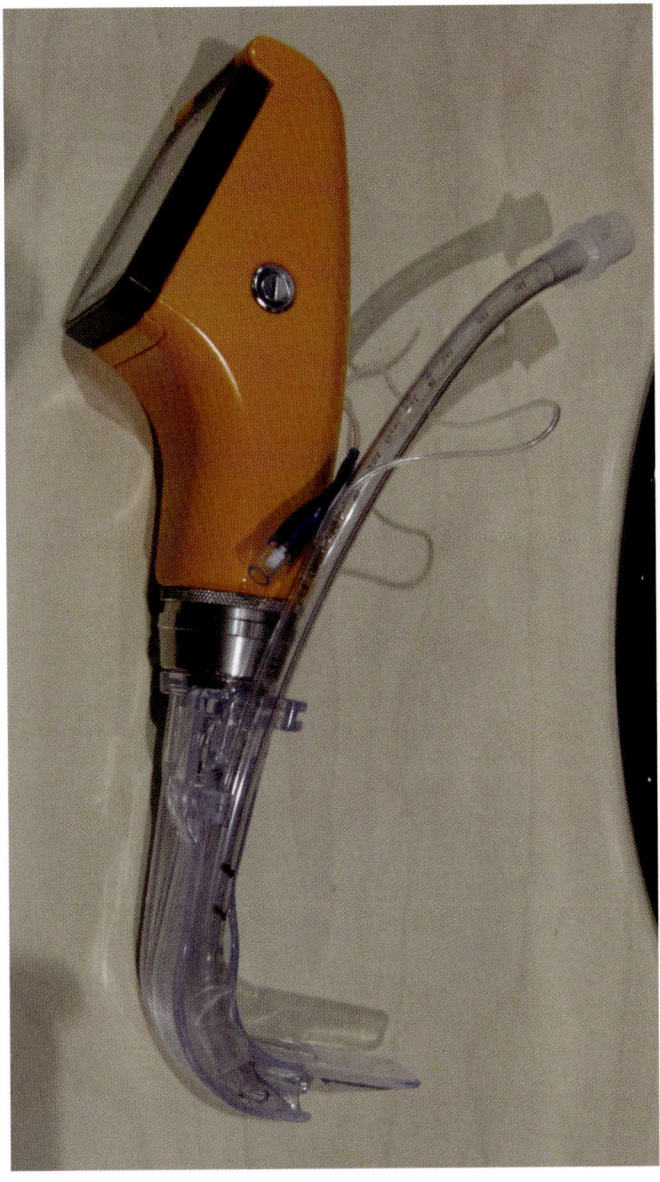

FIGURE 16-8 Pentax AWS® with ETT in channel.

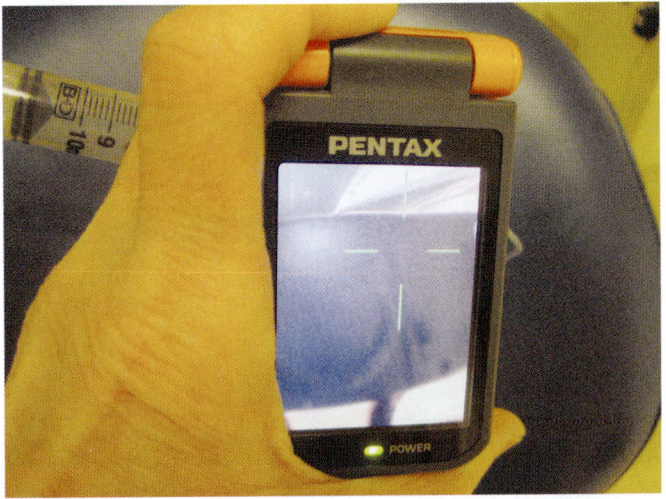

FIGURE 16-10 Crosshairs on video screen align with glottis.

VIDEO LARYNGOSCOPE (INDIRECT AND DIRECT CAPABILITY DEVICE)

C-MAC™ VIDEO LARYNGOSCOPE[6]

Good Stuff (see Figure 16-11)

- Introduced in 2009; angled D-blade just came out (2010), so the jury is still out.
- Thin steel blade just like a Macintosh
- Lots of sizes
- Large video monitor

Tricky Stuff

- Quite broad, rectangular handle is a bit odd to hold.
- C-blade length may impinge on the patient's chest.

Indirect Technique

Similar to other VLs.

Direct Technique

Similar to rigid Macintosh DL:
- Use it like a MacDL (except that Big Brother can watch the video).
- Hey! Keep an eye on the teeth, too; it is made of steel!

Concerns/Complications
With All Video laryngoscope Use

- VL intubation isn't always a slam-dunk: The ETT may impinge anteriorly due to tenting of the neck by angled blades. This is less likely if you don't insert the VL so far in, so that the larynx doesn't stay at the total top of the screen and just get an intubatable view.
- Regular laryngoscopy trauma: VL is less likely to cause damage to lips, teeth, or intraoral structures due to less mucking around, since the camera view is so much better. Especially likely if the VL is plastic.

- ETT cuff may rupture: Uncommon, but it's caused by looking under direct vision for maybe a nanosecond as the ETT just enters the mouth and then shooting your concentration to the video screen while simultaneously shoving the ETT into the patient's mouth. Meanwhile, as the ETT goes by, the teeth can score the cuff and you end up with a leak. What a bummer; particularly sad if it was a difficult intubation!
  - Preventative measure: Eyeball the ETT going past the teeth into the mouth.
- Palate and tonsil perforation: Similar cause, but a more rare effect. It's due to blindly inserting ETT into the mouth while watching the video screen. No sequelae so far. However, unless you have a specific request for body piercing, it's best to avoid this.
  - Preventative measure: Same thing; once you see the laryngeal view, keep the VL steady and stop looking at the video screen. Observe the ETT as you insert it into the patient's mouth and hug the tongue, aiming the ETT midline and caudad toward the imagined VL tip (this also prevents cuff rupture on teeth). *Note: Use of most VL devices has the potential for ETT perforation if we're fixated on the video screen and forget to observe the ETT's entry into the mouth.*
- Environmental issue: Are disposables really good for our environment? And what about the chemicals for cleaning devices that aren't disposable? Has anybody done a study to see which is worse?

Things to Remember and Other Tips

- A third hand: This is always good for any intubation, particularly if a difficult airway is present, to help with BURP, tongue pull, jaw thrust, pulling stylets, or whatever.
- Obesity: Don't ramp up; vamp up! Stop stuffing blankets under patients and struggling to pull them out after intubation! Just put your patient in a reverse Trendelenburg position or back-up position on the OR table until the patient's external auditory meatus is at the level of his/her sternal notch.[7] Get a footstool so that you are at a comfortable height. Postintubation, zoom the OR table back to "level." You'll save effort, OR time spent on ramping/unramping (money), and laundry (more money); blankets may cost 75 cents to wash, which is not a lot, but six blankets per patient is $4.50 wasted.
- Smaller ETT: For potentially difficult intubations, use ETT that are one to two sizes smaller.
- Defogger: Apply on any device that doesn't have an intrinsic defogger.

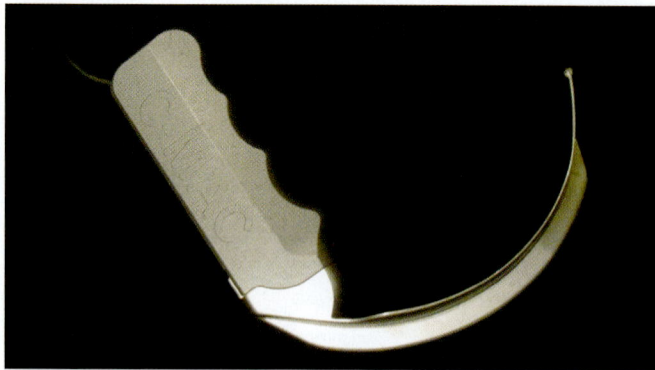

FIGURE 16-11 CMac™ VL D-blade.

- Yeow, pain! Watch out for pinched skin with the disposable Pentax AWS® blades as you slide them in place—yours!
- Stylet choice is irrelevant: If needed, malleable stylets are as good as any, plus you can bend them.
- Watch the ETT! Can't repeat it often enough. Watch the ETT as it enters the patient's mouth.
- Retromolar insertion: Use this approach to insert ETT from the corner of the mouth and then hug forward on the tongue, aiming mediocaudally. This also helps prevent the ETT from getting bent into an S-shape by the incisors.
- Plastic: intuitively sounds pretty good in comparison to cold, hard steel.
  - So, instructors, be wary of watching the "teaching" video while your newbie is using that cold, hard steel near the teeth. If the newbie is watching for the glottis and you are looking at the screen, who's protecting the teeth?
  - And suppose it's a difficult airway patient and your experienced trainee and you are both looking at the video. Then, who's protecting the teeth?
  - If you aren't watching, the dentist might be!
- Good view of larynx but can't pass the ETT? Is there a solution?
  - Try backing the VL out by little bits and see if the larynx moves posteriorly.
  - Try to get the ETT toward the bottom of the larynx, where the entry is wider.
  - When in the glottis, hang onto the ETT as someone slowly removes the stylet.
  - Try rotating ETT clockwise or counterclockwise.
- Crosshairs: You have to use the Pentax® as a Miller blade, lifting the epiglottis; otherwise you can't align the loaded ETT with the glottis.
- Coordination: Think you're having problems looking at the video screen and maneuvering the ETT in place? That's how the surgeons feel during their video games.
- Where'd it go? Watch out for the lighter weight, portable VLs (McGrath®, King Vision®, and Pentax AWS®) because they are easier to...hmmm...shall we say the politically incorrect words?...they're easier to steal.

CASES TO ILLUSTRATE THESE POINTS

Hey I'm a Diagnostician, Not Just a Technician!

A 35-year-old, sleep apnea patient who presented for cholecystectomy had been pestered to have an uvulopalatoplasty. His history was negative. On physical examination, other than obesity and a Mallampati II airway with 60 degrees of neck extension, he had no abnormal airway signs. After induction of general anesthesia, examination with a VL revealed excessive intrapharyngeal tissue and redundant perilaryngeal tissue. His palate and uvula were quite normal so it is doubtful uvulopalatoplasty would help. He was glad.

Know When to Turn to Plan B

After more than 300 GVL® uses in all comers (except for extremes who needed awake FOB intubations), only once was there anything but a grade 1 or 2 view and all got intubated. On that one, though, we saw just a rim of epiglottis when my colleague looked in, even with some manipulation on my part. Second look by me revealed the sliver of epiglottis, again. Bingo, goodbye VL! Went to an asleep FOB and everyone was happy.

Teaching Made Easy

July 1... ah, it's a new trainee, who luckily has already seen one intubation, on the Learning Channel. Here's the patient now. Five feet 8 inches, 120 kg, Mallampati 3, interdental distance 6 cm, thyromental distance 8 cm, neck extension 45 degrees out of a possible 80 to 90 degrees, upper lip bite test class 2. Oh look—she has $2000 veneers on every tooth in her head. Excellent! Get me that video laryngoscope and I won't even care if my newbie turns mute. I'll talk the newbie through it and the ETT will zip into place like an arrow—total relaxation!

OPTICAL LARYNGOSCOPE (OL)

Sort of similar to indirect VL, but uses prisms, has an eyepiece, is channeled for ETT, and has a hookup for recording ability.

Indications

Similar to those for VL.

Contraindications

Similar to those for VL:
- Particularly, soiled airway may be problematic as distal optics can get mucked up.

Philosophy

Similar to that for VL except:
- Magnified airway views: Not as sharp as VL.
- Cost: Totally disposable device, so while cheap (about $80), you'll have to decide if number of usages will really end up cheaper depending on how often you use it.

AIRTRAQ® OPTICAL LARYNGOSCOPE[8] (INDIRECT AND DIRECT CAPABILITY DEVICE)

Good Stuff (see Figure 16-12)

- Introduced in 2006
- Less angled with a channel for loading ETT
- Intrinsic defogger
- Lots of sizes
- May be used in vallecula or to lift the epiglottis
- A nonchanneled model helps find the glottis for nasotracheal intubations

Tricky Stuff

- Broad rectangular handle feels a bit odd.
- Mouth opening needs to be ≥1.25 to 1.8 cm

Indirect Technique

Similar to that for VL except:
- Turn on OL for ≥30 to 60 seconds (defogging).
- Load a well-lubricated ETT until the tip is barely seen, in view.

Eyepiece Technique

Similar except:
- Look through eyepiece.

Concerns/Complications With Optical Laryngoscope Use

- Regular laryngoscopy trauma: Damage more likely compared to VL but less than DL
- Optics: Not as high definition compared to VL

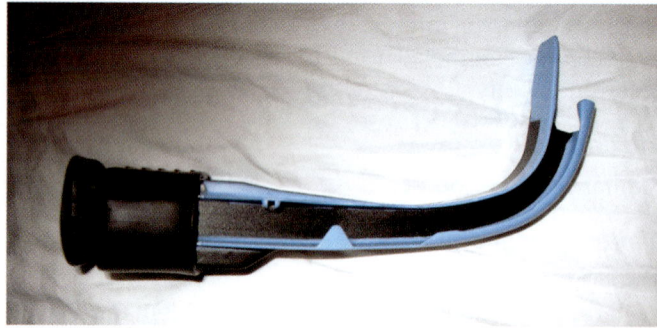

FIGURE 16-12 Airtraq® optical laryngoscope with eyepiece and ETT channel.

OPTICAL STYLETS (OSs)

Lighted, rigid, or semi-rigid steel, stylet-like endoscopes for eyepiece or indirect visual ETT intubation. They have an O_2 insufflation port that helps reduce fogging, are often malleable, and may have recording capability.

Indications

Fewer compared to VL:
- Most elective; certain difficult airway patients, especially with smaller mouth openings
- Useful for assisted intubation through supraglottic laryngeal mask airway (LMA)-type airway devices

Contraindications

Similar to those for VL except:
- Soiled airways (blood, etc.) or airway abnormalities make visuals exceedingly difficult.

Philosophy

Similar to that for VL except:
- OSs are not meant to "open an airway path" by themselves; i.e., often used with DL.
- Learning curve: Steeper than for DL, but their different technical approach makes a less steep learning curve versus that for VL. The smaller field of view of OS is more prone to the dreaded "pink-out" when against mucosa, where nothing is seen and you are "lost in space." They can be used as stand-alone devices, but success is greater with DL.
- Hemodynamic changes: Effects are usually less versus DL, unless you use OS with DL, eh!
- Used as lighted stylets or wands: Why not? They're straight, malleable, and have light.
- Cost: Midprice (up to about $4000)

BONFILS RETROMOLAR INTUBATION FIBRESCOPE™

Good Stuff (see Figure 16-13)

- Lots of sizes
- Mouth opening needs to be ≥ ETT diameter

Technique

- Adjust OR table height according to length of stylet.
- Slide and "lock" the lubricated ETT to cover tip of OS.
- Use defogger.
- Lift up the mandible to open the mouth.
- Insert the system preferably retromolar or else midline at about 30 to 45 degrees cephalad.

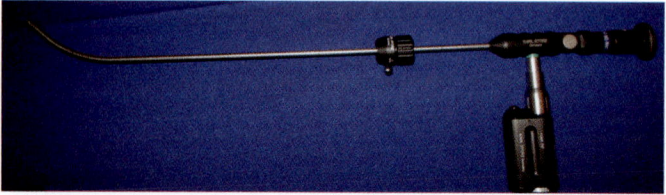

FIGURE 16-13 Bonfils® OS with eyepiece and movable ETT stop.

- Stabilize the system against the upper jaw.
- Visualize landmarks from a distance through the eyepiece, staying off the mucosa.
- Enter the glottis and push the ETT through the vocal cords.
- May need DL to help

LEVITAN FPS SCOPE™

Good Stuff (see Figure 16-14)

Similar to OS except:
- Greater malleability

Tricky Stuff

- Fixed ETT stop, so you have to cut the ETT to 28 cm, to make it fit properly.
- Only one size

Technique

Similar to that for OS

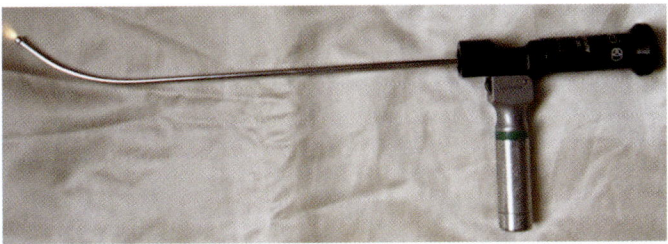

FIGURE 16-14 Levitan™ OS with eyepiece (nonmovable ETT stop).

SHIKANI SOS OPTICAL STYLET™

Good Stuff (see Figure 16-15)

Similar to OS except:
- Lots of sizes and shorter angled device allows easier manipulation.

Technique

Similar to that for OS.

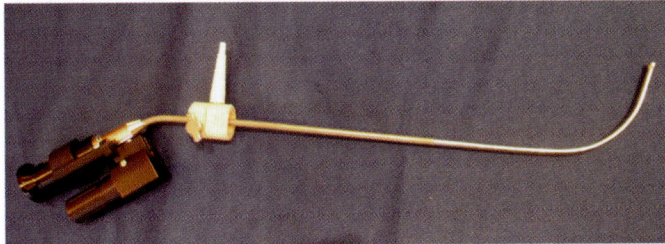

FIGURE 16-15 Shikani™ OS with eyepiece and movable ETT stop.

CLARUS® VIDEO SYSTEM

Good Stuff and Technique (see Figure 16-16)

Similar to OS except:
- Has LCD screen mounted
- Alternative red LED light for transillumination

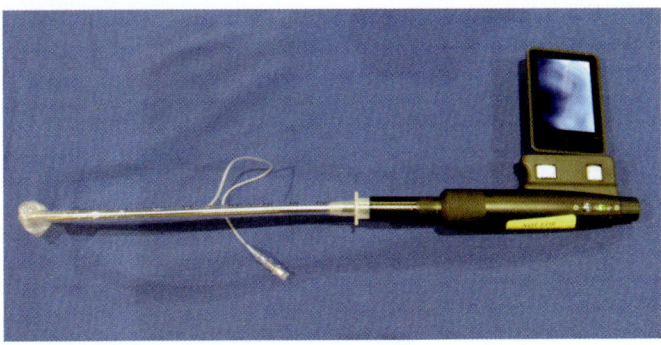

FIGURE 16-16 Clarus® Video System OS with ETT.

VIDEO RIFL®

Good Stuff (see Figure 16-17)

Similar to OS except:
- Flexible tip stylet articulates (anteriorly only) by a squeeze of a lever (Figure 16-18)
- Or ETT lies within a flex blade channel whose tip likewise articulates by lever squeeze.
- Has LCD screen mounted

Tricky Stuff and Technique

Somewhat similar except:
- Device has several parts.

Concerns/Complications With Optical Stylet Use

Regular laryngoscopy trauma: Compared to DL is not documented. But watch out if you can't see!

Learning curve: Not as steep as for VL but steeper than for DL. Needing a stool and having to use an OS in conjunction with DL is more complex; makes you want three hands.

Oxygen insufflation to prevent fogging may be dangerous: Reports of pneumothorax and gastric rupture have occurred with other airway devices!

Things to Remember and Other Tips

- Defogger: Is a must
- Have step stools available: if table height with OS is too high
- Clockwise, counterclockwise, and up-down motions: often help

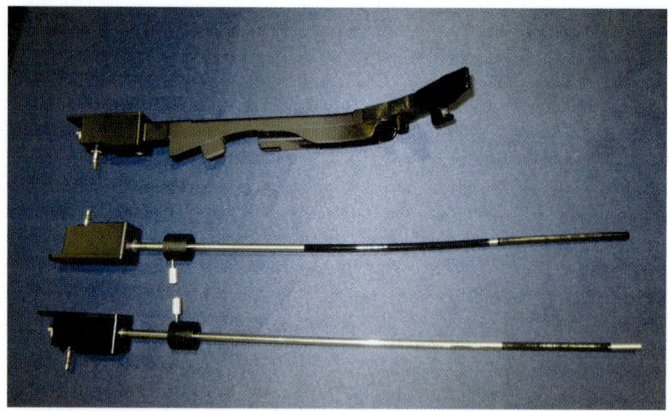

FIGURE 16-17 Video RIFL® OS with flex blade and stylets.

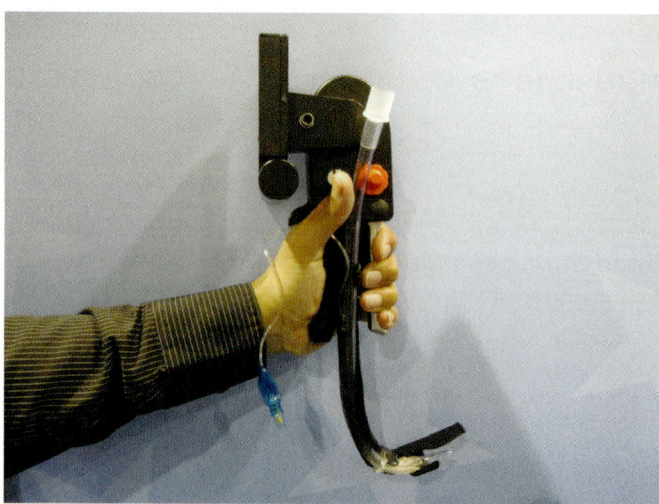

FIGURE 16-18 Video RIFL® OS with ETT in channel, articulating-tip lever being grasped.

LIGHTED STYLETS (LSs)

Lighted, malleable stylet-like devices using transillumination in the neck region to perform ETT intubation.

Kind of like these... makes you feel like Luke Skywalker.

Indications

Similar to OS except:
- Soiled airways: yes! Transillumination through blood, no prob... Like a scuba light!

Contraindications

Similar to OS.

Philosophy

Similar to OS except:
- Extremely fast learning curve: Oddly, intubation times may be longer in easy airways, even with experience or shorter in anticipated difficult-intubation patients.
- Super-cheap: $40
- Don't believe everything you read: Burns from LS bulbs have never been reported, but don't tempt fate by sticking the bulb beyond the ETT tip, anyway.

BOVIE AARON SURCH-LITE™[9]

Good Stuff (see Figure 16-19)

Similar to OS except:
- Malleable semi-rigid plastic stylet-like wand
- Size ≥ 5.5 mm ETT

Technique

Similar to OS except:
- Slide and fix a lubricated ETT onto Surch-Lite™.
- Insert the system, bent at 90 degrees midline or retro-molar rotating midline.
- Darken the room lights.
- Stabilize system against the upper jaw.
- Advance until you see a pretracheal glow.
- Advance until the glow moves very brightly caudally.
- Insert the ETT farther into the trachea.

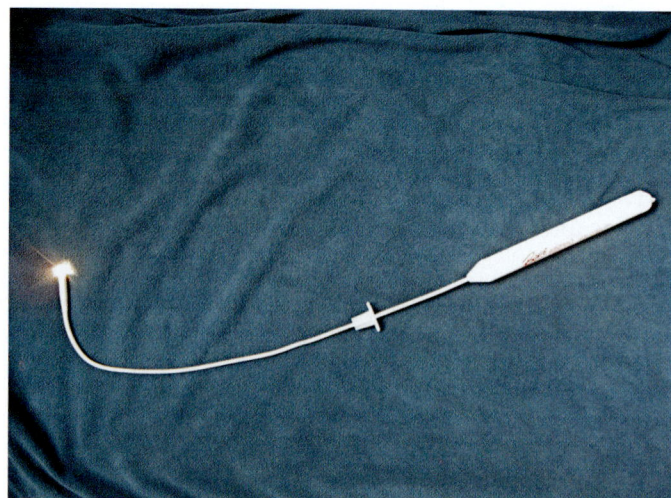

FIGURE 16-19 Bovie Aaron Surch-Lite™ Lighted stylet and movable ETT stop.

Concerns/Complications With Lighted Stylet Use

Regular laryngoscopy trauma: Less damage compared to DL.[9]

Things to Remember and Tips

- Pretest brightness: Shine through the patient's cheek to simulate degree of pre-tracheal glow.
- Glow off to one side: Pull out slightly and re-advance by rotating away from that side.
- Glow dimmer, localized anteriorly: Pull out of submental area and reinsert posteriorly.
- Glow very dim: same, but angle it out of the esophagus until pretracheal glow is seen.
- Obese patients: really tricky! Spread neck skin to sides; thins out the midline tissues.
- Practice and teaching tidbit: With an FOB or OS, just turn off the room lights. Watch for the glow—too cool! If you don't have a video screen, you can instruct the trainee (who is looking through the eyepiece) where to go if experiencing "pink-out."

TRAUMA: A CASE STUDY

A young man was driving home after throwing an anniversary get-together for his aunt and uncle. All of a sudden, someone ran a red light. Aunt and uncle never made it. Oddly enough, he'd been NPO for 10 hours in order to have surgery the next morning, wanting to avoid nausea. Loose and broken teeth everywhere, which would have been problematic even for the most delicate of VL or DL approaches. Choices were between a nasal fiberoptic intubation or intubation via left retromolar optical stylet. The idea was to save him from a tracheotomy. It worked perfectly; no neck scars for him (Figure 16-20).

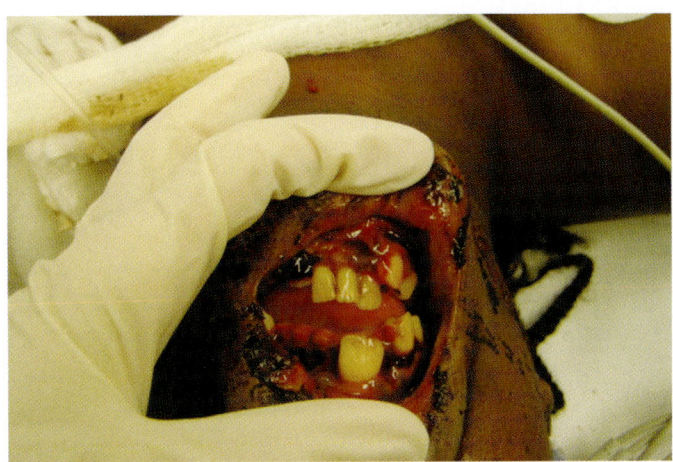

FIGURE 16-20 Loose, broken, and missing teeth.

CONCLUSION

Welcome to the 21st century where airway management "gizmos" are being produced exponentially and the best choices available for airway management are mandatory. Anxious? Well, no one is comfortable with any skill until it's done a number of times. Even paraphernalia for intravenous insertion was once a challenge and probably thought of as a "gizmo." See Web sites or devices on the Internet for instructional videos. Join workshops. The upshot is that VLs are skyscrapers in comparison to the other triple-deckers. But even the triple-deckers have lots of advantages over the lowly, on-the-brink-of-retirement, rigid laryngoscope (RL). What's required before total takeover? A "gizmo" cost adjustment—and within the past year, two were taken.

Sorry to see the demise of the RL? Not really. Ultrasound is facilitating decades-old rudimentary regional anesthetic techniques. Endoscopic procedures blanket surgical fields. What's your prediction for airway management in 10 or 20 years? I say hang on to your RL in case you go on a medical mission or need a good paperweight. And, for flexible fiberoptic/endoscopic bronchoscope enthusiasts, no worries! VLs won't replace 'em. Both are phenoms at asleep or awake airway control in the majority of patients, but nothing goes around corners or down holes like a friendly snake. So keep up your fiberoptic skills and open yourselves up to the stress-free world of videolaryngoscopy and other "gizmos."

REFERENCES

1. Crosby ET, Cooper RM, Douglas MJ, et al. The unanticipated difficult airway with recommendations for management. *Can J Anaesth* 1998;45:757–776.
   Landmark article reviews airway and device management.

2. Mort TC. Emergency tracheal intubation: complications associated with repeated laryngoscopic attempts. *Anesth Analg* 2004;99:607–613.
   Classic study on all the dangers of persistent intubation attempts with a rigid laryngoscope.

3. Cooper RM, Pacey JA, Bishop MJ, McCluskey SA. Early clinical experience with a new video laryngoscope (Glidescope®) in 728 patients. *Can J Anaesth* 2005; 52:191–198.
   Large numbers of patients in this study illustrated the improved view obtained with GlideScope® VL, whereby 99% of all patients had Cormack-Lehane grade 1 or 2 views.

4. Ayoub CM, Kanazi GE, Al Alami A, Rameh C, El-Khatib MF. Tracheal intubation following training with the GlideScope® compared to direct laryngoscopy. *Anaesthesia* 2010;65:674–678.
   Novices who practised with VL on mannequins, had subsequent clinical advantage with DL intubation success in

live patients in comparison to live-patient success rate of novices taught with DL on mannequins beforehand.

5. Asai T, Enomoto Y, Shimuizu K, Shinguu K, Okuda Y. The Pentax-AWS® video-laryngoscope: the first experience in one hundred patients. *Anesth Analg* 2008;106:257–259.
   Successful intubation occurred in the first or second attempts (96 and 2, respectively), while the remaining two patients were unable to be intubated with the Pentax VL due to concern for dental anatomy or impaction of ETT on arytenoids.

6. Cavus EMD, Kieckhaefer JMD, Doerges VMD, Moeller TMD, Thee CMD, Wagner KMD. The C-MAC™ videolaryngoscope: first experiences with a new device for videolaryngoscopy-guided intubation. *Anesth Analg* 2010;110:473–477.
   This article found the following results with C-Mac™ VL use in patients: tracheal intubation had higher success rates.

7. Rao S, Kunselman AR, Schuler HG, DesHarnais S. Laryngoscopy and tracheal intubation in the head-elevated position in obese patients: a randomized, controlled, equivalence trial. *Anesth Analg* 2008;107(6):1912–1918.
   Why "ramp" and "un-ramp" patients when we're all living in a push-button world? This study shows equally good views and fast times for intubation between the "ramp" method and putting the back of the OR table up until the external auditory meatus was across from the sternal notch.

8. Park SJ, Lee WK, Lee DH. Is the Airtraq® optical laryngoscope effective in tracheal intubation by novice personnel? *Korean J Anesthesiol* 2010;59(1):17–21.
   Good learning curve study for all you newbies out there. A single experienced laryngoscopist graded the Cormack-Lehane views. Seventy-four patients were divided into two groups (one using Airtraq® and one with Mac DL). Thirty-seven medical student novices participated in both groups. Findings: With the Airtraq® the success rate at first attempt at intubation was higher, time to intubation was lower, attempts were fewer, adverse effects were less, and student usage was felt to be easier.

9. Rhee KY, Lee JR, Kim J, Park S, Kwon WK, Han SH. A comparison of lighted stylet (Surch-Lite™) and direct laryngoscopic intubation in patients with high Mallampati scores. *Anesth Analg* 2009;108(4):1215–1219.
   Sixty patients were divided into two groups. One had LS and the other DL intubation; 96% of the LS group had successful first attempt intubation in comparison to 80% of the DL. Changes in vital signs included elevations in mean blood pressure, 20 torr vs. 38 torr higher in the LS vs. DL groups, respectively. Heart rates in the LS group were about 10 beats per minutes lower.

CHAPTER 17

FIRE! FIRE! IN THE OPERATING ROOM

LALITHA SUNDARARAMAN
CARLOS MIJARES
MICHAEL C. LEWIS

The mind is not a vessel to be filled but a fire to be kindled.

Plutarch

FIRE IN THE OPERATING ROOM: WHERE ARE WE TODAY?

Despite great strides in anesthesia and surgery, the incidence of operating room (OR) fires has changed minimally over the years. There are 50 to 200 fires each year, with as many as 20% associated with serious injury or death. This chapter deals with only three questions. In case of a fire: what to do *and not to do*, when to do it, and when to run.

THE ETERNAL FIRE TRIANGLE

For a fire to start, three components are necessary:
Heat or ignition source, fuel, and an oxidizer[1] (Figure 17-1).

THE IGNITION SOURCES IN THE OPERATING ROOM

- The electrosurgical unit (ESU)
- Lasers
- The ends of fiberoptic light cords

The Oxidizers
- Air
- Oxygen
- Nitrous oxide

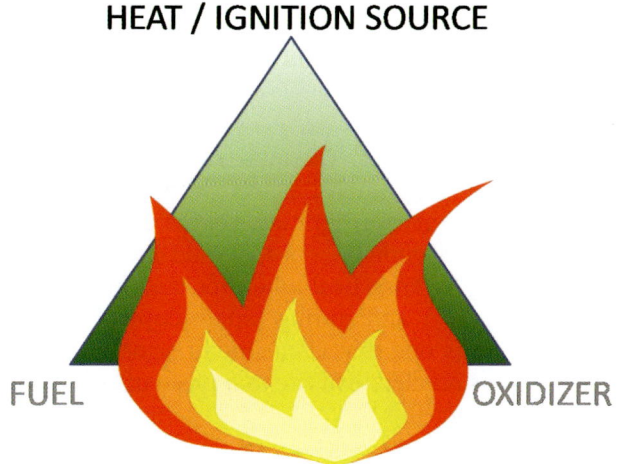

FIGURE 17-1 The core elements that combine to initiate a fire.

Oxygen and nitrous oxide function equally well as oxidizers, so a combination of 50% oxygen and 50% nitrous oxide would support combustion, as would 100% oxygen.

The Fuel
The fuel sources that are virtually omnipresent in the OR include gauze dressings, endotracheal tubes, gel mattress pads, facial or body hair, and paper drapes, which have largely replaced cloth drapes and are much easier to ignite and burn with greater intensity than cloth drapes.[2]

How to Prevent
Don't allow all three of the elements of the fire triad to come together at the same time. The challenge in the

OR is that frequently each of the elements of the fire triad is controlled by a different individual. For instance, the surgeon is frequently in charge of the ignition source, the anesthesiologist is usually administering the oxidizer, and the OR nurse frequently controls the fuel sources. It is not always evident to any one individual that all of these elements may be coming together at the same time. Hence communication becomes vital in this case.[3]

The Toxicants and the Toxic Injuries

Fire in the OR produces not only burns but also several injurious compounds such as carbon monoxide, ammonia, hydrogen chloride, and even cyanide. These toxicants can produce injury by damaging airways and lung tissue, and can cause asphyxia. OR fires can often produce significant amounts of smoke and toxicants, *but may not cause enough heat to activate overhead sprinkler systems.* Hence if enough smoke is produced, the OR personnel may have to evacuate the area. Hence, it is essential to have a pre–thought-out evacuation plan for both the OR personnel and the patient.

Are You In or Out?

OR fires are of two types. The more common type of fire occurs *in* or *on* the patient, especially during high-risk procedures in which an ignition source is used in an oxidizer-rich environment. These would include airway fires (including endotracheal tube fires, and fires in head and neck surgery) and during laparoscopy. The other type of OR fire is one that is *outside* or remote from the patient such as an electrical fire in a piece of equipment, or a CO_2 absorber fire.[4]

So What to Expect and How to Prevent?

General preventive measures for OR fires include:

1. Keep the cautery unit in the holster when it is not being used.
2. Use a nonconductive plastic clamp to attach the cautery to the surgical field.
3. Adjust the cautery settings so that sparks do not occur.
4. Disconnect the power from high-intensity light sources when not in use.
5. Never allow fiberoptic cables to come into contact with flammable materials.
6. Use appropriately protected endotracheal tubes when operating near the trachea during tracheostomy.
7. Never use cautery to enter the trachea.
8. Use air or air/oxygen mixtures in anesthetic gases and avoid using nitrous oxide, especially during bowel surgery.
9. Avoid "tenting" of surgical drapes that would allow accumulation of oxygen.
10. Use water-soluble (rather than oil-based) substances to cover lanugo hair.
11. Avoid alcohol-based skin preparations and petroleum-based eye ointments.
12. Stop supplemental oxygen at least 1 minute before using cautery on the head and neck.
13. Use a properly applied "incise drape" to isolate head and neck incisions from flammable vapors beneath the drapes.
14. Use fire-retardant surgical drapes.
15. Wet all gauze sponges and cotton pledgets during oropharyngeal surgery.
16. Use suction to scavenge the gases from the mouth of an intubated patient during oropharyngeal surgery.

And What About a Laser Fire?

When evaluating the risk of an airway fire, attention must be paid to the type of surgery and to the laser and oxidizers used. Head and neck, plastic, and airway surgeries, in which laser is used, are particularly vulnerable. Red rubber, polyvinyl chloride, and silicone endotracheal tubes all have oxygen-flammability indices (defined as the minimum O_2 fraction in N_2 that will just support a candle-like flame for a given fuel source using a standard ignition source) of <26% and should be avoided in airway laser surgeries. The LaserFlex™ (Mallinckrodt, Pleasanton, CA) is a flexible metal tube that has two cuffs that can be inflated with saline colored with methylene blue. The methylene blue enables the surgeon to easily recognize if he or she has accidentally penetrated one of the cuffs. The LaserFlex tube is highly resistant to being struck by the laser. If the neodymium:yttrium-aluminum-garnet (Nd:YAG) laser is being used, then the Lasertubus™ (Rüsch Inc., Duluth, GA) can be used. The Lasertubus has a soft rubber shaft that is covered by a corrugated silver foil that is in turn covered in a Merocel sponge jacket. In order to provide maximum protection, the Merocel must be kept moist with saline.

There are a number of basic safety precautions that should be taken whenever a laser is used in surgery. Since laser light can be reflected off any metal surface, it is important that all OR personnel wear protective goggles that are specific to the type of laser being used. The anesthesiologist needs to be aware that the laser goggles may make it difficult to read certain monitor displays. In addition, it is important that the patient's eyes be covered with wet gauze or eye packs. OR personnel should also wear high-filtration masks because the laser "plume" may contain vaporized virus particles or chemical toxins. Finally, all doors to the OR should have warning signs that a laser is in use, and all windows should be covered with black window shades.

Guidelines Specific to Laser Surgery Are As Follows

1. Use a combination of intravenous sedation and localized nerve blocks without supplemental oxygen during facial skin resurfacing.
2. Limit the laser output to the lowest acceptable power density and pulse duration.
3. Place the laser in "standby" mode when it is not in use.
4. Remove laser foot switches so they are not accidentally activated.
5. Use a metal, laser-safe endotracheal tube if laser surgery is being performed with endotracheal anesthesia.
6. Place moist towels around the patient's face and neck prevent ignition of the surrounding drapes.
7. Use metal (rather than plastic) corneal protectors to prevent thermal injury to the cornea.
8. Never allow laser fibers to be clamped to surgical drapes (clamping can break the fibers, causing ignition of the laser fiber sheath).

And the Remote Fires?

Remote fires may be due to faulty equipment, which can be prevented by frequent checks to see if they are compatible with American Society for Testing and Materials (ASTM) and fire safety guidelines. Remote fires can also be due to the CO_2 absorbent. Though halogenation confers nonflammability, sevoflurane and desiccated CO_2 absorbent (either soda lime or Baralyme) can undergo exothermic chemical reactions that have been implicated in several fires that involved the anesthesia breathing circuit. Avoiding absorbent in high-risk cases or use of absorbent without a strong alkali such as Amsorb™ is recommended.

GENERAL PRINCIPLES OF RESPONDING TO AN OR FIRE

Remember the acronym ERASE: *e*xtinguish, *r*escue, *a*ctivate, *s*hut, and *e*valuate.

In sequence: First, the team should generally attempt to extinguish a fire on, in, or near the patient. Depending on the situation, this may include the use of saline or a CO_2 fire extinguisher. If the initial attempts at extinguishing the fire are unsuccessful, the patient and all other persons at risk should be rescued and the OR evacuated, if possible, and the fire alarm should be activated. Once the OR is emptied of personnel, the doors should be shut and the medical gas supply to the room should be shut off. The patient should then be evaluated, and any injuries should be appropriately managed.

In brief, the following guidelines should be implemented for prevention of OR fires:[5]

- Prepare
  - Train personnel in OR fire management, assign to each member, his or her, task in case of fire.
  - Practice responses to fires (fire drills).
  - Check and ensure ready availability of anti-fire equipment.
  - Determine during a time out if a fire hazard exists and prepare accordingly.
- Prevent
  - Allow flammable skin preparations such as iodophor and DuraPrep to dry before draping.
  - Adjust surgical drapes to avoid buildup of oxidizer.
  - The anesthesiologist collaborates with team throughout the procedure to minimize the oxidizer-enriched environment near an ignition source.
    - Keep O_2 concentration as low as clinically possible.
    - Avoid N_2O.
  - The surgeon must be informed if the oxidizer and ignition source are in proximity to each other.
  - Moisten gauze and sponges that are near an ignition source.
- Be vigilant
  - Look for early warning sign of a fire (e.g., pop, flash, or smoke).
  - Stop the procedure, and each team member immediately carries out his or her assigned task.
- Manage
  - *Simultaneously* remove the endotracheal tube and stop gases; disconnect circuit.
  - Pour saline into the airway.
  - Remove burning materials.
  - Mask ventilate patient, assess injury, consider bronchoscopy, and reintubate.
- Fire *on* the patient
  - Turn off gases.
  - Remove drapes and burning materials.
  - Extinguish flames with water, saline, or fire extinguisher.
  - Assess patient's status, devise care plan, and assess for smoke inhalation.

- Failure to extinguish
  - Use CO_2 fire extinguisher.
  - Activate fire alarm.
  - Consider evacuation of room: close door and do not reopen.
  - Turn off medical gas supply to the room.
- Risk management
  - Preserve the scene.
  - Notify the hospital risk manager.
  - Follow local regulatory reporting requirements.
  - Treat fire as an adverse event.
  - Hold fire drills.

ABOUT FIRE EXTINGUISHERS

Fire extinguishers are divided into three classes, A, B, and C, based on the types of fires for which they are best suited. Class A extinguishers are used on paper, cloth, and plastic materials. Class B extinguishers are used for fires when liquids or grease are involved. Class C extinguishers are used for energized electrical equipment. A single fire extinguisher may be useful for any one, two, or all three types of fires. Probably the best fire extinguisher for the OR is the CO_2 extinguisher. This can be used on class B and C fires and some class A fires. Other extinguishers are water mist and new environmentally friendly fluorocarbons that replaced the halon fire extinguisher. Finally, many ORs are equipped with a fire hose that supplies pressurized water at a rate of 50 gallons per minute. Such equipment is best left to the fire department to use, unless there is a need to rescue someone from a fire. In order to effectively use a fire extinguisher, remember the acronym PASS: *p*ull the pin to activate the fire extinguisher, *a*im at the *b*ase of the fire, *s*queeze the trigger, and *s*weep the extinguisher back and forth across the base of the fire. When responding to a fire, the acronym RACE is useful: *r*escue, *a*larm, *c*onfine, *e*xtinguish. Clearly, having a plan that everyone is familiar with will greatly facilitate extinguishing the fire and minimize the harm to the patient and equipment.

CONCLUSION

Fires in the OR are largely prevented by anticipation and preparation; good communication and team work between the OR nurse, surgeon, and anesthesiologist, wherein each person knows his or her assigned role; and regular drills and simulations.

REFERENCES

1. Rinder CS. Fire safety in the operating room. *Curr Opin Anesth* 2008:21:790–795.
   This article elucidates the elements of the fire triad and their interaction to produce a fire.
2. Spigelman AD, Swan JR. Skin antiseptics and the risk of operating room fires. *ANZ J Surg* 2005;75:556–558.
   This article elucidates the most important fuels, namely skin antiseptics used by anesthesiologists and surgeons alike in various procedures and how to safely use them.
3. Daane SP, Toth BA. Fire in the operating room: principles and prevention. *Plast Reconstr Surg* 2005;115:73e.
   This article discusses the importance of communication and other steps in fire prevention.
4. Ehrenworth J, Seifert HA. Electrical and fire safety. In: Barash PG, Cullen BF, Stoelting RK, et al., eds. *Clinical Anesthesia*. Philadelphia: Lippincott Williams and Wilkins; 2009:165–191.
   This is an excellent chapter delineating when a fire occurs and how to manage it.
5. American Society of Anesthesiologists. Practice advisory for the prevention and management of operating room fires. *Anesthesiology* 2008;108:786–801.
   The guidelines for prevention and management of operating room fires!

CHAPTER 18
KIDDIE AIRWAY

JAMIE WINGATE
MARK ROSSBERG
DEBORAH SCHWENGEL

Behold the child, by nature's kindly law,
Pleased with a rattle, tickled with a straw.

Alexander Pope
An Essay On Man
1733, way before kids wanted Wii's and X-Boxes

INTRODUCTION

It has been said before and we will say it again: kids are not just small adults. There are differences in anatomy and physiology that are important to pediatric airway management. There are some valid reasons to be afraid of babies, especially newborns and premies: they don't follow the rules of physiology you are familiar with in adults. That is one reason pediatric anesthesiology is a true subspecialty. The top three reasons for cardiac arrest in children are airway, airway, airway!

ANATOMY AND IMPLICATIONS FOR AIRWAY MANAGEMENT

- Head
  - Prominent occiput in infants and younger children that tends to flex the neck
  - Automatically in the sniffing position without placing anything under the head, although a foam head ring helps to keep the head from rolling to the side or flexing
  - Positioning for airway management (mask ventilation, intubation, etc.)
    - Use a shoulder roll in children under age 2 because it prevents the neck from flexing. The infant's large head and tongue, mobile epiglottis, and anterior larynx makes intubation easier with the infant's neck neutral (rather than extended).
    - Consider the use of a pillow under the head in children over age 2 for the sniffing position (Figure 18-1 and 18-2).
- Nose
  - Narrow nasal passages
  - Responsible for 50% of total airway resistance[1]
- Mouth
  - Large tongue
  - There is loss of muscle tone during anesthesia and sedation, predisposing to upper airway obstruction.
  - Potentially loose teeth:
    - Clutzy laryngoscopy can cause deposition of a tooth in the trachea or stomach.
    - One should consider electively removing very loose teeth after induction and prior to laryngoscopy.
    - A newly missing tooth that cannot be found can be located on neck/chest x-ray (and this should be done prior to emerging the patient) (Figure 18-3).
- Epiglottis
  - Long and folded (classically called omega-shaped)
  - Hanging angle of epiglottis is more acute in infants.
  - These features make viewing the glottis more difficult and therefore the epiglottis is usually lifted directly out of the way during laryngoscopy (Figure 18-4).
  - Straight blade (Miller or Wis) is most commonly used in babies simply because it is placed posterior to the epiglottis and lifts it directly. Mac blades, when placed in the vallecula, are less desirable because they rely on the rigidity of the median glossoepiglottic fold (not a rigid structure in an infant), but Mac blades can be used like a straight blade to lift the epiglottis directly.

- Larynx
  - At C1-C3 in the infant, C5-C6 in the older child and adult. This can make for the impression of an "anterior" larynx and more difficult view in young infants. The larynx is not really anterior, but the combination of the higher larynx, smaller mandible, and fatter tongue makes it seem "anterior."
  - Vocal cords slant anteriorly making their view more difficult; they're also concave (as opposed to the straighter ones in adults). This angulation makes the view of the glottis different and might create some challenges in intubation.
  - Pediatric patients have a highly cartilaginous larynx, as opposed to the more well-developed ligaments in adults. This means that the arytenoid cartilages are very prominent and the vocal cords are similar in texture and color to the surrounding larynx and are therefore less apparent. You will often see a pink vertical opening rather than the white ligamentous glottis you see in adults (Figure 18-4).
- Trachea
  - This should be obvious: the younger the child, the narrower the trachea. Based on Poiseuille's law: $R = \frac{l8v}{\pi r^4}$ ($l = length$, $v = viscosity$, $r = radius$). We know that airway resistance is inversely proportional to the fourth power of the radius of the trachea. Therefore, there is higher resistance to gas flow in the tracheas of younger children, and placing a small endotracheal tube increases that resistance by adding length and decreasing diameter. So choose the largest endotracheal tube (ETT) that can safely fit (has a reasonable leak, ideally 15 to 25 cm H_2O pressure).
  - Not so obvious is that the cricoid cartilage is the narrowest part of the pediatric airway (in adults it is at the level of the vocal cords); the cricoid cartilage is a complete ring, so the ETT must be sized to fit the subglottic space (Figure 18-5).
  - Also obvious: pediatric tracheas are short. The neonatal trachea is approximately 4 cm in length, and around 2 cm for a premie. This is not abnormal compared to the size of the body, but it is just simply short and therefore easy to displace the tube. Neck extension may lead to extubation. Neck flexion may cause endobronchial intubation. Remember: the tube goes where the nose goes. This is not intuitively obvious, so you must understand that the cervical spine acts as a fulcrum, not the trachea. It is very important to reconfirm ETT placement after positioning for the surgical procedure.
- Neck
  - Short
  - Trachea lacks rigidity secondary to poorly developed cartilage; you can easily obstruct it when using cricoid pressure.
  - Because of the large occiput, the neck is more prone to flexion and airway obstruction.

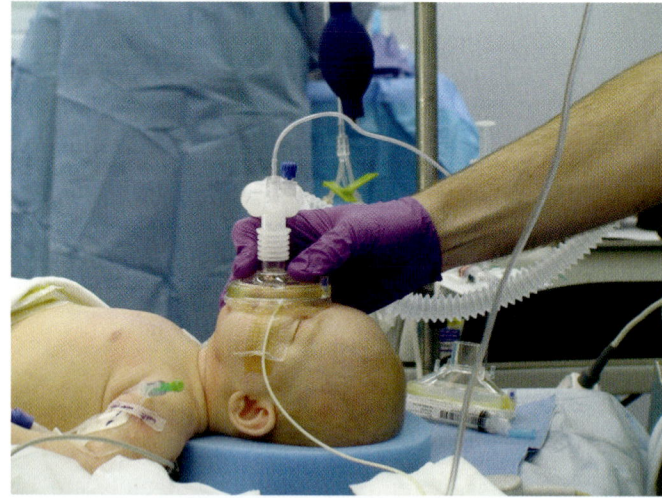

FIGURE 18-1 The infant's prominent occiput produces the sniffing position without anything under the head. A head ring is used to stabilize the head and prevent flexion.

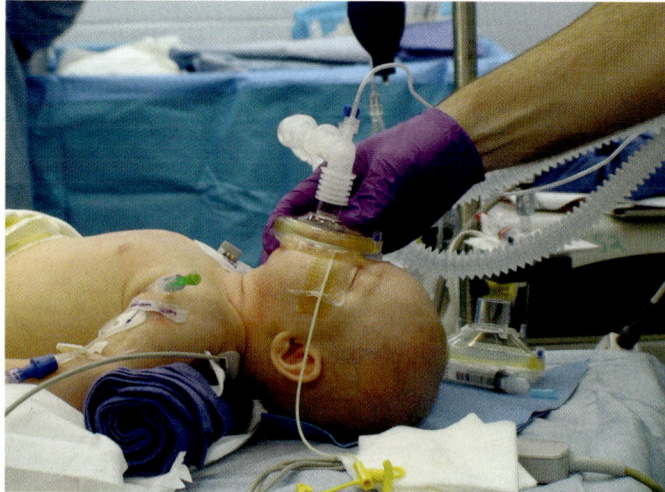

FIGURE 18-2 Neck extension and optimal position for mask ventilation and intubation, using a shoulder roll.

Chapter 18 KIDDIE AIRWAY

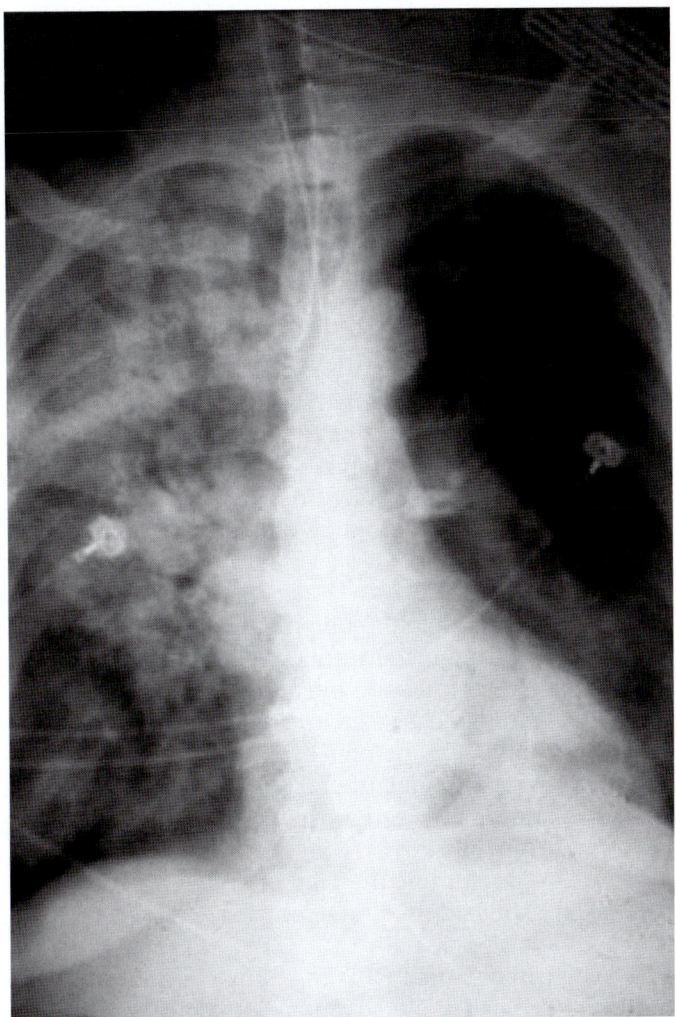

FIGURE 18-3 Chest x-ray showing a tooth in this patient's left mainstem bronchus. The tooth was loose at baseline and dislodged during laryngoscopy.

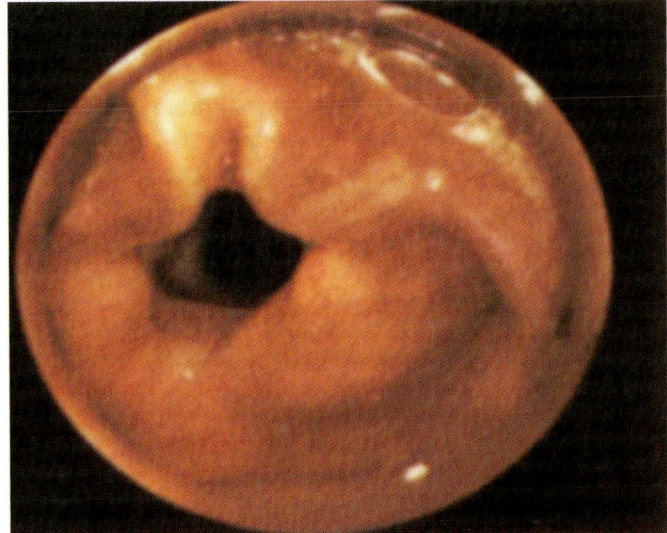

FIGURE 18-4 Infant larynx on the above, compared with the adult larynx below. Note the omega-shaped epiglottis and the prominent arytenoids cartilages of the infant larynx. (Courtesy of Lauren D. Holinger, MD. *Smith's anesthesia for infants and children,* 6th ed. St. Louis: Mosby, with permission.)

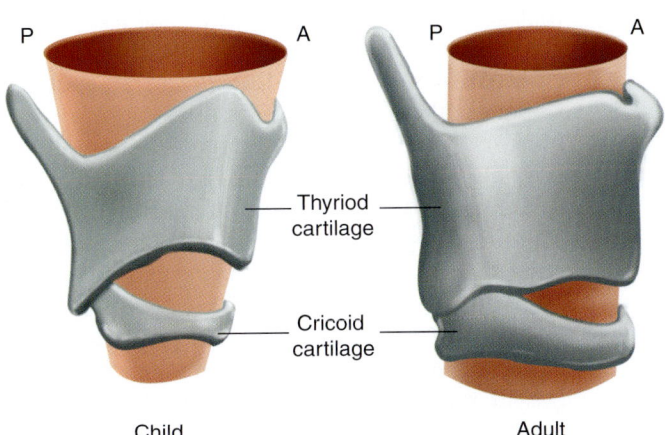

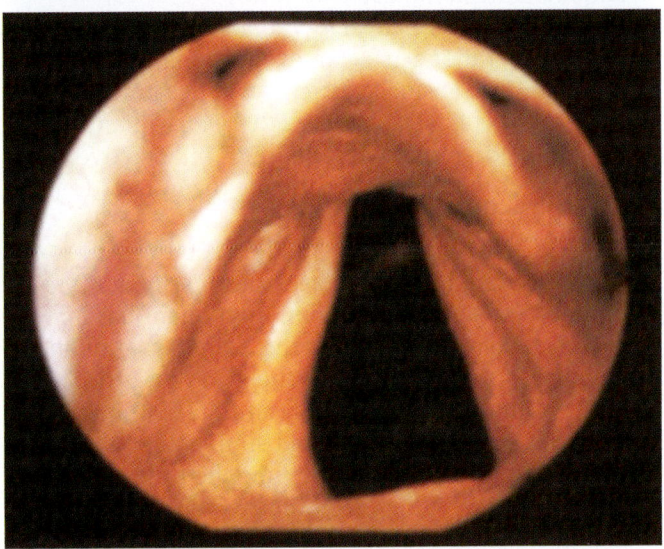

FIGURE 18-5 The cricoid ring is the narrowest portion of the pediatric trachea, up to the age of 8 to 10; the glottis is the narrowest portion of the adult airway and the trachea is cylindrical. (Drawn by Kelly Brenan Rothschild).

PHYSIOLOGY AND IMPLICATIONS FOR AIRWAY MANAGEMENT

Cardinal rules in medicine are to maintain physiologic balance such as supply and demand. Oxygen supply and demand can easily become unbalanced in infants under anesthesia. To understand this, you must know something about oxygen consumption and oxygen reserves.
- Oxygen consumption
  - Infants have a job in life and that is to grow and develop, so it is no surprise to learn that their oxygen consumption is higher than in adults. Depending on the age of the persons compared, infants consume oxygen at a rate two to three times that of adults. Oxygen consumption is highest in the first 6 months of life.
- Functional residual capacity (FRC)
  - FRC is the large capacity (almost half of total lung capacity) that acts as an oxygenation gas tank. When FRC is small, patients will desaturate faster. Newborns have a smaller FRC. Older infants and children maintain their FRC in an active way but when you anesthetize them, FRC drops significantly.
- The oxygen consumption–to-FRC ratio explains the desaturation we often see when caring for infants in the operating room. If an infant has an oxygen consumption that is three times that of an adult and an FRC when anesthetized that is 0.5 of the adult, the infant will desaturate six times faster than an adult. Plain and simple, that is why some infants are blue by the time the tube goes through the cords. It doesn't mean you are a lousy laryngoscopist; it is just physiology at work. Then make the kid sick and it can get a whole lot more interesting....

EQUIPMENT

In adults, one or two sizes fit all. In children all equipment needs to be appropriately sized in order to be effective. You must always be prepared with a whole array of sizes in case your planned blade or tube just isn't the right fit.
- Mask sizes
  - This is the most crucial skill for airway management.
  - Refer to Figure 18-2 for positioning and technique.
  - Masks come in at least four or five sizes; each is labeled for the corresponding age group.
  - Always have multiple mask sizes available, as each patient may not have facial features consistent with the mask size suggested for a patient of that age.
  - Appropriate mask size is important to ensure a seal around the face and to facilitate mask ventilation (Figure 18-6).
- Laryngoscope blades
  - Premie or newborn: Miller 0 or 1
  - 1 month to 1 year: Miller or Wis 1
  - 1 year to 2 years: Miller 1 or MacIntosh 2
  - > 2 years: MacIntosh 2 or Miller 2 (Figure 18-7)
- ETTs
  - Appropriate-size ETT relates to the patient's age, not weight
  - Common ETT sizing formula: size = (age/4) + 4
  - The formula only works well between ages 2 and 10. The rest you just have to memorize (sorry), and even then some patients do not read the rule book; those with larger or smaller airways might end up getting more than one laryngoscopy to find the right fit.
- Uncuffed ETT
  - Premie: 2.5 to 3.0 uncuffed ETT
  - Full-term newborn: uncuffed 3.0 to 3.5 ETT
  - 1 to 6 months old: uncuffed 3.5 ETT
  - 6 months to 2 years uncuffed 4.0 ETT
  - 2 years old: uncuffed 4.5 ETT
  - 4 years old: uncuffed 5.0 ETT
  - For ages between those listed, you would extrapolate.
  - 5 year old: uncuffed 5.5 or cuffed 5.0
  - If using a cuffed tube, downsize the calculated tube size by 0.5.
- The use of cuffed ETTs in young children is still debated.[2] The advantage of using a cuffed ETT is that it reduces the need for repeat laryngoscopies to upsize uncuffed ETTs with excess leaks, and it allows the anesthesiologist to regulate the leak pressure. This may minimize airway trauma and tracheal ischemia if you don't overinflate the cuff.
- ETTs with microcuffs
  - High-volume and low-pressure cuffs provide superior sealing of the trachea with pressures that don't promote tracheal mucosal ischemia.
  - Tracheal mucosal perfusion pressure is less in children than in adults.[3] Cuff pressures should be set at 20 cm H_2O pressure or less.
  - Longer ventilation with nitrous oxide is possible before cuff pressures exceed safe limits when using the microcuff tubes.[4]
  - The tubes also provide improved sizing of the cuffs that fit well between the cricoid ring and the carina.
  - For an informative discussion of the history of endotracheal tubes and the development of the microcuff tubes, we recommend the reading found at the following Web

site: http://www.vap.kchealthcare.com/media/62958/clinical%20article_new%20advances%20in%20pediatric%20intubation.pdf
- ETT depth is governed by the 1-2-3/7-8-9 rule for infants. If the patient weighs 1 kg, the ETT should be 7 cm from the lips, 8 cm for 2 kg, and 9 cm for 3 kg. Alternatively, depth = ETT diameter × 3. The ETT should pass 1 to 2 cm beyond the infant's glottis. Nasal intubation requires adding 20% to the ideal depth for oral tube placement.
- Laryngeal mask airway (LMA) sizes
  - They are available in seven sizes in the classic LMA and are sized by weight; just look at the package.
  - Size 1 for kids <5 kg, neonate, or premie
  - Size 1½ for 5 to 10 kg, infant-toddler
  - Size 2 for 10 to 20 kg, toddler-preschooler
  - Size 2½ for 20 to 30 kg, preschooler-school age
  - Size 3 for 30 to 50 kg, large child
  - Sizes 4 and 5 for adults (Figure 18-8)
- Airway adjuncts
  - Nasal airway
    - Choose the size by measuring it from the child's nostril to the tragus distance.
    - Contraindicated in basilar skull fractures, cerebrospinal fluid (CSF) leaks, or coagulopathy.
    - Can use a small ETT as a nasal airway or ventilate through a normal-sized ETT placed above the glottis; just measure it from nostril to tragus and cut it to fit the patient.

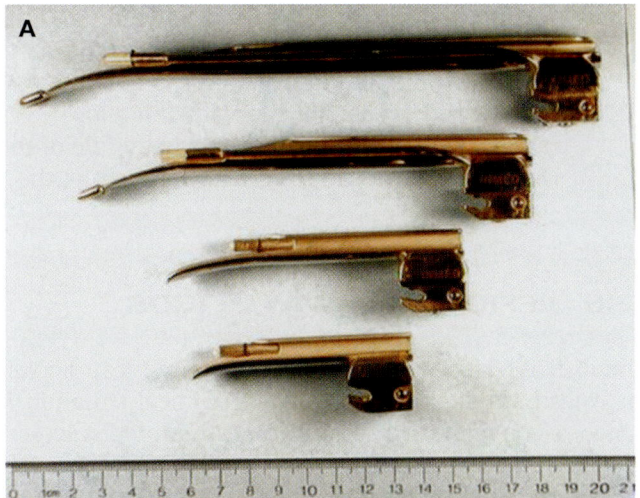

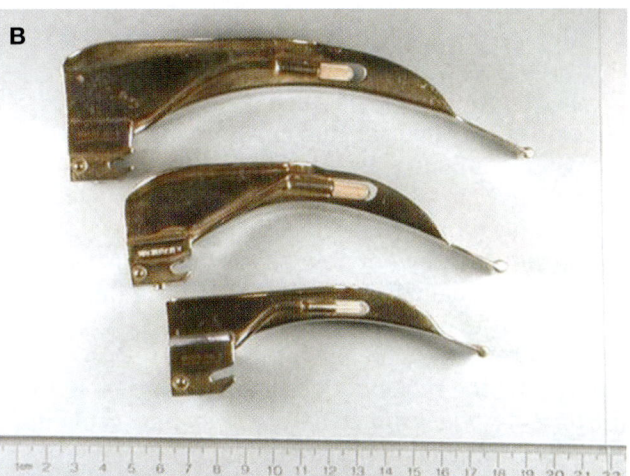

FIGURE 18-7 (A) Miller blade sizes. (B) Mac blade sizes.

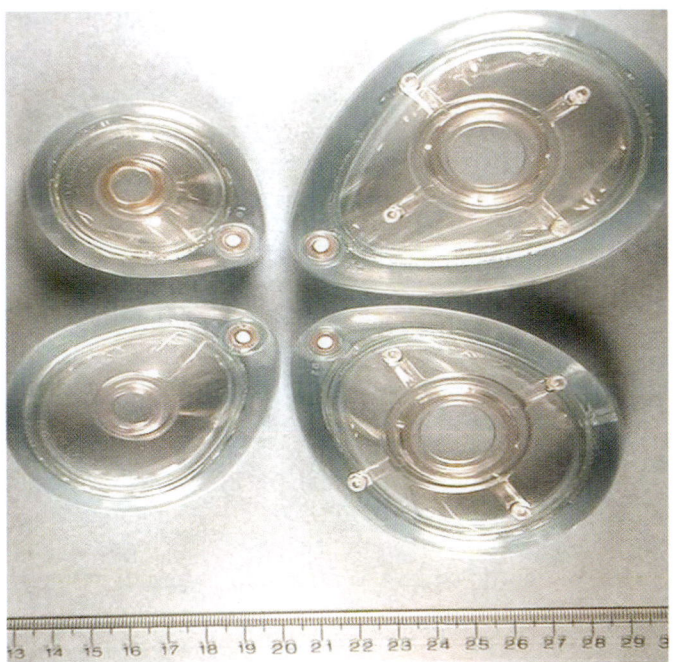

FIGURE 18-6 Mask sizes.

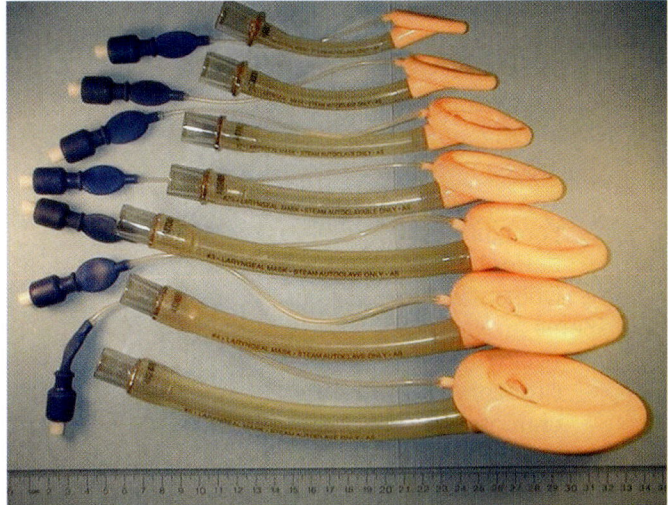

FIGURE 18-8 LMA sizes.

- Oral airway
  - Sizing: If it's too long, it will press on the epiglottis and fold it posteriorly to cover the larynx and obstruct the airway. If it's too short, its curve will compress the middle of the tongue and force it posteriorly to obstruct the upper airway.

THE DIFFICULT AIRWAY IN KIDS

The difficult airway is defined by the American Society for Anesthesiologists (ASA) as "the clinical situation in which a conventionally trained anesthesiologist experiences difficulty with face mask ventilation of the upper airway, difficulty with intubation, or both."[5]

- When
  - May be expected or unexpected
  - Discuss airway plan with surgeon; have ear, nose, and throat (ENT) specialist present if needed.
  - Management of patients in whom intubation will be difficult differs by determining whether patients can be easily mask ventilated or not.
  - Patients who have been easily intubated previously may not now be easy to intubate. Similarly, patients who may have been difficult in the past may no longer be so difficult.
- Airway diseases: who and what
  - Beyond the scope of this chapter, but they're listed for your review/interest (and they may show up when you take the boards).
  - Airway abnormalities that make mask ventilation or intubation difficult:
    - Apnea (central or obstructive) or sleep disordered breathing
    - Cleft lip/palate
    - High-arched palate
    - Narrow intermaxillary distance
    - Laryngomalacia
    - Subglottic stenosis (congenital or acquired)
    - Choanal atresia
    - Micrognathia
    - Tracheoesophageal fistula
    - Trauma or burns to the airway
    - Foreign body aspiration
    - Retropharyngeal abscess[6]
    - Obesity
  - Some airway syndromes to know:
    - Beckwith-Wiedemann syndrome: large tongue
    - Crouzon, Apert, Pfeiffer syndromes: craniofacial abnormalities
    - Down syndrome: large tongue, atlantoaxial subluxation
    - Goldenhar syndrome: unilateral micrognathia
    - Hunter, Hurler, Morquio syndromes (mucopolysaccharidoses): deposition of mucopolysaccharides in airway soft tissue; gets worse with age
    - Pierre-Robin syndrome: micrognathia; worse in infancy
    - Treacher-Collins syndrome: micrognathia; worse in infancy
    - Always be wary of someone with ear deformities or microtia.
    - Be suspicious of someone with hand anomalies.
    - There are many more out there. If the child has a "syndrome," look it up so you know the range of anomalies and possibly what to expect.
- How to manage
  - Start with the basics and decide how to induce the patient. You will usually not have the luxury of keeping the patient awake for airway management as you do with adults. Most children will not be able to cooperate with instructions.
  - Consider keeping the patient breathing spontaneously with either volatile anesthetics or intravenous anesthetics.
  - If the patient can be mask ventilated, proceed to your next step.
  - If the patient cannot be mask ventilated, consider placing an LMA, proceeding to laryngoscopy or surgical airway. Follow the ASA difficult airway algorithm, using equipment appropriate for the size of your patient.
- Airway management devices for children with difficult airways are the same or similar to those used for adults, but there might not be a small enough size for the smallest patients. There are some devices that are available in infant sizes:
  - Frova®: Intubating stylet by Cook, is the pediatric equivalent of the Eschman stylet but it is hollow with a removable stylet, and oxygen can be delivered via a jet ventilator adaptor or an Ambu-type adaptor. It will accommodate an ETT as small as 3.0 (Figure 18-9)
  - Fiberoptic bronchoscope (FOB)-assisted intubation is done the same as in adults, only with smaller scopes. The problem with the smallest scopes is that they don't have suction channels, and therefore a view obscured by secretions can be annoying and require frequent scope cleaning (Figure 18-10).
    - Suctioning alongside the FOB can help, or blowing oxygen alongside can also help keep secretions off of the tip of the scope and might help the patient to maintain oxygenation.
    - FOB through an LMA is another option. The LMA allows for the option of intermittent ventilation during the procedure as well. Although it is not optimal to give positive pressure ventilation through the LMA, it is

reasonable to do so until the airway is secured with an endotracheal tube.
- Place the LMA and then thread the FOB through the ETT and drive the scope through the LMA toward the glottis (Figure 18-11).
- Advance the ETT into the trachea.
- Confirm ventilation.
- Remove the LMA by holding the ETT with alligator forceps or inserting another ETT into the tracheal tube. Hold the ETT in place while removing the LMA.
- Confirm ventilation again.
- Check tube placement with the FOB.
- Secure the ETT.
• Airtraq® is a single-use Mac-like optical laryngoscope in which the ETT is advanced

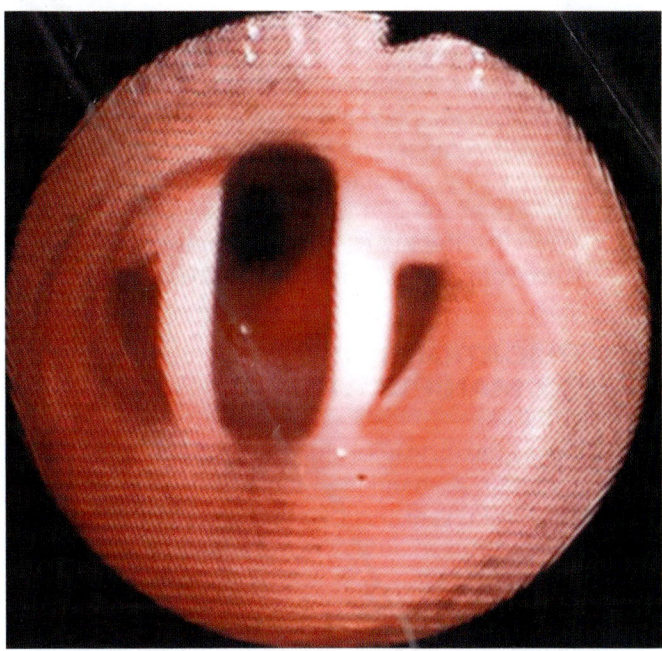

FIGURE 18-11 A view of the larynx through an LMA.

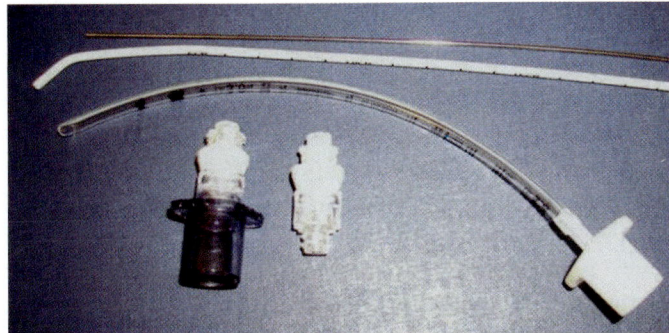

FIGURE 18-9 The Frova® intubating introducer showing its stylet, jet ventilator adapter, and Ambu bag adaptor, all next to a 3.0 ETT.

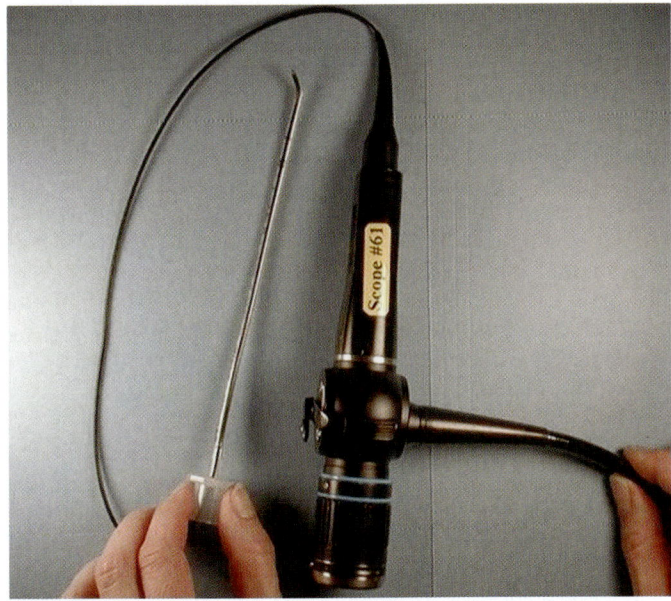

FIGURE 18-10 A 2.2 mm ultrathin bronchoscope through a 3.0 ETT. The scope has no suction channel.

through a guide channel on the side of the scope. A disadvantage is that resistance to passing the ETT can be either from inadequate lubrication of it or from an incorrect angle of placement (and therefore could result in airway injury if more force is used). It is also less useful in patients with a small mouth opening.
  − To view the Airtraq® device go to: http://airtraq.com/airtraq/portal.portal.action
• Glidescope® features single-use Mac-like laryngoscopy blades of many sizes with a reusable video baton. The steep angulation of the blade tip has been shown to produce a better view of the glottis; however, time for ETT insertion may be longer than with direct laryngoscopy.
  − For more information about the glidescope go to http://verathon.com/language/en-us/products/glidescope.aspx
  − To see a video of a glidescope being used to intubate an infant go to: http://www.youtube.com/watch?v = SK3tLEKQGMg&playnext = 1& list = PLB5CEB1FFBA007E82
• Storz DCI has a Miller-like blade but with small height; therefore, it is very useful in infants with limited mouth opening. It does, however, require that the blade tip is close to the glottis.
  − To view the Storz videolaryngoscopy system and some video clips go to: http://vam.anest.ufl.edu/airwaydevice/storz/index.html
• Truview PCD® is a small laryngoscope with an adapter for oxygen insufflation that significantly prolongs the time before the infant desaturates.

It has not, however, been studied in children with difficult airways.
- To view the Truview device go to: http://www.truphatek.com/p-80/
- McGrath video laryngoscope has the advantage of being very portable but with a smaller video screen than some of the other systems.
  - To view the McGrath device go to: http://www.lmana.com/mcgrath/index.html

COMPLICATIONS OF AIRWAY MANIPULATION

- Trauma to the airway could make further manipulation or ventilation more difficult or impossible. Prevent this by optimizing intubating conditions prior to airway instrumentation.
- Laryngospasm
  - Due to stimulation of the superior laryngeal nerve causing spasm of the laryngeal muscles and adduction of the vocal cords preventing air entry into the glottis.
  - It may occur at any time, but especially on induction or emergence, just after extubation or during ventilation with a mask or LMA.
  - Risk factors include light plane of anesthesia during airway manipulation, exposure to smoke at home, and recent upper respiratory infection (URI).
  - Diagnose it by the inability to ventilate.
  - Treat with positive-pressure ventilation.
  - Laryngospasm that is not relieved by positive pressure may require treatment with IV or IM succinylcholine. This can be associated with bradycardia. Therefore, atropine is often coadministered.
  - Resolution is heralded by the ability to ventilate. Remember, if the child is crying or phonating, his vocal cords are open
    - To view a video of laryngospasm go to: http://www.fauquierent.net/voice/misc/laryngospasm.mov
- Postextubation stridor or croup can be caused by the use of an ETT that is too large. Check for a cuff leak with positive-pressure ventilation to prevent this complication.

SHARING THE AIRWAY WITH THE SURGEONS

- The cardinal rule is always, always, always discuss your airway management with the surgeons when you will be sharing the airway, and if you think airway management could be challenging, have the surgeons in the room for induction and possibly prepared for a surgical airway.
- Cleft lip/palate repair: Use an RAE tube to stay out of the surgeons' way and avoid kinking of the ETT.
- Tonsillectomy: Use an RAE tube to stay out of the surgeons' way and avoid kinking of the ETT.
- Retropharyngeal or peritonsillar abscess drainage: RAE or straight ETT; discuss with the surgeon before you place it.
- Endoscopy for foreign body (FB) removal: If the FB is in the esophagus, place the ETT and then hold or secure the ETT tightly, as the endoscope may dislodge it during the procedure. If the FB is in the trachea or bronchus, it is often preferable NOT to intubate the trachea and let the surgeons go right in with the rigid bronchoscope. Sometimes the FB can be plucked out quickly. Other times you might need to ventilate through the ventilating bronchoscope. Jet ventilation is sometimes useful for these cases. Be prepared for anything and everything!
- Suspension microlaryngoscopy: You'll probably mask ventilate the patient in between passes of the scope or laser treatments, etc. Consider the use of total intravenous anesthesia (TIVA), e.g., propofol.
- Beware of the risks of possible airway fire when cautery or laser is used in the airway; you must limit the inspired oxygen concentration to < 30%. Nitrous oxide can also sustain a flame.

REFERENCES

1. Principato JJ, Wolf P. Pediatric nasal resistance. *Laryngoscope* 1985;95:1067–1069.
2. Weiss M, Dullenkopf A, Fischer JE, Keller C, Gerber AC, and the European Paediatric Endotracheal Intubation Study Group. Prospective randomized controlled multicentre trial of cuffed or uncuffed endotracheal tubes in small children. *Br J Anaesth* 2009;103(6):867–873.
3. Dullenkopf A, Schmitz A, Gerber A, Weiss M. Tracheal sealing characteristics of pediatric cuffed tracheal tubes. *Pediatr Anesth* 2004;14:825–830.
4. Dullenkopf A, Gerber A, Weiss M. The microcuff tube allows a longer time interval until unsafe cuff pressures are reached in children. *Can J Anesth* 2004;51(10):997–1001.
5. Practice Guidelines for Management of the Difficult Airway: An updated report by the American Society of Anesthesiologists Task Force on Management of the Difficult Airway. *Anesthesiology* 2003;98:1269–1277.
6. D'Agostino J. Pediatric airway nightmares. *Emerg Med Clin North Am* 2010;28:119–126.

SUGGESTED READING

Finder JD. Airway clearance modalities in neuromuscular disease. *Paediatr Respir Rev* 2010;11:31–34.
Thevasagayam M, Rodger K, Cove D, Witmans M, El-Hakim H. Prevalence of laryngomalacia in children presenting with sleep disordered breathing. Laryngoscope 2010;120(8):1662–1666.

CHAPTER 19
SURGICAL AIRWAY

WENDY DALEY
JOHN DENNY
GEORGE P. BATSIDES
NEIL STOCKMASTER

When you sit to dine with a ruler, note well who is before you and put a knife to thy throat.
Proverbs 23:2
(The Anesthesiologist's Emergency Airway Arsenal)

INTRODUCTION

What Is It?
- Cricothyrotomy, aka cricothyroidotomy
- Creating an opening in the cricothyroid membrane (CTM), the space between the anterior inferior border of the thyroid cartilage and anterior superior border of the cricoid cartilage, and securing an artificial airway in the opening

INDICATIONS

- Help! You need an immediate airway because you cannot establish an orotracheal or nasotracheal airway and can't ventilate the patient.[1]
- Although this can't ventilate, can't intubate (CVCI) situation is to be avoided at all costs, even the most compulsive anesthesiologists cannot guarantee they will not run into it (and not from it!).
- If you are in a CVCI, consider the Guidelines for Management of the Difficult Airway, published by the American Society of Anesthesiologists (ASA).
- In this situation, most practitioners would quickly try to salvage a CVCI by inserting the laryngeal mask airway (LMA). Recognize that since these are supraglottic ventilatory devices, they will NOT fix all CVCI situations. Thus, it's pretty sweet to be comfortable with another rescue technique.
- With any technique, the time to bust out your moves is NOT on a blue 350-pound patient.
- Get familiar with the technique before the oximeter tone is so low that only your dog can hear it!

CONTRAINDICATIONS

- If you can, avoid cricothyroidotomy when the patient has sustained massive trauma to the larynx or cricoid cartilage.[1]
- Here are clinical situations that warrant a second thought, although when you have a patient in front of you in CVCI, you won't spend too much time on these points:
  - Intubated translaryngeally for more than 3 to 7 days: higher chance for developing subglottic stenosis
  - Preexisting laryngeal diseases (cancer, acute/chronic inflammation, epiglottitis, and neck masses): distorts normal neck anatomy
  - History of coagulopathy or bleeding diathesis should give pause to the anesthesiologist faced with this challenge.[2]

WHY

- KISS principle: Keep It Simple, Stupid
- Faster, simpler, less prone to cause bleeding, and most importantly, dear reader, QUICKER than tracheotomy
- By using the more exposed cricothyroid membrane, we avoid more difficult exposure associated with a traditional trach. This all translates into a quicker lifesaving procedure for the patient!

LOCATION, LOCATION, LOCATION!

Real estate is prime. A needle in the *thyro*hyoid membrane would not make for a happy anesthesiologist and patient.

- The CTM lies subcutaneously and midline in between the thyroid cartilage and the cricoid cartilage.
- Start with the patient's neck extended to expose the CTM.
- Try to avoid neck extension if there is evidence of trauma to the head or neck. It should not take significant extension to get good exposure.
- The thyroid cartilage (Adam's apple) is the most prominent landmark on the neck.
- The cricothyroid membrane lies 1 to 1½ finger breadths below the thyroid cartilage.
- The cricoid cartilage is the next cartilaginous structure below the thyroid cartilage.[2]
- Keep in mind the superior cricothyroid vessels cross the upper third of cricothyroid membrane in a horizontal manner. *Vessels are not your friends.* Avoid them (Figure 19-1).
- In cases where the normal anatomy cannot be identified, start by placing the small finger of the right hand in the suprasternal notch.
- Work your way up in a stepwise fashion with each adjacent finger touching the one below it.
- The index finger should end up on or near the cricothyroid membrane (CTM).[2]
- Fortunately for us, the vocal cords lie 1 cm above the CTM, and so are rarely injured (Figure 19-2).

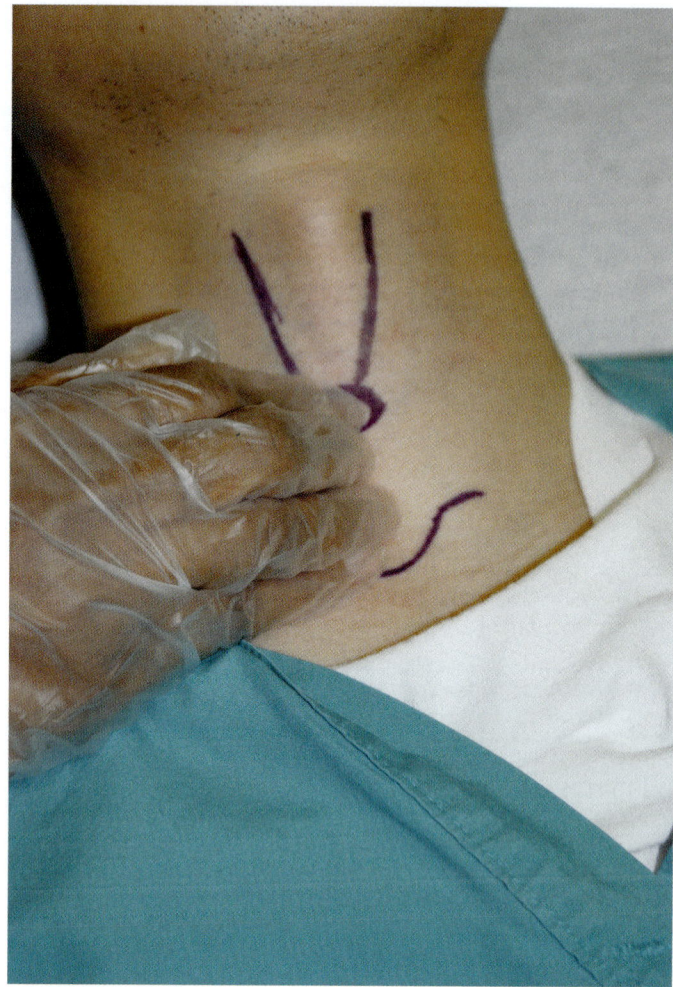

FIGURE 19-2 The pinky finger is at the sternal notch. Each consecutive finger is placed above the prior finger. The index finger ends up on the CTM.

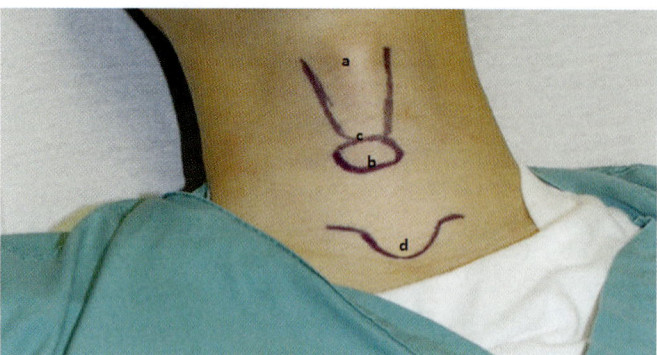

FIGURE 19-1 (a) Thyroid cartilage is the prominent structure in the upper midline of the neck. (b) Cricoid cartilage is beneath the thyroid prominence. (c) CTM lies between the thyroid and cricoid cartilages. (d) The sternal notch is the most inferior structure in the figure.

TECHNIQUE AND EQUIPMENT

OK, now that we have the anatomy, let's get that airway in! There are multiple techniques and equipment for placing an emergency airway. Here are the basic techniques and commonly used equipment for each.

TRANSTRACHEAL CATHETER VENTILATION

- A temporizing measure when an immediate airway is needed.
- It buys you and the patient TIME for placement of a more permanent airway.

- The patient will be oxygenated, although adequate ventilation is NOT ensured.
- Requires a special high-pressure system to provide adequate ventilation: hospital wall outlet O_2 without regulator set at a flow of 15 L/min, or an emergency jet ventilator (Mercury Medical).
- If these are lacking, an Ambu bag can temporarily be used.
- Surgical cricothyrotomy can then be performed.
- Requires insertion of a catheter over a needle.
- Additional benefits are that the anesthesiologist can breathe again.

Equipment[3]

Always have your equipment ready just in case the patient's clinical situation suddenly deteriorates. If time permits, universal precautions will never hurt you or the patient; so go on, get those sterile gloves, gown, and mask. For this technique, all you need are standard hospital materials:

- Large-bore needles 14-, 16-, 18-gauge (G)
- 10 mL syringe half-filled with normal saline
- 3 mL syringe without plunger
- Ambu bag
- Size 7.5 endotracheal tube adapter that attaches to a 3 mL syringe without plunger
- Suture or tracheostomy tie
- Some extra stuff if time permits: chlorhexidine, sterile drape, 1% lidocaine with syringe for local injection

Technique[3]

- If (rarely!!) the clinical situation permits, prep the site with chlorhexidine, inject 1% lidocaine subcutaneously into the site, and drape the site.
- Stabilize the larynx by holding the thyroid cartilage in between the first and third finger.
- With the index finger palpate the CTM.
- With a 10 mL syringe filled with 5 mL of saline attached to the needle hub, direct the needle through the lower border of the CTM in a caudad direction. *Remember who your friends are; stay away from the upper border of the CTM.*
- Aspirate while inserting until air bubbles through the normal saline. Air bubbles confirm tracheal position. If you don't see air bubbles, reposition and start again.
- In this situation the anesthesiologist looks like a kid who has just discovered how to blow bubbles. Refrain from overexcitement, you have more to do.
- Advance the catheter over the needle until the hub sits securely on the skin. Flexible catheters are prone to kinking! One hand must hold the hub at skin to prevent this. Cook Medical makes a very robust, wire reinforced catheter just for this purpose (Figures 19-3 and 19-4).
- Preferably, use an emergency jet ventilator now.
- Connect a Luer lock to the hub of the catheter.
- One person MUST be dedicated to holding the catheter in place at the skin so that it does NOT kink or migrate. If using a 16-G catheter and a 50-psi O_2 source, delivering inspiration of 1 to 1.5 second only will typically deliver 400 to 750 cc tidal volume. Be sure to allow for egress of O_2 by also using oral and nasal airways (Figures 19-5 and 19-6).
- If you don't have a jet ventilator, you can at least temporarily oxygenate (although not ventilate) the patient by connecting to an Ambu bag. This may buy time for a more definitive airway. However, this is much inferior to the above technique of jet ventilation through a catheter, and is only TEMPORARY!
- Disconnect the syringe and connect the hub of the catheter to the 3 mL syringe minus the plunger with the 7.5 endotracheal tube adapter attached. Be careful; if you accidentally let go of the hub, you can lose your tracheal position and end up subcutaneously. Don't let go of the hub!
- Connect the adapter to the Ambu bag. Because of good old Poiseuille's law, there is so much resistance through that small catheter that you probably WON'T see bilateral chest rise and fall, but you will hopefully at least hear the pulse oximeter rise in pitch, and a noncyanotic patient should also relieve your tachycardia and keep your pants dry.
- Make sure all of your work is not for naught. Hold the catheter in position until a more definitive airway can be secured.

Complications[3]

- A kinked catheter won't allow for adequate ventilation; it is preventable by using kink-resistant Teflon catheters and keeping the hub exclusive; only one person is in charge of holding the hub.
- Barotrauma can occur with a high ventilation rate, not allowing for adequate expiration; prevent by decreasing frequency and allowing adequate expiratory time.
- Subcutaneous emphysema: minimize by using kink-resistant Teflon catheters, keep the hub exclusive, and use a commercially available cricothyroidotomy catheter with attached flanges for securing the catheter, applying pressure over the puncture site for a few minutes to prevent air leak after catheter removal.

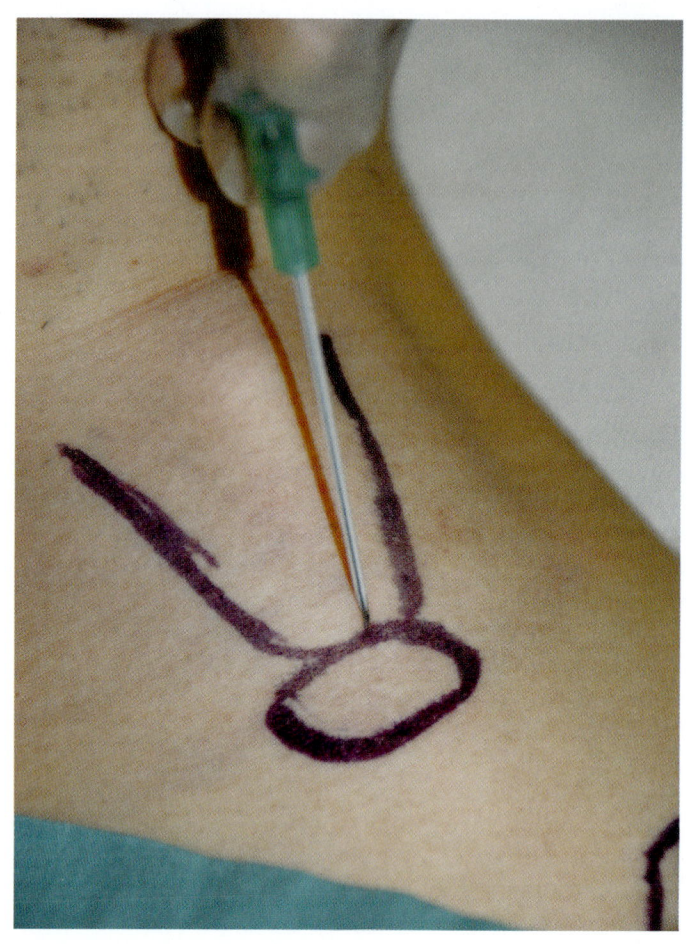

FIGURE 19-3 An 18-G needle attached to a 10-mL syringe filled with 5-mL normal saline (NS) is directed at the CTM in a caudal direction.

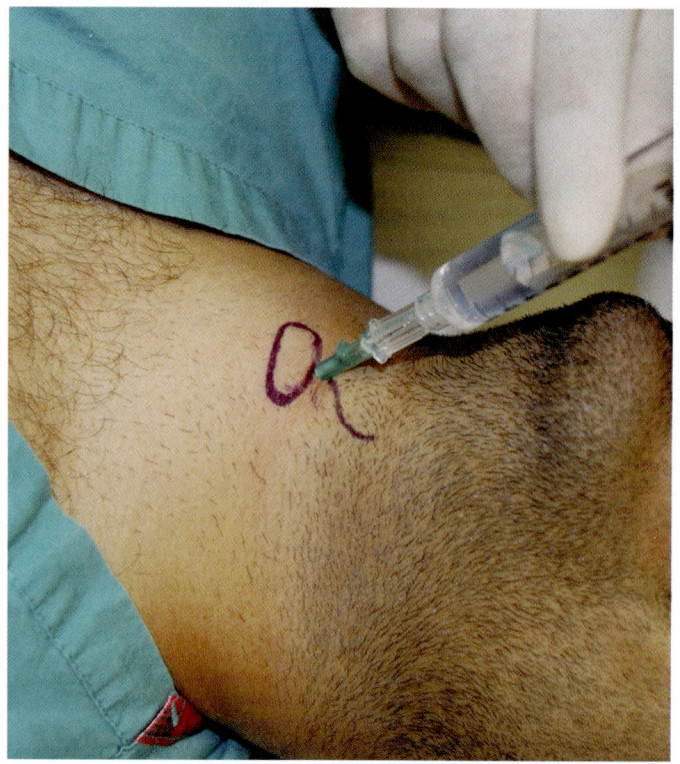

FIGURE 19-4 An 18-G hub sitting firmly on the skin with a 10-mL saline syringe showing air bubbles aspirated from the needle in the trachea.

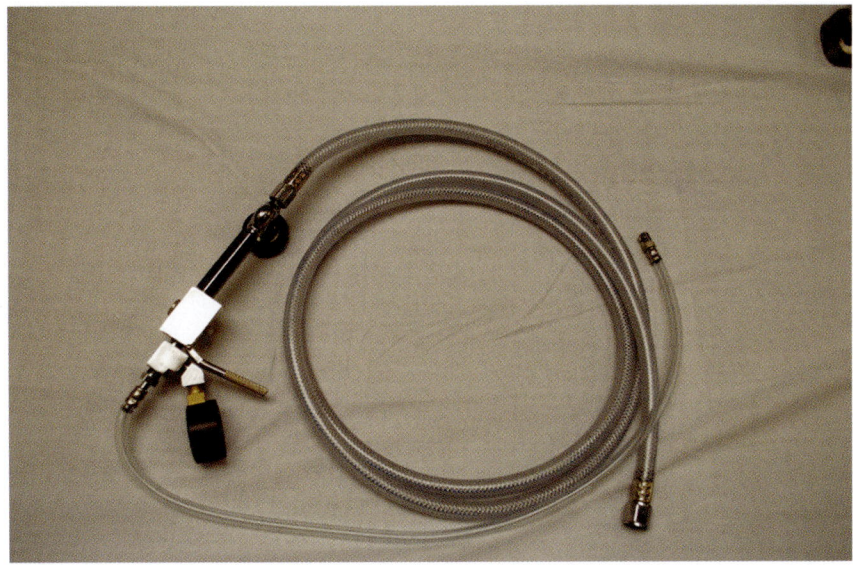

FIGURE 19-5 Jet ventilator.

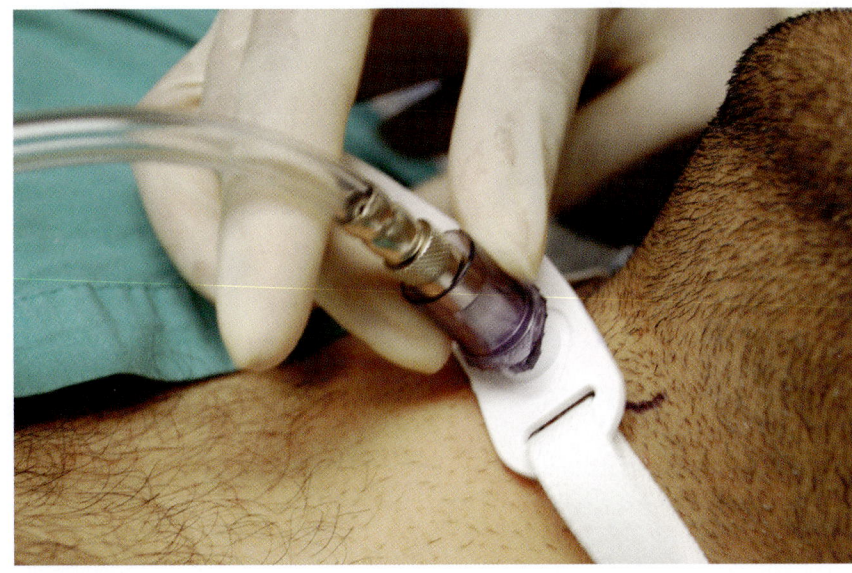

FIGURE 19-6 Jet ventilator attached to an airway catheter used in the percutaneous dilational technique described below.

PERCUTANEOUS DILATIONAL CRICOTHYROTOMY

- Requires a skin incision with introduction of a guidewire inserted through a needle or catheter through the CTM.
- A dilator is introduced and a catheter threaded over a guidewire.
- Allows for insertion of a larger diameter airway to allow for ventilation with conventional ventilators.

Equipment

Different kits are available in each hospital system, e.g., Melker Emergency Cricothyrotomy Catheter set, Portex Mini-Trach II, Pertrach, and Tri-anim sets. For this demonstration the Arndt Emergency Cricothyrotomy Catheter™ set (Cook Medical) will be used:

- 5 mL syringe with normal saline
- 18-G introducer needle
- 180-G catheter introducer needle

- 0.038 inch-diameter stainless steel guidewire with flexible tip
- 9-French airway catheter with dilator
- Connecting tube
- Scalpel blade (Figures 19-7 and 19-8)

Technique

- If (rarely!) the clinical situation permits, prep the site with chlorhexidine, inject 1% lidocaine subcutaneously into the site and drape the site.
- Stabilize the larynx by holding the thyroid cartilage in between the first and third finger.
- With the index finger palpate the CTM.
- Make a 1- to 1.5-cm vertical incision in the lower border of the CTM. Remember, those vessels on the upper border of the CTM are not your friends.
- Advance the 18-G introducer needle with attached syringe into the incision site in a caudad direction.
- Aspirate while advancing. Aspiration of free air confirms airway placement. If you don't see air bubbles, reposition your needle.
- Now advance the guidewire through the catheter several centimeters.
- Remove the introducer needle while leaving the guidewire in place.
- Advance the dilator, tapered end first, into the connector end of the airway catheter and secure at the hub by the female Luer lock connector.
- Advance this assembly over the guidewire until the proximal stiff end of the guidewire is completely through and visible at the handle end of the dilator.
- Advance the airway over the guidewire while removing the guidewire and dilator simultaneously. Fix the catheter in place with the tracheostomy tape strip.
- Connect the airway catheter to Y-tubing and a ventilating source (Figures 19-9, 19-10, 19-11 and 19-12).

Complications

- Subcutaneous emphysema
- Hemorrhage: apply direct pressure to control bleed

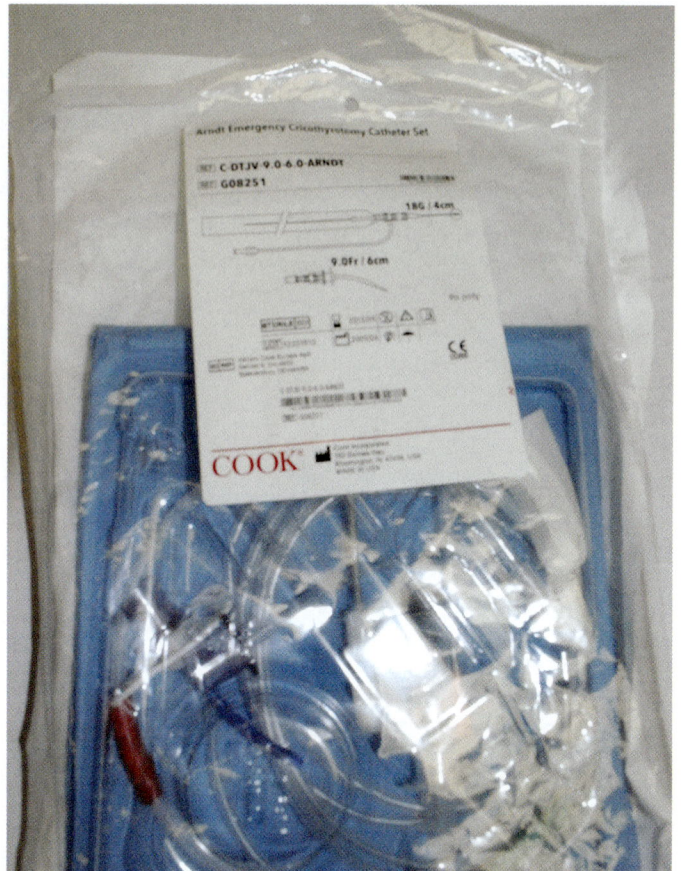

FIGURE 19-7 Arndt Cricothyrotomy Kit package.

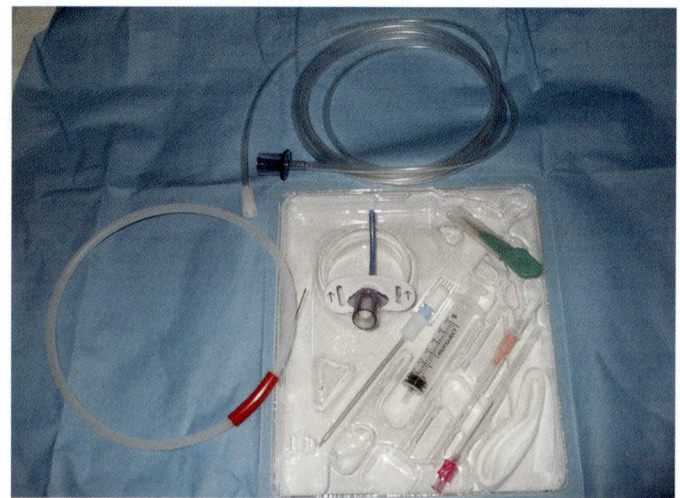

FIGURE 19-8 Arndt Cricothyrotomy Kit.

Chapter 19 SURGICAL AIRWAY

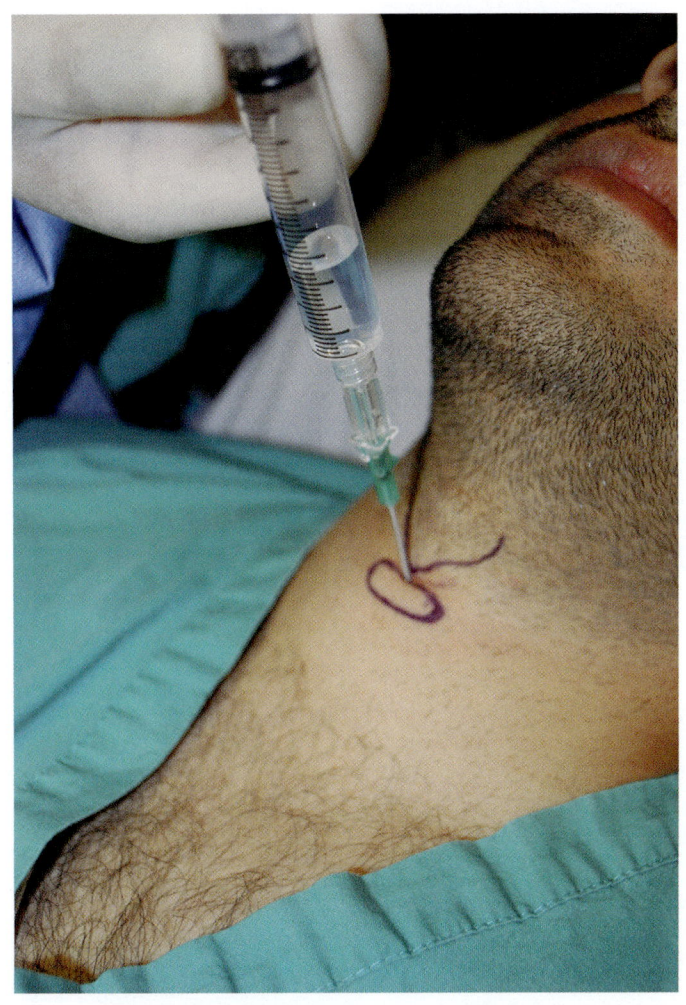

FIGURE 19-9 An 18-G needle and saline-filled syringe directed caudally at CTM. Note that the Arndt 18-G introducer needle is not depicted here.

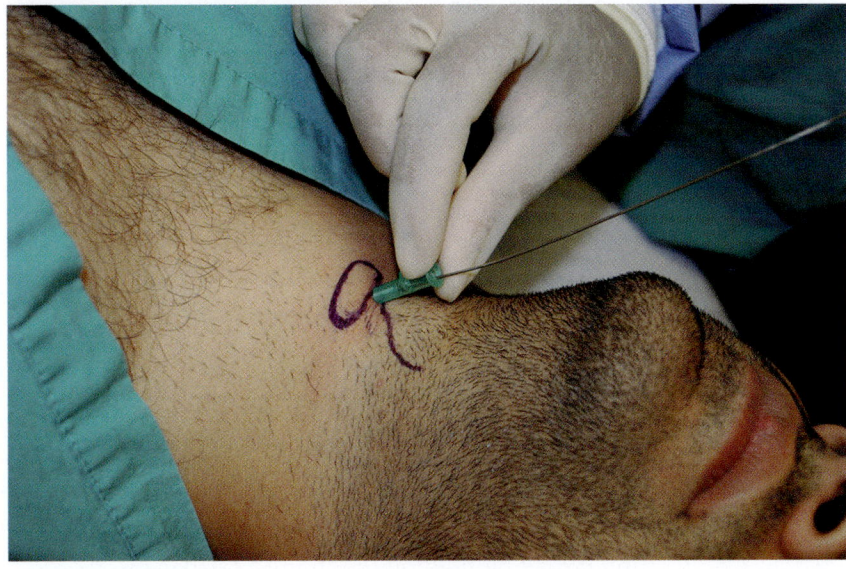

FIGURE 19-10 Guidewire being inserted through the 18-G hub into the cricothyroid membrane. Note that the Arndt 18-G introducer needle is not depicted here.

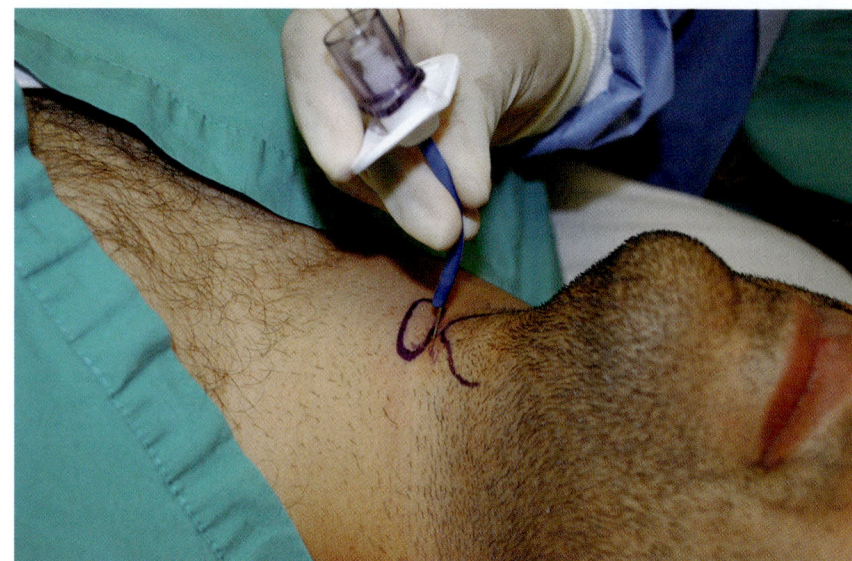

FIGURE 19-11 Dilator and catheter directed over guidewire through the CTM.

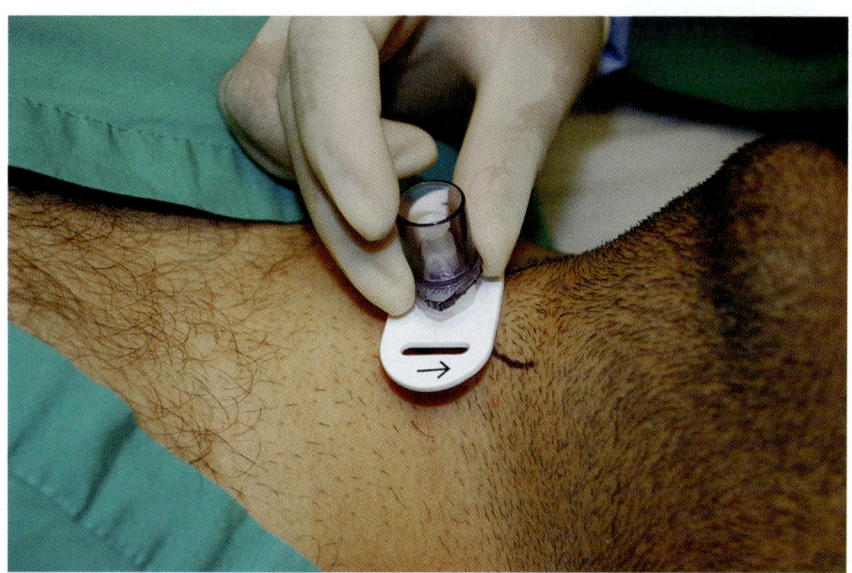

FIGURE 19-12 Airway catheter positioned on skin.

SURGICAL CRICOTHYROTOMY

- Use of a scalpel to create an opening between the skin and cricothyroid space to place an endotracheal tube (ETT) or tracheostomy.
- Allows for ventilation with conventional ventilators

Equipment[1]
- Tracheostomy tube
- Scalpel with No. 10 or 11 blade
- Curved hemostat
- Trousseau dilator
- Tracheal hook
- 10 mL syringe
- Suture

Technique[1]
- If (rarely) the clinical situation permits, prep the site with chlorhexidine, inject 1% lidocaine subcutaneously into the site, and drape the site.
- While standing on the patient's right side, stabilize the larynx by holding the thyroid cartilage in between the first and third finger.
- With the index finger, palpate the CTM.

- Use the scalpel to make a vertical 2.5-cm incision into the subcutaneous tissue.
- Use the hemostat to make a dissection into the subcutaneous tissue.
- Make horizontal incision though the CTM.
- Extend the incision laterally in both directions.
- Keep the scalpel within the incision until the tracheal hook is inserted and the distal portion of the trachea is pulled up.
- Remove the scalpel only when the hook is in place. Insert the dilator and open the membrane vertically.
- Insert the tracheostomy tube.
- Remove the obturator.
- Inflate the balloon.
- Tie the tracheostomy in place.
- Attach the tracheostomy to a Y-piece and connect to a ventilating source.
- With all airways check for bilateral chest rise and fall, auscultate, and use an easy cap, and an end-tidal CO_2 detector, if available.

Complications[1]

- Hemorrhage: apply direct pressure to control bleed. You may need to ligate major vessels.
- Esophageal perforation: try to prevent by only going as far as 1.3 cm deep
- Subcutaneous emphysema: limit the length of the horizontal incision.

THE SURGICAL AIRWAY

Tracheostomy: A Brief Historical Perspective

Tracheostomy, or more precisely, tracheotomy, has for centuries been the surgical gold standard of airway control. Opening the trachea in the neck to improve airflow and release humors is portrayed on Egyptian tablets dating to 3600 BC. The first documented attempt at tracheostomy is often credited to Asclepiads of Persia in 100 BC. In 160 AD, Galen elegantly described the central role of the trachea by noting that "by blowing air through a reed into the trachea, airflow is noted in the bronchioles." However, the first successful tracheostomy to treat acute airway obstruction secondary to a laryngeal abscess was reported by Antonio Musa Prasovala, an Italian physician, in 1546 (Figure 19-13).

For the next several centuries, the procedure grew in clinical acceptance slowly, and was mainly employed during emergencies related to infections or inflammation of the upper airway. In fact, George Washington, the first president of the United States, is widely believed to have died from acute bacterial epiglottitis. One of the physicians tending President Washington, Dr. Elisha Cullen Dick, suggested performing a tracheostomy in an attempt to relieve the president's pending respiratory failure, only to be overturned by two other physicians, Dr. Gustavus Brown and Dr. James Craik, the president's personal physician, who felt the procedure was too dangerous.

Tracheostomies became much more commonplace during the diphtheria epidemics of the 1800s. It was during this timeframe that the first successful tracheostomy was reported in a child. Trendelenburg first suggested the use of cuffed tracheostomy tubes in 1869. In 1909, Dr. Chevalier Jackson refined the surgical technique, moving the entry point from the proximal trachea to the fourth or fifth tracheal ring, in an attempt to avoid subglottic stenosis, which was increasingly common during the polio epidemic. Since this time, tracheostomy has transitioned from an emergent procedure to treat pending airway collapse to an elective procedure for airway stabilization in ventilator dependent patients (Figure 19-14).

Who Should Perform

General surgeons; trauma surgeons; ear, nose, and throat (ENT) specialists; and thoracic surgeons.

Indications

Chronic and acute respiratory insufficiency, head and neck trauma and head and neck surgery, emergency airway control (cricothyroidotomy is preferable here; see above).

Open Tracheostomy: Sometimes Bigger Is Better!

- Location: operating room or ICU (well lit, please)
- Positioning: supine with neck slightly hyperextended (baring any neck trauma or fusion); arms tucked and shoulder roll placed (Figure 19-15)
- Thyroid cartilage and cricothyroid membrane are identified.
- Landmarks: thyroid cartilage, cricothyroid membrane, and sternal notch identified (and marked if need be) (Figures 19-16, 19-17 and 19-18)
- In cases of large breasts or extreme amounts of adipose tissue, taping of soft tissue for exposure may be required. Exposure is everything! Chin to mid-sternum prepped. Pulse oximeter placed and functioning. End tidal CO_2 monitor available and functioning.

Procedure

- Clearly identify landmarks. A 2- to 3-cm incision is made one finger breath above the sternal notch (in general). Cautery at low settings is used to transect subcutaneous tissue and platysma. Self-retaining retractor are placed, and strap muscles are identified and incised vertically in the midline. Palpation of trachea should be performed through each step (layer) to confirm midline location.

- If straps are not identified properly, muscle bleeding or bleeding from anterior jugular veins may occur. Please note that the anterior jugular veins can bleed briskly and can be clipped or ligated with impunity. After straps are separated, the thyroid isthmus may be seen; if so, it should be elevated cephalad (for those of you educated in California, this means toward the head).
- To elevate the thyroid isthmus, a peanut is used; any midline vessels are clipped or cauterized, and the gland is gently teased upward. If need be (and this is rare) it can be divided. The trachea is again palpated to ensure midline location (we can't overemphasize this).
- The pretracheal fascia is incised, and the second and third tracheal rings are identified. The trachea may be cleaned off a bit laterally for better exposure (Figure 19-19).
- Good exposure here is key! A self-retaining retractor and hand-held retractors are necessary. A good assistant with three hands is key (see above). Not to mention a good headlight. We find this one operation that we will not perform without a headlight.
- It is also important that all the appropriate equipment be on the surgical field.
- A tracheal hook is placed in the first ring, and it is elevated slightly cephalad and toward the ceiling.

At this point, if you are worried about a difficult postoperative airway, two Prolene stay sutures are placed through the trachea adjacent to the lateral aspects of the future ostomy. These are ultimately air knotted and tagged to the skin with Steri-Strips later. (Important aside: these can be very useful in the early postoperative period (first 2 weeks) if the tracheostomy becomes dislodged. In an emergency the sutures can be pulled up gently at the bedside to help deliver the trachea toward the wound so that it can be safely recannulated).
- Once the trachea is exposed and elevated via the hook, the anesthesia teas is alerted so that the ETT tape is cut and so that they are alerted to the timing of the tracheal incision. Good communication is imperative here (Figure 19-20).
- Important point to remember: loss of an airway is **as** dangerous as dropping a knife on the aorta. In either case, death will ensue, if it is not remedied quickly! A knife and Alice clamp or tooth forceps are then used to excise a small rectangular segment of the middle of the third tracheal ring.
- The third tracheal ring is ideal; however, in certain cases it's too low and the first or second needs to be

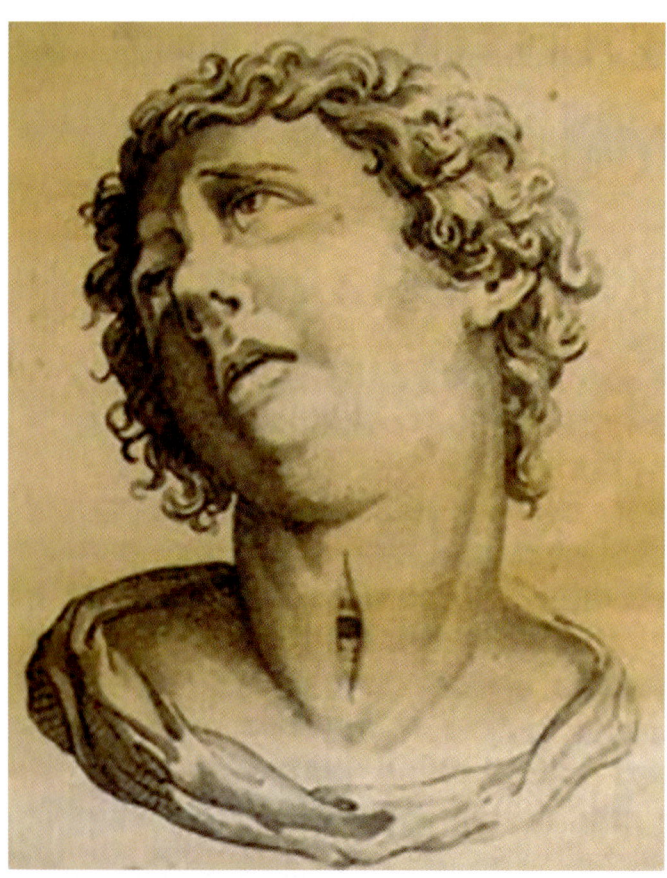

FIGURE 19-13 Historical neck picture 1.

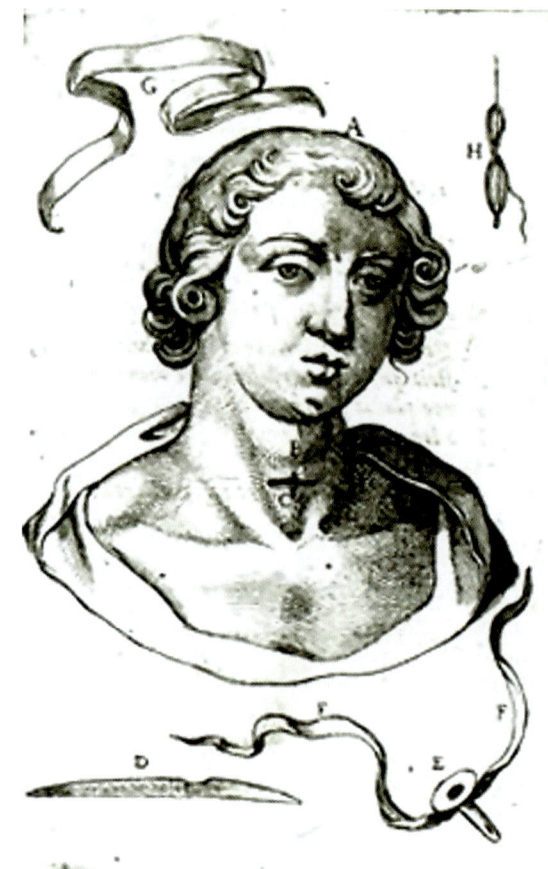

FIGURE 19-14 Historical neck picture 2.

incised. Remember: too low can put the patient at risk for the dreaded tracheoinnominate fistula.
- Alert the anesthesia team that the balloon of the ETT will likely be ruptured. Occasionally, if there is brisk bleeding from the edges of the trachea, ventilation is held and light cautery can be used on the edges (try to avoid flames) (Figure 19-21).
- The assistant must maintain a firm hold of the tracheal hook. A tracheal three-prong dilator is used to dilate the ostomy. The trach tube (which is prelubricated and the balloon pretested) is brought into the field as the ETT is pulled back under direct vision.
- Suction here is imperative to clear the trachea of any secretions. Once the tube is just above the stoma, the trach is inserted, gently rotating it as it passes through the stoma. Great care is taken to avoid a pretracheal mediastinal track. The tracheal hook, good lighting, and a well-dilated trach stoma help avoid this potentially devastating complication.
- Once the trach is placed, the obturator is removed and the inner cannula inserted. The patient is placed on the vent via the trach, the cuff is inflated, and end-tidal CO_2 is monitored as well as the pulse oximeter and heart rate.
- Critical points to remember: If there is any doubt in placement and the monitors are telling you the trach is not in, auscultation may help. If there is still a question, the trach must be removed and the ETT readvanced until the problem is identified. Remember: CO_2 is the most sensitive indicator, and saturation is second (this may take a while to rebound); bradycardia is an ominous sign and should be acted upon quickly, by obtaining a safe air way, either by recannulation if easy, re-intubation, or even cricothyroidotomy.

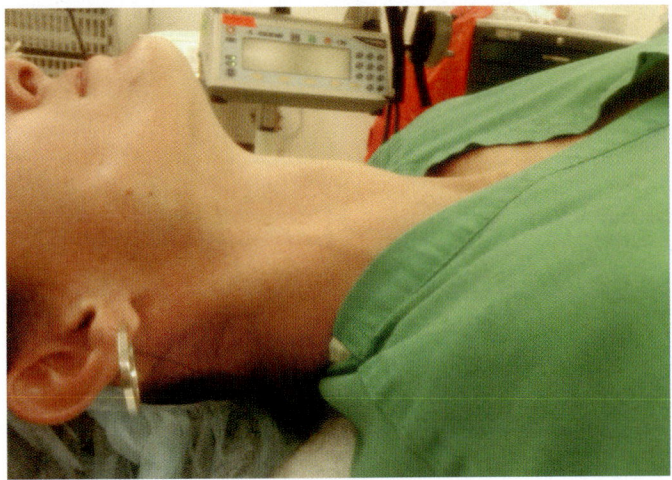

FIGURE 19-15 Neck positioning (hyperextended).

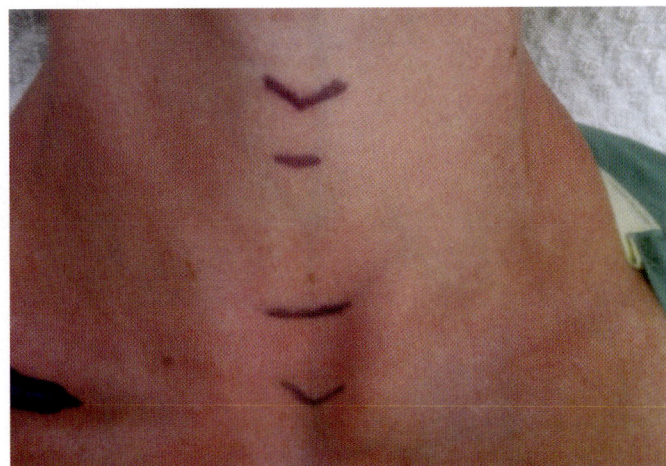

FIGURE 19-17 Marking of anatomical landmarks.

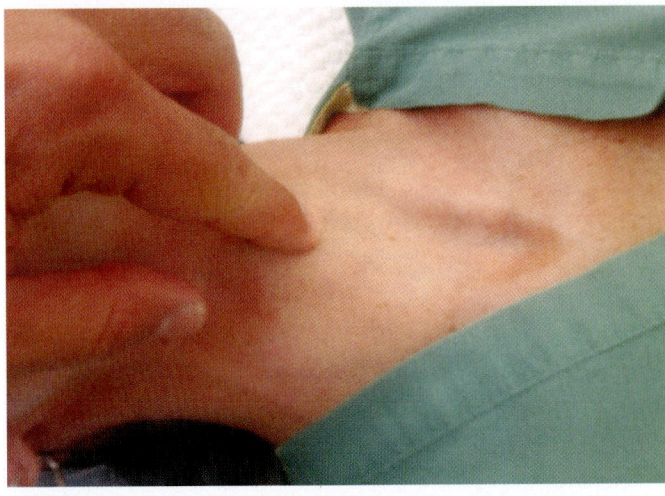

FIGURE 19-16 Palpation of anatomical landmarks.

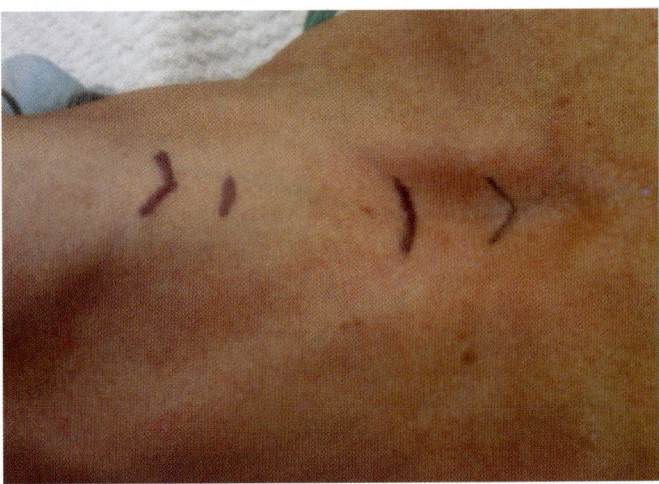

FIGURE 19-18 Marked anatomical landmarks 2.

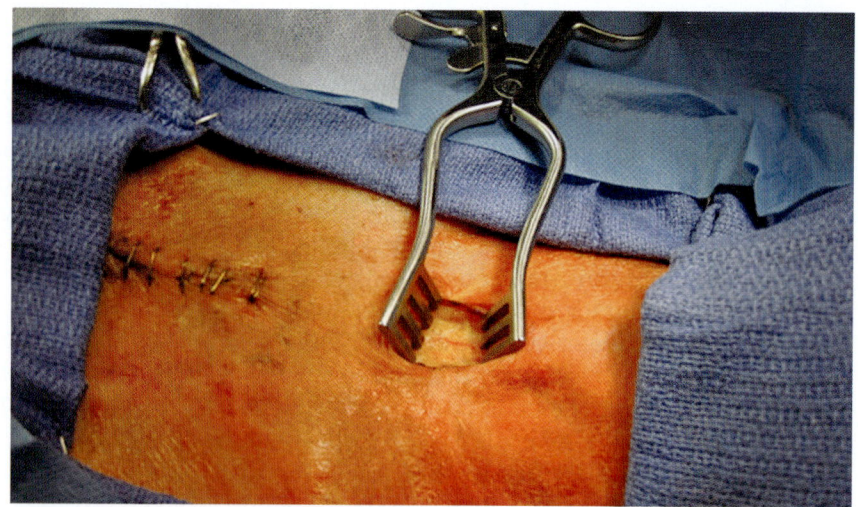

FIGURE 19-19 Tracheal exposure with self-retaining retractor.

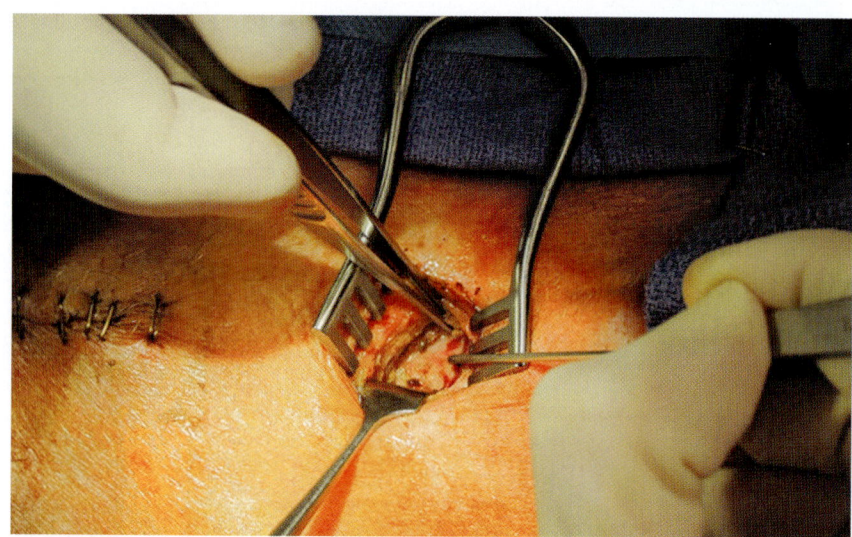

FIGURE 19-20 Excision tracheal ring and hook elevation.

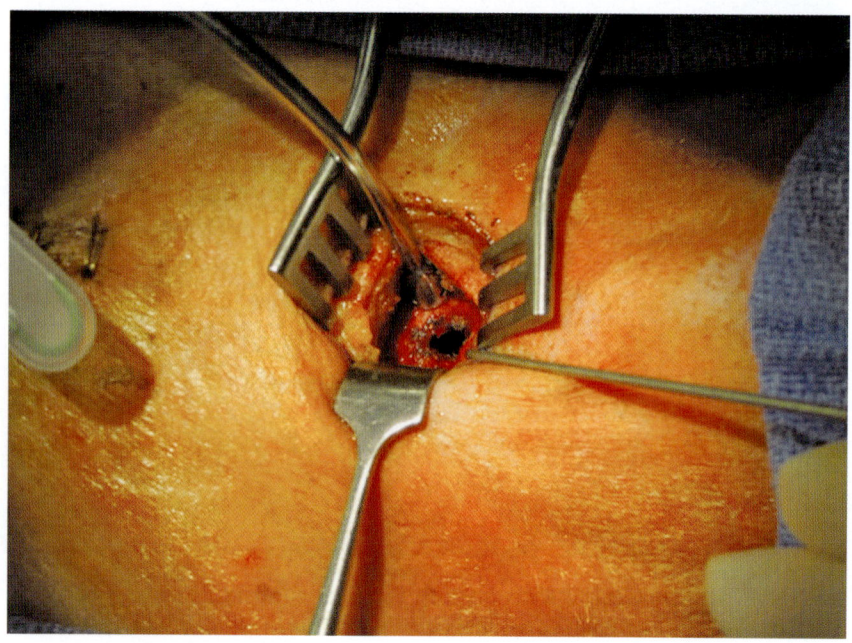

FIGURE 19-21 Application of tracheal hook.

PERCUTANEOUS TRACHEOSTOMY

- Similar setup and positioning as open tracheostomy. Please ensure all percutaneous equipment is in package and functional, and bronchoscopy cart available (bronchoscopic guidance is preferable). Sometimes the "minimally invasive" percutaneous tracheostomy procedure can lull one into a false sense of security (Figure 19-22).
- The airway is obviously a serious issue and should be treated as such! The "it's just a trach" attitude can kill. There is no role for cowboy surgeons or anesthesiologists in airway management.
- Preparation is key. All OR staff should be attentive and prepared for the worst.
- Authors' soap box: Although this procedure is often done electively in intensive care units, we do not agree with this approach. Loss of just one airway in that type of setting will convince you as well. Please try your best not to be part of that.
- Landmarks identified (see above). Area anesthetized with lidocaine/Marcaine. A 1 to 2-cm transverse incision is made (same location).
- The catheter introducer needle (with a 5-cc saline-filled syringe) is inserted into the midline of third tracheal ring. If no bronchoscope is available, the syringe is aspirated as the needle is inserted. Once brisk bubbling of air is encountered, the catheter is advanced and the needle withdrawn. This should be reconfirmed by refilling the syringe and reaspirating. A nice continuous stream of air/bubbles should be seen. Easier yet is stepping into the modern age and using a bronchoscope! In this case, as the needle is advanced, the patient is bronched simultaneously; once the needle is visualized in the trachea, via the bronch, the catheter is advanced and needle withdrawn.
- The 0.052-inch guidewire is thus inserted. This can be visualized going down the trach (a nice concept).
- Next, the guiding catheter is passed over the wire and inserted up to the skin level positioning mark. At this point, a series of well-lubricated dilators can be passed or the single Ciaglia Blue Rhino dilator passed (preferable) over the wire up to the skin level guide.
- Please note the trach (8 or 6 Shiley) is also prelubricated prior to this and loaded on the largest single dilator (Figure 19-23).
- The end-tidal CO_2 monitor must be ready (or EZ cap CO_2 detection monitor if you are doing this in a cave and dislike the patient).
- The Blue Rhino dilator is removed, leaving the wire in place, and the dilator with the loaded (lubricated) trach is passed into the airway.
- Subsequently the wire and dilator are removed with one easy pull while the trach is held firm on the skin and the trach cuff inflated. The patient is placed on the ventilator and CO_2 is confirmed. The trach is then secured (four-point suturing and trach fastener).

Modified Open Technique: Authors' Choice

- Positioning and prep are identical to the open procedure.
- Landmarks and incision are identical.
- Platysma transected and strap muscles are incised vertically in the midline.
- Similar to the open procedure, self-retaining and handheld retractors are necessary.

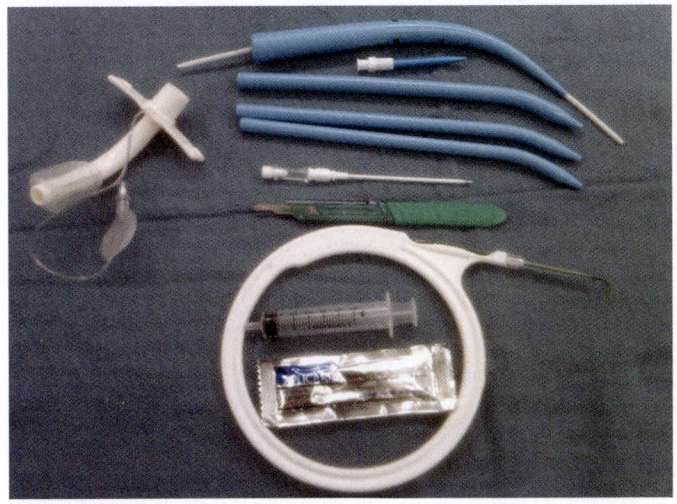

FIGURE 19-22 Percutaneous tracheostomy kit.

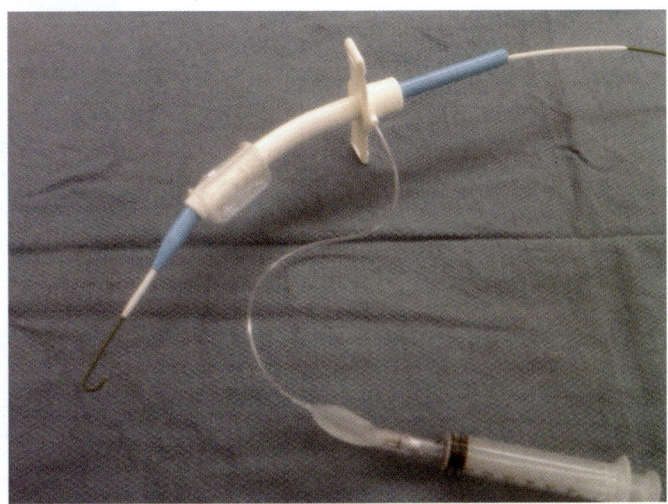

FIGURE 19-23 Trach loaded on dilator.

- The thyroid isthmus is elevated if need be, and the pretracheal fascia is incised. The tracheal hook is used to elevate and expose the third ring.
- As in the classic open tracheostomy, a small portion of third ring (preferable) is excised. (The anesthesia team has been notified and the guidewire is ready up in the field.) (Figure 19-24)
- The wire is passed directly into the trachea, once the ETT is pulled back (under direct vision). Please note: good suction and lighting are imperative here (Figure 19-25).
- The Blue Rhino single-stage dilator is passed over the wire up to the skin level mark. The dilator is then removed, leaving the wire. This can all be done rather quickly (when necessary the ventilator can be held for this step, to minimize heavy airway secretions and optimize visualization) (Figure 19-26).
- Subsequently, the preloaded and lubricated dilator and trach unit are thus passed into the airway (Figure 19-27).
- The dilator and wire are removed, the inner cannula is inserted, and the patient is placed on the ventilator via the tracheostomy. End-tidal CO_2 and pulse oximeter are checked. Mind you, we are not telling anesthesiologists how to do their job, but the ETT should be left in place (just above tracheostomy, in the airway) until a stable airway is confirmed and sutured in place (Figure 19-28).

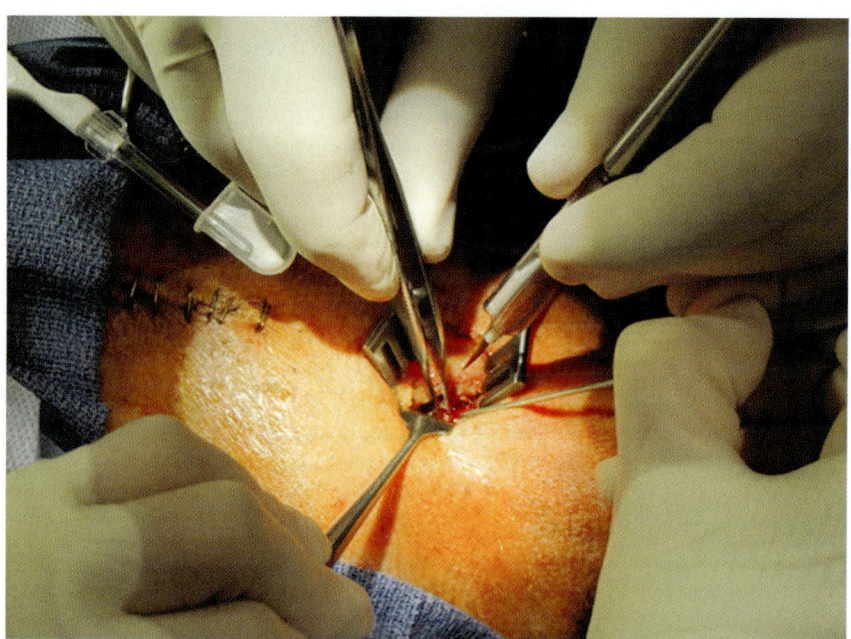

FIGURE 19-24 Excision of tracheal ring.

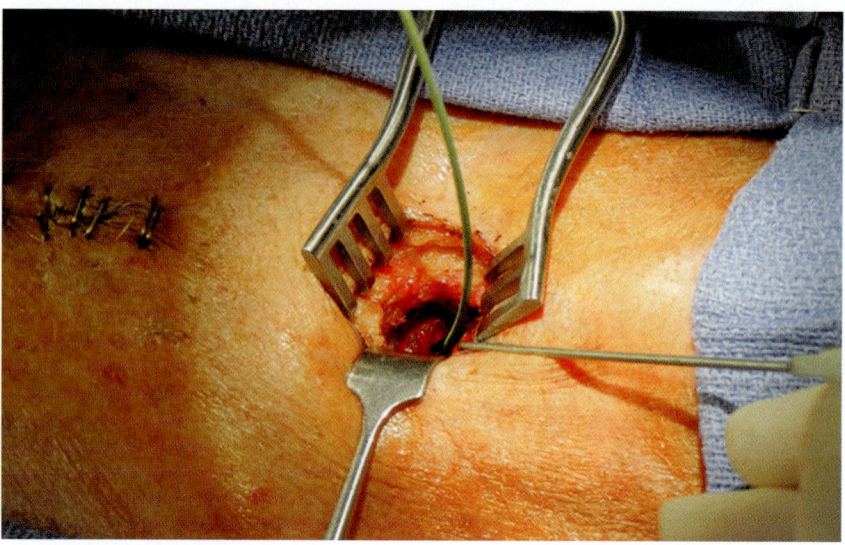

FIGURE 19-25 Insertion of tracheal guidewire.

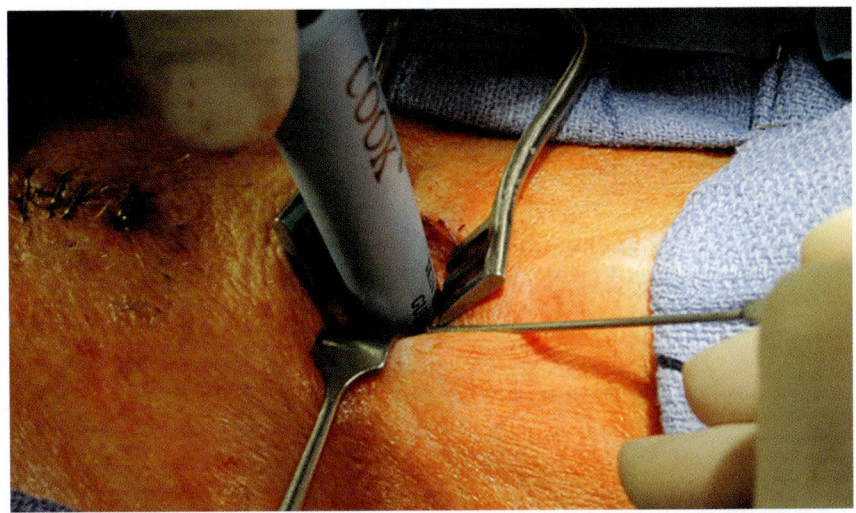

FIGURE 19-26 Tracheal dilatation over guidewire.

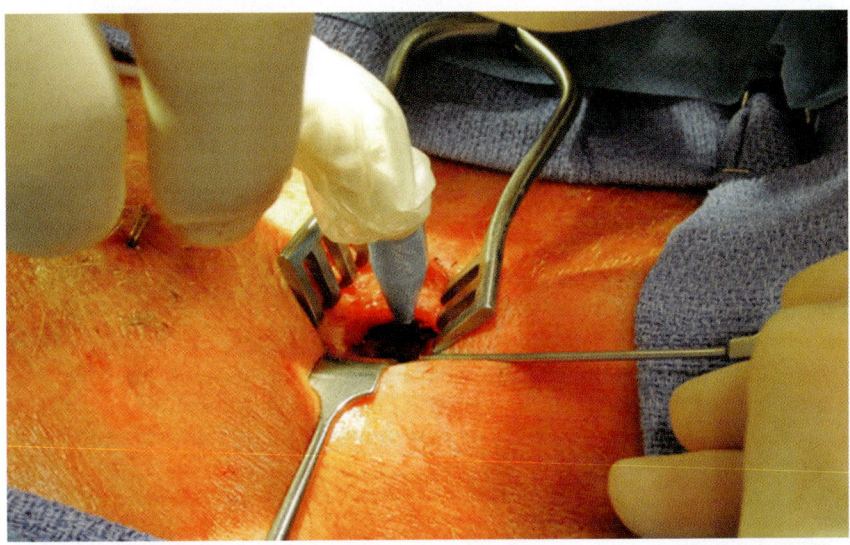

FIGURE 19-27 Insertion of trach/dilator over guidewire.

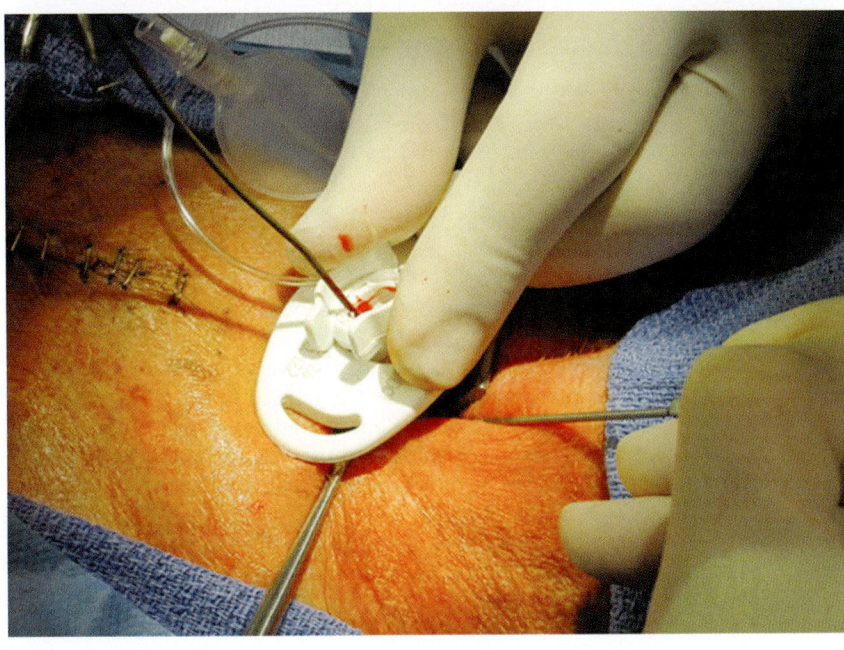

FIGURE 19-28 Removal of dilator and guidewire.

- The trach is sutured at four points and a tracheal fastener is placed around the neck. The goal here is to make it safe when the patient is moved/treated later on in the ICU or the ward.
- We like the "open" guidewire and dilator technique. It seems to minimize the occurrence of false pretracheal passages.
- We believe the single-pass dilator technique, rather than the old three-pronged dilator, minimizes sharp edges and thus minimizes trach cuff tears.
- We also believe that the "modified" open technique, if done properly, will minimize not only airway loss but also bleeding complications (i.e., the thyroid is mobilized if needed, not just dilated and cannulated).

TRACHEOSTOMY COMPLICATIONS

Bleeding

- Bleeding after a tracheostomy can result from a multitude of sources, from the mundane skin edge to the dreaded tracheoinnominate fistula.
- The first priority during the evaluation for postoperative tracheostomy hemorrhage is to assess the patency and correct location of the tracheostomy tube. If any question arises, the patient should be orotracheally intubated immediately.
- Next, posttracheostomy bleeding is assessed by observing the amount and location of bleeding, i.e., endoluminal or around the tracheostomy tube. Skin edge or soft tissue bleeding can often be easily controlled with local maneuvers, such as electrocautery, wound packing, or suture control.
- Endoluminal hemorrhage should be assessed with bronchoscopy to evaluate for tracheal erosion, endoluminal lesions/masses, or evidence of fistula.
- If exsanguinating hemorrhage is noted endoluminally and a tracheoinnominate fistula is suspected, immediate orotracheal intubated is performed, followed by arteriography or other imaging modality, if time permits, ideally in the operating room. If not, then emergent digital compression is performed by occluding the innominate artery against the underside of the sternum while preparing for emergent sternotomy and direct surgical ligation, and soft tissue interposition with possible vascular reconstruction.

Airway Fires

- During elective and emergent airway procedures, the presence of concentrated oxygen raises the risk of operative site/airway fire. These can, and should, be best avoided by thoughtful and consistent communication between surgeons and anesthesia providers.
- Announcing that the airway is nearly exposed should prompt minimization of concentrated oxygen, as tolerated by patient factors. Additionally, extreme care must be utilized with the use of electrocautery to enter or control hemorrhage associated with the trachea.

ACKNOWLEDGMENT

Special thanks to Jennifer Mohr, for posing for our photos.

REFERENCES

1. Hsiao J, Pacheco-Fowler V. Cricothyroidotomy. *N Engl J Med Videos in Clinical Medicine* 2008;358:e25. http://www.nejm.org.libproxy.umdnj.edu/doi/full/10.1056/NEJMvcm0706755
   Good video showing cricothyroidotomy.
2. Melker R, Kost K. (2007). Benumof's airway management: principles and practice. In: *Percutaneous dilational cricothyrotomy and tracheostomy.* Philadelphia: Mosby Elsevier; 2007, pp 640–678.
   Details equipment for cricothyrotomy.
3. Mittal MK. Needle cricothyroidotomy with percutaneous transtracheal ventilation. *UptoDate Online* 2010;18.2. http://www.uptodate.com/home/content/topic.do?topicKey=ped_proc/11574#
   Details indications, risks and the procedure for needle cricothyroidotomy.

SUGGESTED READING

Gaufberg SV, Workman TP. New needle cricothyroidotomy setup. *Am J Emerg Med* 2004;22(1):37–39.
Summary of cricothyrotomy procedure and ventilation techniques.
Graamans K, Pirsig W, Biefel K. The shift in the indications for the tracheostomy between 1940 and 1955: an historical review. *J Laryngol Otol* 1999;113(7):624–627.
Morens DM. Death of a president. *N Engl J Med* 1999;341(24): 1845–1849.
Ridley RW, Zwischenberger JB. Tracheoinnominate fistula: surgical management of an iatrogenic disaster. *J Laryngol Otol* 2006;120(8):676–680. Epub 2006 May 19.
Rogers ML, et al. Airway fire during tracheostomy: prevention strategies for surgeons and anaesthetists. *Ann R Coll Surg Engl* 2001;83:376.
Stock CR. What is past is prologue: a short history of the development of the tracheostomy. *ENT J* 1987;66(4):166–169.

CHAPTER 20
SMOOTH AWAKENING

MICHAEL WONG
RENU CHHOKRA

A **smooth** sea never made a skillful mariner.

English proverb

WHAT IS SMOOTH AWAKENING?

Awakening from anesthesia: promptly, smoothly, without fighting and without pain for the patient and yourself.

Other Names
- Controlled emergence
- Elegant emergence
- Gradual awakening

Often Confused with
- Deep extubation

Points of Difference

In deep extubation, the patient is still asleep, not responding to stimuli, but breathing regularly and taking good tidal volumes. (Remember, in this state, the patient may obstruct or aspirate. Thoroughly suction the patient prior to extubation and have an oral/nasal airway handy). NEVER extubate deep patients with a full stomach or patients who are difficult to ventilate or intubate. Otherwise, you may find yourself in a disaster with only you to blame!

In smooth awakening, the patient is awake, following commands, and breathing spontaneously without residual muscle relaxant and with well-controlled pain.

Every patient deserves smooth awakening.

So why extubate deep? The endotracheal tube (ETT) is one of the most stimulating factors in awake extubations; deep extubation eliminates this potential source of agitation, so it is often confused with smooth emergence.

TECHNIQUE TO SMOOTH AWAKENING

A smooth landing requires careful planning and preparation. Don't wait till the drapes are down.

Recovery of Spontaneous Ventilation

This should be the first step. You should start when the surgeon does not require muscle relaxant, in other words when incision closure starts and the fascia is closed.

Remember CO_2 is the gas of life. It stimulates the respiratory center and makes us breathe in the absence of paralytic and centrally acting respiratory depressants.
- Building CO_2 is achieved by hypoventilating the patient.
- Use your favorite method: synchronized intermittent mandatory ventilation (SIMV) or switching to a bag. Really, any way that hypoventilates and builds CO_2 is acceptable.
- Building CO_2 does not mean dropping oxygen saturation (SaO_2)! Spontaneous ventilation can be achieved while maintaining saturation if adequate FiO_2 is used.
- Starting spontaneous ventilation does not mean you are decreasing the anesthetic gases. Keep the patient asleep (Figure 20-1).

Anesthetics

Keep your eyes on the surgeon's hands. Titrate anesthetic gases with closure of procedure. Remember, anesthesia administration is an art and we are the artists, so create a masterpiece!

Suctioning

Perform pharyngeal suctioning while the patient is still deep. The airway is very sensitive, so suctioning while in a light plane will induce coughing and bucking and a surgeon yelling at you. The endotracheal tube cuff is below the cords, so adequate suctioning should extend down to the hypopharynx. Everything in the airway should be done gently; otherwise, you'll traumatize the mucosa and end up with a bloody, ugly airway (Figure 20-2).

Minimizing Coughing and "Bucking" on the ETT

1. Meds
   a. Intracuff lidocaine:[1]
      Typically 4% lidocaine solution can be injected into the ETT cuff, which then diffuses across into the tracheal mucosa. This will decrease irritation from the ETT. Studies have shown improvement in longer cases, >1.5 hours, especially in smokers. For cases <1.5 hours, some studies have shown no improvement, however. Inflation of the cuff should be the same as usual, to 20 to 30 cm H_2O to minimize irritation to mucosa. Lidocaine ointment 5% may also be slathered on the outside of the ETT prior to placement both to lubricate the tube and to anesthetize the airway.[2]
   b. Intratracheal lidocaine:[3]
      This is a topical lidocaine, often 4% solution as well, administered via several methods. Laryngotracheal anesthesia (LTA) 360 kits are premade and ready to be inserted inside of the ETT tube with an attached 5-mL syringe of 2% lidocaine. Atomizers or an angiocath may be attached to a syringe filled with lidocaine solution as well, if LTA is not available.
   c. Intravenous lidocaine:
      IV lidocaine decreases airway reactivity.[3] Any preparation is acceptable, often administered 1 to 1.5 mg/kg a few minutes before extubation.
   d. Intratracheal versus IV lidocaine[4]
      No significant difference has been found between the two. Basically, choose whichever you would like to or utilize multiple techniques as long as you're cognizant of total dose.
   e. Decreasing airway irritation by ETT:
      Proper inflation of the cuff is important. High pressures will occlude capillaries in the tracheal mucosa and may cause ischemia, leading to irritation and pain. Nitrous oxide diffuses into the cuff, so the cuff should always be checked several times to deflate as needed (Figure 20-3).

2. Analgesia: a pain-free patient is a happy patient
   a. Nonnarcotic:
      Nonnarcotics are underused. These medications, as long as they are not contraindicated, are not only effective but lack the respiratory depressant effects of narcotics. Examples: acetaminophen, nonsteroidal antiinflammatory drugs (NSAIDs), local anesthetics injected by surgeon.
   b. Narcotic:
      Narcotics are the go-to drug for pain control. There are a myriad of drugs available. As long as they are dosed appropriately, they are interchangeable unless specific side effects or metabolites are significant because of patient comorbidities, e.g., active renally excreted metabolite of morphine morphine-6-glucuronide for end-stage renal disease (ESRD) patients. IV fentanyl is also commonly used to treat emergence delirium in children.
      - Remifentanil: Potent, short acting. Has been shown to decrease cough on emergence in cases, e.g., thyroidectomies, where manipulation around airway is highly stimulating.
      - Goals/end points in dosing: Narcotics will increase tidal volumes and decrease respiratory rates. Titrate the narcotics to a respiratory rate of 15 to 20. This may not be possible in patients who are difficult to ventilate/intubate or have severe respiratory disease.

3. Dexmedetomidine[5]
   Dexmedetomidine is a relatively newly used agent that can often be very useful. It is an α_2-agonist. It is a sedative with no respiratory depressant effects. This means that a patient may wake up sedated but still breathing well.

4. Bronchodilators
   If patients are asthmatics or have chronic obstructive pulmonary disease (COPD), they may need to receive some bronchodilator like albuterol prior to extubation.

5. Antiemetics
   Patients may experience severe nausea postanesthesia due to both surgical as well as anesthetic factors. Vomiting at the very least is uncomfortable for the patient and inconvenient for you, but it may also result in aspiration with all its possible complications. A 5-hydroxytryptamine (5-HT$_3$) blocker such as ondansetron has minimal side effects and is effective. Dexamethasone may be administered at the beginning of the case. Metoclopramide, a dopamine antagonist, also prevents nausea as well as increases gastrointestinal (GI) motility, which may be important in diabetics with gastroparesis.

Chapter 20 SMOOTH AWAKENING

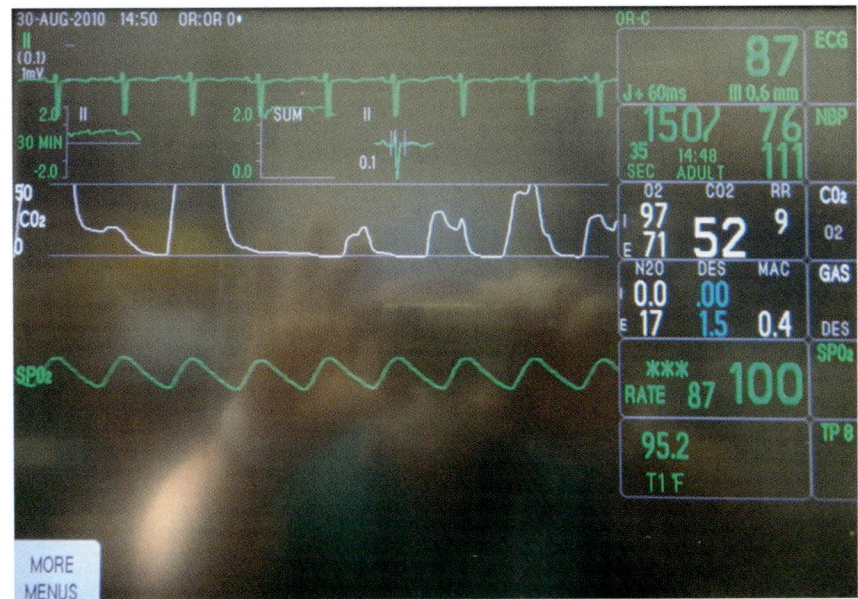

FIGURE 20-1 The capnograph pictured shows a patient beginning to breathe after building up carbon dioxide. It is the second wave form in this figure.

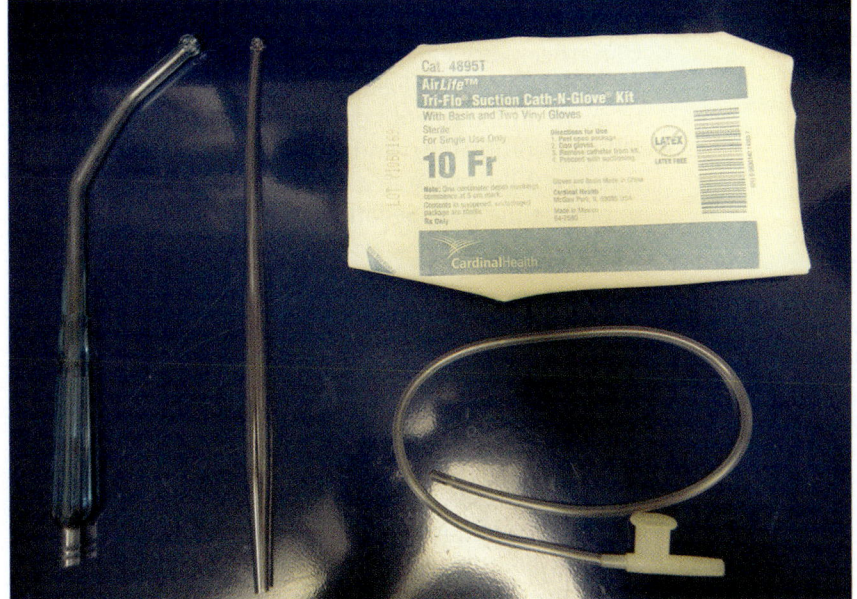

FIGURE 20-2 Several suction catheters. The blue Yankauer suction tip is typically used for adults. The clear tip is smaller in diameter and is used in pediatrics. The soft suction catheter can be used for anyone, and is particularly useful for suctioning within the ETT.

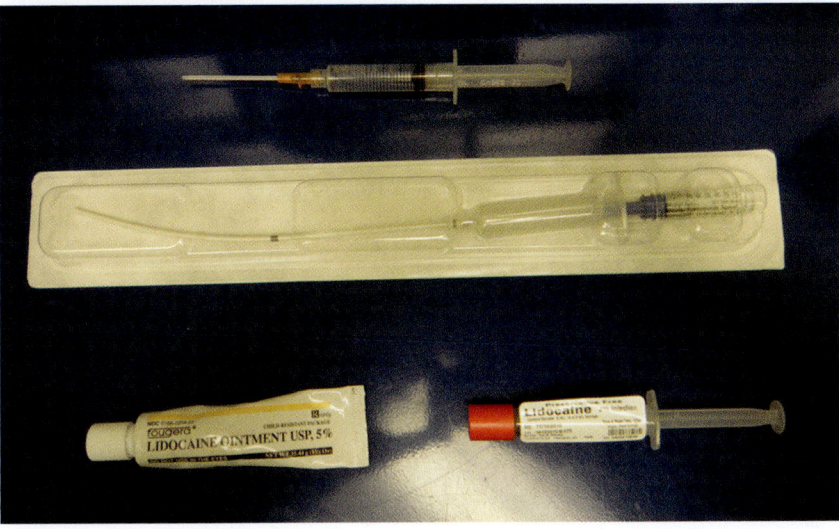

FIGURE 20-3 Different preparations of lidocaine. Top: lidocaine solution in a syringe with a 14-gauge Angiocath attached. Middle: laryngotracheal anesthesia (LTA). Bottom left: lidocaine ointment, which can be placed on the outside of the ETT. Bottom right: IV lidocaine.

6. Reversal of muscle relaxant:
   Twitches must be carefully monitored intraoperatively so that there is at least one twitch prior to reversal. Neostigmine should be given with glycopyrrolate; otherwise, severe bradycardia will ensue. With one twitch, 90% of neuromuscular junction acetylcholine receptors are still occupied. Two twitches means 80% of receptors are occupied, three twitches 75%, and four twitches about 70%. The best indicator is sustained tetany for greater than 5 seconds without fade, which is about 60% receptor occupancy. Sustained head lift or strong hand grip for over 5 seconds represents 60% occupancy as well.

   Now that the patient is breathing regularly and following commands it is time to take out the breathing tube if extubation criteria are satisfied.

7. Extubation Criteria[6]
   a. Level of consciousness: awake and following commands
   b. Avoid light anesthesia, aka "stage 2": disconjugate gaze, breath holding, coughing, not following commands
   c. Volumes: vital capacity ≥10 mL/kg, tidal volumes ≥6 mL/kg
   d. Cuff leak: The airway becomes edematous after 3 to 4 L of crystalloid. Additional factors are the prone position, steep Trendelenburg, long operative times, and surgical airway edema.
   e. Negative inspiratory force (NIF): This is checked by removing the bag and occluding its attachment site with something like your palm, and then asking the patient to take a vital capacity breath. The maximum negative inspiratory pressure should be greater than 25 cm H_2O.[4]

CHALLENGES TO SMOOTH EXTUBATION

Patient Factors

- Obesity: Obesity makes smooth extubation more difficult in several ways. First, patients may be more difficult to intubate or ventilate, so the patients must be fully awake before extubation, often coughing/bucking on the tube. They are often more difficult to ventilate throughout the case because of the pressure from the soft tissue. Postextubation breathing is often more difficult as well, not to mention that the patients have likely developed atelectasis intraop. Abundant adipose tissue during extremely long procedures means more anesthetic is deposited peripherally and the patients will have a slower wakeup. Patients are also more likely to suffer from obstructive sleep apnea (OSA).
- Obstructive sleep apnea: Patients with OSA will obstruct easily with sedation. They also have a higher threshold for breathing, so more CO_2 must be built up. However, excessive CO_2 may cause narcosis. Narcotics should therefore be used minimally if problems are expected.
- Chronic obstructive pulmonary disease (COPD) and asthma: Careful auscultation of the lungs should be done to assess for wheezing. Preoperative nebulizers, e.g., β_2-agonists and anticholinergics, may be useful. Inhalers can be used intraoperatively as well. The relationship between CO_2 and breathing is similar to that in OSA.
- Smokers: Patients who smoke have increased airway reactivity, increased sputum production, decreased ciliary function, higher carboxyhemoglobin, and thus a left-shifted oxyhemoglobin dissociation curve. All of these will make a smooth extubation more difficult.
- Geriatrics: Very elderly patients will have decreased muscle mass and weaker respiratory muscles, leading to more difficulty with extubation.
- Difficult intubation/ventilation: These patients must be fully awake and meet extubation criteria prior to pulling the ETT. Sedation should be minimized.

COMPLICATIONS

- Airway obstruction: Obstruction may result from bronchospasm, the tongue flopping back, or a loss of pharyngeal tone secondary to anesthetics or paralytics. Patients will have paradoxical breathing: retraction, exaggerated abdominal movement, collapse of chest wall, and abdominal protrusion with inspiration.[3]
  - Treatment: jaw thrust, chin lift, oral/nasal airway, constant positive airway pressure (CPAP), reintubation
- Laryngospasm: This is a forceful involuntary spasm of laryngeal musculature via the superior laryngeal nerve.
  - Treatment: positive pressure (up to 40 cm H_2O), jaw thrust, IV or IM succinylcholine with mask ventilation or reintubation
- Bronchospasm: Bronchospasm results from abnormal spasming of bronchial smooth muscle leading to airway obstruction.
  - Treatment: deepening anesthetic, bronchodilators, positive pressure ventilation
    - Paralytics will not be useful because they do not act on smooth muscle.
- Negative pressure pulmonary edema: occasionally a patient who has strong respiratory muscles might

bite down on the tube, causing complete obstruction while taking a very large breath. The large negative intrathoracic pressure results in a sudden pulmonary edema, causing severe pulmonary distress. An oral airway or bite block will prevent obstruction of the ETT by biting.
- Treatment: positive pressure mechanical ventilation with positive end-expiratory pressure (PEEP); supportive care in the ICU if necessary.
- Nausea/vomiting (N/V): Surgical stimulus or anesthetics may be the cause. N/V can cause straining, tachycardia, and hypertension.
  - Treatment: adequate antiemetics, recognition of risk factors
- Aspiration: If patients vomit, they may aspirate.
  - Treatment: immediately place the patient's head down, turn the face to the side, and suction thoroughly. If respiratory distress ensues, reintubation and mechanical ventilation may be necessary.
- Coughing/bucking on ETT: This may cause tachycardia, hypertension, increased intracranial pressure (ICP), increased intraocular pressure (IOP), possible wound dehiscence, and bleeding.
  - Treatment: lidocaine, adequate analgesia

CONCLUSION

Every patient deserves a smooth awakening, and everyone in the OR will appreciate it. Careful planning and a watchful eye will result in a happy ending for your anesthetic.

REFERENCES

1. Bahk J, Lim Y. Use of intracuff lidocaine during general anesthesia response. *Anesth Analg* 2001;92(4):1075–1107.
   A study of the effects of intracuff lidocaine versus saline or air for decreasing airway irritation.
2. Estebe J, Dollo G, LeCorre P. Alkalinization of intra-cuff lidocaine and use of gel lubrication protect against tracheal tube-induced emergence phenomena *Br J Anaesth* 2004;92(3):361–366.
   Determination of whether or not alkalinization of intracuff lidocaine improves its effects.
3. Jee D, Park SY. Lidocaine sprayed down the endotracheal tube attenuates the airway-circulatory reflexes by local anesthesia during emergence and extubation. *Anesth Analg* 2003;96(1):293–297.
   A study of the effects of LTA kits' effects in reducing airway irritation.
4. Venkatesan T, Korula G. A comparative study between the effects of 4% endotracheal tube cuff lidocaine and 1.5 mg/kg intravenous lidocaine on coughing and hemodynamics during extubation in neurosurgical patients: a randomized controlled double-blind trial. *J Neurosurg Anesthesiol* 2006;18(4):230–234.
   A comparison between intracuff lidocaine and IV lidocaine.
5. Lee Y, Wong S, Hung C. Dexmedetomidine infusion as a supplement to isoflurane anaesthesia for vitreoretinal surgery. *Br J Anaesth* 2007;98(4):477–483.
   The benefits of dexmedetomidine used to decrease strain on extubation.
6. Barash P, Cullen B, Stoetling R. *Clinical anesthesia*, 6th ed. Philadelphia: Lippincott Williams & Wilkins; 2009, pp 769–770.
   A standard reference in anesthesiology, with definitive criteria to meet for successful extubation.

CHAPTER 21

SHOW ME THE MYCOBACTERIUM!— TB PROTECTION

RAINA LOURENS
THERESA L. HARTSELL

"She's beautiful, but consumptive."
Dr. Bernard Gallagher,
Dr. Chris Gallagher's grandfather,
commenting on how slender his future
wife was the first time he saw her.

INTRODUCTION

Tuberculosis remains an international health crisis. As an added bonus, it now comes in drug-resistant forms. Protecting yourself, staff, and equipment while providing skilled yet compassionate patient care represents a serious challenge to the anesthesiologist in the perioperative period. Oh, and don't forget the patients you're meeting for the first time in code/emergency airway situations or in the trauma bay!

MYCOBACTERIUM BASICS

- Keep in mind that the term *Mycobacterium tuberculosis* (MTB, TB, tubercle bacillus, white plague, the consumption) encompasses a family of bacterial strains and a continuum of disease.
- Remember to distinguish between infection and disease. Infection refers to exposure and the subsequent development of a latent illness; it's possible to have exposure without any sequelae (thank goodness!). Disease, in contrast, involves active lesions (most commonly pulmonary) and the coughing and spewing of particles, which in turn expose (and potentially infect) others.
- One third of the world is infected with TB. Latent TB infection is asymptomatic, and affected persons are not infectious. Five to 10% of those infected with *M. tuberculosis* will develop active TB from a latent infection.
- A bit about Bacillus Calmette-Guerin (BCG): BCG is an isolate of *Mycobacterium bovis* rendered nonpathogenic via serial in vitro passage. BCG is the only vaccine against tuberculosis, and its use remains common in countries with endemic TB. It does not prevent infection or disease, but rather offers some protection against severe manifestations such as meningitis and hematogenous dissemination. It is often given to infants in endemic areas. Patients with a history of BCG vaccination will commonly have some reaction to tuberculin skin testing, although a smaller reaction than infected patients.
- A tuberculin skin test (TST) is the most common way to determine whether or not a person is at least infected with MTB; it cannot distinguish latent infection from active disease. Interpretation of TST reactions can be confusing to practitioners who don't regularly interpret them.
  - Skin tests are administered via the Mantoux method: 0.1 mL of tuberculin purified protein derivative injected intradermally, results read as millimeters of induration 48 to 72 hours after placement, interpretation of positive tests based on specific population. Skin tests improperly placed will give false results.
  - Interferon-gamma release assays are blood tests that measure the amount of interferon-gamma released (hence the name) by host lymphocytes when incubated with *M. tuberculosis* antigens. Interpretation is less subjective than for TST

(read as positive, negative, or indeterminate) and is not affected by BCG vaccination.
- Active disease is diagnosed through sputum analysis and chest x-ray. Sputum analysis involves microscopy for acid-fast "red snappers" and culture. Cavitary lesions are classic findings on chest x-ray, although nonspecific nodules, infiltrates, and pleural effusions can also be seen.

PREOPERATIVE: MYCOBACTERIUM PROFILING

- During the preanesthetic evaluation, identify individuals at risk for TB infection: people who are HIV-positive, homeless, immigrants from countries with endemic TB, prisoners, or substance abusers.
- Inquire about symptoms of active disease during the review of systems: fever, night sweats, weight loss, persistent cough, blood-tinged sputum.
- Consider medical conditions that increase the risk of both infection and disease: HIV, diabetes, chronic renal disease, malnutrition, alcohol, and tobacco abuse.
- Ask about contacts with sick people and exposure of the patient to high-risk populations.
- Look for pertinent signs: you don't want to be the one to miss cavitary lesions on chest x-ray; if you do, the cavitary lesions for sure won't miss you!
- Promptly mask symptomatic patients, find a respirator for yourself, and initiate airborne infection isolation.
- There are three general types of respirators: (1) disposable particulate respirators, (2) powered air-purifying respirators, and (3) supplied-air respirators.
  - A fit-tested disposable particulate respirator (also called a filtering facepiece, e.g., N95 mask) is the *minimum* required respiratory protection. Fit-testing is important to make sure the mask is effective (you're not wearing it just to look stylish!), and you should either keep your fit-tested mask or remember the size/model number that's right for you. It should fit snuggly around your nose and mouth (Figure 21-1).
  - Additional protection such as a powered air-purifying respirators (PAPRs) can be used in aerosol-generating situations, including laryngoscopy, intubation, suctioning—all those things that anesthesiologists like to do! These devices use a blower to force ambient air through filters into a faceshield and provide the added benefit of mucous membrane protection. PAPRs are also recommended for people with facial hair or those unable to be fit-tested to a disposable mask. (People who are sci-fi actor wannabe's are also fair game.) (Figure 21-2)

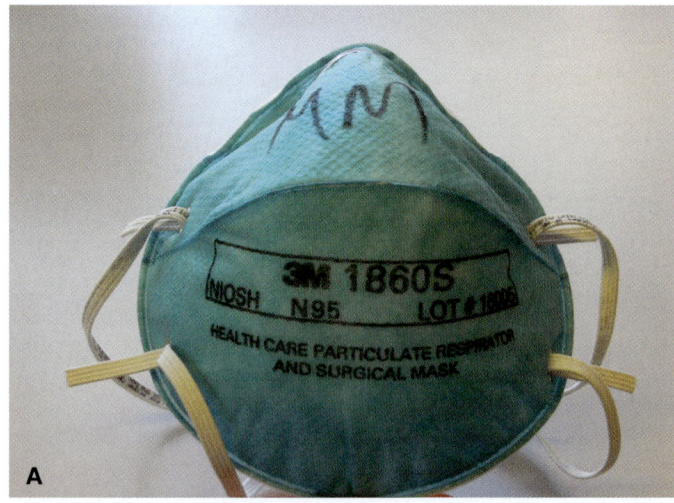
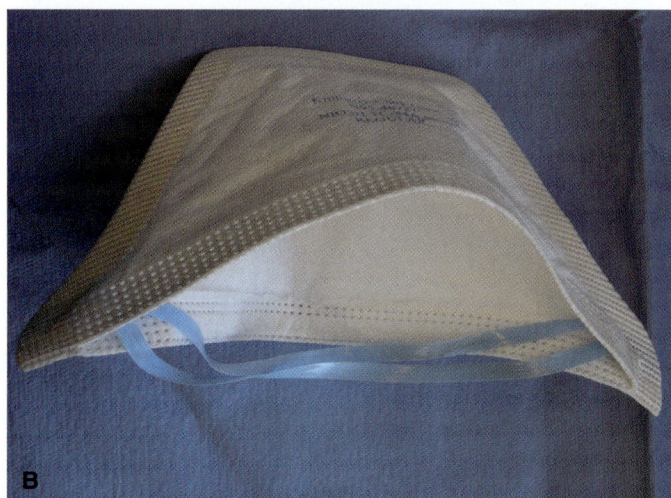
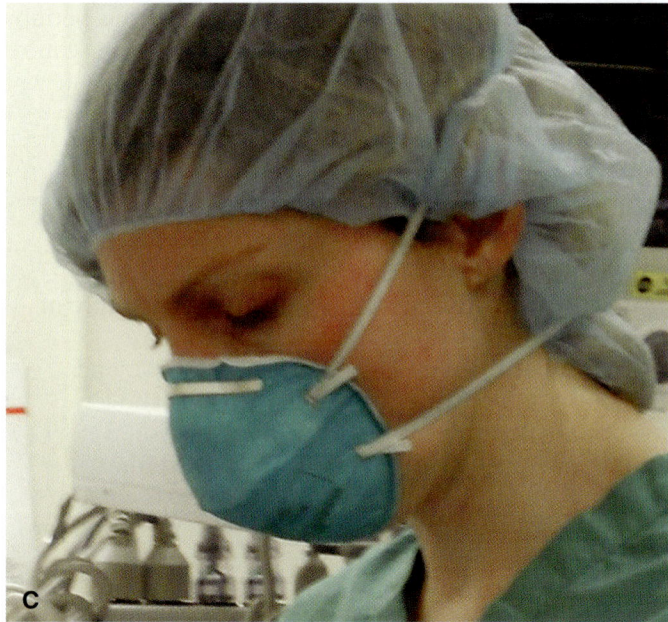

FIGURE 21-1 (A, B) Two disposable N95 particulate respirator masks. (C) A well-fitted N95 mask.

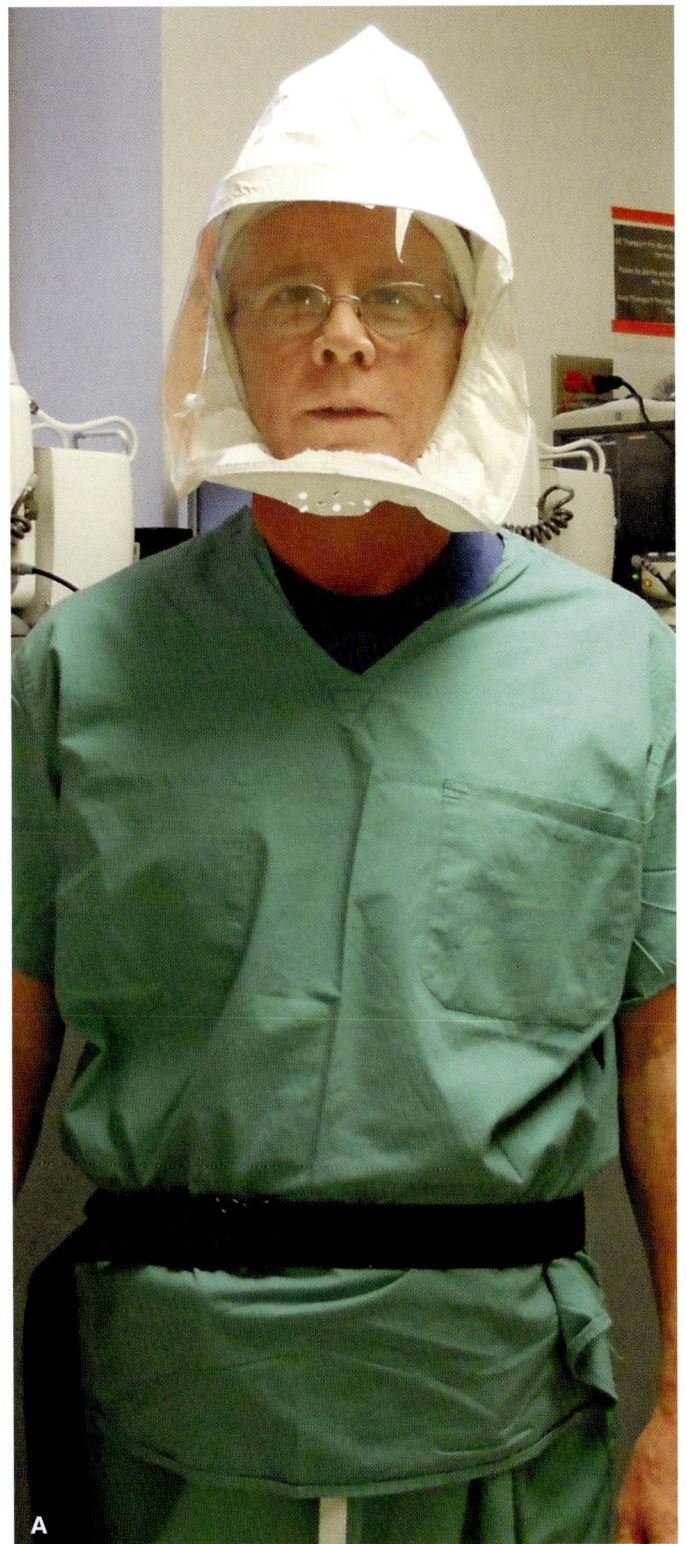 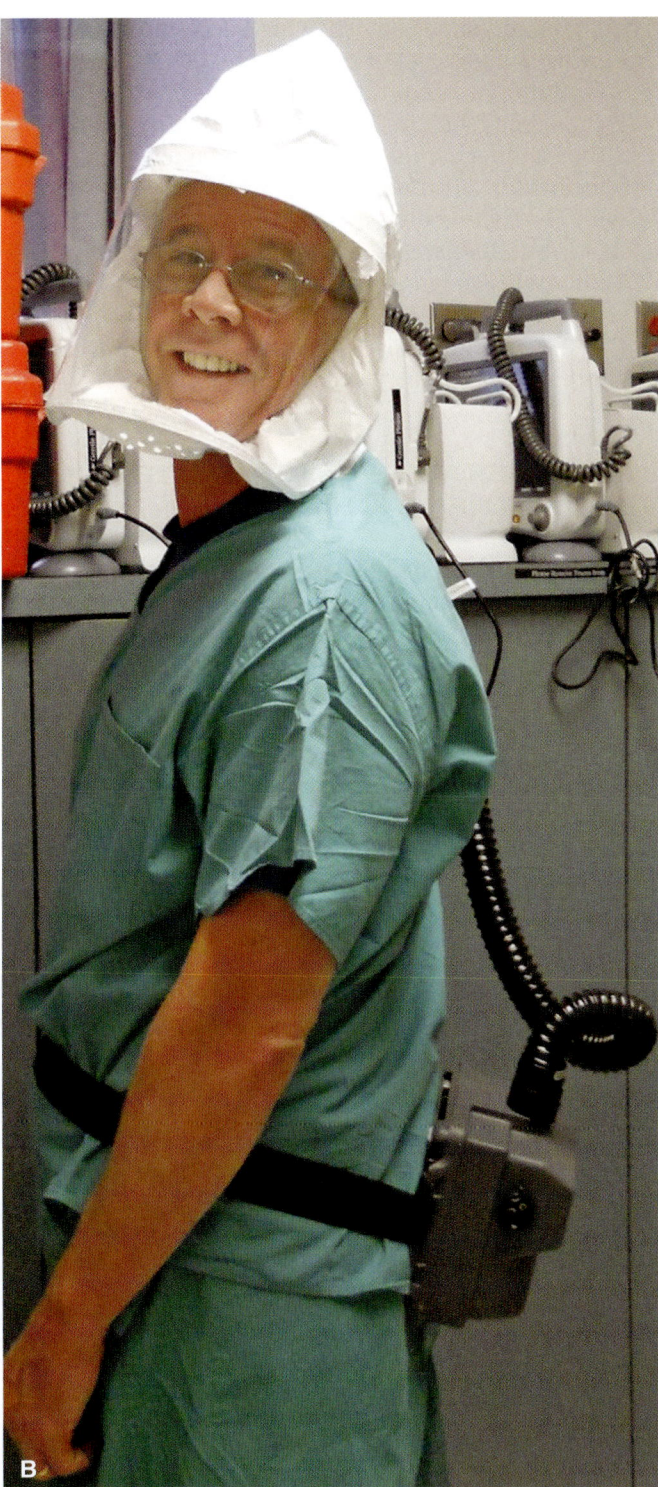

FIGURE 21-2 (A) How to outfit yourself with a powered air-purifying respirator (PAPR). (B) Side view of the PAPR, showing the air pump and how it is worn.

- Supplied-air or "airline" respirators deliver an outside source of compressed rather than ambient (contaminated) air. They are beneficial in areas with a high level of contaminants in which air filtration is not possible.
- If the clinical picture is suspicious for active TB, airborne infection isolation should be initiated. Specifically, airborne precautions mandate rooms with (1) documented negative air pressure relative to surrounding areas, (2) six to 12 air changes per hour, and (3) high-efficiency filtration of room air or venting outdoors.
- Consult infectious disease or contact local infection control services for further help.

INTRAOPERATIVE: MYCOBACTERIUM VERSUS THE MACHINE

- Attempt to minimize exposure of both persons and space. Postpone elective surgeries! Involve the smallest number of staff possible and outfit all with fit-tested particulate respirators. If possible, perform procedures at the patient's bedside in an isolation room with negative air pressure. If an operating room is required, schedule the case as the last procedure of the day to allow adequate time for air exchange and cleaning. Clear the room of unnecessary equipment. Place a surgical or procedure mask on the patient during transport or whenever negative air pressure is not maintained. Use disposable equipment whenever possible.
- Active MTB particles are contained within droplet nuclei that can remain suspended in air for several hours. The minimum dose required for infection is unknown, but has been estimated to be as low as a single bacterium. Yikes!
- Studies have shown aerosolized MTB can move through the expiratory limb of the anesthesia circuit, pass through the soda lime canister, and enter into the inspiratory gas flow.
- Transfer of infectious bacilli within the circle system is prevented by placement of heat and moisture exchange (HME) filters between the proximal end of the endotracheal tube and the Y-piece of the breathing circuit or on the expiratory limb. Specialized HME filters have an integrated bacterial and viral filter with an efficiency of 99.99%. These single-use filters should be replaced between patients or every 24 hours. There are many commercially available HME filters of two basic designs: mechanical and electrostatic. The former provide a physical barrier with efficacy dependent on pore size; the latter use electric charges to capture their prey (Figure 21-3).

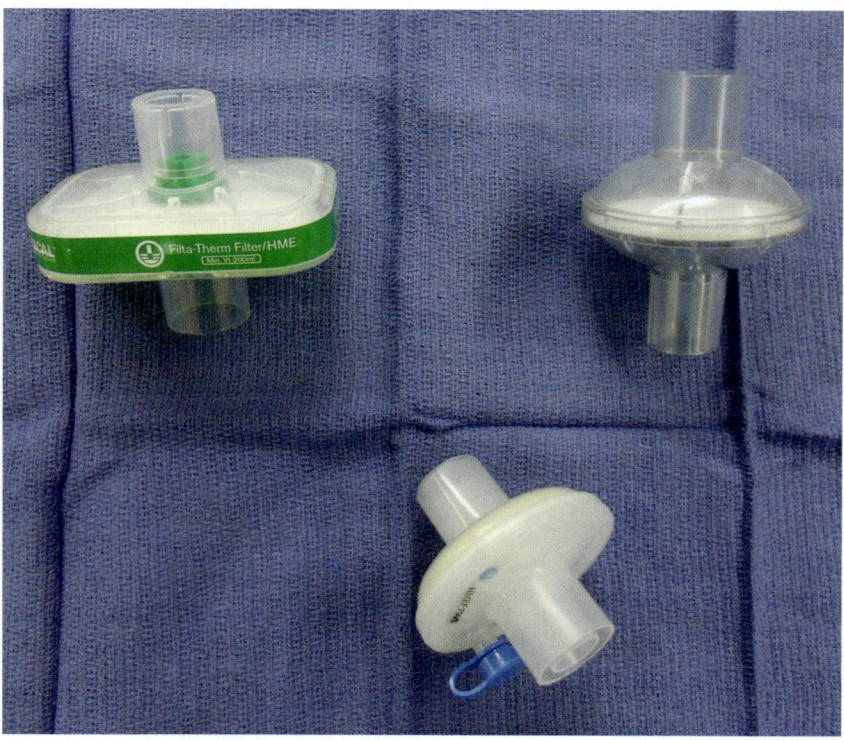

FIGURE 21-3 Examples of heat and moisture (HME) filters.

- Although a fit-tested particulate respirator is sufficient for most situations, be especially vigilant of protection during aerosol-generating procedures, e.g., bronchoscopy, intubation, and suctioning. Consider a PAPR during these procedures for additional mucous membrane protection. Keep in mind that endotracheal tubes make especially good conduits for the transmission of respiratory pathogens.

POSTOPERATIVE: ADIOS TUBERCULOSIS

- Continue all airborne infection isolation precautions. Preferably, the patient should be recovered in a negative air pressure isolation room; at a minimum, a surgical mask on the patient and fit-tested respirators on all surrounding staff members are required.
- HME filters on the anesthesia machine should be followed by HME filters on ventilators in ICU settings.
- Different filters offer differ levels of humidification. The ability to provide humidification is more important with prolonged mechanical ventilation than with short stints in the operating room.
- HME filters typically add a small amount of dead space (>35 mL for adults, 10 to 35 mL for children). This is likely negligible in routine anesthesia cases; however, it should be considered when weaning from the ventilator is difficult in ICU patients.
- Decontaminate the anesthesia machine, including disposal of the soda lime canister, at the completion of the case. Single-use anesthesia circuits are preferred; however, old-school reusable circuits can be decontaminated with ethylene oxide gas.
- Treatment of MTB is a complicated venture, with variability in drug regimens based on predominant strains, patient factors, and potential for hepatotoxicity. Treating clinicians don't haphazardly throw antibiotics at tuberculosis.
- The preferred treatment for latent TB infection is isoniazid for 9 months. This regimen is up to 90% effective in preventing the development of active disease, even in HIV-positive populations.
- The preferred treatment for active disease is divided into initial and continuation phases. In general, the first 2 months (initial phase) are a four-drug regimen of isoniazid, rifampin, pyrazinamide, and ethambutol. A usual continuation phase is an additional 4 months of isoniazid and rifampin, although patients with cavitary lesions and positive sputum culture after the initial phase can be prescribed a continuation phase of 7 months.

CONCLUSION

TB is prevalent and potentially underrecognized in the perioperative period. Keep MTB in your mind's eye of the differential diagnosis for pulmonary infection and chronic disease. If you slap on an N95 and have the patient tested, you might save yourself from 9 months of isoniazid, or worse.

SUGGESTED READING

Centers for Disease Control/National Institute for Occupational Safety and Health. *TB respiratory protection program in health care facilities: administrator's guide.* NIOSH Publication No. 99-143. Atlanta: CDC; 1999.

Centers for Disease Control and Prevention. Guidelines for preventing the transmission of Mycobacterium tuberculosis in health-care settings, 2005. *MMWR* 2005;54(RR-17).

Centers for Disease Control and Prevention, Division of Tuberculosis Elimination, 2010. http://www.cdc.gov/tb/.

Curtis AB, Ridzon R, Vogel R, et al. Extensive transmission of Mycobacterium tuberculosis from a child. *N Engl J Med* 1999;341(20):1491–1495.

Dellamonica J, Boisseau N, Goubaux B, Raucoules-Aimé M. Comparison of manufacturers' specifications for 44 types of heat and moisture exchanging filters. *Br J Anaesth* 2004;93(4):532–539.

Dye C, Williams BG. The population dynamics and control of tuberculosis. *Science* 2010;328(5980):856–861.

Huebner RE, Schein MF, Bass JB Jr. The tuberculin skin test. *Clin Infect Dis* 1993;17(6):968–975.

Langevin PB, Rand KH, Layon AJ. The potential for dissemination of Mycobacterium tuberculosis through the anesthesia breathing circuit. *Chest* 1999;115(4):1107–1114.

Neil JA. Perioperative care of the patient with tuberculosis. *AORN J* 2008;88(6):942–958.

Olmsted RN. Pilot study of directional airflow and containment of airborne particles in the size of Mycobacterium tuberculosis in an operating room. *Am J Infect Control* 2008;36(4):260–267.

Russell DG, Barry CE 3rd, Flynn JL. Tuberculosis: what we don't know can, and does, hurt us. *Science* 2010;328(5980): 852–856.

Van Wormer LM. Tuberculosis: the latest. *CRNA* 2000;11(1): 15–19.

World Health Organization. *Global tuberculosis control: a short update to the 2009 report.* Geneva: World Health Organization; 2009.

CHAPTER 22

INTUBATIONS OUTSIDE THE OPERATING ROOM

HEATHER NIXON

The most successful people are those who are good at plan B.

James Yorke

INTRODUCTION

Ultimately, anesthesiologists are specialists and consultants. We are the "airway experts," and as such are often called all over the hospital to perform intubations or airway maneuvers. We are asked to step out of the controlled environment of the operating room into very foreign and often chaotic environments. The potential to do harm is high, and one should not take this role lightly. In fact, some of the most catastrophic stories I have encountered or personally experienced have involved intubations in the intensive care unit. There are some basics you need to know. This chapter addresses how you should prepare for off-site intubations, the basics of situation assessment, and optimization of your environment.

CODE BOX: PREPARATION IS EVERYTHING!

Welcome to the "code box." This box differs in size and contents in every institution. In fact, sometimes it is actually a bag. If you are expected to carry the code or airway pager, you need to know where this box is and what it contains. Before your shift begins, you should check its contents to make sure you do not arrive at an emergency with an empty box. You would be surprised how many of your colleagues will forget to restock this bag after a long night on call (Figure 22-1).

To stock the bag, think of the things you need to have in the operating room for an intubation (Figure 22-2).

Endotracheal Tubes of Various Sizes

These tubes should include at least one 8.0-mm tube or greater.
- If a patient is experiencing respiratory distress, the team may plan to perform a bronchoscopy after intubation.
- Many adult bronchoscopes will not fit down an endotracheal tube less than 7.5 mm and also permit adequate simultaneous ventilation.
- It's an incredibly disappointing experience to successfully intubate a high-risk patient and then discover that you need to change the tube. Spare yourself and intubate with a large tube unless you have a reason to not do so.

Laryngoscope and Blades

- Check these at the beginning of your shift. A dead battery can equal a dead patient.
- It is often more important to have a MAC 4 and a Miller 2 than the smaller versions of these blades. It is easier to pull your blade back than to extend its reach. Ideally, you have all four.

Syringes and Needles

You will need a syringe to inflate the pilot balloon and you will need syringes to draw up drugs.

Oral Airways

You may need these to help you ventilate.

Advanced Airway Supplies

These vary, but I would recommend a bougie, an intubating laryngeal mask airway (LMA), and a regular LMA. Some institutions now have portable glidescopes (a video screen enabled intubating device) that can be taken to codes.

- It is not practical to carry a fiberoptic scope with you to every airway. However, if you suspect you will need it, you should take it with you.
- Some code boxes will also be stocked with cricothyrotomy kits.
- Review your difficult airway algorithm!

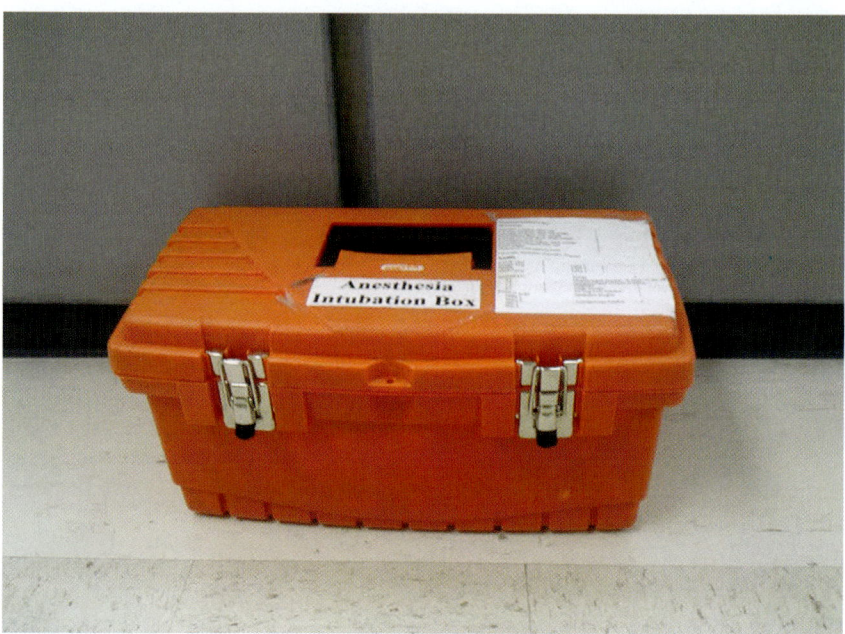

FIGURE 22-1 Code box: ready to go.

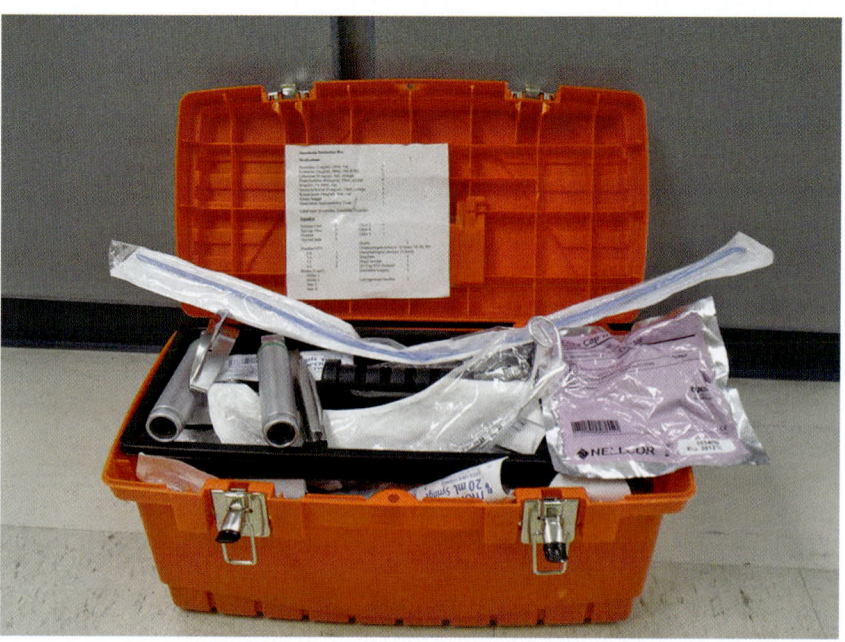

FIGURE 22-2 Code box: opened with supplies.

End Tidal CO_2 Detector

- In the operating room, our ventilator supplies the end tidal CO_2 confirmation. Off-site, you must rely on your clinical assessment of placement, lung sounds, chest wall rise, and sometimes an end-tidal CO_2 detector. This is a little device that attaches to the end of your endotracheal tube and will change from purple to yellow in the presence of carbon dioxide. This can be a confirmatory test for intubation.
- Beware: If the patient is in cardiac arrest when you arrive, you may not get end-tidal CO_2 when you successfully intubate the trachea, and therefore no color change will occur. No cardiac output equals no end-tidal carbon dioxide. If you intubate King Tut, you will not get a color change.
- Often, other health care providers will be very concerned that there is no change in color because they believe this means you have placed the tube in the esophagus. If you are concerned about the placement, you might want to leave the tube in place and perform a direct laryngoscopy to confirm placement between the cords. Likewise you can use the fiberoptic scope to confirm placement. However if you are convinced your placement is proper, you might gently remind the service that they need to address the cardiac output. Delay of treatment for hypoperfusion to confirm tube placement is never acceptable (Figures 22-3 and 22-4).

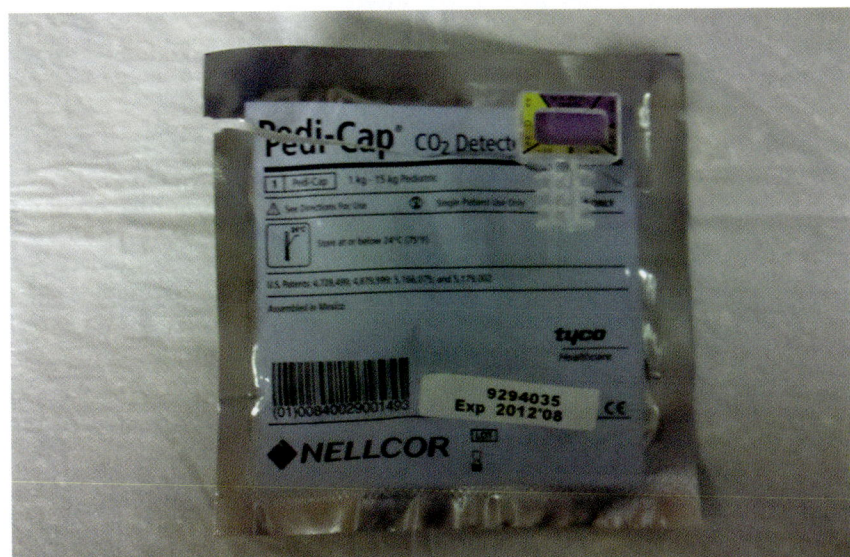

FIGURE 22-3 A sample of the pediatric version of the end-tidal carbon dioxide detector (E_TCO_2).

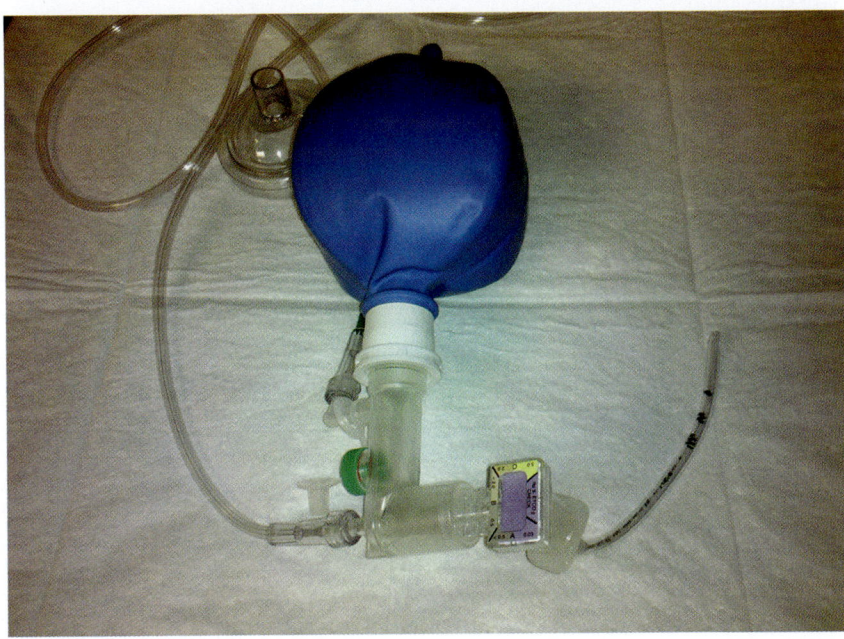

FIGURE 22-4 The E_TCO_2 detector attached correctly between the Ambu bag and the endotracheal tube. The screen is purple and will turn gold when E_TCO_2 is detected.

Tube Exchanger

- This is a long, thin semi-flexible tube that you will place through an existing endotracheal tube to act as a track for placement of a new tube. Generally, we do not use this device in the operating room. The key to the tube exchanger is that it allows you to ventilate (albeit poorly) the patient by attachment of oxygen to the end of the tube.
- *Do not administer continuous high flow oxygen* through this device. Imagine a continuous inflow of air to a balloon without the ability of air to egress; eventually the balloon will pop. So will the lungs, resulting in a tension pneumothorax.
- Similarly, you need to measure the tube exchanger next to an endotracheal tube before inserting it. Many exchangers have measurements on the side, but some do not. You want to place the exchanger at the end of the preexisting endotracheal tube, not much beyond it. If you aggressively advance the exchanger, you can cause damage to the trachea, bronchus, or lung. In addition, if the patient is lightly anesthetized, you will elicit coughing and bucking. It is no fun to have a patient with creepy crawlies in their lungs start coughing in your face. (See the previous chapter on acid-fast creepy crawlies.)

Drugs

- Institutions vary on drugs of choice and who is responsible for obtaining these medications. In some hospitals, the anesthesiologists bring their own medications. In other places, nurses retrieve the medications for the anesthesiologists. Know your institution's practice.
- Just remember, sick patients often tank after intubation so also have some vasopressors available.
- Finally, take what you need. Do not overburden the code box with too much equipment. You have to carry this box, and extra weight means extra time. In addition, if you stuff the box with thousands of tubes, you will have a harder time finding what you need when you get there.

ASSESSMENT OF THE SITUATION

Clinical judgment and the ability to quickly assess your environment are critical. If you are receiving a phone call or page for an intubation, try to get any information about the scenario that you can. More information equals one trip with all the correct equipment.

Some airway questions to ask:
- "Is the patient in a c-collar or halo?"—especially in the neurosurgical ICU (fiberoptic anyone?).
- "Is the patient a known difficult airway?"
- "Has this patient been intubated previously in this hospitalization?"

If a panicked nurse says, "We need the patient intubated now!" do not press for details; you will not get them. Most likely this poor soul was the only one available to call you because she is not involved with the patient care; she does not know anything about the patient.

Arriving at any code or urgent situation is always daunting. Take a deep breath, sort through the chaos, and follow the advice from "House of God"—first, take your own pulse.

The absolute most important thing you need to do is to determine the urgency of the situation. Any scenario can be triaged into one of three categories: emergent, urgent, or elective.

The Emergency Situation

You have to do what you have to do.
- If the team is doing chest compression, this is an emergency.
- If the patient is totally unresponsive, this is an emergency.
- If the patient has an oxygen saturation in the 60s, this is an emergency.
- The good thing about an emergency is that you must do something. There is not a lot to argue about or discuss.
- Enter the room and start preparing for intubation while you ask questions.
  - Remember the mnemonic **SOAP**:
    - **S** = suction; immediately ask a nurse to set up suction. If there is a nasogastric tube in place, have the nurse put it on continuous suction and set up a second suction for you.
    - **O** = oxygen; make sure there is an Ambu bag with a source of oxygen.
    - **A** = airway; take out all the equipment you need to intubate.
    - **P** = pharmacy; determine what you want to give the patient, if anything, and draw it up.
  - Ask the team the **AMPLE** mnemonic:
    - **A** = allergies
    - **M** = medications, specifically narcotics (is this an opioid overdose?)
    - **P** = pertinent past medical history; screen for ability to rapid sequence—last K+, burn victim, muscular dystrophy, crush injury, paralysis, stroke. Cardiac history? Surgical history? Bowel obstruction? DNR/DNI? Does the patient have head trauma or coagulopathy that might preclude nasal intubation?
    - **L** = last oral intake, including when the tube feeds were shut off
    - **E** = events leading to situation

- Now, this advice is good and helpful, but in a real-life scenario, there will be chaos. Trying to find someone who knows the patient history can be difficult. Do your best and try to use the nurses to set things up. You should focus on your equipment and delegate the suction, oxygen, IV check, and bed positioning to someone else, who will most likely be happy to have a job and direction.
- Special situation: If you have to intubate a patient receiving chest compressions, tell the team to continue compressions while you set up. Get to the head of the bed with all your equipment and get ready to intubate. Ideally, you do not want to interrupt chest compression, so if possible intubate the patient as compressions are being performed. If this is not possible, ask the team to hold compressions while you perform your direct laryngoscopy, and as soon as you get your laryngoscope out of the mouth ask the team to resume compressions. If you are having trouble establishing an airway, *do not delay compressions*. Come out, mask ventilate, and reassess.

The Urgent Situation: Dangerous Territory

- As consultants, anesthesiologists are often asked by other health care providers to perform services. Intubation is one of these services. Although a surgical or medical team may "order an intubation," we are the experts and you must remember that your knowledge about the airway or potential problems with intubation is far greater than other physicians.
- Often other primary services will make the decision to intubate a patient and will call the anesthesia team to get it done. Intubations, however, are not without risk, and it is incumbent on us as experts to voice our concerns. Simply put, do not get bullied into intubating a patient quickly if you are concerned about safety. In an urgent situation, your assessment shows that the patient needs an airway but there is time to set up and do it in a more controlled manner.
- If you need advanced airway equipment, you can call for it before proceeding. If you need another skilled pair of hands, call before you proceed. Also, if NPO status is questionable and the patient does not need to be intubated emergently, it may be prudent to wait until it is more favorable. Likewise, if a patient has a bowel obstruction, make sure there is a nasogastric tube. Again, do not trust the service to optimize the patient before you arrive.
- Succinylcholine—the tough decision. In an emergency situation you might have to trust a medical history or a potassium level that someone tells you, or the patient might not require paralysis for intubation. If the patient can wait for intubation, confirm the information yourself. It is a humbling experience to proceed with a rapid-sequence intubation on a patient who had a recent stroke because the medical resident said, "The patient does not have any contraindications to succinylcholine." Similarly, remember that deconditioning from a prolonged hospital stay can also put patients at risk for hyperkalemia from succinylcholine.
- Ultimately, in the urgent situation you must trust your own instincts and come up with a plan that is safe. Treat this patient as an operating room patient and tailor the drug regiment and airway supplies as necessary.

The Elective Situation: The Truly Absurd

- You are called to computed tomography for a patient in "respiratory distress." If you enter the room and the patient is saturating 100% on room air and is talking easily, take pause. You have a right to evaluate the patient and if you feel the intubation is not medically necessary, call an anesthesiology attending and talk to the service. You do not want to be obstructive, you do not want to deny care, but you must never take an unnecessary risk with someone's life. If the scenario does not seem right to you, get help and get more information.
- One of my colleagues was called to the neurosurgical ICU to perform an intubation on a patient so that magnetic resonance imaging (MRI) could be performed. In other words, they wanted to administer heavy sedation to the patient and needed an airway. The patient had a questionable airway and recent oral intake. The primary physicians did not understand the real risk of aspiration or a lost airway. In addition, the service never even asked the cooperative patient if he could lie still during an MRI. Do not trust other services to even have a rudimentary understanding of the airway exam or intubation risks.
- In another example, the airway team was called to intubate a patient for "blood pressure control" in a patient who had received an endovascular abdominal aortic aneurysm (AAA) repair. The story was that the patient needed to be intubated in order to be sedated, which was the plan for blood pressure control. True, he had a great-looking airway. On closer evaluation, however, he was on chronic Valium and had not received any Valium in the previous 48 hours. Oh, and no effort at pharmacologic blood pressure control had been instituted either. The take home message here is: assess the entire situation in these cases, not just the airway. The intubation may be totally unwarranted.
- Another unfortunately common scenario is the request for a tube exchange. You will get called because "the cuff is leaking." Health care providers

are often concerned because the oxygen saturation might be low as well. This usually occurs in the ICU setting and can be a frustrating experience for an anesthesiologist. Take care to examine the patient's ventilator; if the peak airway pressures are adequate and the patient is receiving an appropriate tidal volume, there is probably not a leak. A small leak is fine as long as the patient is adequately ventilating. The low oxygen saturation is most likely a problem with the patient, not the tube. Remember, switching a tube can result in airway disaster and should only be undertaken if there is a need. If you do replace the tube, make sure you deflate the pilot balloon several times before pulling the tube. If the respiratory therapists or nurses were concerned about a leak, they may have repeatedly inflated the cuff to decrease the leak and a large quantity of air may be present in the cuff. You can cause significant damage to the airway by pulling an inflated cuff.

OPTIMIZING YOUR ENVIRONMENT

When you intubate outside the operating room, you are in foreign territory, and the equipment and personnel are not familiar. Personnel outside the operating room often do not know how to assist you. You need to ask for exactly what you want.

Patient Positioning for an Off-Site Intubation

Here are the things you need to know (Figure 22-5):
- First, move the bed away from the wall; you need room to work.
- Second, the board on the head of the ICU bed is removable; remove it if you want to reach the patient (Figure 22-6).
- Most ICU beds are soft to prevent ulcers; have the staff deflate it to make it more rigid.
- Remove the soft pillow from behind the patient's head.
- You need to plug in the bed to make adjustments to height, angle, etc.
- It is wise to ask the team to help move the patient up in the bed so that you can reach.
- Some patients will not tolerate the supine position; their oxygen saturation will plummet. So, it might be preferable to intubate all patients at a 30- to 45-degree angle with the head of the bed slightly elevated; theoretically, this limits the passive flow of aspirate.
- If a cervical collar or halo is in place, ask the service if it can be removed. And get ready for a fiberoptic intubation. Anecdotally, I remember a case of a lost airway in the neurosurgical ICU because no one ever thought to ask the service to remove the halo. It was a very bad outcome.

Room Environment

- Make sure all your monitors are attached and you check baseline vitals.
- Have everything you need close to the head of the bed.
- Ask anyone who is not actively participating in patient care to leave the room.
- Have the IV close to you with a dedicated injection port available (Figure 22-7).

Assumptions You Are Always Safe to Make

- You will need full personal protective gear including a face mask, gloves, and gown.
- These do not need to be sterile; they are to protect you, not the patient. Blood or vomitus in the face will ruin anyone's day.
- As previously discussed, you need suction—two suctions if your patient has a nasogastric (NG) tube, one dedicated for continuous NG suction. Start this prior to inductions. You may find liters of fluid just waiting to be aspirated.
- Your patient should generally be assumed to have a full stomach, full rapid sequence when possible.
- You are most likely the only person who knows how to correctly apply cricoid pressure.
- It is advisable for you to place someone else's hand in the correct position and ask him or her to hold it in place until you say to release the position.
- If the airway is really bloody, ask for a second suction setup; one alone may not be sufficient. One suction can get clotted easily if blood is involved.
- Patients are generally sicker and require less medication for intubation than healthy patients.
- You need to get consent for intubation if the patient or family can give it. You do not want an assault charge on your permanent record.
- If things are not going well, call for help as soon as you can. It will take a while to get it. Also, limit the potential for people to misquote you. For example, if you need the nurse to call your attending to bring the fiberoptic scope, say, "Call this number and tell them to bring the fiberoptic scope now" instead of, "Well, tell them that I am having difficulty and I might need the fiberoptic scope because it is a poor view, but I can ventilate." Have you ever played the telephone game? The shorter your message, the more likely it will be passed on correctly.

Chapter 22 INTUBATIONS OUTSIDE THE OPERATING ROOM

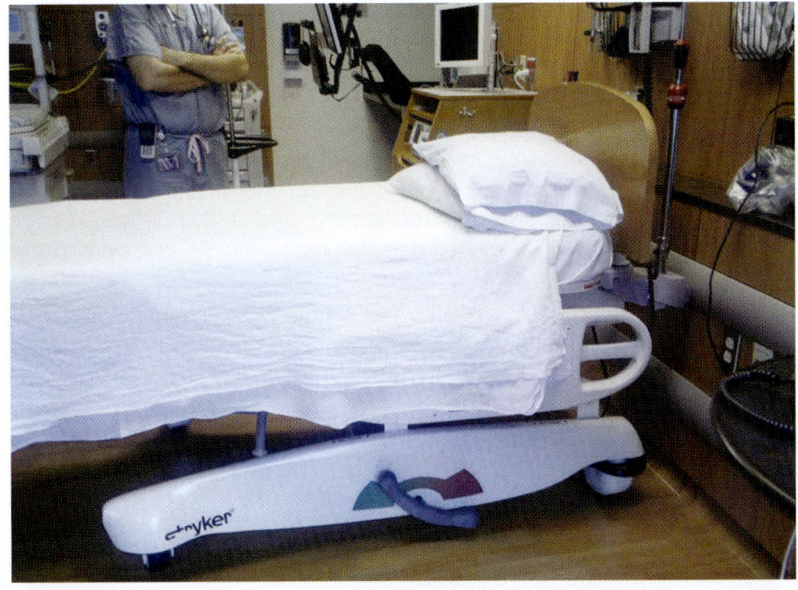

FIGURE 22-5 When you arrive, this is what the bed often looks like.

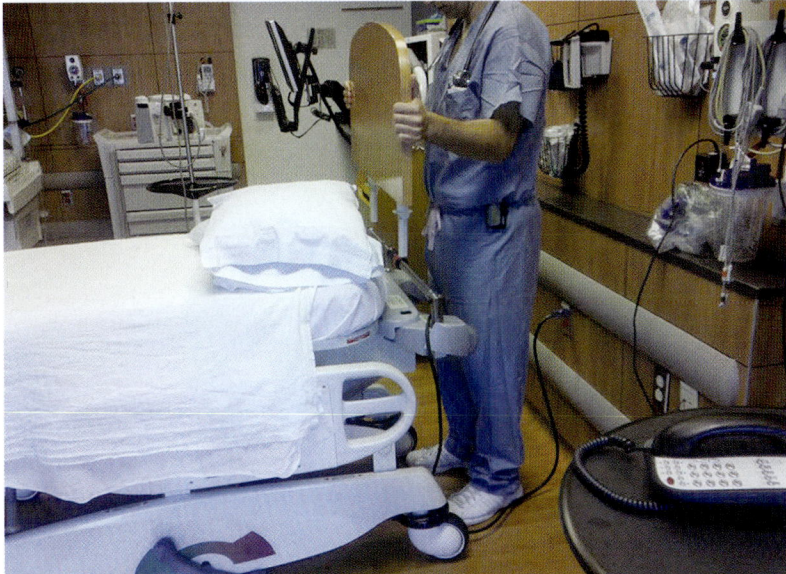

FIGURE 22-6 The bed pulled away from the wall and the headboard removed.

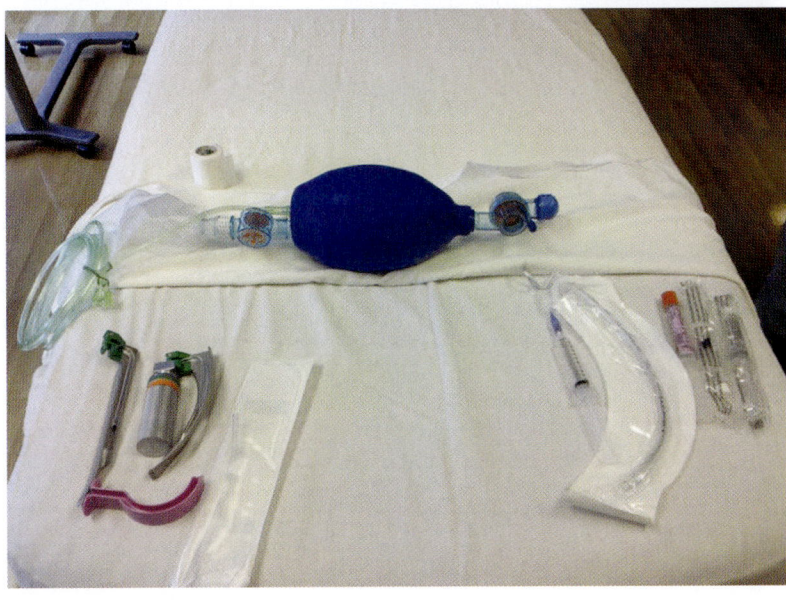

FIGURE 22-7 All the equipment you should have handy at the head of the bed.

CONCLUSION

Off-site intubations can be scary and dangerous. Patients are usually very sick and have little reserve to tolerate mistakes. You need to quickly assess the situation, direct others to assist you, and stay organized. A little preparation, triage, and optimization go a long way. Most importantly, never be afraid to call for help.

SUGGESTED READING

Jaber S, Amraoui J, Lefrant JY, et al. Clinical practice and risk factors for immediate complications of endotracheal intubation in the intensive care unit: a prospective, multiple-center study. *Crit Care Med* 2006;34:2355–2361.

Identifies high rates of immediate and severe complications associated with ICU endotracheal intubations. Patients with acute respiratory failure and shock were at highest risk for complications. Recommend protocols for critically ill patients.

Needham DM, Thompson DA, Holzmueller CG, et al. A system factors analysis of airway events from the Intensive Care Unit Safety Reporting System (ICUSRS). *Crit Care Med* 2004;32:2227–2233.

Analysis of an ICU adverse event reporting system identified that most airway events were preventable and resulted in physical injury, increased hospital stays, and family dissatisfaction. Adequate ICU staffing and skilled assistants were identified as factors that decreased severity of events. Bring help if you think you will need it!

Porhomayon J, El-Solh AA, Nader ND. National survey to assess the content and availability of difficult-airway carts in critical-care units in the United States. *J Anesth* 2010;24:811–814.

Survey to identify the availability of equipment and content of difficult airway carts in ICU settings in the U.S. Found that 70% of ICUs surveyed had difficult airway carts in the ICU and only 50% had the difficult airway algorithm attached. Bring what you need (it might not be there) and know the difficult airway algorithm.

For stories and advice from peers, go to forums.studentdoctor.net.

CHAPTER 23
NASOGASTRIC TUBE PLACEMENT: THE AGONY AND THE ECSTASY

ASHER EMANUEL
THOMAS CORRADO
CHRISTOPHER GALLAGHER

INTRODUCTION

Though being one of the simplest procedures, placement of a nasogastric tube (NGT) has the potential of making you sweat the most, as it is fraught with troubleshooting and possible complications. Your vascular lines may take you less time to get going than a misplaced NGT.

INDICATIONS

- Gastric drainage/decompression in bowel obstruction, to improve operating conditions (e.g., laparoscopy) and full stomach prior to intubation
- Gastric lavage in drug overdose, poisoning, and GI bleeding
- Enteral feeding or administration of medications

CONTRAINDICATIONS

- Severe facial trauma or recent sinus surgery—the possibility of cribriform place disruption resulting in nasocranial intubation! In this situation, an orogastric (OG) tube would be an alternative.
- Extra caution in coagulopathic patients, those with esophageal varices, and friable mucosa (i.e. pregnant women).

COMPLICATIONS

- Aspiration, tissue trauma and pressure necrosis, esophageal perforation and retropharyngeal abscess, endotracheal placement, pneumothorax, and even intravascular placement (it has happened!). One case reported inadvertent placement of an NGT into the eustachian tube of a child! Also don't forget: every other bad thing you can imagine happening can in fact happen.
- In adults, tube errors vary from 1.3% to 50%.
- Partially anesthetized or awake patients may gag and vomit during placement. Keep suction equipment ready and wear protective gear.

EQUIPMENT

- Personal protection (e.g., gloves, gown, etc.)
- NG/OG tube of appropriate size
- 60-mL catheter tip irrigation syringe
- Water-soluble lubricant
- If the patient is awake, lidocaine jelly 2% or an atomizer with lidocaine 4%. Benzocaine spray can also be used to anesthetize the pharynx. But don't overdo it, as methemoglobinemia is a real risk when using benzocaine.
- Adhesive tape

- Suction equipment
- Stethoscope
- Ice chips or cup of water for an awake patient
- Emesis basin
- pH strips
- End-tidal CO_2 detector

PROCEDURE

Gather and prepare the equipment. When removing the tube from its packaging, check that the connector between the tube and suction equipment ("the football") is not misplaced, as it often is.

1. Wear nonsterile gloves.
2. If patient is awake, explain the procedure, show the equipment and make sure the patient agrees to the procedure.
3. Sit an awake patient up for optimal alignment of the neck, esophagus, and stomach.
4. Examine the nostrils and begin with the one that appears wider. Also, if patient is awake, ask which nostril is easier to breathe from.
5. Measure tube from the bridge of the nose to the earlobe and then to a point halfway between the end of the xiphoid and the navel. Note the markings along the tube and at the nostril; ideally this is how far the tube should be placed. In females the tube should pass 8 to 9 cm and in males 9 to 11 cm. If the patient's belly is prepped and sterile, make your best estimate and avoid contaminating the field.
6. Apply lidocaine or benzocaine in the nostril and back of the throat to make for a much more pleasant experience in the awake patient.
7. Lubricate 2 to 4 inches from the end of the tube.
8. Note the natural curvature of the tube and use it to your advantage by making the convexity of the tube approximate that of the posterior pharynx.
9. Flex the patient's neck or, in an anesthetized patient, lift the jaw.
10. Ideally, the tube should enter almost perpendicular to the face at the nostril rather than directly downward (Figure 23-1).
11. Have the awake patient swallow ice or water and advance as the patient swallows.
12. Continue to advance the tube until the mark is reached.
13. If any resistance is met, do not use force. Rather, attempt rotating the tube 180 degrees and continuing to advance.
14. If you continue to have trouble advancing or further resistance is met, refer to the troubleshooting section of this chapter (see below).
15. If any of the following occurs, immediately withdraw the tube: the patient coughs, a sudden change occurs in the capnograph in an intubated patient, the ventilator alarms go off or the bellows suddenly fall flat and don't rise (this may suggest endotracheal placement and a possible breach around the cuff), or the tube coils in the patient's mouth.
16. Confirmation:
    - The most reliable way of confirming placement is a chest x-ray. This is a must if you plan on injecting anything through the tube.
    - If an x-ray is not possible yet, DO NOT administer anything through the tube until an x-ray is possible. The next most reliable confirmation test is to aspirate the tube and look for the presence of gastric contents. This would appear yellow or green, except in GI bleeding. The pH would be less than 6.
    - If the pH is higher than 6, the NGT may be in the lungs or in the intestine.
    - Unreliable results for pH testing will be found in any patient with pernicious anemia, on H_2-blockers, full stomach, medications, or HIV positive.
    - Auscultation for epigastric sounds by insufflating through the tube is the least reliable method to confirm tube placement and may be positive even if the tube is in the lungs.
    - There are some tubes that can be confirmed using an electromagnetic transceiver. Although more effective than aspiration or auscultation, its usefulness is limited to institutional availability. Check with your institution, as there may be set policies regarding confirmation of NGT placement.
    - Capnography or CO_2 detectors are reliable for ruling out endotracheal placement as long as the tube is not kinked.
17. Secure the tube with adhesive tape along the nose. Be sure to leave some slack so as not to compress the skin. This may lead to ischemic necrosis.
18. Place the tube to drain by gravity or low intermittent suction, according to your needs.
19. Document the procedure and how you confirmed placement in the patient's chart:
    - NGT placed in right lower lobe of lung.
    - NGT placed in stomach.

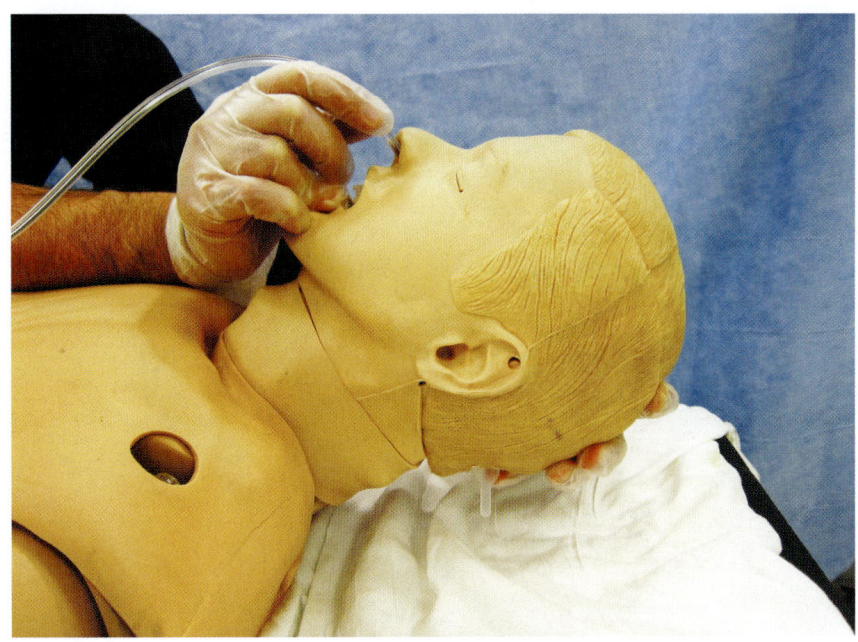

FIGURE 23-1 Positioning of head during placement of nasogastric tube.

TROUBLESHOOTING AND CLINICAL PEARLS

The pyriform sinuses and the arytenoid cartilage are the most common sites for impaction to the advancement of the NGT (Figure 23-2). Here are some maneuvers to keep the tube approximated to the posterior/lateral pharyngeal wall and facilitate smooth passage:

- Digital assistance with a gloved finger can keep the tube from coiling in the pharynx and steer it into the esophagus.
- Neck flexion to align the neck-esophagus axis can be very useful.
- Forward displacement of the larynx (reverse Sellick maneuver) is better done on an anesthetized patient.
- Direct laryngoscopy and Magill forceps can help facilitate passage of the tube into the esophagus under direct visualization (Figures 23-3 and 23-4). This can also be used when placing an orogastric tube. The GlideScope or other airway visualization devices may be useful here as well (Figures 23-5 and 23-6).
- Placing the tip of the tube in ice for a few minutes can help enhance its natural curvature, which can then be used to your advantage.
- Remember that x-ray is the gold standard for confirmation of tube placement and must be done prior to infusing anything into the tube.
- A cuffed endotracheal tube (ETT) does not necessarily prevent the NGT from entering the lungs.
- If the tube must be inserted into an awake infant, have the infant suck on a pacifier.
- If you are using a Univent, make sure to label the endobronchial blocker as something through which you CANNOT feed. This is not the stuff of legends, as rookie ancillary staff may not know the Univent and can mistake the endobronchial blocker for a feeding tube.

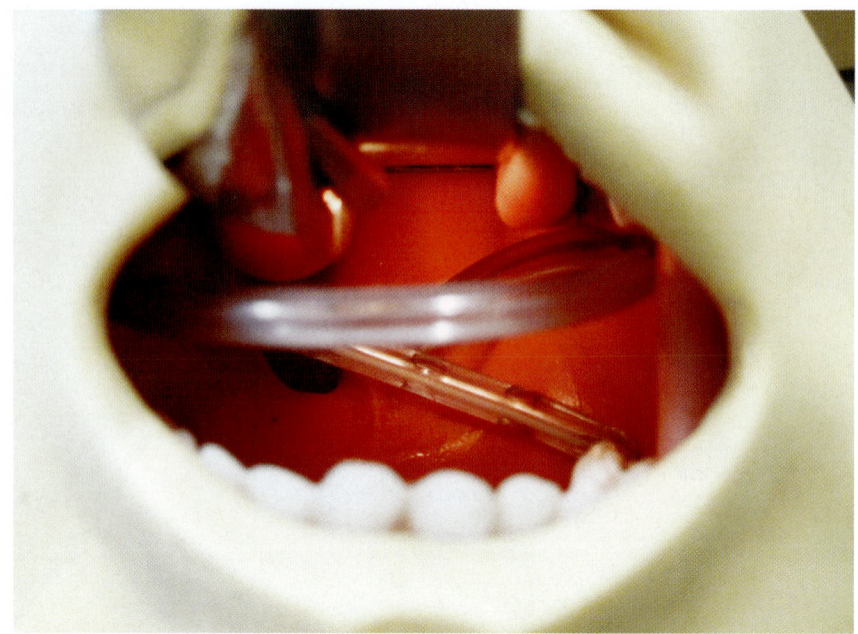

FIGURE 23-2 Nasogastric tube coiled inside the mouth.

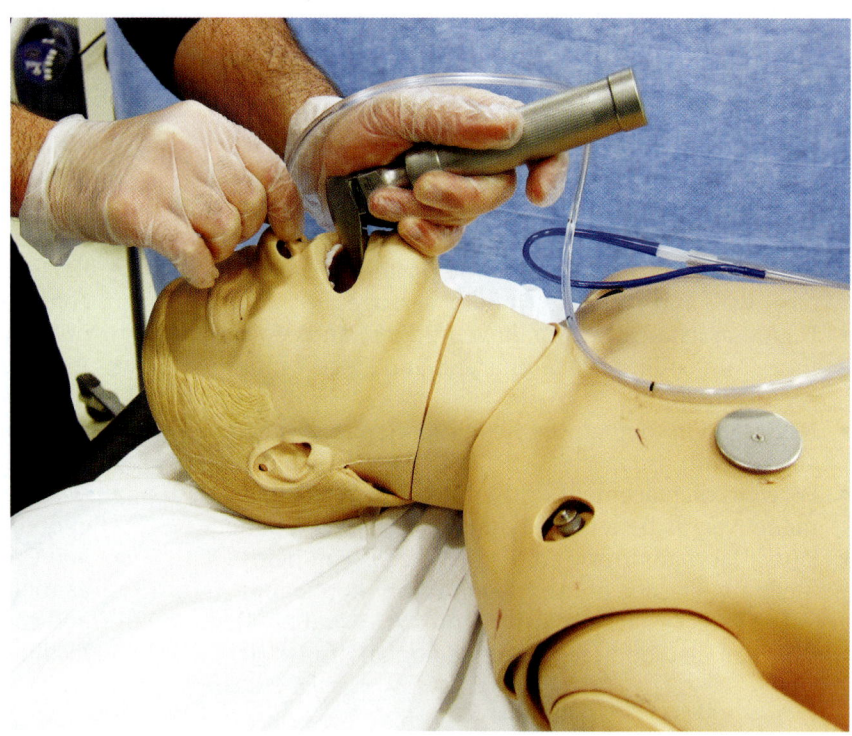

FIGURE 23-3 Using direct laryngoscopy to aid in visualization of nasogastric tube into esophagus.

Chapter 23 NASOGASTRIC TUBE PLACEMENT: THE AGONY AND THE ECSTASY

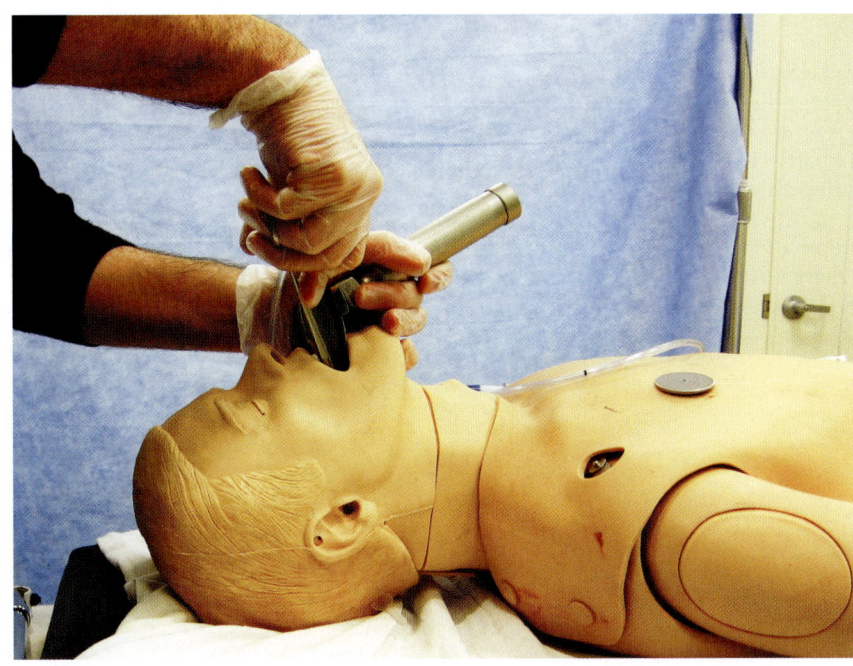

FIGURE 23-4 Using direct laryngoscopy combined with McGill forceps to assist in advancement of nasogastric tube into esophagus.

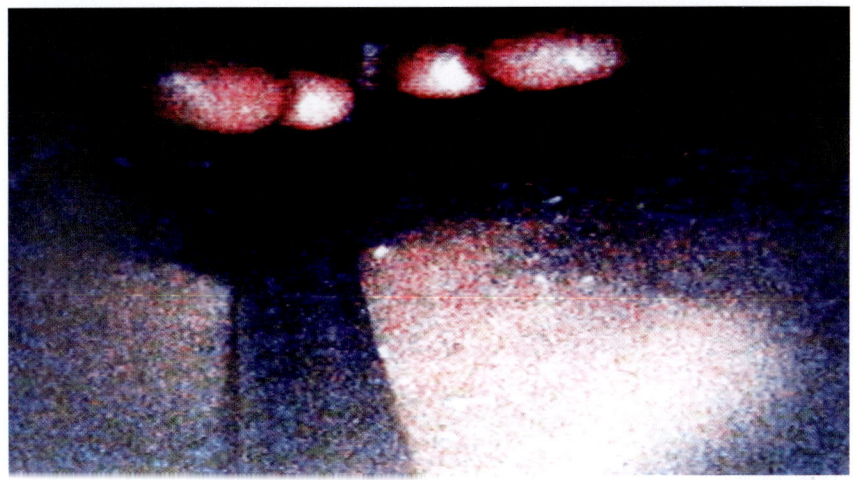

FIGURE 23-5 Video laryngoscope images showing nasogastric tube entering the esophagus.

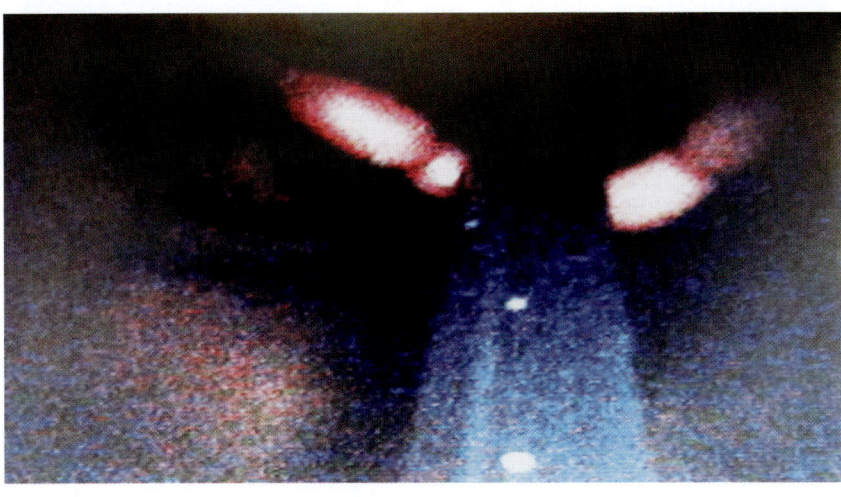

FIGURE 23-6 Video laryngoscope image showing nasogastric tube passing above the posterior arytenoids and entering the trachea.

SUGGESTED READING

Agarwal A, Gaur A, Sahu D, Singh PK, Pandey CK. Nasogastric tube knotting over the epiglottis: a cause of respiratory distress. *Anesth Analg* 2002;94(6):1659–1660.

Araujo-Preza CE, Melhado ME, Gutierrez FJ, Maniatis T, Castellano MA. Use of capnometry to verify feeding tube placement. *Crit Care Med* 2002;30(10):2255–2259.

Freij RM, Mullett ST. Inadvertent intracranial insertion of a nasogastric tube in a non-trauma patient. *J Accid Emerg Med* 1997;14(1):45–47.

Metheny NA, Meert KL, Clouse RE. Complications related to feeding tube placement. *Curr Opin Gastroenterol* 2007;23(2):178–182.

Roubenoff R, Ravich WJ. Pneumothorax due to nasogastric feeding tubes. Report of four cases, review of the literature, and recommendations for prevention. *Arch Intern Med* 1989;149(1):184–188.

Wynne DM, Borg HK, Geddes NK, Fredericks B. Nasogastric tube misplacement into Eustachian tube. *Int J Pediatr Otorhinolaryngol* 2003;67(2):185–187.

PART IV
BACK

CHAPTER 24
SPINAL ANESTHESIA

ALEXANDER M. DELEON
AMREESH MAHIL

Opera is when a guy gets stabbed in the back and, instead of bleeding, he sings.

Ed Gardner

INTRODUCTION

- Spinal anesthesia was first administered in 1899 by August Bier (the same guy as the Bier block). Dr. Bier and his assistant administered spinal anesthetics to each other with the use of cocaine and a technique described by Heinrich Quincke (who had a needle later named after him), and after striking the tibia with a hammer and pulling on a testicle, the experiment was considered a success and spinal anesthesia was born (true story).
- Not only was this Bier guy lucky enough to discover such a widely used anesthetic technique, leading to great fame, he also had the pleasure of discovering (and experiencing) one of the most widely whined-about complications, the postdural puncture headache.

INDICATIONS

- Surgery involving only the lower body (up to about the midabdomen) lasting up to 2 hours.
- Although neuraxial techniques (including spinal anesthesia) have been described for a wide range of surgical procedures, including thoracic, abdominal, lower extremities, breast, laparoscopy, anal, and even coronary artery bypass graft (CABG) surgery, factors such as patient comfort, surgeon preference, and anesthesiologist preference limit the use of spinal anesthetics.
- Common indications for spinal anesthesia are surgeries involving the knees (total knee replacements and knee arthroscopies), hips (open reductions of fractures and total hip replacements), C-sections, cervical cerclages, and postpartum tubal ligations.

CONTRAINDICATIONS

- Patient refusal
- Severe coagulopathy (which puts your patient at risk for a spinal hematoma; it ruins your day and your patient's day as well)
- Localized infection at the site of spinal insertion
- Mass in the spinal column (e.g., from metastatic cancer)

Relative Contraindications

- Preload-dependent cardiac lesions (think aortic stenosis)
- Previous spine surgery (this is more important for epidurals than spinals)
- Hypovolemia (who isn't at least a little hypovolemic after all that fasting?)
- Elevated intracranial pressure (could theoretically cause herniation)

EQUIPMENT AND PERSONNEL

- Spinal kit (Figure 24-1)
- Gloves, cap, mask
- Sterile prep solution (may be included in kit)
- Blood pressure cuff, pulse oximeter
- An assistant to help with patient positioning
- A chair or stool to rest patient's feet on

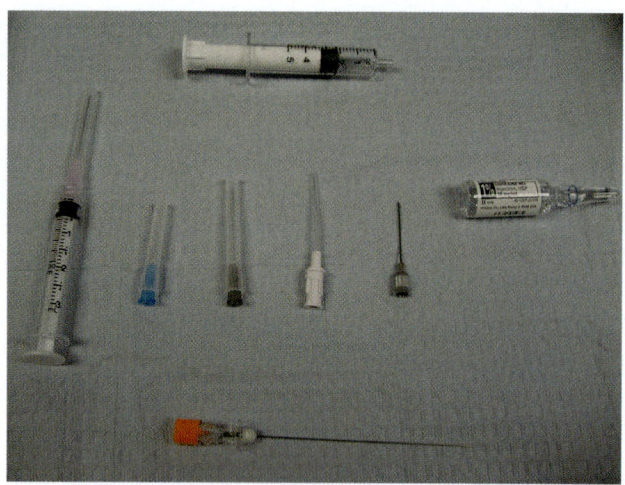

FIGURE 24-1 Typical contents of a spinal kit: a 25-G spinal needle, a syringe for the spinal drugs (*top*); a syringe for local infiltration; (*from left to right*) a 25-G needle for skin, a 22-G needle for deeper skin, a filter needle for drawing up the spinal drugs (it removes bits of glass that might have broken off when the vial was opened), a 3-cm-long introducer needle; local anesthetic for skin; and a spinal needle (*bottom*).

PHILOSOPHY OF SPINALS

- Although your average internist/cardiologist may believe that a patient who cannot tolerate general anesthesia may tolerate spinal anesthesia better (there is no evidence to support this), spinal anesthetics are not "safer" than general anesthetics.
- Some patients, when faced with the decision of general anesthesia or spinal anesthesia, may believe that general anesthesia takes away their sense of control and thus prefer spinal anesthesia.
- Some patients, when they hear that we need to place a "breathing tube" for general anesthesia, suddenly don't mind the prospect of a small needle in their back.
- Although not a guarantee of avoidance of the airway (a spinal may become high, fail, or wear off), you are more likely to avoid the airway with a spinal compared to a general anesthetic. Thus, patients with anticipated difficult airways, severe asthma, or obstructive sleep apnea may be better candidates for spinal anesthesia versus general anesthesia. (Note: It is controversial to do a regional in the face of a difficult airway. It's a no-brainer on labor and delivery, but outside of that the answer is not as clear.)
- Although a spinal may not shorten recovery time, patients will usually feel more awake during the recovery period compared to general anesthesia.
- Pregnant patients have different reasons for benefiting from spinal anesthesia versus general, which are beyond the scope of this discussion, but to simplify, spinals may be safer in the pregnant population due to avoidance of the pregnant woman's airway, which may be more edematous and difficult to secure.

SPINAL HISTORY AND PHYSICAL

- Ask about bleeding disorders, easy bleeding or bruising, anticoagulant/antiplatelet agent use (follow the American Society of Regional Anesthesia guidelines for neuraxial anesthesia and anticoagulation: www.asra.com).
- Preexisting neurologic conditions such as multiple sclerosis (some association with spinal anesthesia and relapse) make the use of a spinal anesthetic problematic.
- History of scoliosis, scoliosis repair, or other back surgeries. If a patient has scoliosis, placement may be difficult, yet neither scoliosis nor previous back surgeries are generally considered contraindications to spinal anesthesia.
- Physical examination may indicate scoliosis or difficult palpation of landmarks, and may lead you to advise a patient to accept general anesthesia rather than potentially suffer through a difficult spinal placement.

TECHNIQUE: CHOOSE YOUR DRUGS WISELY

- The patient wants a spinal for the knee scope procedure. Now it is time to decide what you plan to inject through that spinal needle. The five decisions regarding the spinal drug choice you need to make are:
  1. Drug choice
  2. Baricity
  3. Dose
  4. Adding an opioid
  5. Epinephrine or not
- Which drug to choose? The choice of drug depends on how long the surgery is going to last. Similarly, the decision of the addition of epinephrine depends on the duration of the surgery.
- In order from shortest to longest duration of action, the common choices are lidocaine, mepivacaine, bupivacaine, and tetracaine.
- Both lidocaine and mepivacaine are associated with a higher incidence of transient neurologic symptoms (TNS; see Complications, below) compared with bupivacaine.

- The downside to using bupivacaine simply to avoid TNS is that although the duration of surgical anesthesia may only be on the order of 1 hour longer compared to lidocaine, the time until a patient is able to urinate (and thus go home) may be 2 to 3 hours longer than with lidocaine.
- After deciding which local anesthetic to use, the next question is what baricity to use. Baricity is defined as the density of a local anesthetic solution compared to the density of cerebrospinal fluid (CSF) at 37°C.
- Thus, hyperbaric local anesthetics will flow caudad when a patient sits and cephalad when a patient lies flat (due to the lordosis of the spine in the lumbar region). Use of a hyperbaric drug allows for a thoracic level to be obtained, which is especially useful for C-sections (where a T4 level is desired). The downside to using hyperbaric drug is that with a thoracic level comes a higher incidence of hypotension.
- Isobaric local anesthetic will tend to stay closer to the level of insertion. Usually about a T10 level is obtained. Such a level is ideal for both hip and knee surgeries, and decreases the risk of hypotension.
- Hypobaric solutions are rarely used.
- Epinephrine (a vasoconstrictor) is added to prolong the duration of action of a local anesthetic.
- Adding epinephrine to bupivacaine at a dose of 100 to 200 µg will increase the duration of block by greater than 50% and will also increase the time until urination by a considerable amount.
- Addition of fentanyl (15 µg) or sufentanil may improve the quality of the block. In other words, you may get more bang for your buck with a lower dose of local anesthetic. The addition of these drugs may allow you to use less local, and thus less hypotension will result.
- Addition of morphine (150 µg) to a spinal anesthetic will provide about 12 hours of postoperative analgesia, but you'll need to monitor the patient for respiratory depression for >12 hours after the procedure. For this reason, morphine is discouraged for ambulatory surgery (see Suggested Reading, below).

TECHNIQUE: KNOW THE ANATOMY

- The spinal cord in adults terminates at L1, and thus spinal anesthetics are often performed below this level.
- A line joining the upper boarder of each iliac crest crosses L4; therefore, the L3-4 interspace is above this line and the L4-5 space is below this line.
- The layers that are crossed in order to reach the dura are skin, subcutaneous fat, supraspinous ligament, interspinous ligament, ligamentum flavum, and dura.

TECHNIQUE: PATIENT SEATED

- Have the patient sit with the legs hanging off the side of the bed and have your assistant stabilize the patient.
- Monitor the patient's blood pressure and pulse ox throughout the procedure.
- Have the patient curl the back like a cooked shrimp with the shoulders relaxed and the chin close to the chest.
- You may want to feel the spinous processes prior to placing your sterile gloves and prior to prepping the back so as to better focus your prep (Figures 24-2 and 24-3).
- The iliac crests mark the L4 vertebral body, and therefore the L3-4 space is above this landmark. Since the spinal cord ends at L1, usually L3-4 is a good starting point for your initial attempt at placement (Figure 24-4).
- Once you have an idea of where to start, prep the back with your prep solution starting in the center and making concentric circles.
- Then place the drape with the target in the center.
- Draw up your local anesthetic intended for the spinal dose using the 5 mL syringe and the filter needle. If you choose to add fentanyl (usually 15 µg) or epinephrine (100 to 200 µg), you may have an assistant inject those into your syringe using a small needle (such as the ones used for purified protein derivative [PPD] tests or insulin administration).
- Inject local anesthetic into the skin using the 25-gauge (G) (the blue needle pictured). You may choose to use a second needle to inject local anesthetic (such as a 22-G needle), but keep in mind that it is possible to nick the dura with the longer 22-G needle (Figures 24-5 and 24-6).
- Place the introducer needle at an angle almost perpendicular to the skin, but with a slightly cephalad trajectory (Figures 24-7 and 24-8).
- The spinal needle is then inserted through the introducer needle. You will notice resistance to insertion once the spinal needle exits the tip of the introducer. Continue to advance the spinal needle until a "pop" is felt, which indicates puncture of the dura (Figures 24-9 and 24-10).
- Remove the stylette and the spinal needle, and observe CSF return. Once the CSF is about to drip from the hub, attach the spinal local anesthetic needle (Figure 24-11).
- Aspirate CSF, which will appear as a swirl within the syringe, and then inject the local anesthetic dose. Some choose to aspirate incrementally to ensure continued flow (Figure 24-12).
- Remove the needle, drape, and lay the patient on his or her back.

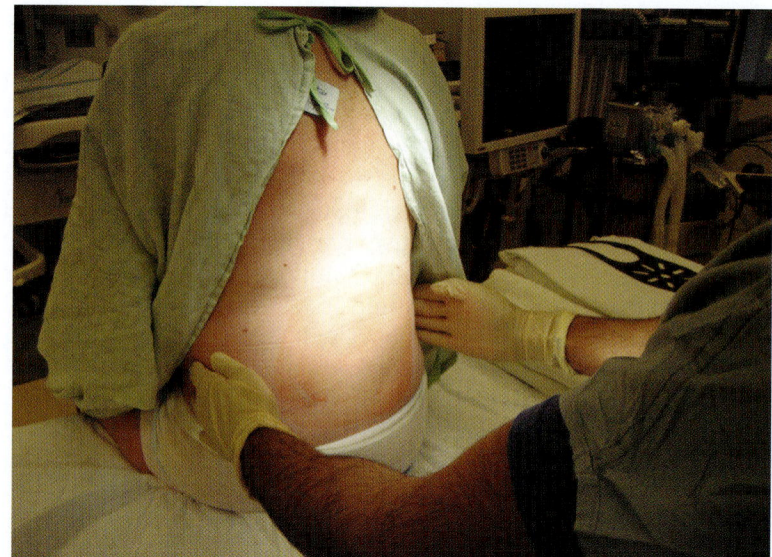

FIGURE 24-2 The first step after proper positioning and monitoring is to palpate the iliac crests (prior to putting on your sterile gloves).

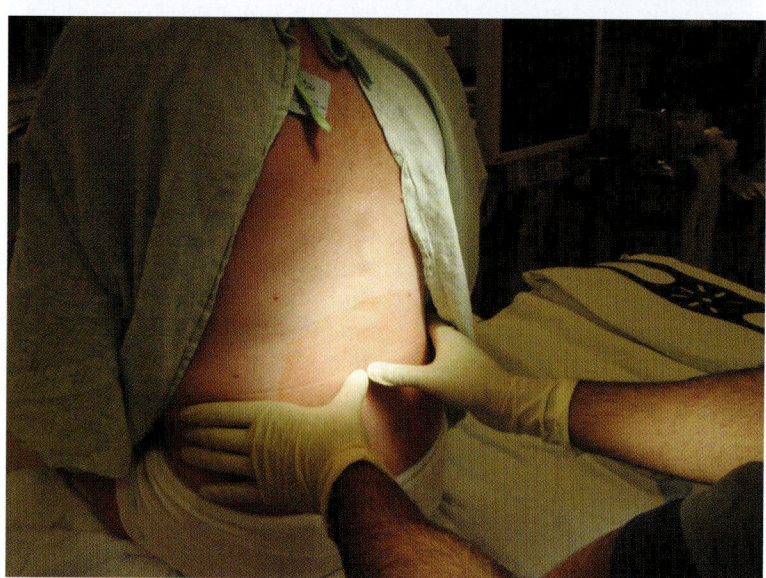

FIGURE 24-3 With your fingers on the iliac crests, you can now locate the L3-4 interspace with your thumbs. You may choose to mark this space by slightly indenting it with your finger nail.

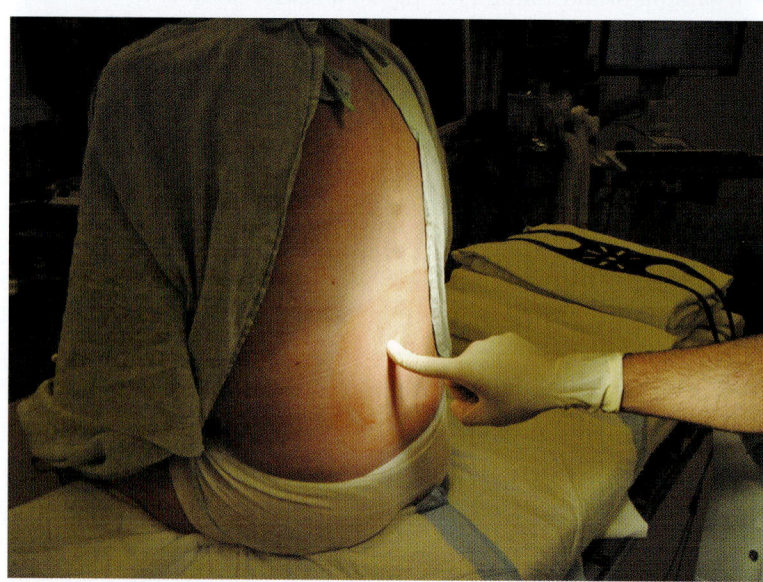

FIGURE 24-4 Indenting the L3-4 interspace with a fingernail.

Chapter 24 SPINAL ANESTHESIA

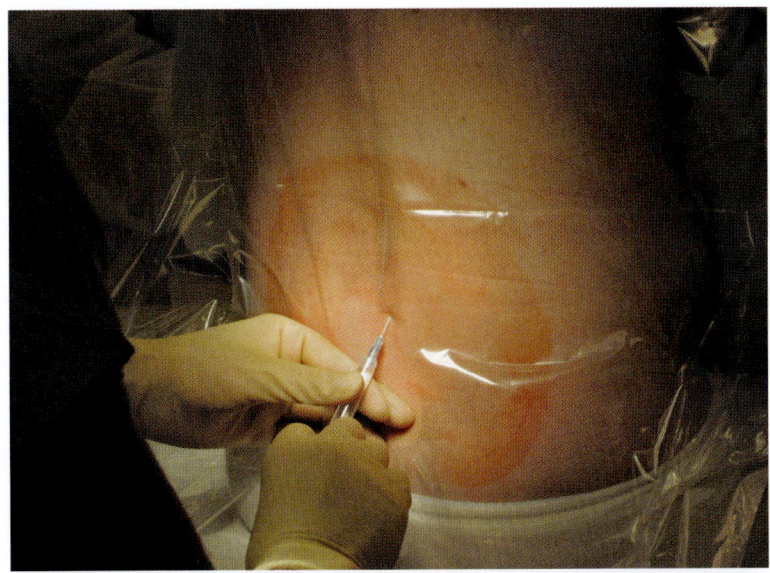

FIGURE 24-5 Once the area is prepped and draped, a small-gauge needle (25-G) is used to inject local anesthetic into the skin.

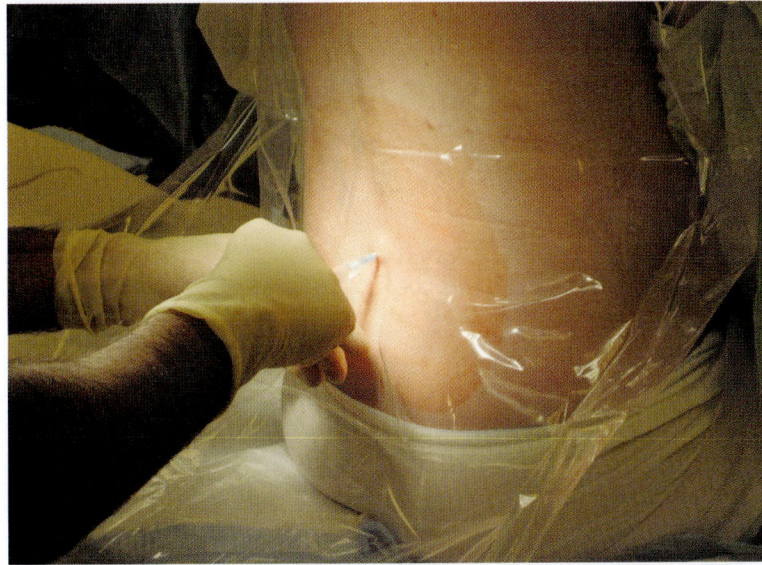

FIGURE 24-6 The 25-G needle is then inserted deep. Resistance to injection when the needle is inserted helps to confirm the needle placement into the interspinous ligament. This is the trajectory that your introducer needle should take.

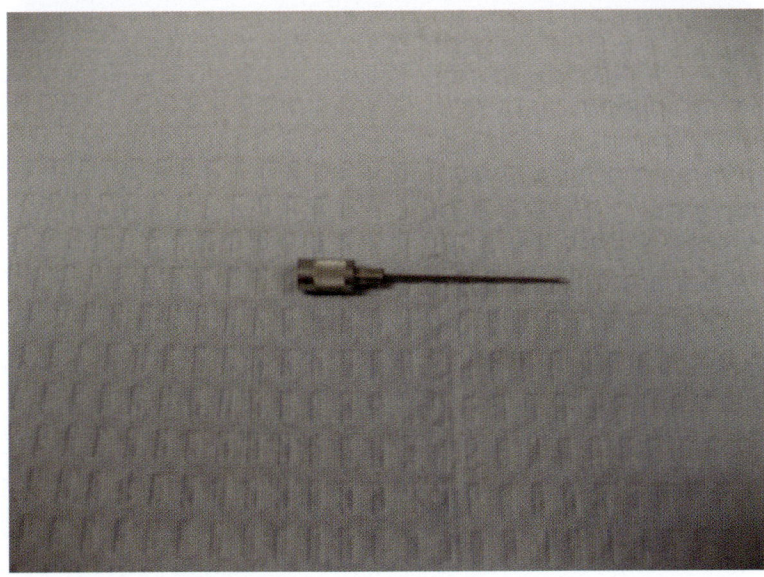

FIGURE 24-7 Introducer needle. The purpose of the introducer needle is to allow easy insertion of the spinal needle. The spinal needle tip is blunt and thus would be difficult to insert through the skin. Also, given the relatively flimsy nature of a 25-G spinal needle, an introducer helps to direct the spinal needle into the interspinous ligament. Most of us have heard of a colleague who has seen CSF come through this needle; therefore, beware of burying this in patients who are extremely thin (that colleague might be you).

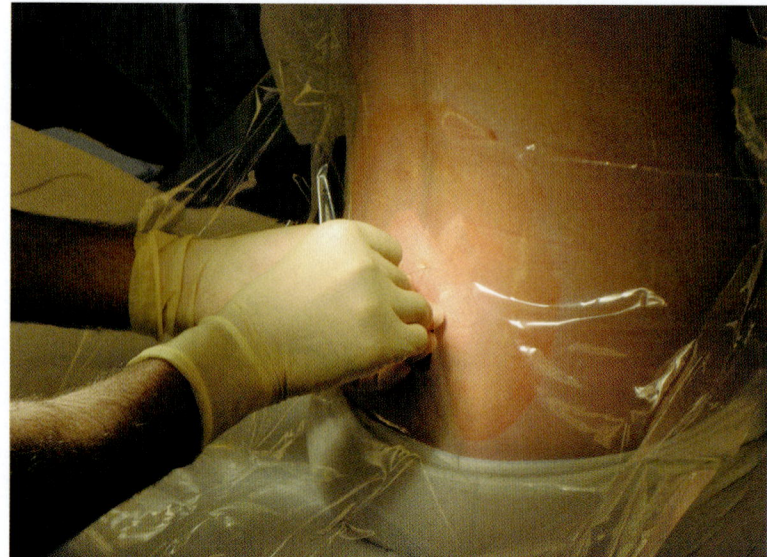

FIGURE 24-8 Introducing the introducer needle. The goal is to place this needle into the interspinous ligament. The needle direction should be horizontal to the ground (usually about 15 degrees cephalad due to the patient leaning slightly forward).

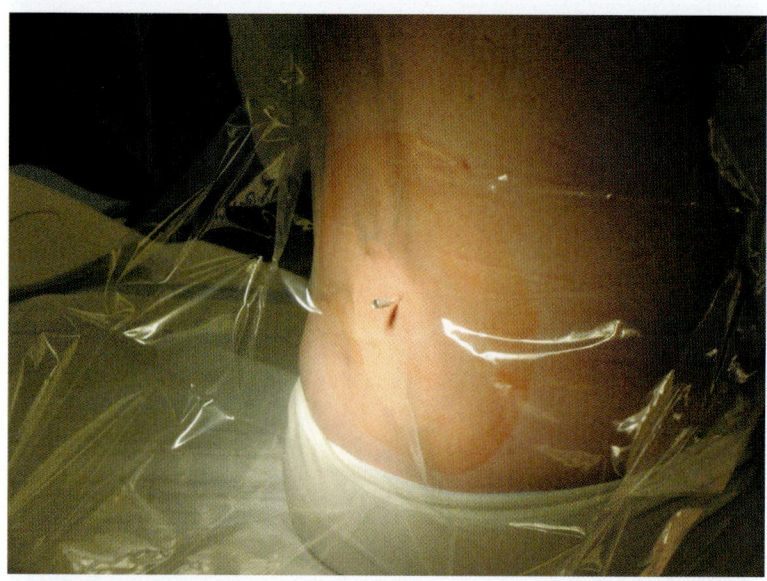

FIGURE 24-9 Introducer needle is inserted.

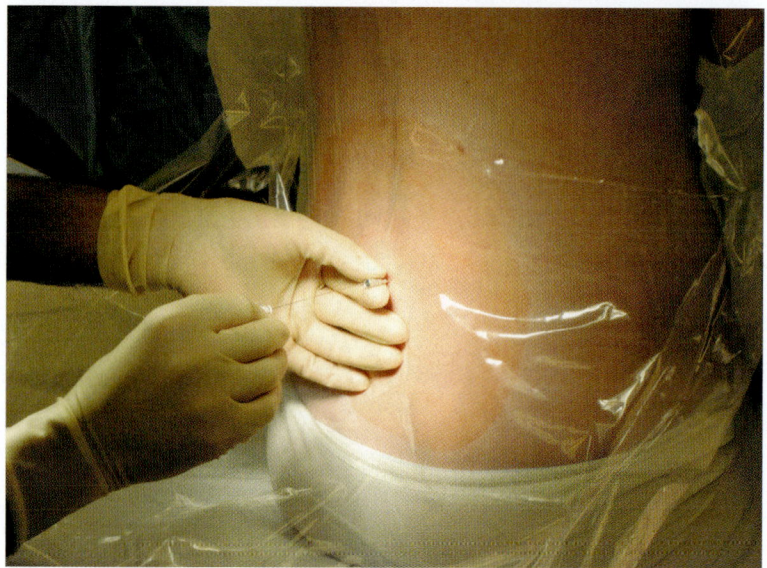

FIGURE 24-10 Insert the spinal needle through the introducer. You will notice resistance to insertion once the spinal needle exits the tip of the introducer. There is no need to check for CSF until you feel the characteristic "pop" of penetration of the dura. Many beginners feel that they need to check for CSF after ever 2 mm of insertion, but this is a waste of time and prolongs the time that the needle is in the patient's back.

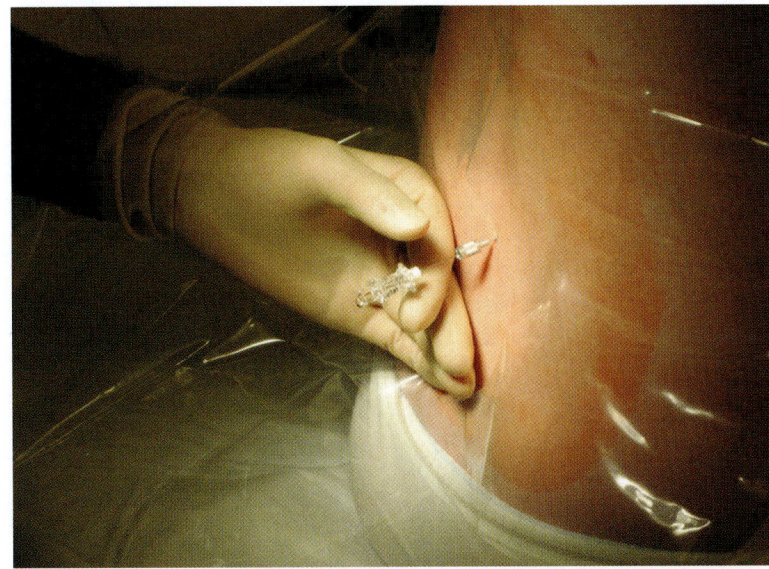

FIGURE 24-11 CSF will return slowly (remember this is only a 25-G needle). Wait until the first drop of CSF is about to exit the hub, then attach the syringe of local spinal anesthetic. The goal is not to inject air intrathecally (this could possibly cause a headache from a pneumocephalus).

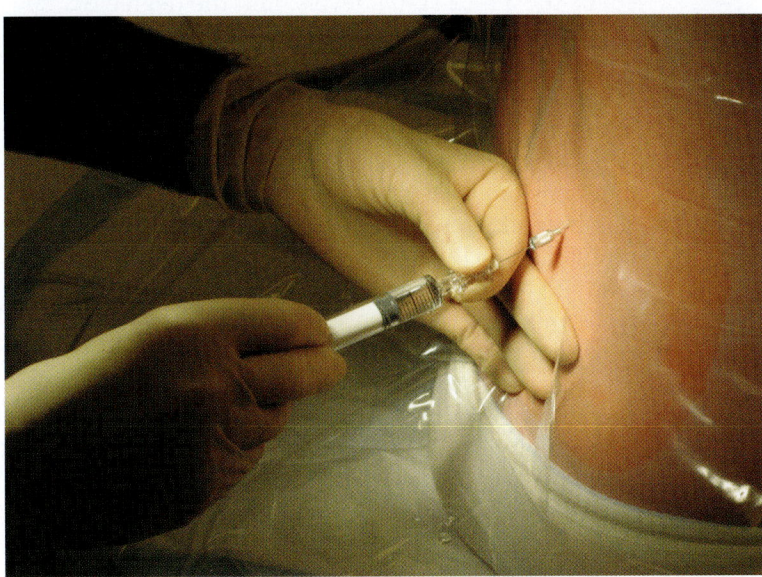

FIGURE 24-12 Finally, aspirate to ensure that the needle tip did not dislodge. Inject the local anesthetic. Some clinicians will aspirate in the middle of the injection and at the end to ensure that CSF still flows (and thus know that the patient received the entire dose). The act of aspirating in the middle may actually cause you to move the needle, and I personally omit the mid-injection aspiration.

TECHNIQUE: PATIENT IN LATERAL POSITION

- Some patients do better in the lateral position such as a patient with a hip fracture who cannot sit up. For this reason it is worthwhile to be skilled in performing spinal anesthetics also in the lateral position.
- The landmarks and technique for lateral spinal placement are similar to those for the sitting placement.
- Although you attempt to have the patient's hips perpendicular to the floor, often the patient's up hip is rotated forward and thus you may need to angle your needle slightly downward (about 10 to 15 degrees).

REDIRECTION: HITTING BONE

- When you hit bone, and you are pretty sure you are midline, you are likely to be contacting spinous process. If your needle has contacted the superior edge of the inferior spinous process (which is often the case), a 15- to 20-degree cephalad redirection is indicated.
- When redirecting, be sure to withdraw the spinal needle out of the tip of the introducer. Then withdraw the introducer needle about 2 cm (does not need to be withdrawn from the skin) and reinsert the introducer followed by the spinal needle.

- If you contact bone, you may ask the patient if they feel the needle to the left, right, or in the middle. You may be contacting lamina (lateral to midline) and thus will need to redirect left or right.
- If you contact bone immediately after inserting the spinal needle (at a very shallow depth), you might be in the middle of a spinous process. In this case you should consider removing the needles and starting 1 to 2 cm above or below the original insertion spot.
- If you continue to contact bone despite multiple redirections, consider trying a new interspace.

PARESTHESIA: TO INJECT OR NOT?

- A patient may jump and complain about an "electrical sensation" down the leg. This is very disconcerting to beginners, and many worry that they will paralyze the patient if they inject. Some clinicians would suggest that you don't even check for CSF if a patient experiences a paresthesia; rather, you should remove the spinal needle and proceed in a different location.
- An observational study[1] found that in 86.7% of patients experiencing a paresthesia on spinal needle insertion, CSF was observed in the needle hub. The authors concluded that when a transient paresthesia occurs during spinal needle placement it is appropriate to stop and assess for the presence of CSF in the needle hub, rather than withdraw and redirect the spinal needle.
- So if you get a paresthesia, check for CSF. If CSF is present, inject slowly. If the paresthesia returns, consider stopping your injection and placing the spinal in a different spot. If the paresthesia does not return, you are in the clear.

COMPLICATIONS (THINGS THAT WILL GIVE YOU A HEADACHE)

- Transient neurologic symptoms occur after spinal anesthesia and are described as pain in the gluteal region radiating to both lower extremities. The incidence has been reported as approximately 14% when lidocaine is used, which is seven times more common than with bupivacaine, prilocaine, or procaine. When mepivacaine is used, the incidence is similar to that with lidocaine. Some clinicians avoid lidocaine completely to preclude this complaint, yet TNS is easily treated with nonsteroidal antiinflammatory drugs (NSAIDs), such as ibuprofen, and is rarely severe. I recommend warning patients that they may have a backache (if I'm going to use lidocaine), and that if they do have this backache, take ibuprofen.
- Postdural puncture headaches (PDPHs) are reported to range from 0% to 14.5% with a 25- to 27-G pencil point needle. Our experience is that they occur less than 1% with spinal anesthetics. The headaches may last up to 7 to 10 days.
- Other devastating complications that may lead to permanent nerve injury such as epidural hematoma and abscess are thankfully rare (on the order of 1 in 200,000).

SIDE EFFECTS

- The biggest side effect of spinal anesthesia is hypotension. The sympathetic nervous system spans the T1-L2 spinal levels, and the degree of hypotension correlates to the height of the block.
- Thus a T4 level will give you more hypotension than a T10 level. Using isobaric solutions for lower extremity surgery (where a high thoracic level is not needed) may help to decrease the risk of hypotension.
- The potential for hypotension is a big reason to monitor the patient closely after a spinal and be ready to treat hypotension with fluids, pressors, and positioning.
- A patient may have a subjective sensation of shortness of breath after a spinal is placed due to loss of proprioception of the chest muscles. Check grip strength (C6-8) to reassure yourself that the phrenic nerves (C3-5) are intact.

CONCLUSION

- Why do attendings always seem to be moving so fast when they are doing spinals? The secret is that each pass with the needle should be extremely quick (yet controlled), and they can make 10 passes in the time it takes a beginner to make two. A big part of the successful spinal placement is trial and error, so make deliberate redirections each time your needle contacts bone.
- Patients who get hypotensive from a spinal often complain first of nausea. When a patient has nausea immediately after a spinal, you may choose to treat with pressors rather than grabbing the antiemetic of choice.
- Finally, tell patients before the spinal is placed that they may have a headache afterward. I don't try to scare them away from a spinal, but the last thing

you want is for postdural puncture headache patients to claim that they wouldn't have gotten a spinal if they knew this could happen (and this has happened to me).

REFERENCE

1. Pong RP, Gmelch BS, Bernards CM. Does a paresthesia during spinal needle insertion indicate intrathecal needle placement? *Reg Anesth Pain Med* 2009;34(1):29–32.
   This article addresses the association between paresthesias and proper intrathecal needle placement.

SUGGESTED READING

Hartmann B, Junger A, Klasen J, et al. The incidence and risk factors for hypotension after spinal anesthesia induction: an analysis with automated data collection. *Anesth Analg* 2002;94(6):1521–1529.

Hypotension is a very common side effect after spinal anesthesia. This article identifies the risk factors for spinal anesthesia induced hypotension.

Horlocker TT, Burton AW, Connis RT, et al. Practice guidelines for the prevention, detection, and management of respiratory depression associated with neuraxial opioid administration. *Anesthesiology* 2009;110(2):218–230.

Respiratory depression with administration of neuraxial opioids has implications over decisions regarding choice of opioids and postoperative monitoring.

Horlocker TT, Wedel DJ. Neurologic complications of spinal and epidural anesthesia. *Reg Anesth Pain Med* 2000;25(1):83–98.

Patients may ask questions about neurologic complications/risks associated with neuraxial anesthesia, and this is a good article discussing the topic.

Horlocker TT, Wedel DJ, Rowlingson JC, Enneking FK. Executive summary: regional anesthesia in the patient receiving antithrombotic or thrombolytic therapy: American Society of Regional Anesthesia and Pain Medicine Evidence-Based Guidelines (third edition). *Reg Anesth Pain Med* 2010;35(1):102–105.

Given that the most often mentioned contraindication for neuraxial anesthesia is coagulopathy, it benefits you to have read through the entire document. This panel reconvenes periodically and updates are posted on the Web site www.asra.com.

Zaric D, Christiansen C, Pace NL, Punjasawadwong Y. Transient neurologic symptoms after spinal anesthesia with lidocaine versus other local anesthetics: a systematic review of randomized, controlled trials. *Anesth Analg* 2005;100(6):1811–1816.

This is an in-depth article about the relationship between types of local anesthetics and incidence of transient neurologic symptoms.

CHAPTER 25
EPIDURAL, LUMBAR

SOFIA GERALEMOU
RANY MAKARYUS
ROBERT KYUREGHIAN
ROBIN J. SCHILLER
JOY SCHABEL

INTRODUCTION: EPIDURALS ARE GREAT

Epidurals can be used for a wide variety of cases, from foot cases to orthopedic cases to vascular cases. Epidurals can also be used in combined general-epidural cases, using the epidural for postoperative pain relief as well as intraoperative management (e.g., thoracic surgeries). So the epidural can do what most spinals can do, plus the catheter stays in for redosing, to be used after the procedure—all kinds of wonderful things.

But who are we kidding; the most frequent use of epidurals is on the labor deck. "Yea, I have heard the voice of woman in travail," says the Good Book, and, if you are an anesthesiologist, "Yeah, ye too will hear the voice of woman in travail." And they will be asking for pain relief from "the grievous burden of birth."

And that means you.

And that means an epidural.

INDICATIONS

- Delivery of local anesthetic to provide anesthesia
- Delivery of local anesthetic to provide analgesia
- Delivery of narcotic to provide analgesia
- Delivery of local anesthetic to provide sympathetic block (for preeclamptic patients committed for delivery)
- In a few special cases, delivery of other medications for analgesia (clonidine, for example)
- Placement of epidural steroids for pain relief
- Placement of epidural devices for chronic pain relief (these last two more in the realm of a pain textbook)

CONTRAINDICATIONS

- Coagulopathy
- Infection at the site
- Systemic infection (relative contraindication; for example, the pregnant patient with chorioamnionitis is at low risk of getting an epidural abscess from the systemic infection, and an epidural should be placed early to have in place if she should need a C-section entailing a risk of infection, but a functioning epidural makes her a safer C-section in case of a sudden need to cut, so you may place the epidural even in the face of an infection)
- Mass in the back, such a metastatic cancer (CA). Keep in mind the cancers that often spread to the back, such as prostate CA.
- Ongoing neurologic problems (relative contraindication; a pregnant patient with a lot of sciatica may benefit from the safety of a well-placed and functioning epidural, even though you are loathe to instrument the back of someone who has chronic back pain)
- Increased intracranial pressure. You could get a wet tap, then the patient could herniate.
- Hypovolemia (where the sympathectomy could bring the blood pressure to zero)
- Stenotic valve lesion (where the sympathectomy could finish the patient off, but even this is relative, since you could argue that you could dose very slowly, watch the volume status, and still pull this off in a safe fashion. It's hard to make absolute statements in the world of medicine!)

EQUIPMENT

- Epidural kit, operator's choice
- Someone to watch the patients and hold them in good position (crucial, crucial, crucial)
- On OB, a fetal heart monitor that's sending a good, reliable signal (don't place an epidural if you're not picking up a good signal, the baby could get in trouble and you'd never know it)

BEWARE THE ALREADY-IN EPIDURAL

- Have a low threshold to repeat the test dose. People wiggle around, and the epidural may have fallen out.
- Of particular danger is this scene: You get a wet tap, thread a catheter into the CSF, use the epidural as a continuous spinal, and then you get relieved and somehow the message doesn't get related. Then someone forgets, gives an epidural dose through a continuous spinal—and now *TOTAL SPINAL!* Communication with colleagues and nursing staff is essential.

PHILOSOPHY

- Outside of the OB setting, you can sedate patients when you place epidurals.
- When you sedate patients, don't overdo it. You need their cooperation to be still and direct you if you are having trouble getting in the space. In this situation, you can ask the patient, "Where do you feel the pressure of the needle?" If the patient replies, "On the right," then aim to the left. The patient also needs to be awake enough to report or react to a paresthesia.
- We hesitate to place epidurals in the patient under general anesthesia (the exception being a kiddie caudal), because a patient under general anesthesia cannot report to you that you have nailed a nerve root.
- If you do have to give a sedative to a pregnant patient, then let the pediatricians know it since they may have to support the baby's ventilation.
- On OB, when you place the epidural, you have to keep your third eye on the fetal heart rate at all times, or deputize the holding person to watch it.
- Do your best to keep the patients from extending their backs pre-epidural. When that doesn't work, give a demonstration and frequent reminders during the procedure. Then do your epidural work between contractions when the patient will lean forward. She'll tell you when a contraction is starting. You may be able to strike a deal with her and you'll stop and let her wiggle and breathe through it.
- On OB, if you see trouble coming (very large patients, potential bad airway, preeclampsia), get your epidural in early, even if that means you just place the catheter, but don't run a continuous infusion catheter; test it. Remember, you are working hard to prevent the following disaster:
  - Fetal trouble
  - Back to OR
  - Stat C-section
  - No time for a regional or can't get it in under pressure
  - Induce general anesthesia
  - Lose the airway
  - Catastrophe
- No kidding, no kidding this happens, so put on your proactive shoes and get ready early on. An epidural that works and that you have confidence in will go a long way toward heading off this very real threat.
- Thoracic epidurals for thoracotomies provide great pain relief, and a thoracotomy is a most painful procedure. So this is one regional technique we encourage patients to accept.
- If you are placing an epidural for a vascular or orthopedic case, think carefully about dosing with heparin and Lovenox, and think carefully about when you will pull the catheter out. If, for example, an abdominal aortic aneurysm (AAA) turns into a bloodbath and the patient develops a coagulopathy, then make sure the coagulation system is back to normal before you remove the catheter.
- If you ever get a hint of epidural trouble such as a hematoma or abscess, drop everything! Get neurosurgery and get a study (MRI or CT) right away! *Don't let someone else* take care of this! Don't send orders and hope they'll get done! Don't continue your normal workday! Absolutely make this the number-one priority in your life—this minute, this second. A short stretch of time separates complete recovery from complete paralysis and you have got to make it happen!

EPIDURAL HISTORY AND PHYSICAL

- Ask about and look for the contraindications to an epidural.
- Easy bleeding and bruising? On Plavix? On Coumadin? Lovenox?
- If patients are on aspirin, that's OK, as long as they aren't on all sorts of anticoagulants.

Chapter 25 EPIDURAL, LUMBAR

- Systolic murmur no one heard about before? Get an echo and make sure they don't have aortic or mitral stenosis.
- Look at the back for masses, infections, and old scars from surgery.
- Does the patient have preexisting numbness or weakness? Back pain?

TECHNIQUE

- All the wizardry you employ to find the space between the bones for a spinal, apply here.
- Palpate the back, getting a feel for where the spinous processes are. If time is precious, then omit this step to save time. You will be palpating again after the patient is prepped and draped.
- Look again at a model of the vertebrae, so your mind's eye will be able to navigate the twists and turns and avoid bone.
- Feel the space with your bare hand and make a dent in the skin with the hub of a needle, which often gives you a better first shot.
- You can go midline or paramedian, keeping in mind that the paramedian approach is a little more likely to get you into a blood vessel.
- For a lumbar approach, go L3-4 or L4-5, as you do for a spinal. For a thoracic approach, you can place the epidural almost anywhere; the idea is to make sure you will cover the area of the incision.
- For the thoracic approach, the higher you go in the thorax, the steeper the angle. The lower you go in the thorax, the shallower the angle. Thus, a low thoracic epidural is not much different from a high lumbar.
- You can place epidurals with the patient sitting or lying on his or her side, just as with a spinal.
- Place your local midline for the midline approach.
- Place your local 1 to 2 cm lateral and caudad for a paramedian approach.
- Place the epidural needle through the same hole made by local skin wheal. No patient needs to have more than one scab his or her back.
- Attach a syringe filled with air or saline. This syringe should be a special epidural syringe that has an easy-slide plunger that will give you a good feel for the loss of resistance. We think glass syringes give the best feel.
- You can use air or saline; however, bear in mind that saline and CSF look the same, and if there's any question that you have a wet tap, a syringe that was previously filled with air, now filled with fluid, will leave little doubt as to what has transpired. (See Air vs. Saline, below, for pros and cons.)
- Advance the needle slowly, applying pressure to the plunger, until you feel a give. This is hard to describe in words, and it's something you just have to do to get the Aha! feeling.
- Don't advance any more. You are close to CSF and a wet tap.
- Remove the syringe and look out for warm CSF telling you that you got a wet tap.
- Inject 5 cc of saline to help prevent IV insertion.
- Advance the epidural catheter into the epidural space. Leave it about 3 to 5 cm in the space.
- Placing the catheter too shallow runs the risk of the catheter pulling out.
- Placing the catheter too deep runs the risk of getting into a nerve foramen and getting one-sided block or getting intravascular.
- The catheter should go easily.
- Once the catheter is in, pull the needle back. Never pull the catheter back through the needle, because you may sheer the catheter off.
- Discard the needle, and secure the catheter.
- Make sure you use a transparent dressing because you will want to inspect the site.
- Aspirate the catheter, looking for blood (a red substance) or CSF (a clear substance). If you get either of these, remove the catheter and start over.
- Alternately, if you get CSF, you can use this as a continuous spinal catheter, but make sure everybody knows! Label everywhere. the catheter, the infusion pump, even the infusion tubing! An epidural dose of local anesthetic delivered into the CSF is a vast overdose, and will result in a high spinal, respiratory arrest, and circulatory collapse.
- The above-mentioned three items are not good things.
- Your test-dose solution will consist of a quick-onset local anesthetic, and usually 1:200,000 epinephrine. The typical test does is 3 cc of lidocaine 1.5% with epi 1:200,000.
- Give the test dose of local anesthetic, looking for signs of intra-CSF injection (you get a complete block similar to a spinal) or an intravascular injection (ringing in the ears, funny feeling, tingling around the mouth, or tachycardia).
- If the test dose is negative, then the catheter is probably in. You will not be 100% sure this is so until you get a sensory block after dosing the catheter.
- Keep in mind, though that every dose you give is a test dose, and that a catheter that was in the right place may now be in the wrong place. Have a healthy respect for epidurals, and always look at them as maybe, just maybe, not still in the epidural space (Figures 25-1 to 25-10).

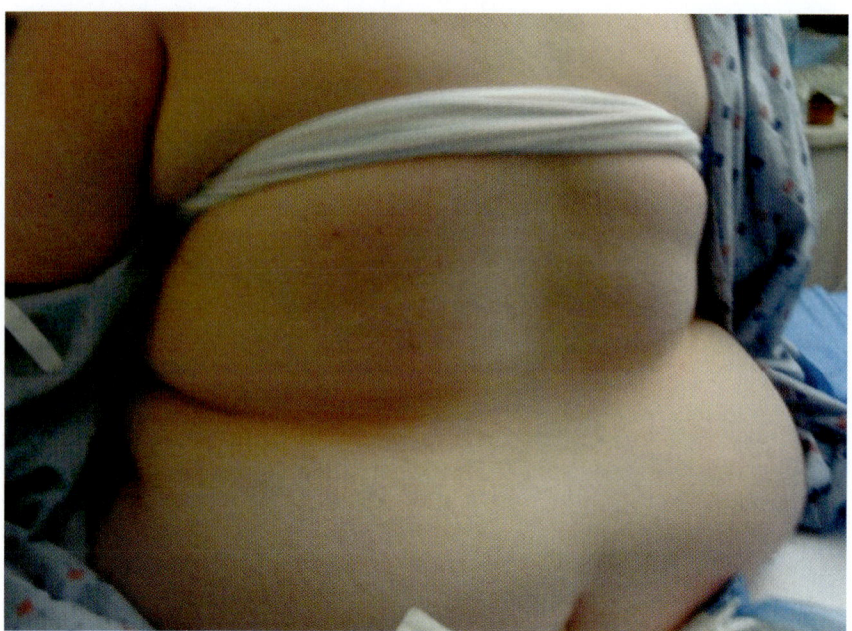

FIGURE 25-1 Sitting position.

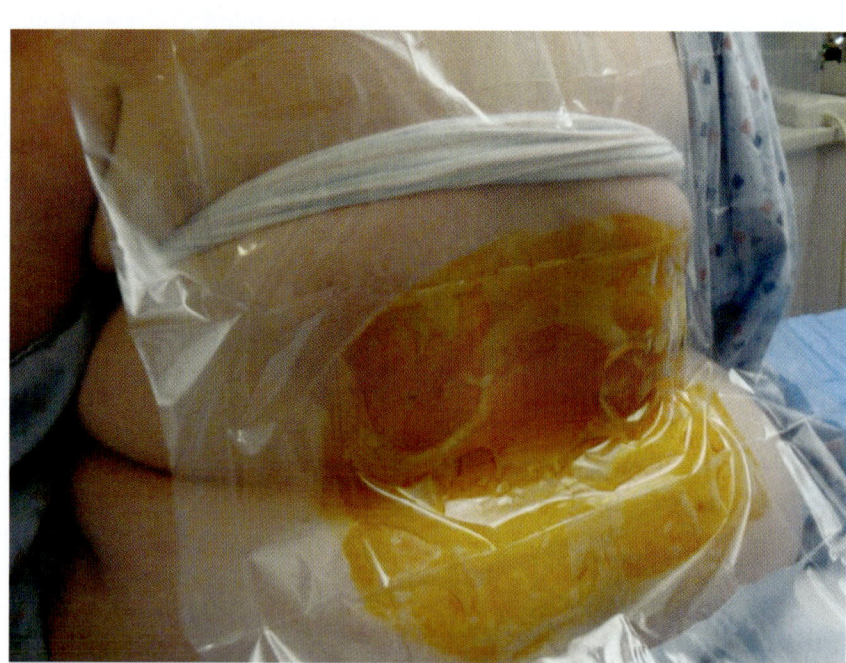

FIGURE 25-2 Prepped and draped.

Chapter 25 EPIDURAL, LUMBAR

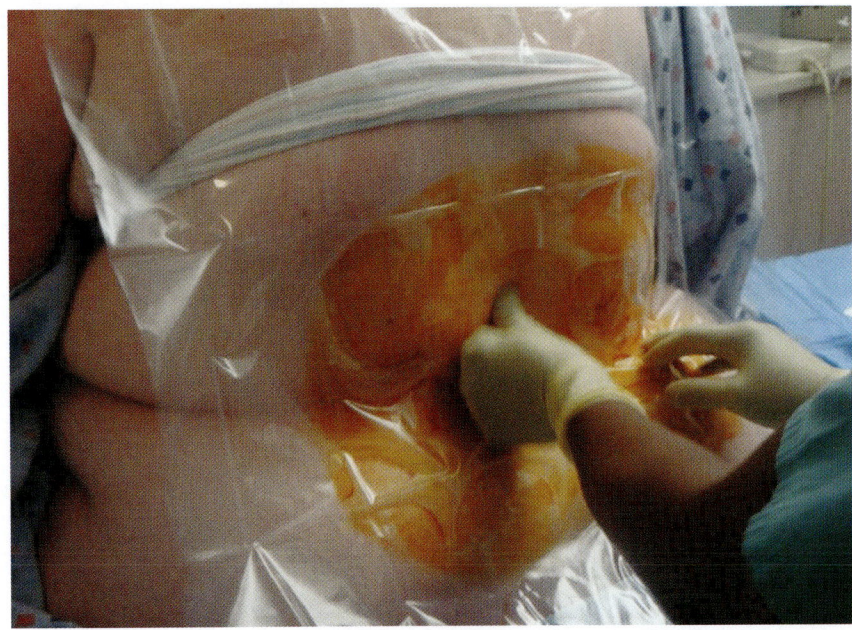

FIGURE 25-3 Feel the spinous processes to establish midline.

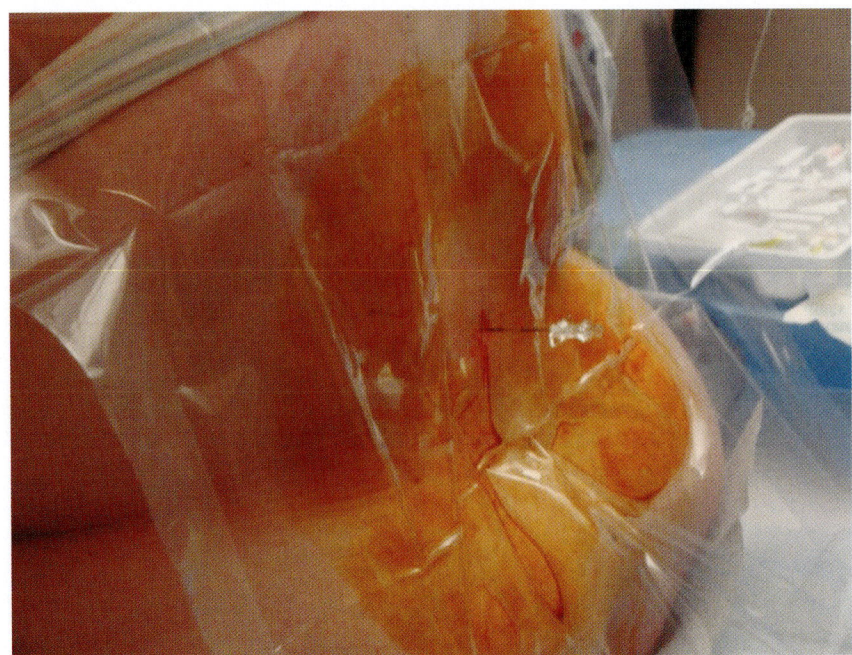

FIGURE 25-4 Tuohy needle seated in supra/interspinous ligament.

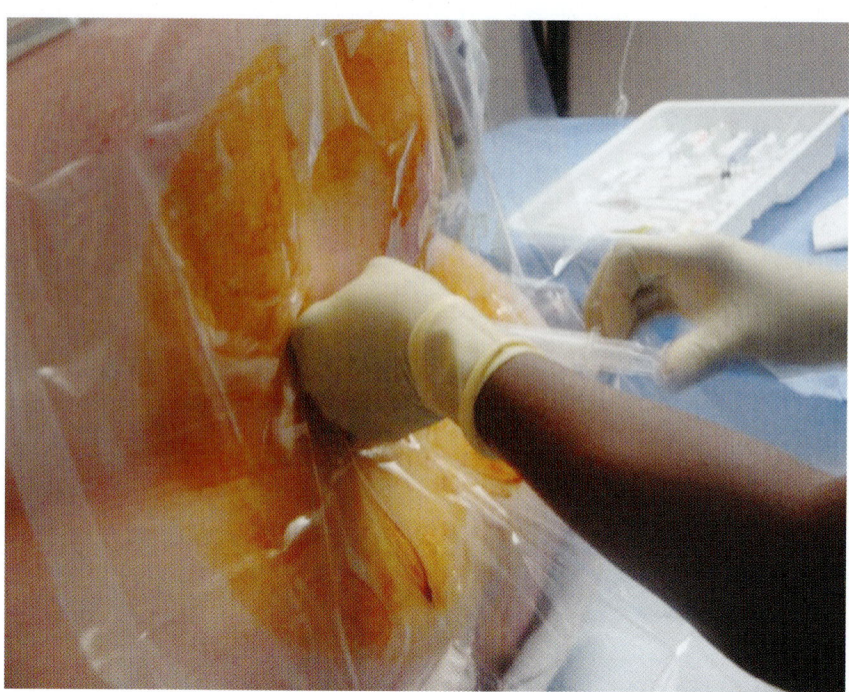

FIGURE 25-5 Glass syringe/LOR technique.

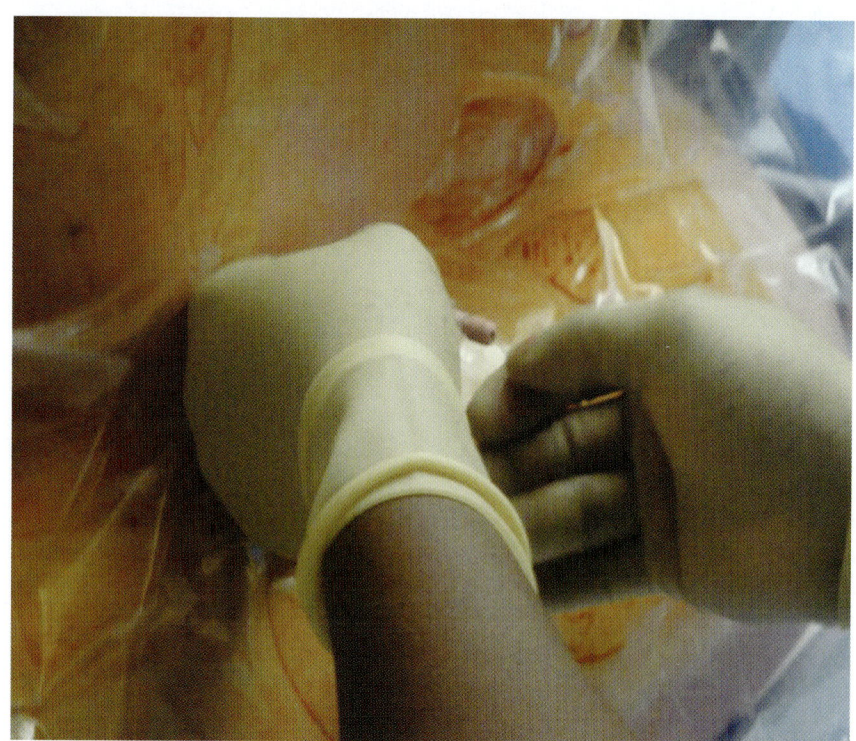

FIGURE 25-6 Threading the catheter.

Chapter 25 EPIDURAL, LUMBAR

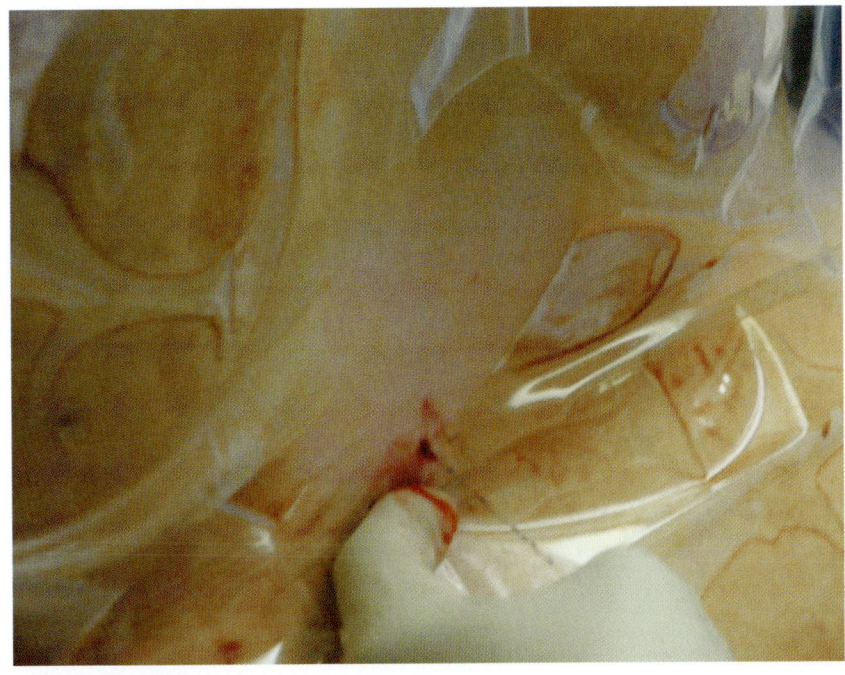

FIGURE 25-7 Pulling the catheter back to the appropriate depth.

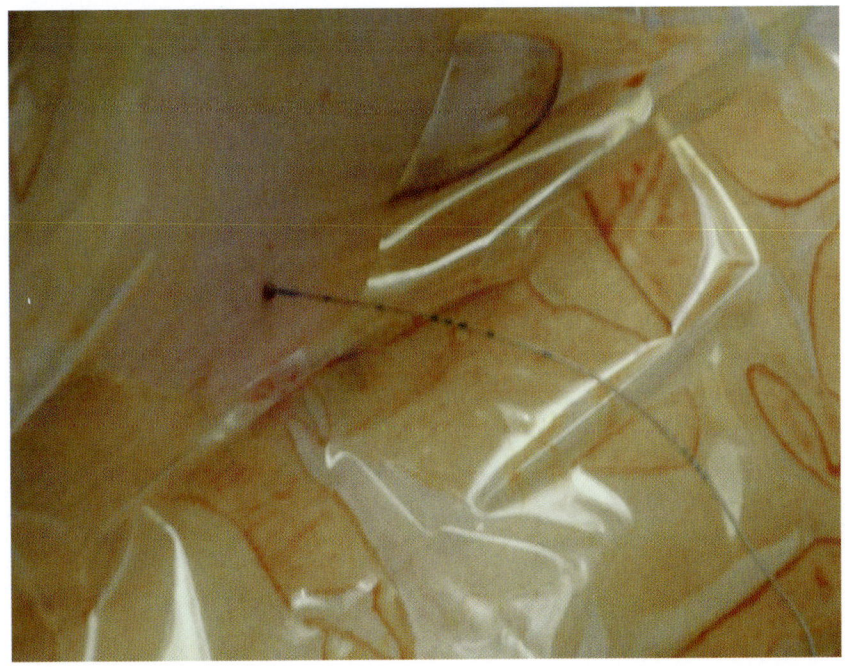

FIGURE 25-8 The catheter in place.

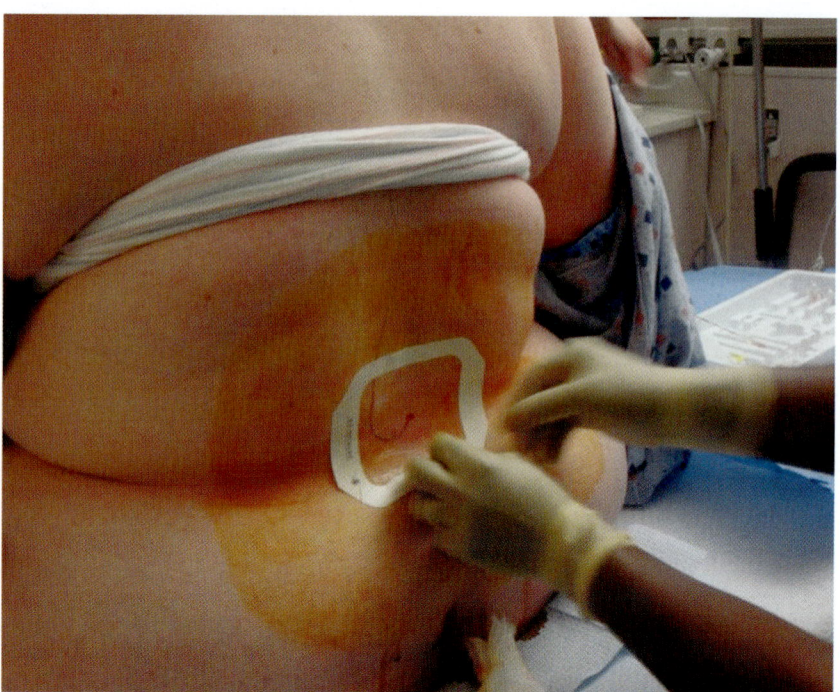

FIGURE 25-9 Securing the catheter with a Tegaderm.

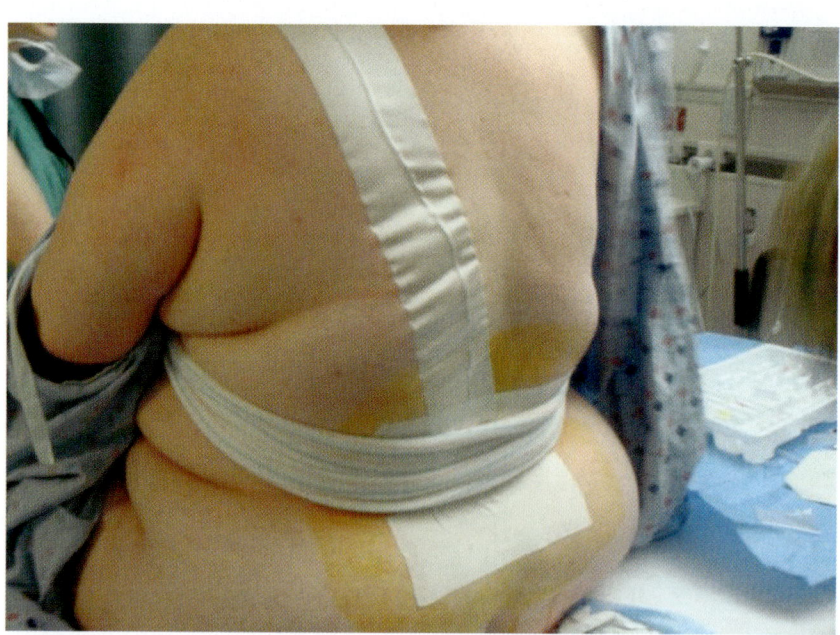

FIGURE 25-10 All done! (after we had a negative test dose, of course).

AIR VERSUS SALINE FOR LOSS OF RESISTANCE

- There are advantages and disadvantages of both, but more and more anesthesiologists seem to prefer loss of resistance (LOR) to saline these days.
- Some of the reported LOR air disadvantages include incomplete analgesia, increased chance of pneumocephalus headache caused by intracranial air, and increased risk of venous air embolism.
- One of the main advantages of using LOR air is that wet taps are clear with this technique. There should be no confusion if the clear fluid is saline or CSF if no saline was used!
- Bottom line. Latest reports show that there is no difference in block success whether air or saline was used to locate the epidural space.

ULTRASOUND GUIDANCE

- Bedside ultrasound can be helpful to facilitate epidural placement by identifying the midline, the best interspace, and the presence of scoliosis. Landmarks may be difficult or impossible to palpate in the obese patient. Having a visual map via ultrasound can help you figure out where to go. The OB ultrasound machine works great for this purpose and is typically readily available to those working on labor and delivery.
- On the other hand, it can add procedural time and it is unclear if there is an advantage of using ultrasound over skill alone.
- You must know lumbar spine anatomy for the ultrasound technique to be helpful to you. You need to recognize the images from two approaches: longitudinal paramedian approach and transverse approach. If you do not know what you are looking at, then there is nothing gained by using ultrasound. A detailed step-by-step approach was described by Carvalho[1] in 2008 and is recommended to those wanting to learn the technique (Figures 25-11 to 25-15).

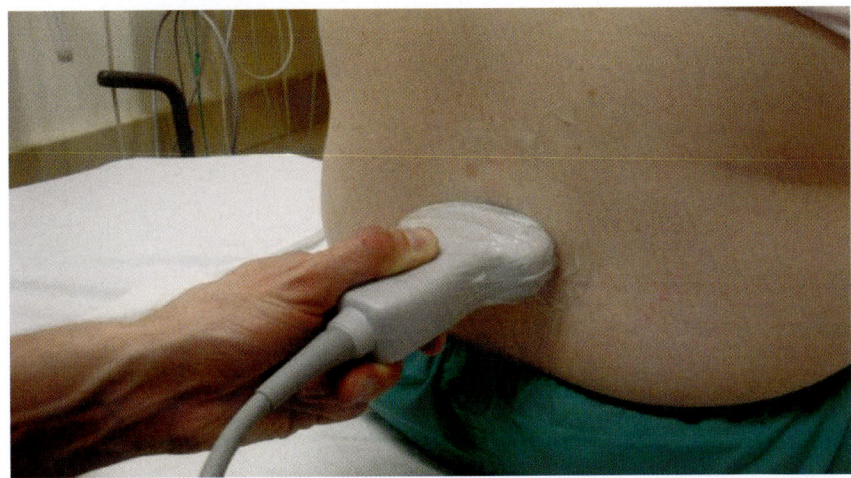

FIGURE 25-11 Put probe over space to see spinous process in center of screen.

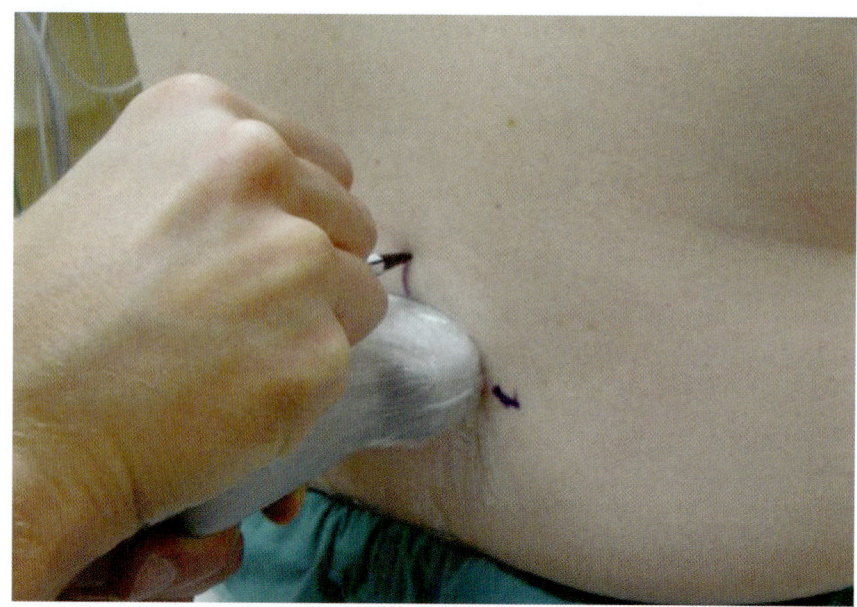

FIGURE 25-12 Mark the lateral and middle portion of the probe.

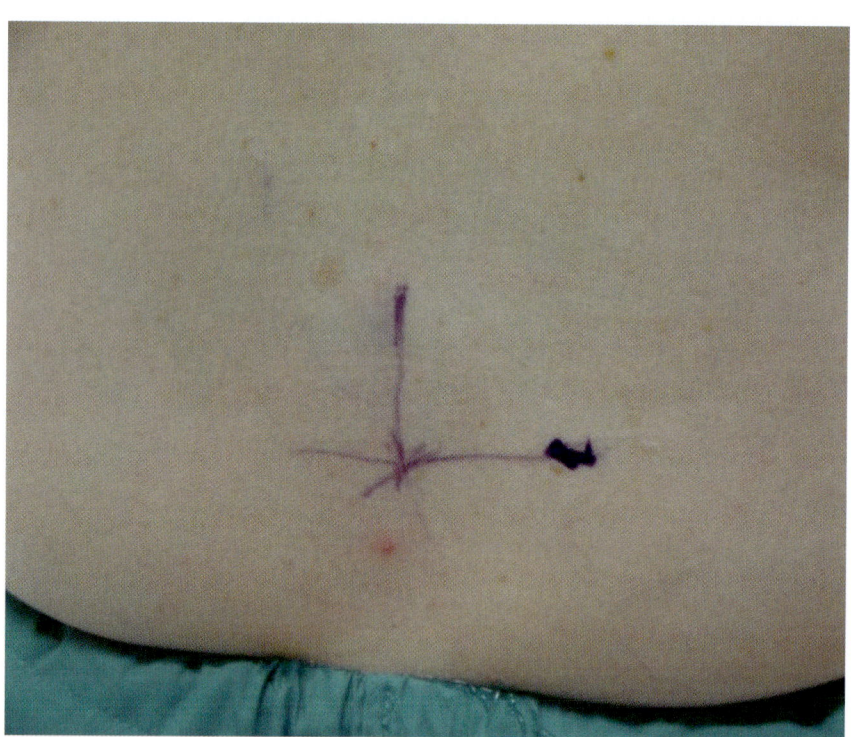

FIGURE 25-13 X marks the spots.

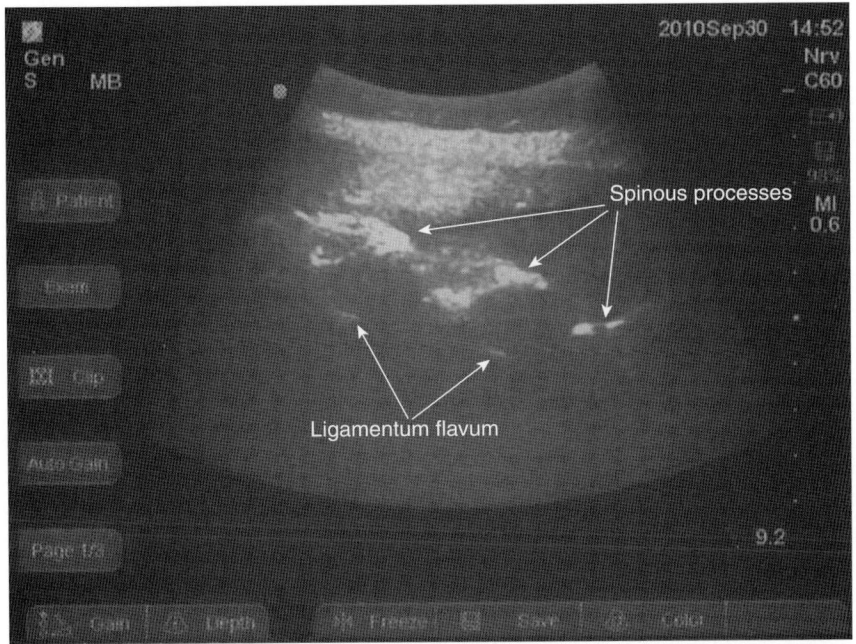

FIGURE 25-14 The longitudinal paramedian approach shows you the best interspace to choose. Place the ultrasound probe vertically about 3 cm to the left of the spine in the sacral area and angle the probe slightly toward the spine. You should see a bright line, which is the sacrum. Move the probe cephalad and you should see a saw-like image. The saw teeth are the articular processes and the spaces between the saw teeth are the interspaces. Below the interspace, you can then see white bands that represent the ligamentum flavum and vertebral body. You can then mark the skin at that point to identify the best part of interspace for needle insertion. In sum, this approach shows you the best interspace to choose.

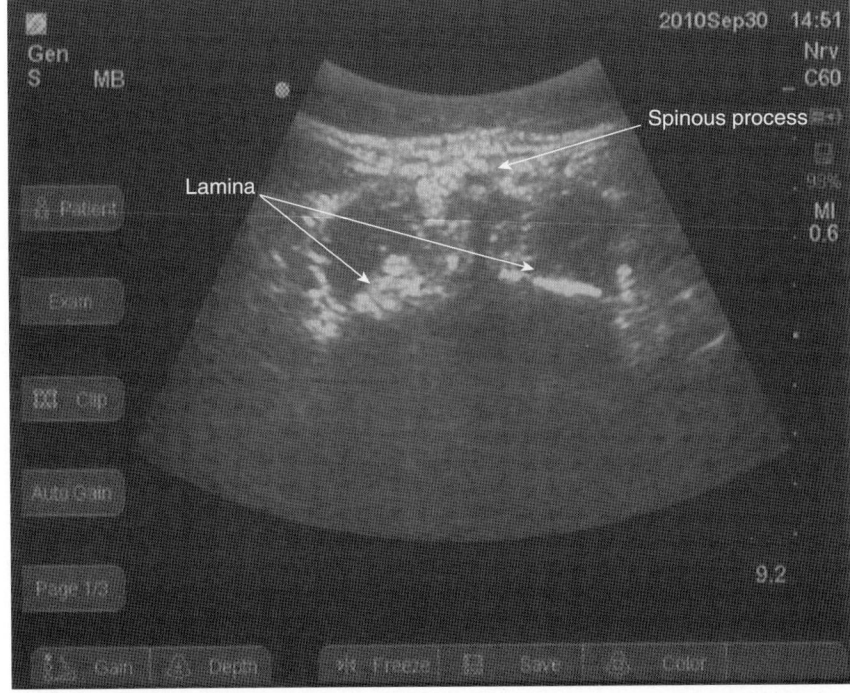

FIGURE 25-15 (A–C) The transverse approach shows you where the midline is. Place the probe horizontally. You should see a white band immediately under the skin, which is the spinous process. By identifying the spinous process, you now know where the midline is. Move the probe slightly up or down and you should see two white bands separated by a dark space. The top white band is the ligamentum flavum and the bottom white band is the vertebral body.

A

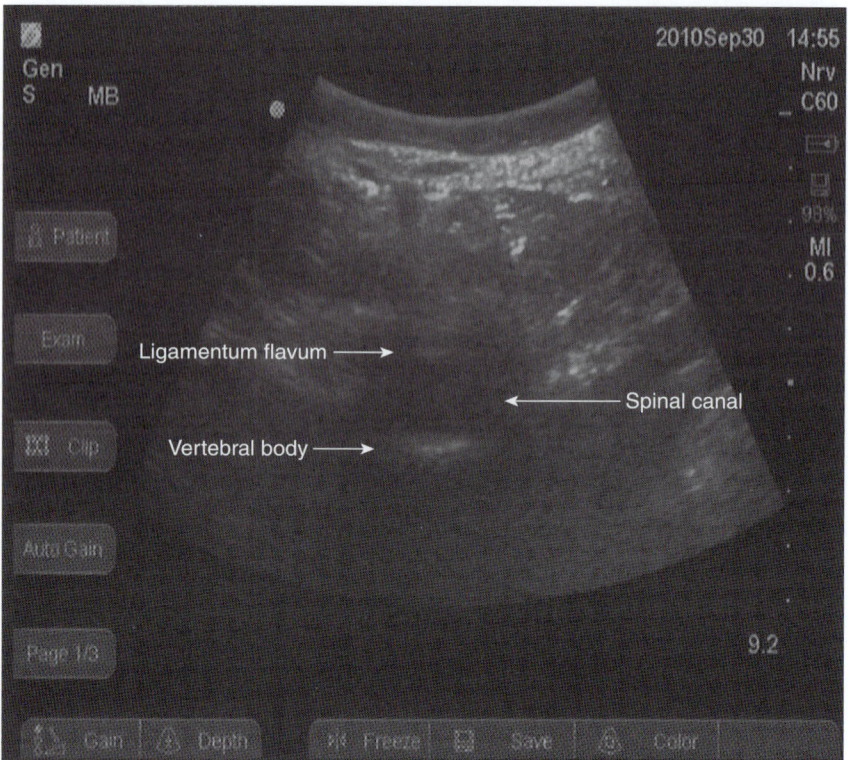

B

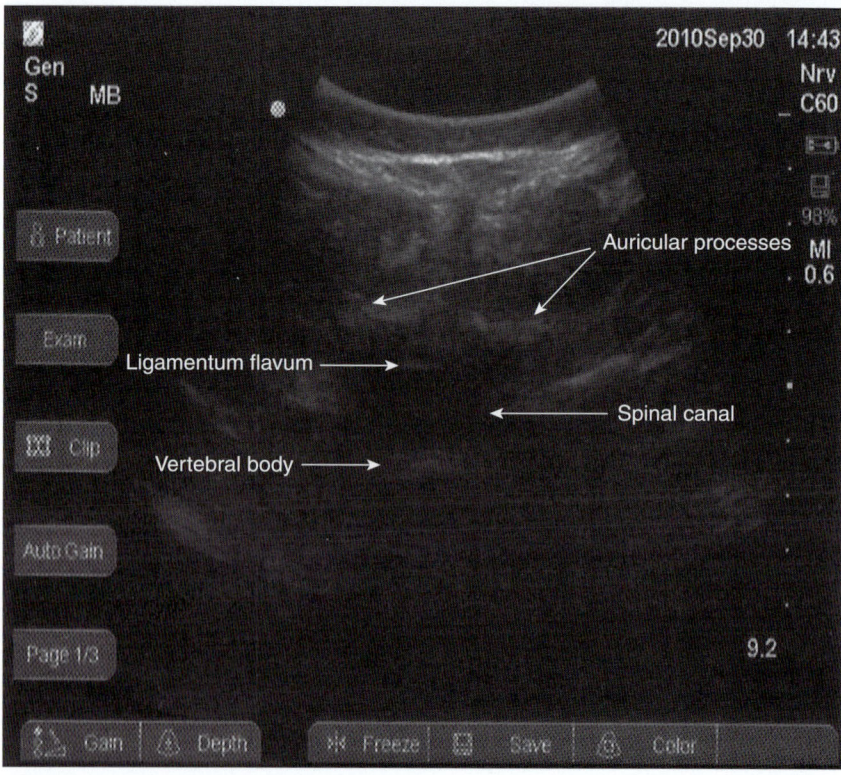

C

FIGURE 25-15 (*continued*) If you can see the two bands clearly, then you may see the image of a flying bat described by Carvalho. You should insert the epidural needle at the skin site where the probe shows you this image best. The articular and transverse processes can also be seen paramedian and above the ligamentum flavum.

GLITCHES

- After you place an epidural in pregnant patients, they should feel relief within a few contractions. If, by the time you finish your paperwork, they are groaning just as loudly with each contraction, troubleshoot the epidural.
- It's faster to redo an epidural than to hem and haw about how it might be in, and let's just give it some time.
- Ideally, you give just enough analgesia to make the patient comfortable, but not so much that she can't push. Every recipe and concentration in the world has been used.
- The best titration is done at bedside with frequent revisits, going up or down on your dosage depending on the patient's response. Start with as dilute a local anesthetic concentration as possible. A little goes a long way on OB.
- Don't place a labor epidural and disappear. Check up on it, keep abreast of developments, and be ready to dose it to treat breakthrough pain or provide surgical anesthesia.
- Thoracic epidurals can be a little touchy. If you put a lot of local in during a case, and the surgeon does a lot of mediastinal manipulation, you can lose your blood pressure.
- Is it the surgeon? The local anesthetic from the epidural? To make your life easier, wait to put the local anesthetic in when all the mediastinal manipulation is over and the surgeon is closing. There will be less going on, less confusion about what is causing the blood pressure drop, and you should have time for the local to set in and have the patient wake up comfortably.
- With narcotic infusions, be sure and write orders for monitoring and treating respiratory depression (disastrous) and pruritus (bothersome, but rarely fatal).
- If you get a wet tap, either slide in a catheter and use it as a continuous spinal, or remove it and go elsewhere. There is some evidence to suggest that a wet tap with a 17-gauge Tuohy, when used as a continuous spinal with the epidural catheter, will have a lower risk of causing a postdural puncture headache than a hole in the dura which wasn't used as a continuous spinal. Either way, tell the patient and be ready to treat a spinal headache later.

PREPARE YE THE WAY OF THE AIRWAY

As you will do a lot of them in labor rooms, rather than operating rooms, you will have to be like a turtle, carrying your house around on your back. Or, in this case, you will have to carry your house around on that red cart.

Make sure the cart has airway equipment (laryngoscopes, endotracheal tubes, laryngeal mask airways [LMAs], bougies, meds for induction, etc.) and know where the suction apparatus and Ambu bag are in the room. When you get into trouble (a seizure, high spinal, cardiovascular collapse—all possibilities you need to consider), you will need to move like lightning. That is no time to be finding stuff, checking the light on the laryngoscope, or spiking the stylet into an endotracheal tube (ETT).

Remember, every obstetric patient has a potential difficult airway, so have some special "can't-get-it-with-traditional-direct-equipment" around to help you with the airway in case you need to do a laryngoscopy. For example, having a glide scope handy, especially for those anticipated difficult airways, can be a lifesaving measure. To reiterate, if patients suddenly seize and you need to secure their airways, there's no time to say, "Oh, I can't see anything, can you go find me a (fill in the blank)?"

SIT OR SIDE, THE ETERNAL QUESTIONS

As with spinals, you want to make sure that you can do both. You'll see a lot of patients, especially in obstetrics, for whom the sitting position is just not an option. You'll sit the patient up, the fetal heart rate trace will not look reassuring, and you'll have to lay the patient on her side. This should not come as a big surprise. Pregnant patients can get supine hypotensive syndrome from lying flat on their backs. Internal vena cava compression is the culprit. So if you sit patients up and scrunch them forward like a shrimp, that same inferior vena cava (IVC) compression can occur, causing hypotension or placental insufficiency.

There are some other advantages to the side position in pregnant patients. Should something go wrong and the patient loses consciousness, that's a lot easier to manage with the patient already down than with the patient toppling forward on the nurse and ripping out all lines and monitors.

Another less dramatic advantage is, if patients are uncomfortable during contractions, they tend to wiggle and straighten up less when they are on their sides. You're less likely to get lost.

Sitting has the usual advantage. If the patients are heroically enormous, and they are more and more these days, you go up from the buttock crease and over the soft tissue fold to hit the spot. Hit bone? Go up or down, those are the only options you need to consider. With patients lying on their sides with the mattress and their midline sagging, your epidural needle can get lost. If you have an ultrasound machine accessible, this may make all the difference between a failed epidural and the potential need for general anesthesia, with the risk of a lost airway, and a nice stress-free, working epidural.

THE ACTUAL STICK

If there's anywhere that an anesthesia book falls short, it's in describing the feel of the loss of resistance. You can practice before you do it for real, though. Take a needle and give an epidural to an orange. As you advance through the peel, you will feel a give when you get through the peel and into the juicy fruit part of the orange. That is sort of what the loss of resistance is. It's been described as "going through leather." However you describe it, the idea of an epidural stick is always the same. Advance the needle slowly, pressing the plunger of the syringe, until you feel a pop and the plunger slides in effortlessly. Some people advance with constant pressure on the plunger; others push the needle in a little, recheck, then push in a little more, and recheck. Either way is fine.

An alternative technique is the hanging drop technique. You put a drop of fluid in the hub, then advance until the drop sucks in. The epidural space, being a potential space, has a little negativity associated with it. So when you enter it, that drop of fluid goes zip right in there. (It's cool to see it.)

Once you're in the space, disconnect the needle from the syringe. This is when you hold your breath and hope that warm CSF fluid doesn't gush out of the needle, meaning you went too far. If just a little fluid drips out, and it's cool to touch, then that is just the saline and you got a wet tap that you used in your syringe. But if it's body temperature, and it keeps on coming, then it's a wet tap.

Assuming that you are in, inject 5 cc of saline and then thread your epidural catheter so it remains 3 to 5 cm in the space. Thread it in much more, and you may slide out a nerve root and get an uneven block or IV catheter. Slide it in less, and the catheter may come out. The catheter should slide in easily. If you try to force it, then you are engaging in futility.

Remember that the epidural space is a potential space that the patient is born with, waiting for you to come along and pop your catheter into; a lot of practitioners actually inject a small amount of saline, 3 to 4 cc, to expand the potential space into an actual space, which also theoretically makes it easier to slide your catheter in.

Once you slide it in, measure and make sure you're in the correct depth; slide the needle out (making sure you don't pull the catheter out), remeasure and make sure you're still in the correct depth, and then secure the catheter. It is a good idea to secure it so that you can see the entry site and the marks on the catheter. If you cover it with tape, you'll never be able to see if the catheter has migrated in or out when assessing a poor block.

DOSING THE EPIDURAL

Aspirate before every injection, and follow the dictum that every dose is a test dose. If you are intravascular, and you don't pick it up by aspirating (it happens), then make sure when the catheter goes in that you never give a fatal dose. Give a few cubic centimeters, watch the patients, talk to them, see if they're weirding out on you, wait a little, then give a few more cubic centimeters. You will never regret dosing slowly, but you sure will regret dosing quickly.

Beware on OB. Super-stat C-sections require rapid injections of local anesthetics for a quick-onset block, so stay alert for signs of inadvertent IV or intrathecal injection; 3% 2-chloroprocaine is a good choice, as it has a fast onset and offset and will less likely get you into a bad situation.

THORACIC EPIDURALS

Go back to your skeleton and look at the thoracic vertebrae. The lower thoracic vertebrae have lumbar-like spinous processes, pointing straight out. Getting between these spinous processes is no harder than doing a lumbar epidural.

Now look at the higher thoracic vertebrae. Those spinous processes nearly overlap like armor plating! To sneak between them, you either have to go paramedian and sneak in from the side (a tough shot, and if you are off to the side you can drop a lung), or you have to do a super-tough steep angle to creep between those overlapping spinous processes.

Also, if you think about it, if you lace the epidural low, say at T10, and slide it up a few centimeters, it allows for spread of local that can provide pain relief for most thoracic cases. If you are the world's greatest and slickest, by all means put it in real high. If you don't do a lot of epidurals, if you're more of an occasional thoracic epidural type, then make your life a little easier and place them low.

CERVICAL EPIDURALS

Doing one of these for surgical anesthesia is exceedingly rare. Most cervical epidurals in the real world are for pain-relief procedures.

How do you do one of these? The usual, prep and drape sterile technique, administer a local, and then advance the epidural needle as for the other locales. Many pain practitioners don't even do them without being guided by fluoroscopy.

PEARLS

- Have a never-ending respect for every epidural that you, or someone else, places.
- When you arrive at a bedside, never trust any catheter you find attached to a patient—not even yours.
- Test-dose everything, every time.
- Remember, setup and backup won't keep the problems away, but they will stave them off longer.
- An altered sensorimotor examination in a patient with an epidural catheter history (with no medication on board) is an emergency.
- If bleeding and coagulopathy were an issue during surgery or postop, get coags on the patient before you touch the catheter.
- Epidurals, like all regional anesthetic techniques, have a failure rate. Even the slickest hands occasionally have to redo a catheter or two.
- If possible, become familiar with ultrasound-guided technique for epidural placement.
- Airway, airway, airway! Always be ready for general anesthesia and remember, a glide scope may bail you out of dangerous situations.

REFERENCE

1. Carvalho JCA. Ultrasound-facilitated epidurals and spinals in obstetrics. *Anesthesiol Clin* 2008;26:145–158.
   A comprehensive review of how to use ultrasound to facilitate epidural placement.

SUGGESTED READING

Ayad S, Demian Y, Narouze S, Tetzlaff J. Subarachnoid catheter placement after wet tap for analgesia in labor. influence on the risk of headache in obstetric patients. *Reg Anesth Pain Med* 2003;28:512–515.
Placing a subarachnoid catheter during a wet tap and leaving the catheter in for 24 hours decreased the incidence of postdural puncture headache.

Beilin Y, Arnold F, Telfeyan C, Bernstein H, Hossain S. Quality of analgesia when air or saline is used for identification of the epidural space in the parturient. *Reg Anesth Pain Med* 2000;25:596–599.
Patient who received an epidural placed with LOR to air had more incomplete analgesia than those who had an epidural placed with LOR to saline (36% with air vs. 19% with saline).

Dalens B, Bazin J, Haberer J. Epidural bubbles as a cause of incomplete analgesia during epidural anesthesia. *Anesth Analg* 1987;66:678–683.

Deschamps A. Autonomic nervous system response to epidural analgesia in laboring patients by wavelet transform of heart rate and blood pressure variability. *Anesthesiology* 2004;101(1):21–27.
Indices of parasympathetic and sympathetic activity after neuraxial blockade in laboring patients can be obtained by analysis of both heart rate and blood pressure variability.

Eltzschig HK, Lieberman ES, Camann WR. Medical progress; regional anesthesia and analgesia for labor and delivery. *N Engl J Med* 2003;348:319–332.
Epidural analgesia has been shown to be a safe, widely used, effective means of pain relief during labor and cesarean delivery.

Evron S, Gladkov V, Sessler D. Predistension of the epidural space before catheter insertion reduces the incidence of intravascular epidural catheter insertion. *Anesth Analg* 2007;105:460–464.
Distention of the epidural space with 5 cc of saline before epidural catheter insertion decreased the incidence of accidental IV cannulation and number of unblocked segments.

Higuchi H. Factors affecting the spread and duration of epidural anesthesia with ropivacaine. *Anesthesiology* 2004;101(2):4514–4560.
Epidural anesthesia can have an unpredictable extent and duration. Differences in the surface area of the dura, epidural fat volume, and epidural venous plexus velocity may explain the variability in the extent and duration of epidural anesthesia.

Holte K. Epidural anesthesia, hypotension, and changes in intravascular volume. *Anesthesiology* 2004;00(2):281–286.
One of the most common side effects of epidural anesthesia is hypotension with relative hypovolemia, requiring fluid boluses or administration of vasopressors.

Miller RM. *Miller's Anesthesia*, 6th ed. New York: Elsevier/Churchill Livingston; 2005.
What can you say, I mean—Miller. It's all there. (Once at an American Society of Anesthesiologists meeting many moons ago, a nondescript anesthesiologist crossed out his own name on his name tag and wrote "Ron Miller" on it. Perhaps it was some vain attempt at horning in on Professor Miller's fame and glory. Alas, this sad sack then ran into the famous Dr. Miller in an elevator! Aag! Busted! With complete nonchalance and utter class, Dr. Miller looked at this name tag, raised his eyebrows, and said, "Interesting name.")

Portnoy D. Mechanisms and management of an incomplete epidural block for cesarean section. *Anesthesiol Clin North Am* 2003;21(1):39–57.
When inadequate epidural block becomes apparent during surgery, there are limited alternatives. Depending on the degree of inadequate anesthesia, options include patient reassurance, supplementation with a variety of inhalational and intravenous agents, and local anesthetic infiltration. General anesthesia is typically left as a backup option, but must be considered if the patient continues to have discomfort.

Segal S. A retrospective effectiveness study of loss of resistance to air or saline for identification of the epidural space. *Anesth Analg* 2010;110(2):558–563.

There is no difference in block success whether air or saline was used to locate the epidural space.

Sielenkämper AW. Thoracic epidural anesthesia. more than just anesthesia/analgesia. *Anesthesiology* 2003;99(3):523–525.

Thoracic epidural blockade may be useful in providing protection against splanchnic hypoperfusion under the conditions of ischemia and reperfusion, which may occur during trauma, hemorrhage, or circulatory shock.

Valentine SJ, Jarvis AP, Shutt LE. Comparative study of the effects of air or saline to identify the extradural space. *Br J Anaesth* 1991;66:224–227.

The use of air for LOR led to a greater number of unblocked dermatomes when compared with using LOR to saline.

Visalyaputra S, Rodanant O, Somboonviboon W, Tantivitayatan K, Thienthong S, Saengchote W. Spinal versus epidural anesthesia for cesarean delivery in severe pre-eclampsia: a prospective, randomized, multicenter study. *Anesth Analg* 2005;101(3):862–868.

In severely preeclamptic patients undergoing regional anesthesia, it was found that there was a statistically significant difference in mean arterial pressure, with more patients in the spinal group exhibiting hypotension, in comparison to those who had received epidural anesthesia.

CHAPTER 26

THORACIC EPIDURALS—WHAT'S THE BIG DEAL?

JONATHAN KRAIDIN
KRISTOFFER DE LARA
JOHN LANGENFELD

And the Lord God...took one of his ribs and closed the flesh.

Genesis 2:21
(no mention of a thoracic epidural
for postoperative pain relief)

INTRODUCTION

Thoracic epidurals are really no different from lumbar epidurals. Well, they are a little bit. The angle of approach for entering the epidural space is much steeper; the space between the bones is much smaller; there is a greater risk of entering the dura; the spinal cord is present instead of the cauda equina, increasing the risk for cord injury; and hypotension after the injection of local into the epidural space is more common.

INDICATIONS

- Thoracotomy
- Pectus (Nuss) repair
- Upper abdominal surgery
- Rib fracture
- Postherpetic neuralgia
- Pain from malignancy

CONTRAINDICATIONS (ABSOLUTE)

- Patient refusal
- Coagulopathy
- Anticoagulation
- Hypovolemia
- Infection at the insertion site
- Increased intracranial pressure
- Thrombocytopenia

CONTRAINDICATIONS (RELATIVE)

- Aortic and mitral stenosis
- Sepsis
- Anatomical abnormalities of the vertebral column
- Neurological disease
- Lack of patient cooperation or language barrier
- Operator inexperience

BENEFITS

- Superior pain relief compared to narcotic-based regimens
- Attenuation of the sympathetic response to surgery
- Earlier return of gastrointestinal function with the use of local anesthetic based solutions

RISKS

- An increased risk of infection with catheters left in for more than 2 to 4 days
- Meningitis and arachnoiditis
- Spinal headache from dural puncture
- Nerve root or cord injury
- Back pain
- Epidural hematoma
- Catheter migration into the intrathecal (0.15%) or intravascular (0.07%) space

THE THORACIC EPIDURAL: THE LOW-DOWN

Early on, as new attendings, the easiest way to get a thoracic epidural done was to find someone else to do it. Hey, these things look scary. However, with a good understanding of the anatomy, anyone should be able to perform one safely.

- The spinal canal extends from the foramen magnum to the sacral hiatus.
- The spinal canal is formed from the bony arches posterior to the vertebral bodies.[1]
- The shape and size of the vertebrae differ in the cervical, thoracic, and lumbar segments. The cervical segments are the smallest, the lumbar are the largest, and the thoracic have the steepest caudad angulation of the spinous process.
- This angulation varies depending on the thoracic level, so the operator must vary the angle of the needle from the horizontal plane depending on the level. The spinal cord is solid until the L2 level, where it splits into numerous filaments, forming the cauda equina. The ligamentum flavum varies in thickness depending on the vertebral level.
- The ligamentum flavum is about 5 to 6 mm thick at the lumbar region, while it is only 3 to 5 mm thick at the thoracic level.

So, a quick review, if you are tapped for a thoracic epidural:

- The needle is going to have a steeper trajectory from the plane of the floor.
- You can hit the spinal cord with the needle if you are too aggressive, causing a traumatic cord injury.[2] This is why you have to make small insertion steps with the needle (Figures 26-1 to 26-3).

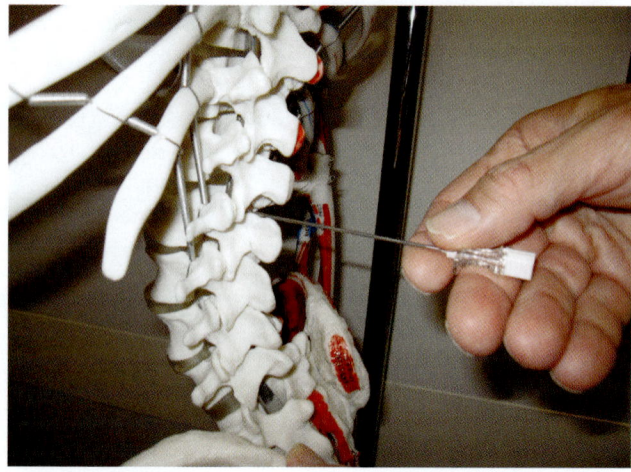

FIGURE 26-1 The needle is close to horizontal at the low-thoracic, high-lumbar region.

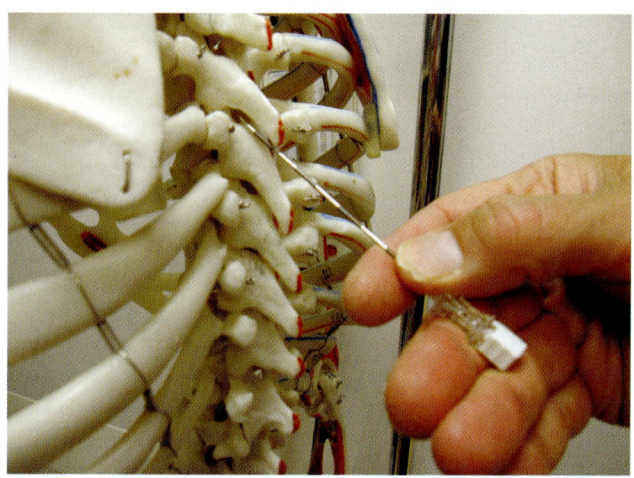

FIGURE 26-2 The needle has a much steeper angle relative to the floor in the midthoracic region.

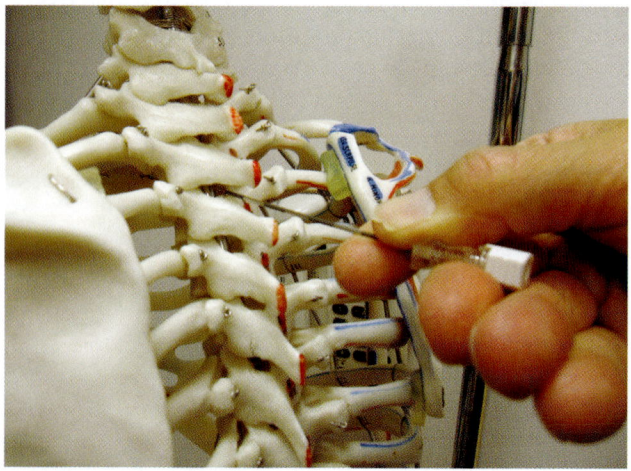

FIGURE 26-3 The needle's angle become more horizontal again at the high thoracic level.

WHERE DO YOU PLACE THE NEEDLE?

- The insertion site depends on what effect you are trying to achieve.
- If this is for a thoracotomy, the surgical incision will be near the T2 to T4 region. Place the needle somewhere between T3 and T6. The scapula is at T7. The most prominent spinous process at the base of the neck is C7. You can use these as landmarks. Remember, you want the catheter to be right next to the action. If you are watching a movie you want good seats. Likewise, you want to deliver your local to the dermatomes that are next to the incision or the broken ribs from the retractors.
- If you are doing the epidural for an upper abdominal procedure, something between T8 and T12 will usually work. If you can't get the catheter close to your ideal location, you can try to make up for this by running a larger volume of a more dilute concentration. However, if the epidural is placed too low, no amount of volume will work well, and the epidural will be useless for pain relief.
- Do not think that you can place a lumbar epidural for an upper abdominal or thoracic procedure and just shove in a lot of catheter with the hope that it will work its way up the vertebral column. Hope is not a method.

PREPARATION

The first thing is to know your patient. Make sure the patient does not have any contraindications for a thoracic epidural.

- When you obtain a history, make sure there is no tendency toward bleeding or easy bruising. Does the patient take garlic, ginkgo, or ginseng supplements (yes, they are anticoagulants)?
- Does the patient have a factor deficiency?
- Does the patient have von Willebrand's disease?
- Check the platelets and coagulation studies.
- Does the patient take Plavix or any anticoagulants?
- Has the patient received low-molecular-weight heparin, or does the surgeon plan to prescribe it after the surgery?

These are examples of things you need to think about. If you feel you are not able to place an epidural, you should consider patient-controlled analgesia (PCA) for postoperative pain relief.

The key thing to remember is not to harm the patient, and an epidural hematoma does not help achieve this goal. Large patient studies note that the risk of spinal hematomas is increased by the concomitant use of anticoagulant and antiplatelet therapy.[3,4] One should be very conservative if a patient is taking a medication that increases the bleeding risk. Let's talk about a few of them.

MEDICATIONS THAT CAN PUT AN END TO THE EPIDURAL SAGA

- You want the patient's international normalized ratio (INR) to be under 1.2. Don't assume that the INR is normal because the Coumadin has been stopped for a week. Check it.
- Systemic heparinization represents an increased risk for epidural bleeding, and needs to be discontinued[5] and the partial thromboplastin time (PTT) rechecked for normalization.
- Low-molecular-weight heparin (LMWH) should not be given 24 hours before or after placing an epidural.
- Original guidelines recommended avoiding thrombolytic drugs within 10 days of inserting a needle through a noncompressible vessel.
- The use of nonsteroidal antiinflammatory drugs (NSAIDs) does not seem to increase the bleeding risk.
- With regard to thienopyridine derivatives, Plavix and Ticlid, you should wait a minimum of 7 to 10 days for the former, and 14 days for the latter after the last dose.
- The use of glycoprotein IIb/IIIa inhibitors such as abciximab, eptifibatide, and tirofiban is also troublesome. Recommendations are to wait 24 to 48 hours for abciximab, and 4 to 8 hours for the other two.
- Personally, I just wait 48 hours if the patient is taking any of these drugs. This simplifies matters considerably.

Now, that is a lot of information, and it doesn't cover everything! To make it worse, the recommendations are always changing as new drugs are added, and other studies are conducted. If you are unsure about the current recommendations for these drugs, go to the American Society of Region Anesthesia's Web site and read them.

One more thought (OK, a few more thoughts):

- Do not perform the epidural on a patient who is asleep. You could hit a nerve root, causing an injury. You can sedate the patient as much as necessary, as long as the patient can tell you that something really hurts as you direct the needle.
- If the patient will not stay still for you to place the catheter, you should abandon the procedure.
- If the procedure is just a video-assisted thoroscopic surgery (VATS), but it might get converted to an open procedure, get consent for the epidural procedure in case you need to insert one postoperatively.

SETUP

- Sit the patient up with a pulse oximeter, blood pressure cuff, and nasal cannula in place. Have the patient rest on a table with the hands outstretched on a pillow. Tell the patient to arch the back like an angry cat. This really helps a lot. Have someone spot the patient in the front to help with positioning and to make sure the patient does not fall. Find the level you want, clean it with alcohol, and inject a good 10 cc of local. Do this before you clean and prep the back, so the local can marinate while you prepare your tray. A numb, comfortable patient will make your task much easier (Figure 26-4).
- Open the kit and put on your mask and sterile gloves. Really clean the area with a wide prep. You don't have to paint a Picasso; you just want a large, clean area. Pour an additional 10 cc of 1% lidocaine without preservative into the tray. During your location of the epidural space you may go through some quasi-loss-of-resistance regions. This will allow you to tighten up these pockets. If you happen to be in the epidural space, the medication is preservative-free, so it is safe to give as an epidural dose. Furthermore, this local allows you to further numb the patient if your initial local was not sufficient.

PREPARE THE HARPOON!

- When time comes to find the epidural space, you have to decide if you feel lucky. Well, do you? Are you going to go for the midline approach, which could technically be easier, but might be thwarted by a very narrow space between very steep spinous processes; or are you going to go for the technically more challenging paramedian approach that offers the potentially larger window to place your needle?
- The midline approach is simple: one, find the midline of the back; two, angle your needle to guide it between the spinous processes; three, carefully insert the needle until you obtain a loss of resistance much like your standard lumbar epidural technique.
- However, it is step two that is the catch. The angle varies with the thoracic level, and the space can be very narrow.
- Use the midline approach for a very high or low thoracic level, unless the patient is tall with a long spine. Taller patients usually have wider spaces.
- When you infiltrate your local, use your 25-gauge (G) needle as a guide for the right angle to get through the processes. If you are not able to get through with a 25-G needle, you are not going to get through with a 17-G Tuohy needle.
- Remember, you are not married to a vertebral level. If one level is troublesome, move up or down and try again. When you direct your needle, keep it perfectly centered. If it deviates off of the midline you will miss the narrow space. You will never hit the epidural space no matter how far you advance the needle past the side of the epidural space, and you will not realize your mistake until the needle comes out of the front of the patient. You will lose style points if this happens (Figure 26-5).
- If you still are not able to get in, you should consider the paramedian approach. With this method you are coming from the side. This is useful if you do not find a path between the spinous processes, or you are unable to maintain a perfect, midline trajectory.
- Find the spinous process and move to either side 1.5 to 2 cm. If the epidural is for a thoracotomy, come in from the side having the surgery. This way, the bulk of the medication is given on the surgical side.
- For beginners, it is simpler to do this in a two-step process. Keep the needle parallel to the floor and come in at 45 degrees from the plane of the patient's back until you hit the intersection of

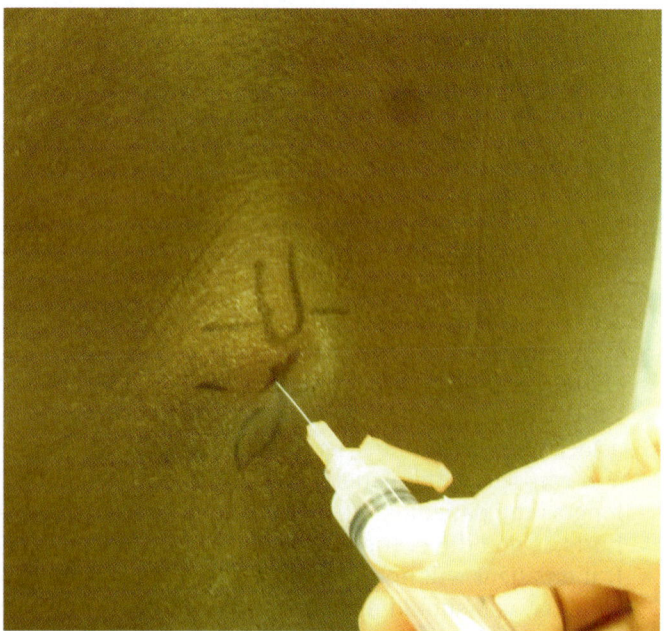

FIGURE 26-4 Be generous with your local. Feel out the space with the needle, but do not go too deep, as you can hit the spinal canal on some patients.

the transverse and spinous processes. Pull the needle back and angle it cephalad 15 degrees. Now advance the needle, checking for loss-of-resistance as you would for any epidural. If you hit bone, come back slightly and redirect the needle more caudally or cephalad until you feel it advance further. Stop if the patient feels pain. You could be hitting a nerve root. Redirect the needle and try again (Figures 26-6 to 26-9).

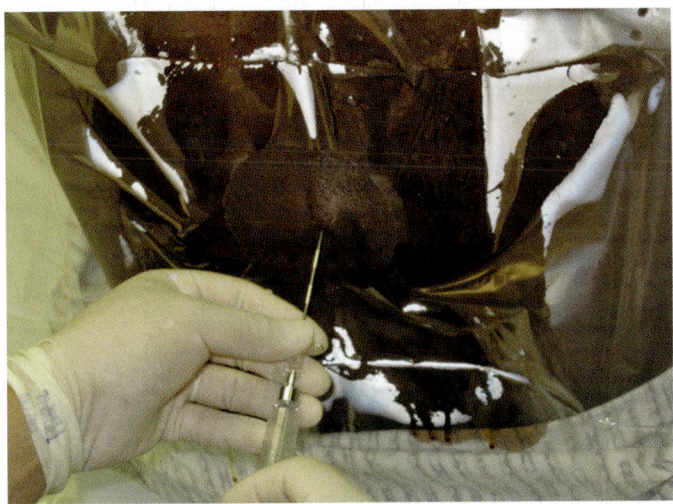

FIGURE 26-5 Midthoracic level, midline approach. This is a much steeper angle than one uses for a lumbar epidural.

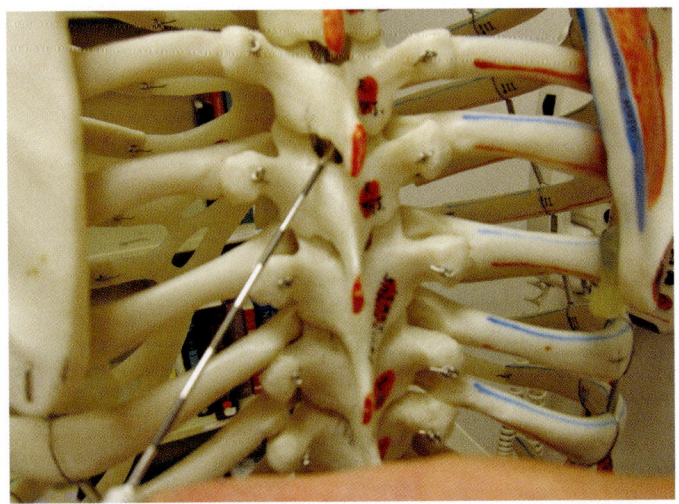

FIGURE 26-6 Approach for paramedian technique viewed from behind.

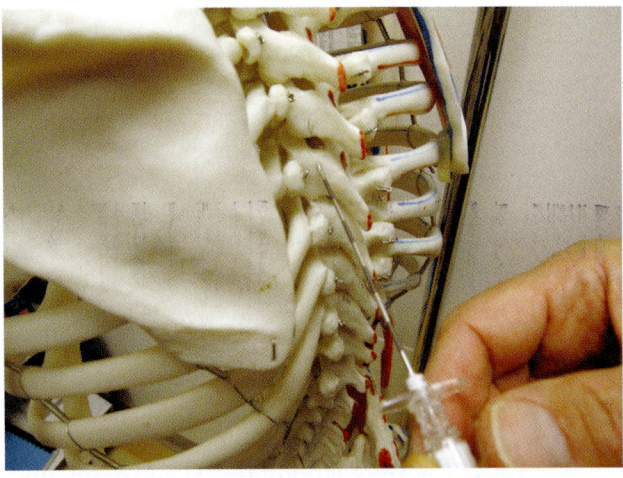

FIGURE 26-7 Approach for paramedian technique viewed from the side.

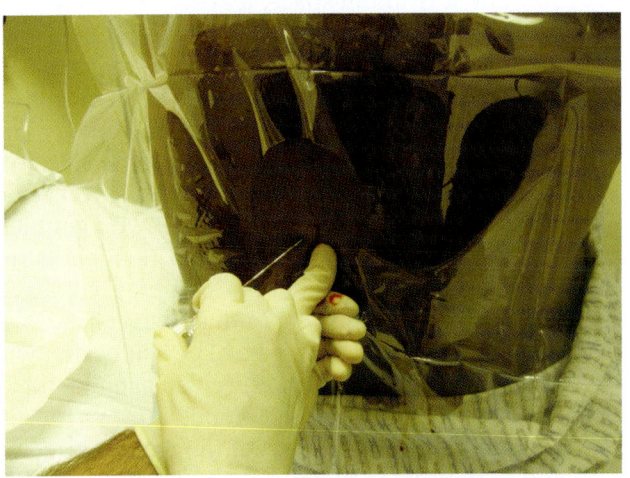

FIGURE 26-8 Paramedian technique viewed from behind.

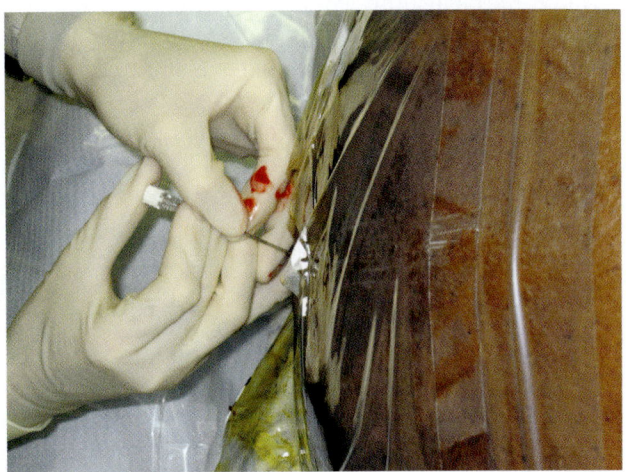

FIGURE 26-9 Paramedian technique viewed from the side.

BE CAREFUL!

- The ligamentum flavum can be paper thin for some elderly patients, unlike the lumbar ligament. You may suddenly find yourself in the epidural space without a great change in the degree of resistance.
- Advance the air-filled syringe and gently tap on the end. After advancing a few centimeters, insert the stylet to ensure there is no tissue plugging the end. If the patient has some discomfort, inject a half milliliter of local anesthetic.
- A comfortable patient is your best friend.
- If you think you have a loss of resistance, see if you can insert your catheter. It should advance easily. If you advance the catheter and it gets stuck, do not try to pull it back through the needle, or you could shear off the end. Instead, remove the needle and catheter together.
- If you think it is in the space, leave it in between 4 and 5 cm within the epidural space. With a standard needle take the number of markings that are still showing on the needle while it is embedded in the patient and subtract this number from 11. The number you get is the catheter depth at the skin that will leave 4 cm in the epidural space. So if you see three markings left on the needle when you get the loss of resistance, subtract three from 11. Eight is the catheter depth at the level of the skin that will leave 4 cm inside the patient's epidural space.
- When you give your test dose of 1.5% lidocaine with 1:200,000 epinephrine, make sure you aspirate for cerebrospinal fluid (CSF) and blood.
- When you inject, check to see if the patient gets a ringing in the ears, a metal taste in the mouth, or the heart rate goes up, indicative of a vascular injection.
- Check to see that the patient's legs do not get heavy, which would suggest a spinal injection.
- Watch for clear fluid leaking from the catheter insertion site at the skin. If you see fluid leaking out when you inject, the catheter is not in the epidural space.
- If you are satisfied with your test dose, secure the catheter to the back.
- If the epidural is for a thoracotomy procedure, secure the catheter on the nonoperative side of the patient.
- Use an OpSite dressing and tape the edges. Make sure not to place tape on the area of the chest where the surgeon will be working.
- If you get a wet tap, you have two options. You can abandon the procedure or you can attempt going at another level. If you get a catheter in at another level you may want to reduce your dosing in case some of the medication gets into the spinal canal.
- What do you do if a VATS becomes a thoracotomy and you did not place an epidural? If a patient does not have a contraindication for an epidural, you should always get a signed consent from a patient having a VATS procedure for an epidural in the event the case becomes an open case. If this is the situation, have the surgeon perform intercostals blocks under direct vision. This will afford the patient some excellent pain relief in the recovery room, allowing you to position the pain-free patient more easily for the definitive epidural procedure. Otherwise, you will have to give the patient, who has a fresh thoracotomy scar with some potentially broken or stretched ribs, a lot of narcotics so you can get a good position.
- Make sure you have a dedicated person holding your postanesthetic patient in the front; otherwise, you might have to perform a craniotomy after the patient falls on the floor.
- If you are unable to sit the patient up, you can attempt the epidural with the patient in the lateral decubitus position.
- When performing a thoracic epidural in the decubitus position, use the paramedian approach. You will find it close to impossible to keep the needle perfectly centered when the patient is bent in all the wrong ways while lying on the side.

DOSING THE EPIDURAL

- Before using the epidural, make sure you aspirate for CSF and blood.
- Your dose depends on the thoracic level of the epidural. Anything below T10 can usually take 10 cc of 0.25% bupivacaine, 0.2% ropivacaine, or 1% lidocaine with 1:200,000 epinephrine.
- When the epidural starts getting above T6, you should decrease your volume, as this can lead to a profound, high sympathetic block, causing hypotension. Usually, 5 to 6 cc is a good start at this level.
- If you dose a thoracic epidural in the middle of a thoracic operation, and the blood pressure drops, it is hard to tell what is the culprit.
- If you are dosing the epidural for a thoracotomy procedure, you can dose it 20 minutes before the end of the procedure.
- You might get a better, faster block of the operative side if you can wait for when you turn the patient supine and immediately dose the epidural.
- If the epidural is working, you should note a significant decrease in the patient's pain.
- One thing the epidural will not block is referred diaphragmatic pain. This manifests as shoulder pain and is best treated with narcotics.

- If you have a thoracic epidural for an esophagectomy procedure, the necessary coverage may exceed the range covered by one epidural catheter, so it is not unreasonable to have a PCA device onboard.
- Sometimes the epidural does not work well, and you may question whether it is working at all. In this case, re-dose the epidural with 5 to 8 cc of 1% lidocaine with epinephrine and watch for an effect.
- Lidocaine is the quickest-acting analgesic, and will allow you to make a rapid assessment.
- The epinephrine will serve as an intravascular marker and limit the systemic absorption of the local anesthetic.
- Check the back to see if the local is leaking out of the back during your injection; also, make sure the catheter has not moved.
- Assess the patient's perception of temperature at various levels to see if you are getting limited or one-sided spread.
- You should also consider a dermatomal spreading pattern suggestive of the catheter residing in one of the dural sleeves. Pull the catheter back a couple of centimeters and re-dose the epidural with 5 cc of 1% lidocaine with epinephrine.
- If the patient does not have any analgesic level or decrease in blood pressure, the epidural is probably a dud. If you're an attending, you can blame the resident; otherwise, pull up your bootstraps and get ready to replace the epidural.

CONSIDERATIONS FOR THE PAIN SERVICE

- It is very important for patients who have had a pulmonary resection and other operations to have good pain relief postoperatively.
- Most patients who require a lung resection have been long-term smokers and have very little pulmonary reserve.
- Patients need to be able to cough postoperatively to keep their airways clear.
- Pain will limit patients' ability to generate a sufficient cough, leading to airway plugging and subsequent pneumonia.
- Pulmonary complications are the leading cause of mortality following a lung resection, which may be preventable with proper pain control.
- A well-functioning epidural catheter is the best means to achieve good pain relief following a thoracotomy.
- The catheter must be placed at the correct level for optimum pain control.
- A common mistake is not to place the epidural catheter high enough.
- When the catheter is at the correct level, the dosage of medication is reduced.
- Thoracic epidurals, like lumbar epidurals, can cause urinary retention.
- Thoracic epidurals, because of their higher placement, are more prone to causing hypotension.
- If the level gets too high, not only will you block the sympathetic outflow, you will block the cardiac accelerator fibers.
- Hypotension must be treated as soon as possible. Run your infusion between 4 to 8 cc/h depending on the level.
- A dilute solution of local anesthetic is sufficient. Typical formulations have 0.0625% bupivacaine with or without fentanyl.
- If the patient does not get hypotensive and still has some pain, you can increase the rate of the infusion by 2 to 3 cc/h.
- If a patient develops hypotension, reduce the epidural rate by half and give a fluid challenge. If this fails, use pressors to increase the blood pressure and consider whether you should remove the epidural catheter. A Foley should remain in place for at least 24 hours after the catheter is removed to prevent urinary retention unless there is a history of urinary problems.
- Lethargy is also a postoperative problem with patients. The team must determine whether the lethargy is from the epidural infusion, especially if fentanyl is part of the infusion mixture, or if it is from other causes such as CO_2 retention, sundowning, or a stroke. The epidural dose is frequently reduced while the patient is being evaluated.
- The epidural should not stay in longer than 5 days because of the risk of infection.
- Before removing the epidural make sure all coagulation studies (PT, PTT, INR, platelets) are acceptable.
- Make sure the patient is not on any anticoagulation or antiplatelet therapy. Remove the catheter slowly and make sure the tip is intact. Document everything with a note in the chart.
- Finally, make sure the patient does not have any muscle weakness, sensory changes, or paresthesias.
- After the removal of the epidural, antithrombolytic therapy can be restarted 2 hours later.
- Prophylactic heparin can be restarted at any time after removal.

REFERENCES

1. Covino BG, Lambert DH. Epidural and spinal anesthesia. In: Barash PG, Cullen BF, Stoelting RK, eds. *Clinical Anesthesia*. 2nd ed. Philadelphia, PA: J. B. Lippincott Company; 1992:811–812.
   This is an excellent section describing the vertebral anatomy.

2. Absalom AR, Martinelli G, Scott NB. Spinal cord injury caused by direct damage by local anaesthetic infiltration needle. *Br J Anaesth* 2001;87(3):512–515.
   The reader should be aware that all procedures carry risks. This article is a good wake-up call.
3. Vandermeulen EP, Van Aken H, Vermylen J. Anticoagulants and spinal-epidural anesthesia. *Anesth Analg* 1994;79:1165–1177.
   One of many articles about anticoagulation and epidurals.
4. Horlocker TT, Wedel DJ. Neuraxial block and low molecular weight heparin: balancing perioperative analgesia and thromboprophylaxis. *Reg Anesth Pain Med* 1998;23:164–177.
   Another article about epidurals and anticoagulation
5. Stafford-Smith M. Impaired haemostasis and regional anaesthesia. *Can J Anaesth* 1996;43:R129–R141.
   This article discusses heparinization with respect to placing epidurals.

CHAPTER 27

MENDING FENCES— THE BLOOD PATCH

DENNIS HALL
ANJANA SAHANI PANJWANI

When the head aches, all the members partake of the pain.
> Miguel de Cervantes Saavedra, *Don Quixote*

If you have a lot of tension and you get a headache, do what it says on the aspirin bottle: "take two aspirins" and "keep away from children."
> Unknown

INTRODUCTION

The anesthesiologist who has never gotten a wet tap hasn't done enough epidurals. In other words, every anesthesiologist who performs epidurals will, at some point or another, get a wet tap. So we all feel your pain the first time you see that clear gush of cerebrospinal fluid (CSF) coming out the hub of your Tuohy needle.

Of course, the patient at the other end of your needle happens to be in active labor, a human moving target, emitting blood-curdling screams with each contraction. And now this. A wet tap.

She sits up the next day and up go the hands to her head: "Aaagh! I've got the worst headache!"

> *I should have been an investment banker.*
> *I should have become an offshore oil driller.*
> *I should have just stayed with my folks and played Guitar Hero in the basement.*
> *I should have done ANYTHING BUT ANESTHESIA!*

It's now postpartum day 2 and the OB resident calls and says the patient cannot perform her activities of daily living because she cannot lift her head. She is so dehydrated from the dry heaves that she is unable to produce milk and her baby is starving. The attorney's office representing this patient calls your chairperson to verify the spelling of your name and address. This is a prime example of Frankenstein's Law, which states, "You make a monster, you keep it."

It is time to mend fences and take care of that postdural puncture headache (PDPH) in our postpartum patient. Time to patch things up with an epidural blood patch (EBP).

PDPH INCIDENCE AND RELATED FACTORS

Postdural puncture headache is the most common adverse effect of dural puncture. Factors that make a PDPH more likely include:

- Needle diameter (area changes by the square of the radius). So, a fat needle is worse than a thin needle. In fact, the incidence of headache after dural puncture with 18-gauge (G) epidural needles has been reported to be up to 80%. For 26-G Quincke needles, the incidence is reported to be between 2% and 12% and <2% with 29-G needles.
- Females get more PDPHs than males.
- Younger people get more PDPHs than older folks.
- The pregnant get more than the nonpregnant.
- The laboring pregnant get more still.
- Cutting needles cause more leakage than equivalent-sized pencil-point needles.
- Cutting needles with the bevel oriented in the plane of dural fibers (rostral to caudal) are thought to cause less CSF leakage than needles with the bevel perpendicular to dural fibers.
- People with a history of PDPHs are thought to be more at risk of a subsequent PDPH.

EPIDURAL BLOOD PATCH MECHANISM OF ACTION

The mechanism of action is not entirely known. However, there are two schools of thought. The more popular theory is that the blood creates a transdural pressure gradient preventing CSF leakage. Or there is also the "Dutch boy finger in the dike" theory of the blood physically plugging the hole(s). In any case, it is well documented that low CSF pressure resulting in traction on the cranial meninges (and sometimes cranial nerves) is the reason for the headache and its many associated symptoms.

EPIDURAL BLOOD PATCH INDICATIONS

- Although EBPs have been rarely used to treat chronic headaches secondary to spinal fluid loss (e.g., surgical, traumatic, idiopathic, etc.), we are really concerned about one indication: a headache that is attributable to the performing of a spinal or epidural. The presence of CSF is not necessary for diagnosis. Headache after a spinal, epidural, caudal, or diagnostic lumbar puncture can either be immediate or will often not be evident for hours or days. However, the incidence of headache in the population at large is about one in six, so your wet tap may be the primary cause, not the problem at all or just the icing on the cake. Here, a neurological examination is needed before the train hits (that is, before you stick a needle somewhere you will wish you hadn't). It may even be necessary to involve one of the doctors who still carry black bags with tuning forks hanging out. After all, the diagnoses of a headache are legion: tumors, toxins, trauma, infections, vascular, neurological, nutritional, congenital, idiopathic, obstetrical (i.e., preeclampsia), and, oh yeah, wet taps.
- In the majority of cases, a PDPH is a self-limiting event. The largest study reported that 72% of headaches resolved within 7 days. Knowing this and conveying this to the patient may affect the choice of treatment, especially in less severe cases (more about this later). Unfortunately, there have been reports of headaches persisting for as long as 6 months even after being treated with an EBP.
- So, if a PDPH is generally a self-limited event, why bother? The answer should be tailored to the individual patient. Is the headache simply a nuisance or a life-altering event? Can the patient perform activities of daily living, care for a newborn, nurse her baby, and participate in this special, fleeting time in her life, or is she sticking needles in a Vermont Teddy Bear dressed in scrubs with your name tag on it?

EPIDURAL BLOOD PATCH CONTRAINDICATIONS

- Patient refusal—YIPPEE! But seriously, would you be surprised or blame her? Recall how much trouble you caused the last time you worked on her back. Hopefully, the headache will resolve itself before she changes her mind. Document the patient's wishes and have a nice day.
- Blood-borne infection—this is the Real McCoy of a contraindication. You don't want to insert fluid that contains microbes and is a great culture medium (septic blood at body temperature) into the epidural space.
- You should probably avoid a blood patch if there is evidence of an ongoing infectious process (e.g., fever, elevated white cell count).
- It is appropriate to perform a blood patch in patients with HIV as long as there are no other active bacterial or viral illnesses present.
- Coagulopathy guidelines should be no different from those for any other epidural (check out the American Society of Regional Anesthesia [ASRA] Web site, www.asra.com, for regional anesthesia in the patient receiving anticoagulants).
- Then there are all the other contraindications to the placement of an epidural, which, in this case, were already considered, since you were doing an epidural when you got the wet tap!

PHILOSOPHY/ALTERNATIVES TO AN EPIDURAL BLOOD PATCH

- PDPH is very distressing to most patients. They can't nurse and care for their baby. Their expectation of a wonderful birth experience has been shattered. Showing concern, explaining the reasons for the headache, the expected time course, and the treatment options available to them will often lessen the patients' fears and stress.
- When getting consent for spinals or epidurals (especially parturients), mention the risk of PDPH. Of course, after you get a wet tap, you need to discuss the possibility of PDPH, assure the patient that you will follow up, and explain the therapeutic options ahead of time.
- The good news about doing an EBP is that for you it's a relatively low-stress situation. The baby is delivered and doing well (usually). Mom's not struggling and suffering during contractions. You're not looking at a crash C-section and maybe a need for general anesthesia, where maybe you'll lose the airway, and your life as you know it will be over. No, you're just doing an EBP in a much less demanding setting.

- Should you go right to an EBP, or should you consider conservative measures? That's a controversial question. Conservative measures include bed rest (shown to have no benefit), analgesics, intravenous hydration, and other medications (e.g., caffeine, sumatriptan, etc.).
- Some people will say to hell with the conservative stuff. Do the patch. It's low risk and usually makes the patient feel better. Jacking Mom on heavy caffeine and IVs prevents her from sleeping, keeps her running to the bathroom all the time, and every time she assumes the upright position she'll be thinking of you.
- The EBP has had a great safety record. However, injecting excessive volumes of blood could theoretically impair spinal cord blood flow. Also, there is the concern of developing an epidural or paraspinous abscess because of the injection of a fantastic culture medium. This has never been reported. Other problems with EBPs include back pain (occurs during the first 48 hours in 35% of patients and persists in 16% of patients for an average of 27 days), bradycardia, cauda equina syndrome, pneumocephalus, and cerebral ischemia.
- The timing of the blood patch is debatable. Studies suggest greater success when the blood patch is delayed for 24 to 48 hours. This, however, may be related to the severity of the headache.
- Prophylactic blood patches are another controversial area. This involves injection of blood or something else, either through a working epidural catheter or doing an EBP prior to the development of a headache. This technique is not widely used, but there are reports of success (statistically, that is, since how would you know in an individual patient?). Given that not all patients will develop a PDPH, some will be needlessly exposed to the risks associated with an EBP. Finally, if injecting blood into an epidural catheter, has a strict aseptic technique been followed the whole time this catheter has been in place?
- There was one report of an immediate total spinal following a prophylactic blood patch. Presumably local anesthetic–laden CSF was pushed cephalad due to compression by the injected blood outside the dura.
- Other alternatives to treat or prevent PDPH: Epidural saline has been used but is ineffective in patients following dural puncture with a 17-G needle, and relief is only temporary. Dextran has been used but has not found widespread acceptance. Gelfoam or fibrin glue has been tried but that junk is difficult to handle. Intrathecal catheter placement following a wet tap with removal after 24 hours has been reported to reduce the incidence of PDPH by promoting an inflammatory response at the dural puncture site (at least in animals). In one small study, the injection of 10 mL of intrathecal saline appeared to decrease the severity of PDPH. Finally, there are reports of significant success in decreasing the need for EBPs by a combination of maneuvers that include re-injecting CSF, injecting 10 cc of saline through the needle, placing an intrathecal catheter, using the catheter for analgesia, and leaving the catheter in situ after delivery.

HISTORY AND PHYSICAL EXAMINATION PRIOR TO EPIDURAL BLOOD PATCH

- Is the headache worse when sitting up? Postural headache is the cardinal feature of PDPH—worse in the upright position within 15 minutes and relief when supine within 30 minutes. In about half of cases, the headache is frontal but may also be occipital, both, or generalized.
- Is there neck pain/stiffness and upper shoulder pain? This can mimic meningitis.
- When did it start? Within the first 2 hours, PDPH will manifest in 38% to 65% of patients. Most cases will be reported within the first 3 days, but headache can occur later in up to 25% of cases.
- If new-onset diplopia is present, we'll bet the farm the patient has a PDPH. The patient may have associated signs suggesting cranial nerve involvement due to traction. Visual disturbances (incidence 14%) involve paresis of cranial nerves III, IV, and VI (92–95%).
- Any hearing changes or tinnitus? These symptoms are related to vestibulocochlear dysfunction. The decrease in CSF pressure is transmitted to the inner ear, disrupting the balance between the endolymphatic and perilymphatic pressures.
- Is there nausea, vomiting, dizziness, ataxia, or loss of appetite? These symptoms are often present in a PDPH.
- How about neurological symptoms such as motor or sensory loss? (This would point to some intracranial or spinal cord pathology.)
- Fever? Suggests infection. Differential: meningitis, chronic or acute sinusitis.
- Hypertension? History of preeclampsia? Remember, 44% of eclamptic seizures occur postpartum without other premonitory signs.
- Is there a history of prior headache?
- Check vital signs, including the fifth vital sign—*pain*. If there is no pain and the headache is gone, then do no harm (i.e., no EBP).
- Do a physical examination to ensure there are no focal findings that would make you question your diagnosis.

EQUIPMENT NEEDED

- Patient in appropriate position and tourniquet on (Figure 27-1)
- Stuff to draw 20 cc of blood in a sterile fashion (tourniquet, 20-cc syringe, needle, prep solution) (Figure 27-2)
- Someone to hold the patient still while you place the epidural (at this point, you're not so worried about fetal heart rates—since the kiddo is out and about somewhere—but mommy can still get vagal and plop over on you).
- An assistant to draw the blood for you is almost mandatory unless your holder can prevent the patient from leaning back/rolling over and pithing themselves on the epidural needle that's now in the epidural space.
- Finally, have masks, hats, sterile gowns, gloves, and an environment that is private and clean. Full battle dress may seem to be overkill, but that's what we would want for one of our family members. Full gowning is not a universal practice for this procedure; it's a suggestion.

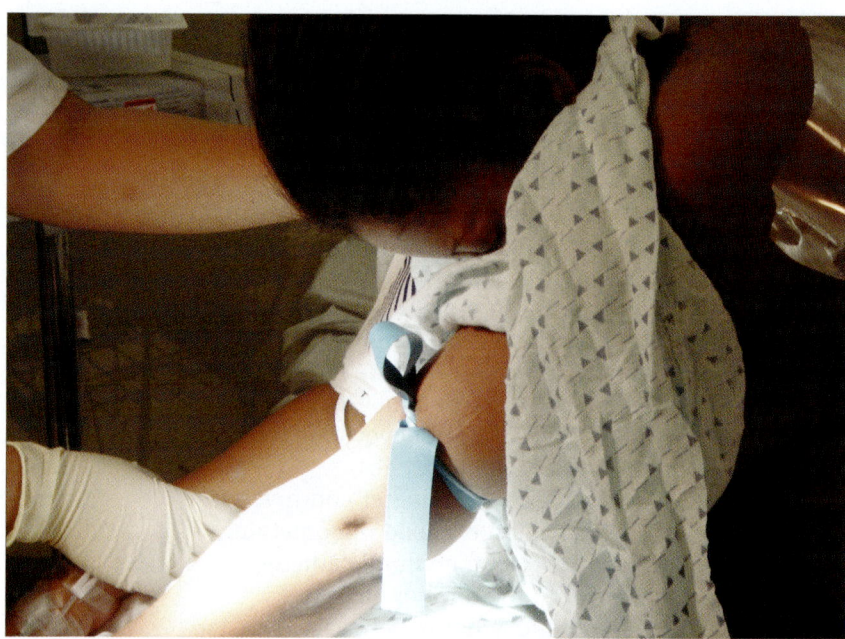

FIGURE 27-1 Patient in appropriate position and tourniquet on.

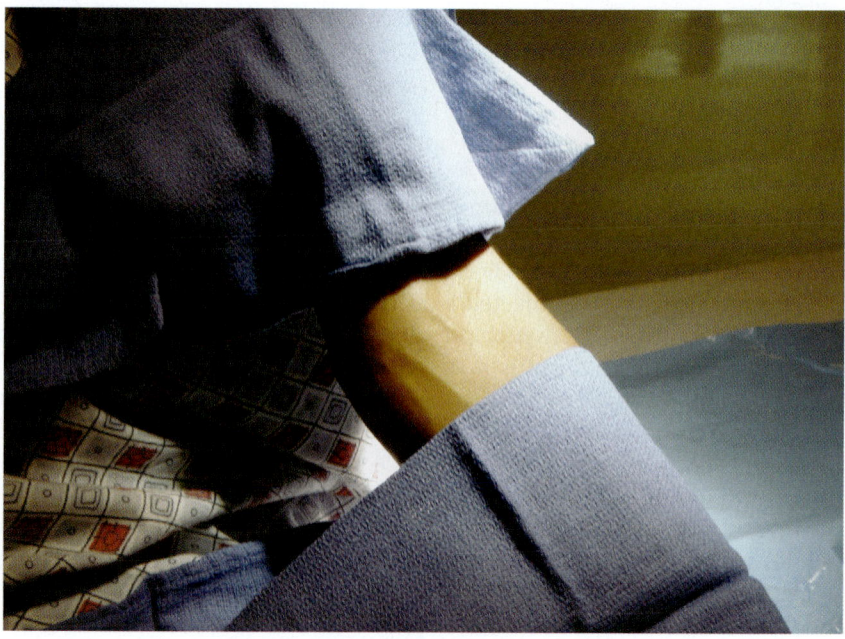

FIGURE 27-2 Venipuncture site prepped sterilely.

TECHNIQUE

Everything should be made as simple as possible, but not simpler.

Albert Einstein

- Have a well-functioning IV in place.
- Make sure you have *SOAP* readily available: *s*uction, *o*xygen, *a*irways, and *p*ressors. In other words, your usual emergency drugs for resuscitation, equipment for airway management, an oxygen delivery system and suction.
- Place the patient in a good position. This is critical; God forbid you blow it and give the patient a second wet tap or just can't get it in. Rule number four of anesthesia (after air goes in and out, blood goes round and round, and oxygen is good): *position and lubrication are everything.*
- Although having the patient in the sitting position is usually easier for the person performing the blood patch, the headache may be so severe you have little choice but to do the procedure with the patient lying on her side.
- At this point, since the baby is out, you can sedate if necessary. However, if the mother is breast-feeding, you will need to take that into consideration.
- Look over where you are going to draw blood. Make sure you will be able to draw 15 to 20 mL of blood from somewhere (Figure 27-2).
- Your assistant should prep the arm and prepare to draw the blood while you are locating the epidural space.
- Choose the interspace at the level of or one level below the original site.
- Do a sterile prep and drape and infiltrate the area with local anesthetic (Figure 27-3).
- Once the epidural space is located, have your assistant withdraw 20 mL of blood in a sterile fashion (Figure 27-4).
- Slowly inject 15 to 20 mL of the blood into the epidural space, or until the patient feels pressure in the back, buttocks, or legs.
- Pull the needle out and take a bow; relief may be almost instantaneous.
- The patient should remain supine for about 1 hour.

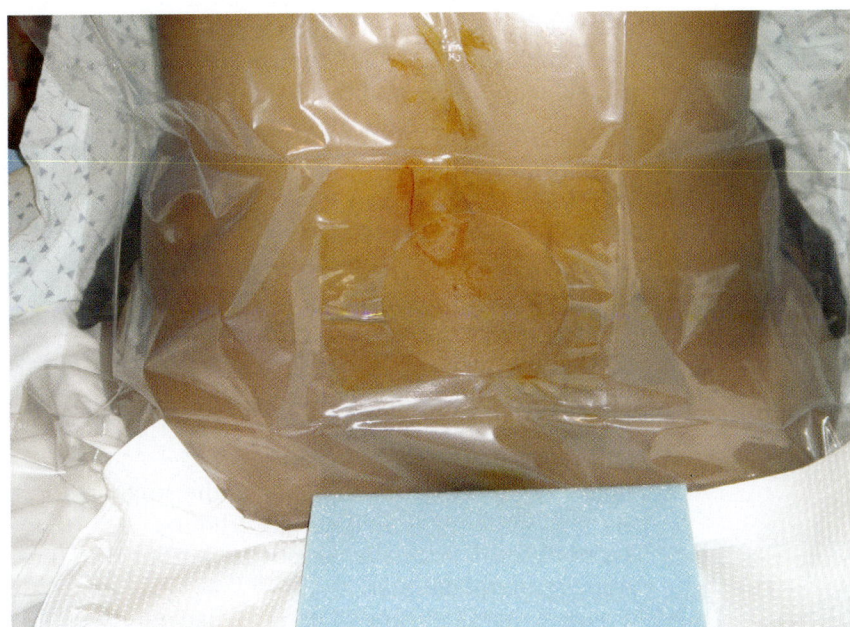

FIGURE 27-3 Sterile field for epidural placement.

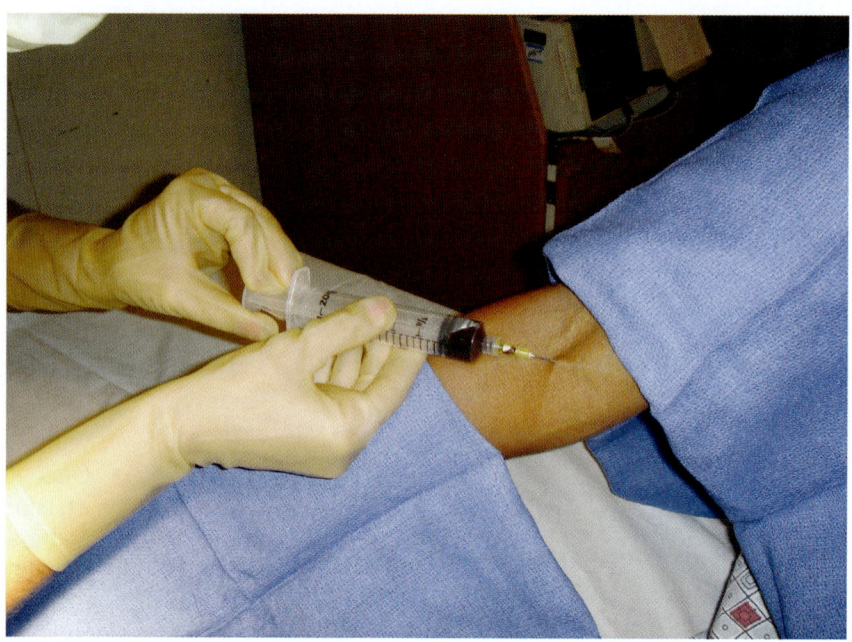

FIGURE 27-4 Sterile blood draw.

WHAT IF

- What if, when trying to do a blood patch, you nail the CSF again (which represents leak from first wet tap)? Then go up a space and try again. If you hit it again, consider counseling and psychotropic meds...for yourself!
- What if you locate the epidural space and can't get blood anywhere? You're in a bad way. Find a vein before you stick the back. Some might consider trying to withdraw blood from the IV. This is not a great alternative since it is doubtful that the IV site and tubing are absolutely sterile. If all else fails, think about using saline as the injectate.
- "Don't get a wet tap!" is about as useful as saying, "Don't double fault" or "Don't miss easy putts." Everyone knows you shouldn't get wet taps. It's not like you do it on purpose. So is there anything you can do to avoid it? Maybe. If you're in an interspace and really floundering—if you can feel the sweat rings forming in your axillae, your arm and shoulder muscles getting tense and starting to cramp, your fingertips holding the needle getting numb, and you're getting so ticked off that your calvarium is about to explode like Mount St. Helen's—then perhaps it's time to reconsider. Pull back. Go to a different interspace. Take a breather. As your frustrat-o-meter goes into the red zone, you are more likely to, as the Doors song goes, "Break on through to the other side." The other side of the dura, that is.
- You know from OB that a general anesthetic has 16 times the risk of a fatal outcome. The patient is *really* both an intubation and a spinal and it looks like they'll be tough. Time is of the essence. You can't get the spinal with a skinny needle. Do you: Go to general anesthesia? Keep floundering with the little needle? Avoid the "let's face it, it's easier to get it in a 22-G spinal needle" for fear of a subsequent headache and the possible need for a blood patch? Go for the bigger needle and get a move on.

CONCLUSION: HALL'S LAWS OF ANESTHESIA

- Air goes in and out.
- Blood goes round and round.
- Oxygen is good.
- Position and lubrication are everything.
- You can't anesthetize a rumor.
- Never trust the surgeon.
- Surgical time is estimated by taking the surgeon's estimate, doubling it, and adding 2 hours.
- The need for IV access is directly proportional to the difficulty in obtaining it.
- At a code, the first thing to do is to take your own pulse.

SUGGESTED READING

Abouleish PJD, Vega S, Blendinger I, et al. Long-term follow-up of epidural blood patch. *Anesth Analg* 1975;54:459–463.
Study finding relief of PDPH in overall 97.5% following blood patch (including those with second blood patch) and procedure safe after 2 year follow up.

Birnbach D, Gatt S, Datta S. *Textbook of obstetric anesthesia.* New York: Churchill-Livingstone; 2000, pp 487–503.
Everything you wanted to know about PDPH but were afraid to ask.

Hughes S, Levinson G, Rosen M. *Schnider and Levinson's anesthesia for obstetrics,* 4th ed. Philadelphia: Lippincott Williams & Wilkins; 2002, pp 415–417.
Text discusses risks associated with PDPH and blood patch.

Kuczkowski KM. Post-dural puncture headache in the obstetric patient: an old problem. New solutions. *Minerva Anestesiol* 2004;70:823–830.
Some steps toward PDPH prevention after the train hits.

Loeser EA, Hill GE, Bennett GM, et al. Time vs. success rate for epidural blood patch. *Anesthesiology* 1978;49(2):147–148.
Answers the question of when to patch.

Turnbull, DK, Shepherd DB. Post-dural puncture headache: pathogenesis, prevention and treatment. *Br J Anaesth* 2003; 91(5):718–729.
Great comprehensive discussion of PDPH and management—from the history to weird and wonderful alternatives to blood patch.

Vandam LD, Dripps RD. Long-term follow-up of patients who received 10,098 spinal anesthetics. Failure to discover major neurological sequelae. *JAMA* 1954;156:1486–1491.
Classic article.

Williams EJ, Beaulieu P, Fawcett WJ, Jenkins JG. Efficacy of epidural blood patch in the obstetric population. *Int J Obstet Anesth* 1999;8:105–109.
Discussion of how well blood patches really work.

CHAPTER 28

KIDDIE CAUDAL EPIDURAL AND PENILE BLOCKS

ZVI JACOB
REBECCA SANGSTER

CAUDAL EPIDURAL SINGLE INJECTION AND CATHETER PLACEMENT

Caudal analgesia is produced by injection of local anesthetic into the caudal canal. This produces block of the sacral and lumbar nerve roots. This block may be given as a single injection or, alternatively, a catheter insertion may be performed for continuous epidural block. Lumbar and low thoracic epidural space can be accessed via the caudal space. The level of the block could be determined by the catheter tip location and the dose of the local anesthetic given. Examples of appropriate surgery include inguinal or umbilical herniorrhaphy, orchidopexy, hypospadias and club foot surgery, and high abdominal or low thoracic areas requiring prolonged effective postoperative analgesia.

PLACEMENT

- Gather your equipment. You will need a pediatric epidural needle and catheter, regular epidural kit, and a 20-gauge (G) Angiocath (Figure 28-1).
- After induction and securing the child's airway, place the child in the lateral decubitus position.
- If you are right handed, the kiddie should be on his left side, and if you are left handed, then place the kiddie on his right side. (It can be done the opposite way, but set yourself up for success!)
- Once the kiddie is positioned, wash your hands and put on a sterile gown and gloves. Prep the patient with antiseptic solution and let it dry while you set up your epidural kit (Figure 28-2).
- It's time to find your landmarks and insert the 20-G catheter, which will be used as the epidural catheter introducer (Figure 28-3).
- Using your thumb, locate the coccyx and then move in a superior direction until you feel a slight divet. Without taking your thumb off the divet, grab and uncap the 20-G catheter and, using a 30- to 45-degree angle, push the Angiocath into the divet until you feel a "give."
- If you are unsure of your position, try to slide the angiocath over the needle; if it does not advance easily you are most likely in the wrong space (Figure 28-4).
- Next thread the epidural catheter into the epidural space to the level of the surgical incision (Figure 28-5).
- Once the catheter threads into the space (it should go smoothly, and if not, this is another sign that your Angiocath may not be in the epidural space), hold the catheter in place and slide the Angiocath out (similar to the epidural needle and catheter in a pregnant women).
- After removing the Angiocath off the catheter, inject a test dose of lidocaine with epinephrine. You may also confirm placement with contrast dye and a fluoro machine (we use diluted Omnipaque 1:1 in normal saline [NS]).
- After catheter placement is confirmed, tape the catheter as securely as possible! Kiddies sure move a lot, so make sure to use lots of tape and Tegaderm.
- Make sure to place a "tape barrier" at the bottom end of the Tegaderm! (Figure 28-6)

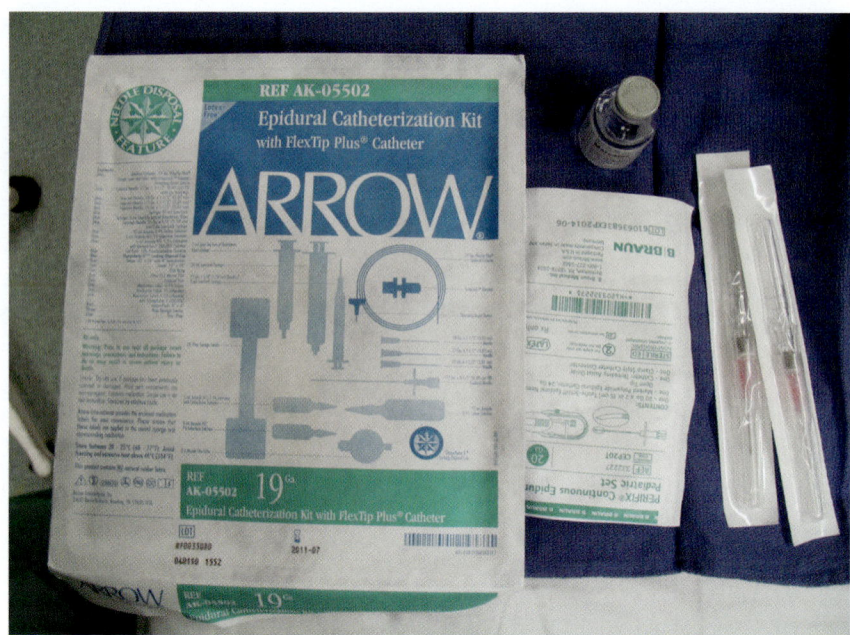

FIGURE 28-1 Equipment required.

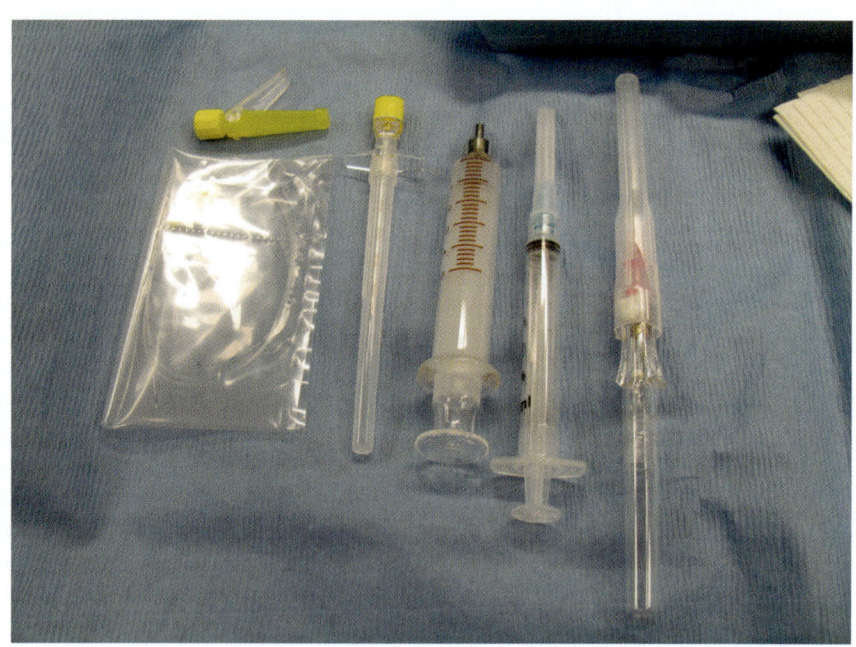

FIGURE 28-2 Epidural kit with all the cool stuff taken out.

Chapter 28 KIDDIE CAUDAL EPIDURAL AND PENILE BLOCKS

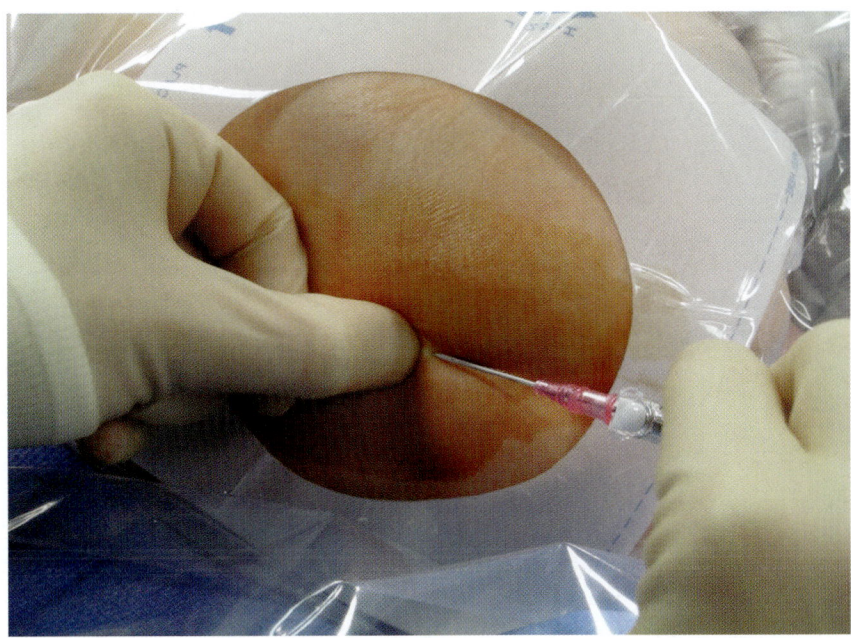

FIGURE 28-3 A 20-G catheter is used as the epidural catheter introducer.

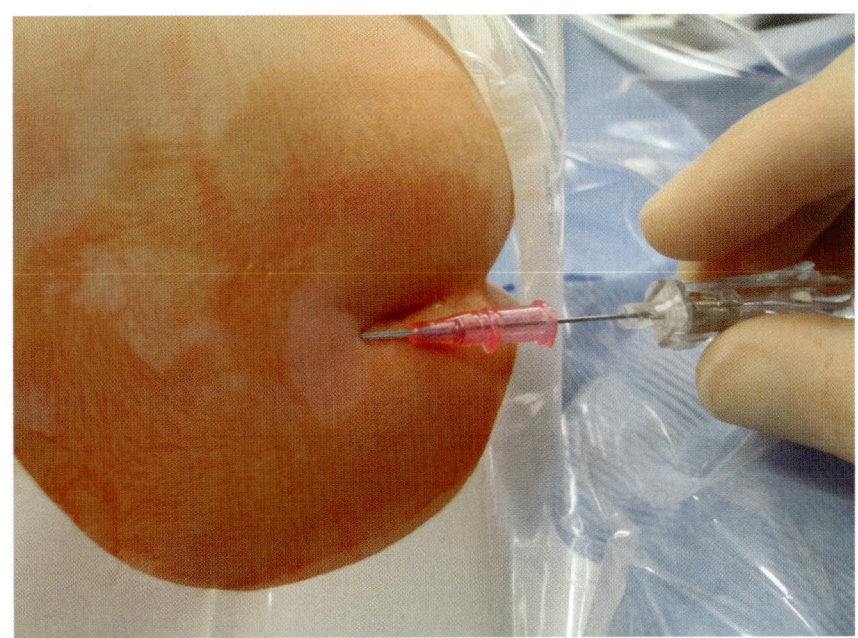

FIGURE 28-4 If the Angiocath does not advance easily, you are most likely in the wrong space.

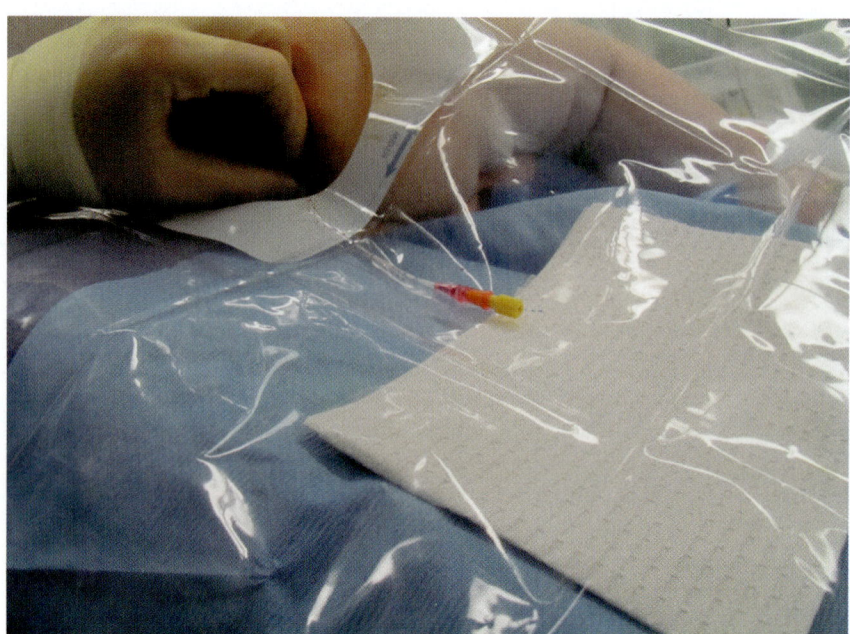

FIGURE 28-5 Thread the epidural catheter into the epidural space to the level of the surgical incision.

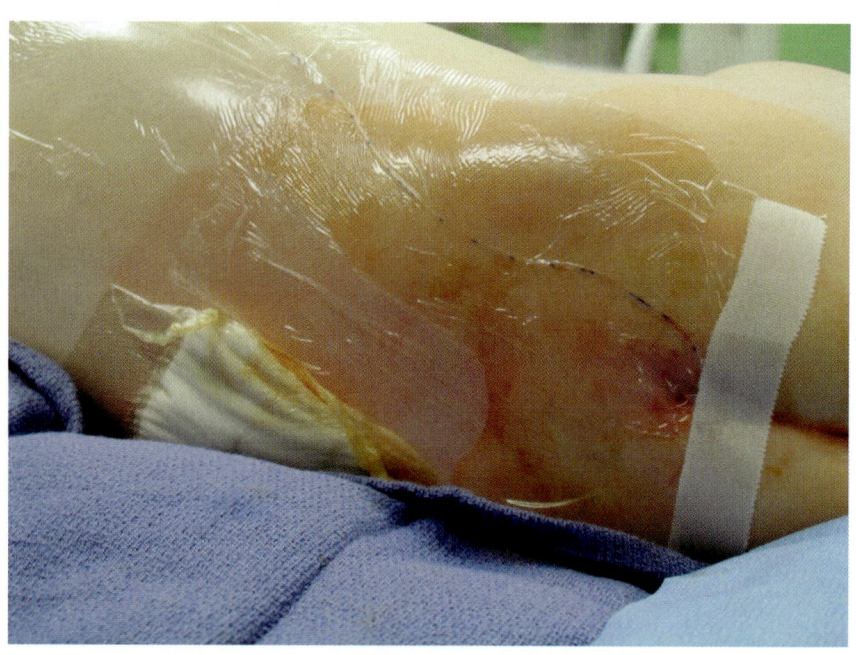

FIGURE 28-6 Place a "tape barrier" at the bottom end of the Tegaderm.

LOCAL ANESTHETIC DOSES

- Body weight is a better correlate than patient age in predicting the spread of local anesthetic following a caudal block.
- Bupivacaine: A single bolus of up to 1 mL/kg of bupivacaine 0.25% (2.5 mg/kg) is acceptable. For continuous epidural infusion, bupivacaine 0.1% at 0.2 to 0.4 mg/kg/h is often used.
- Ropivacaine: For a single-shot caudal block, a bolus of 1 mL/kg of 0.2% ropivacaine is acceptable. For continuous epidural infusion, ropivacaine 0.1% at 0.2 to 0.4 mg/kg/h is often used.

PENILE BLOCK IN A CHILD

- Penile block is used in various procedures, including release of paraphimosis, foreskin procedures, circumcision, and repair of penile lacerations.
- The penis is innervated by the pudendal nerve (S2-S4). This nerve eventually divides into the right and left dorsal nerves of the penis that pass under the pubis symphysis to travel below the Buck fascia to supply the sensory innervation to the penis.
- For this block you will need a local anesthetic agent (no epinephrine, please; we use bupivacaine 0.25%), a syringe, and a small injection needle (Figure 28-7).
- Make sure to do the "time out" prior to proceeding with the block.
- After inducing general anesthesia and securing the child's airway, the child is placed in a supine position.
- Disinfect the base of the penis using alcohol pads.
- Using the smallest fine needle (25-G or a 28-G insulin needle) an intradermal and subcutaneous ring weal is raised around the base of the penis (Figure 28-8).
- For the ventral injection of the para-urethral branches, the penis should be pulled upward and 1 to 2 mL of solution is injected near the base of the penis (Figure 28-9).
- The dorsal nerve is the next to be blocked on each side by injecting 3 to 5 mL of solution into the dorsum of the penis just below but not deep to the symphysis (Figure 28-10).
- Make sure the needle tip lies against the corpus cavernosum; if the needle pierces the corpus cavernosum, pain is experienced and the child will respond by moving. Also blood can be aspirated (Figures 28-11).
- In small infants, smaller volumes are used. Postoperative pain can be relieved by repeated penile block in the awake child.
- The smallest possible needle is used to prevent hematoma formation. If one begins, pressure is applied for 5 minutes to stop it.

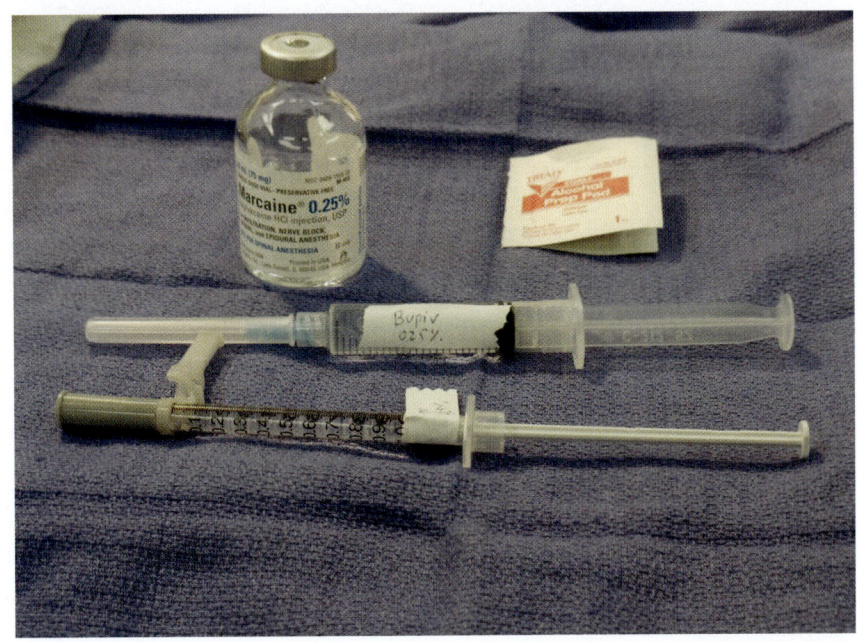

FIGURE 28-7 Equipment you'll need for a penile block.

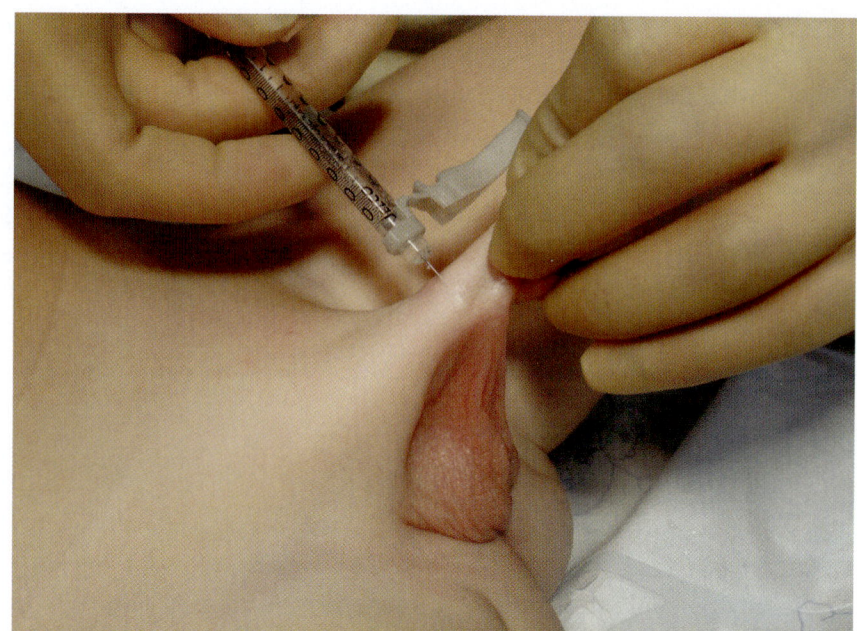

FIGURE 28-8 Using the smallest fine needle (25-G or 28-G insulin needle), an intradermal and subcutaneous ring weal is raised around the base of the penis.

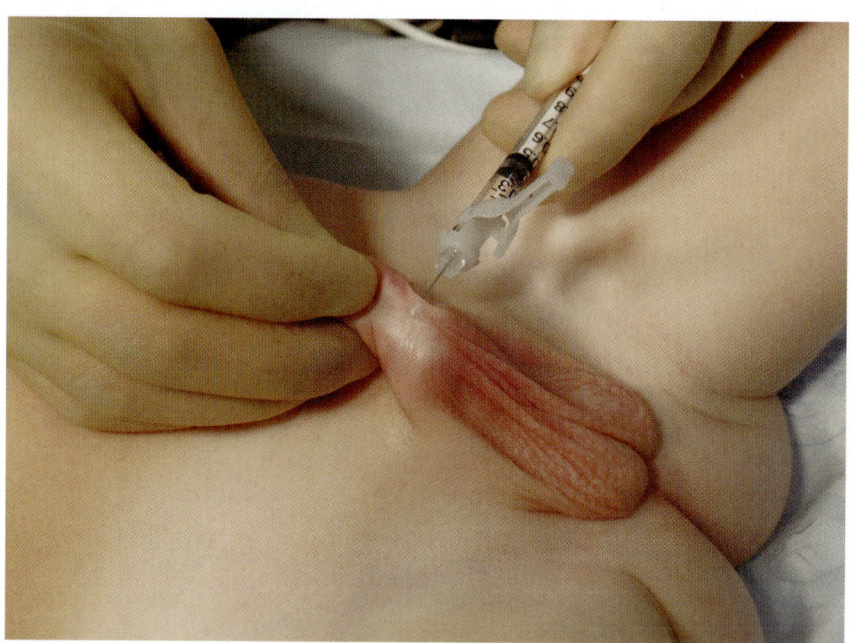

FIGURE 28-9 For the ventral injection of the paraurethral, the penis should be pulled upward and 1 to 2 mL of solution injected near the base of the penis.

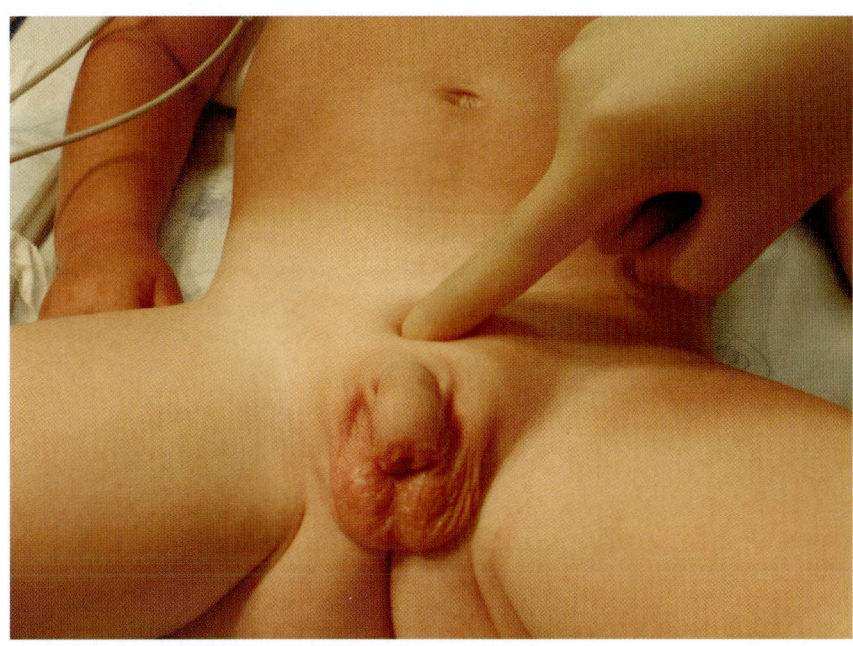

FIGURE 28-10 Palpate the symphisis.

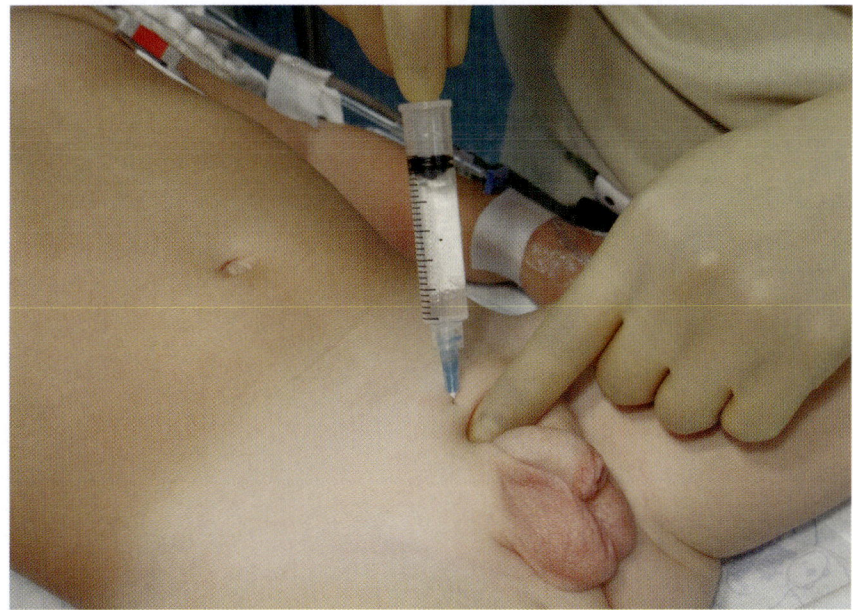

FIGURE 28-11 Injecting the dorsal nerve.

SUGGESTED READING

Bösenberg AT, Thomas J, Lopez T, Huledal G, Jeppsson L, Larsson LE. Plasma concentrations of ropivacaine following a single-shot caudal block of 1, 2 or 3 mg/kg in children. *Acta Anaesthiol Scand* 2001;10:1276–1280.

Breschan C, Jost R, Krumpholz R, et al. A prospective study comparing the analgesic efficacy of levobupivacaine, ropivacaine and bupivacaine in pediatric patients undergoing caudal blockade. *Pediatr Anesth* 2005;15:301–306.

Naja Z, Al-Tannir MA, Faysal W, Daoud N, Ziade F, El-Rajab M. A comparison of pudendal blocks vs. dorsal penile nerve block for circumcision in children: a randomized controlled trial. *Anesthesia* 2011;66:802–807.

Tsui BC, Berde CB. Caudal analgesia and anesthesia techniques in children. *Curr Opin Anesth* 2005;18:283–288.

Valairucha S, Seefelder D, Houck CS. Thoracic epidural catheters placed by the caudal route in infants: the importance of radiographic confirmation. *Pediatr Anesth* 2002;12:424–428.

CHAPTER 29

BLADDER EXSTROPHY—KIDDIE CAUDAL WITH TUNNEL

SHIVANI PATEL
SABINE KOST-BYERLY

A little love to a child and you get a great deal back.
John Ruskin, *The Crown of Wild Olive* (1866)

INTRODUCTION

Bladder exstrophy is a rare congenital disorder due to failure of formation of the anterior abdominal wall, occurring with an incidence of 2 in 100,000 live births. It is four times as common in males as in females. The initial reconstruction comprises either a staged procedure with closure of the abdominal wall within the first few days of life, followed by an epispadias repair several months later, or a complete primary repair. The repair can include pelvic osteotomies if children are older than a few days or if there is a large pelvic diastasis. Postoperatively these children are placed in either modified Bryant's traction or Buck's traction for those with pelvic osteotomy and external fixation for period of 4 to 6 weeks. Proper immobilization is necessary to prevent the distraction forces from causing wound dehiscence or bladder prolapse.[1]

Most neonates undergoing bladder exstrophy repair are otherwise healthy babies. Preoperative goals include preventing infection and maintaining good hydration secondary to increased insensible loss of water.

At the Johns Hopkins Medical Institution, these children undergo modern staged reconstruction, which involves primary closure of the bladder, posterior urethra, pelvis, and anterior abdominal wall. This is performed using combined general and regional anesthesia techniques. After transport to the operating room from the neonatal intensive care unit (NICU), these patients are placed on the operating table covered with a forced-air warming blanket. The operating room temperature is also elevated to decrease heat loss secondary to radiation. Neonates have large body surface area, lack subcutaneous fat and the shivering mechanism to produce heat, which makes them more prone to intraoperative hypothermia. Standard American Society of Anesthesiologists (ASA) monitors are applied. Most of these patients present to the operating room with a peripheral intravenous catheter in place. Neonates tend to desaturate very quickly; hence, preoxygenation prior to induction of anesthesia is necessary.

In the absence of an intravenous access, a mask induction with sevoflurane is performed. Once unconsciousness is established and the ability to ventilate is confirmed, a muscle relaxant such as rocuronium, vecuronium, or pancuronium can be used to facilitate intubation.

NEONATAL AIRWAY

- An appropriate-size mask, generally size 1
- Oral airway
- Two functioning laryngoscopes with Miller straight blade No. 0 (neonates have a long, folded, angulated epiglottis, so the use of a straight blade helps you

lift the epiglottis during laryngoscopy, hence making visualization of the cords easier)
- Endotracheal tubes: 3.0- to 3.5-mm uncuffed endotracheal tube (ETT). The cricoid cartilage is the narrowest part of the neonatal airway. Take care to prevent subglottic edema; always check for leak postintubation.
- Functioning suction catheter
- Laryngeal mask airway (LMA) size 1 (in case you have trouble with ventilation or intubation)
- After endotracheal intubation, confirm presence of tube in the trachea. (Presence of end-tidal CO_2, bilateral chest rise and fall with respiration, auscultation, and presence of fog inside the endotracheal tube with each breath.) The correct position of the endotracheal tube is with the tip lying in the midtrachea. Thus, rule of 1, 2, 3 implies weight in kilograms to the corresponding distance at the lip being 7, 8, or 9 cm or using the formula ETT size × 3.

Once the airway is secured and the eyes are taped to prevent any corneal abrasion, the patient is turned into the left/right lateral decubitus position for placement of tunneled caudal catheter.

"So you are going to put a needle in my back? You better know what you are doing!"

CAUDAL EPIDURAL BLOCKADE

The use of a caudal epidural block has been shown to provide good intraoperative and postoperative analgesia in children. The technique can be performed as a single-shot injection or as a continuous epidural block via placement of the epidural catheter. Both local anesthetic and opioids are used to achieve optimum analgesia.

Technique

1. *Anatomy:* The sacrum is formed by the fusion of five sacral vertebrae. However, the lamina of the fifth sacral vertebrae and partly the fourth fails to fuse in the midline, creating a bony defect posteriorly called the sacral hiatus. This defect is covered by sacrococcygeal ligament. When the patient is placed in the lateral decubitus position, the point of entry into the sacral hiatus can be established by palpating for the sacral cornua (the bony prominence felt as you move the palpating finger away from the coccyx cranially).
2. This procedure is performed *under strict aseptic precautions*, which includes washing the hands, wearing a mask, with or without a sterile gown, sterile gloves, prepping the back with betadine times three or DuraPrep, and the use of sterile drapes to cover the entire patient. Care should be taken to remove residual betadine after catheter insertion, as betadine can lead to significant skin irritation in young children. The FDA has not approved the use of chlorhexidine in children younger than 2 months of age.
3. Once the point of entry is established, a Crawford needle is inserted at a 45-degree angle to the skin and advanced slowly until a characteristic "pop" is felt as the needle penetrates the sacrococcygeal ligament. Then the angle of the needle is dropped (parallel to the skin) and is advanced a few millimeters into the epidural space. The stylet is removed and a 2-mL syringe is attached to rule out aspiration of any blood or cerebrospinal fluid (CSF) (since the dural sac extends to level of S2-3 in children). One milliliter of saline is injected into the epidural space prior to insertion of the catheter to assess resistance and in order to distend the space.
4. The length of catheter insertion is determined by holding the tip of the catheter at the level corresponding to the T10 dermatome on the back extending to the point of entry at the level of the skin. The depth of the needle at which the loss of resistance was encountered is added to the above length. Use of ultrasound guidance or special stimulating epidural catheters (such as Tsui) may facilitate desired segmental positioning.
5. The catheter is then advanced into the epidural space at the determined depth. If the tip of the needle is in the correct space, the catheter threads in very easily. DO NOT REMOVE THE CRAWFORD NEEDLE!
6. When using a commercial kit that allows easy removal of the adapter from the catheter, it is advisable to temporarily attach the adapter now and inject 0.5 to 1 mL of saline into the catheter. (If the catheter is kinked internally, you want to know this now, not after you spend a lot of time creating a tunnel. Be careful not to inject too much saline into the catheter; the more you inject the more you will dilute your anesthetic. For example, 1 mL/kg in a 3-kg neonate is just 3 mL total volume. Wow, these critters are really small!)
7. In order to reduce the risk of catheter colonization, the catheter is tunneled subcutaneously.[2,3] Insert a 22-gauge (G) spinal needle into EXACTLY the same spot as the Crawford needle, aiming subcutaneously to the flank area, emerging just superior of the iliac crest. Now advance a 17-G Tuohy needle from the flank area, using the spinal needle as a guide emerging in the same location as the Crawford needle. Remove the spinal needle. If you have any doubt, gently cut a possible skin bridge between the Crawford and the Tuohy needle using a No. 11 blade. Remove the Crawford needle. Thread the catheter through the Tuohy needle. Remove the Tuohy needle. Slowly retract the catheter until the loop at the sacral hiatus slides below the skin and a dressing is placed over the puncture site.

8. Sterile Steri-Strips and Tegaderm dressing are applied firmly to the site where the tunneled catheter exits on the patient's side, to prevent dislodgment of the catheter. You may also suture the catheter.
9. Once the catheter is in place, a test dose of 0.1 mL/kg of 0.25% bupivacaine with 1:200,000 (5 μg/mL) of epinephrine is injected to rule out intravascular injection as depicted by electrocardiogram changes, such as an increase in heart rate > 10 bpm or a decrease in heart rate in the first minute from baseline or an increase in T-wave amplitude or an increase in systolic blood pressure by 15 mm Hg or more in the first 2 minutes.
10. If the test dose is negative, small incremental doses of 0.25% bupivacaine with 1:200,000 epinephrine are injected into the caudal space to a total volume of 0.5 to 1 mL/kg.

PLACEMENT OF TUNNELED CAUDAL CATHETER (FIGURES 29-1 TO 29-4)

Once the caudal catheter is in place, the patient is turned to the supine position and additional intravenous access is obtained. Either a central venous catheter or a peripherally inserted central catheter (PICC) line is placed. These lines not only help to guide fluid therapy using central venous pressure (CVP) monitoring but also can be used to draw blood for laboratory sampling intraoperatively and during the postoperative period. Having a central venous catheter also helps to provide intravenous hyperalimentation during the postoperative period since feeding might be difficult due to postoperative ileus, and proper nutrition is necessary for adequate healing.

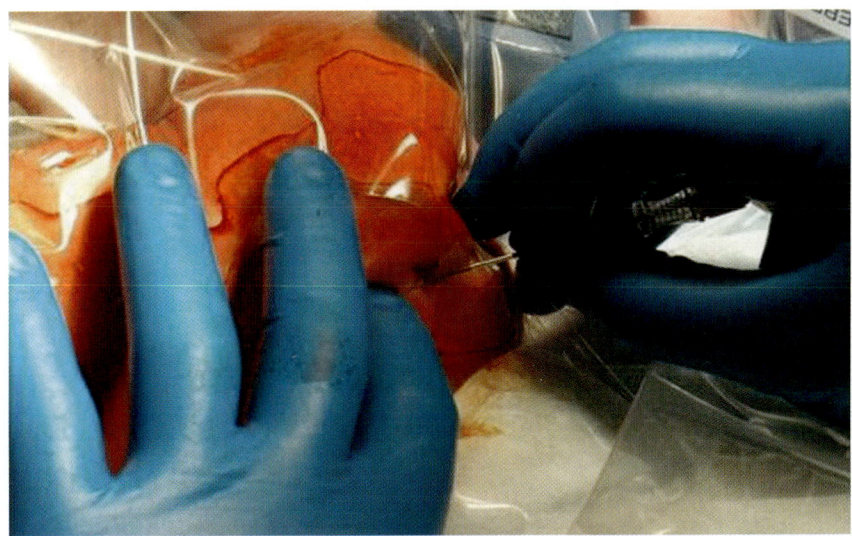

FIGURE 29-1 Insertion of Crawford needle into the epidural space.

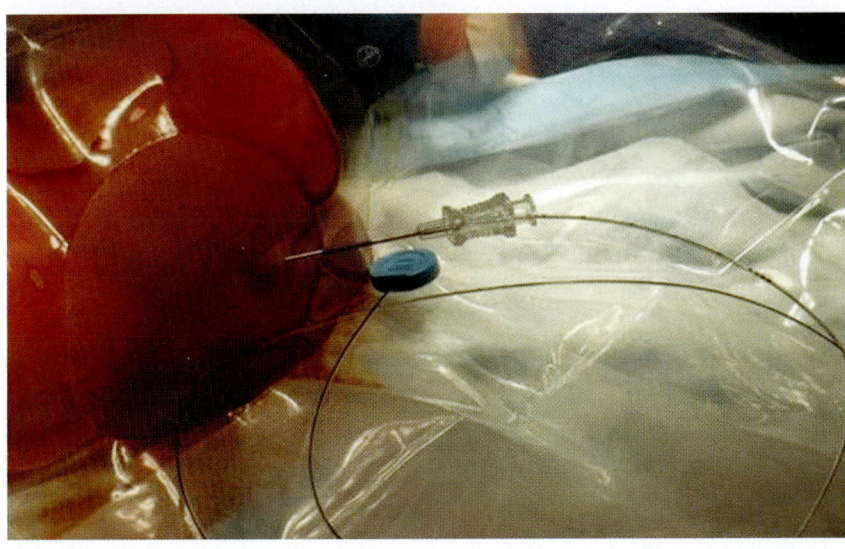

FIGURE 29-2 Insertion of caudal catheter (leave the Crawford needle in place).

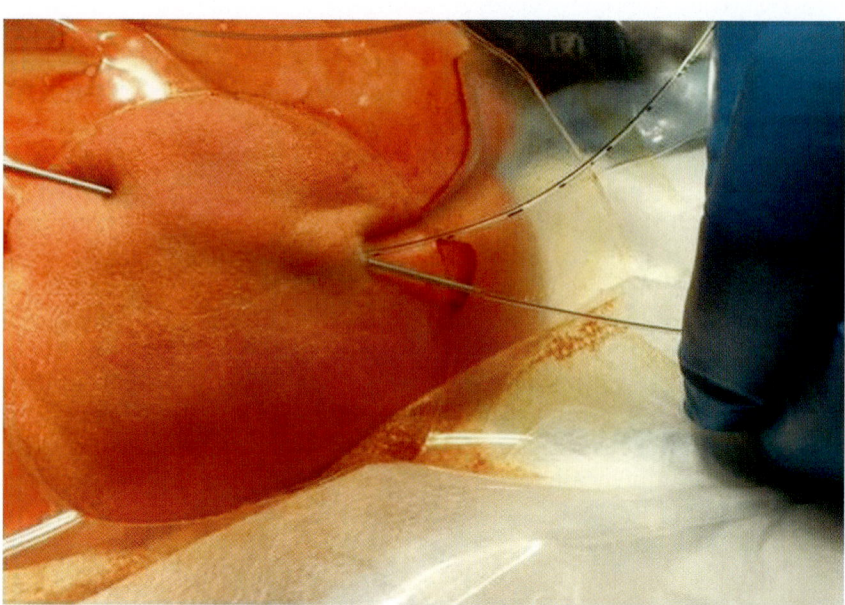

FIGURE 29-3 Tunneling of the caudal catheter.

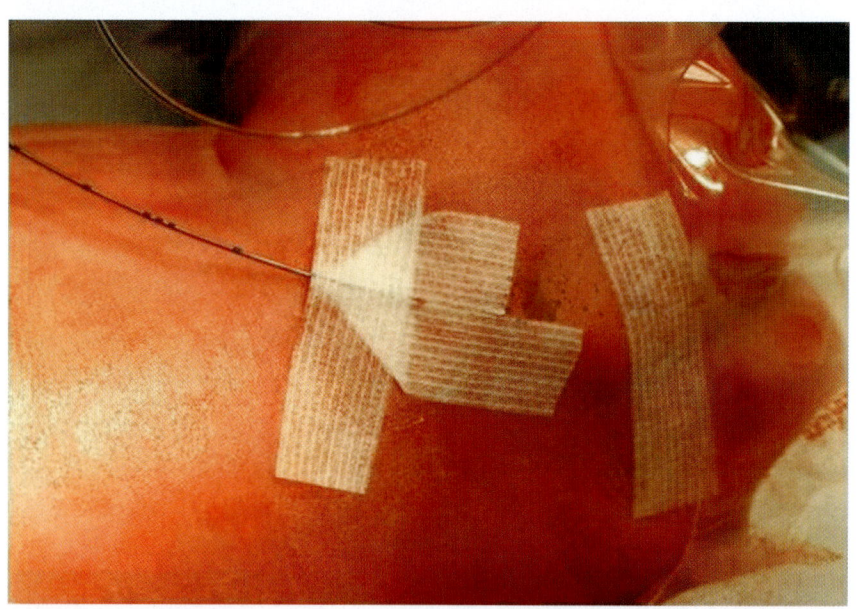

FIGURE 29-4 Securing the catheter.

FLUID MANAGEMENT

This surgery demands meticulous attention to intraoperative fluid administration, particularly in neonates. Replacement of insensible fluid losses is required. If the surgical plan includes pelvic osteotomies, there can be significant blood loss. Placement of an intraarterial catheter is optional.

Fluid replacement is generally determined by preoperative deficit, maintenance needs, insensible loss, and blood loss.

Driving blind

Adequate fluid management is more difficult to assess during bladder surgery as urine output is not available. Only when the surgeon tells you to stop flooding the field then you have overdone it....

Maintenance

Since neonates are more prone to hypoglycemia from the lack of glycogen reserves, some form of dextrose supplementation is necessary. Maintenance fluids are calculated as 4 mL/kg/h. This fluid can be administered via an infusion pump throughout the procedure.

Preoperative Deficit

This deficit generally results from keeping the patient NPO. It is calculated as 4 mL/kg times the number of hours of starvation. Half of it is replaced during the first hour and the remaining half is administered over 2 hours using a balanced salt solution.

Third Space Loss

This depends on the nature of the surgical procedure. In view of exposed intraabdominal contents with bladder exstrophy, the losses can be up to 7 to 10 mL/kg/h and should be replaced with balanced salt solution.

Blood Loss

It is generally difficult to estimate the blood loss in these patients. Due to the relatively small blood volume of a baby or young child, any blood draining into suction container could represent serious losses. Hence, serial monitoring of hemoglobin, CVP, and blood pressure is considered prior to transfusion. Transfusion of 15 mL/kg of packed red cells raises the hemoglobin concentration by 1 g/dL. For neonates always use fresh, cytomegalovirus (CMV) negative, irradiated and washed packed red cells for transfusion. Always warm the blood, since transfusion of cold stored blood can lead to hypothermia. After the transfusion, check for serum ionized calcium levels and, if required, replace with intravenous calcium chloride 10 mg/kg.

MAINTENANCE OF ANESTHESIA

A combination of inhaled anesthetics, muscle relaxant, and regional anesthesia technique is used. Small incremental doses of intravenous opioid may be used to supplement analgesia. Any inhalation anesthetic can be used during the maintenance phase. Avoid the use of nitrous oxide intraoperatively to prevent bowel distension.

Subsequent dosing of the epidural catheter is generally one half to two thirds of the initial dose of bupivacaine 0.25% with epinephrine 1:200,000 every 60 to 90 minutes. Alternatively, an infusion of 0.1% bupivacaine delivering up to 0.2 mg/kg/h in neonates and infants and up to 0.4 mg/kg/h in older children can be employed.

POSTOPERATIVE

At the end of the procedure, depending on the patient's condition, the decision to extubate or not should be made. Older children are transferred to the pediatric intensive care unit (PICU) or to a monitored floor postoperatively; however, younger children are admitted to an intensive care unit.

Patients are followed by a dedicated pediatric pain service team for their entire stay until they are discharged. The success of this surgery depends on close communication among surgeons, anesthesiologists, and the nursing team. A multimodal analgesia approach is used for pain control and immobilization.

Regional Anesthesia

Neonates receive continuous epidural infusion of lidocaine 0.8 mg/kg/h. Fentanyl can be added after a few days if the child has required multiple small doses of fentanyl every day *and* has tolerated them without signs of respiratory depression. Older infants receive either lidocaine 3 mg/mL at 1.5 mg/kg/h (= 0.5 mL/kg/h) or bupivacaine 1 mg/mL at 0.3 mg/kg/h. Clonidine may be added as an adjunct. Its sedative effects are particularly welcome in active toddlers immobilized for several weeks. The combination of local anesthetic, opioid, and α_2-agonist helps to reduce the dose for the individual agent and thereby decreases the risk of toxicity. All local anesthetics are absorbed from the epidural space into the systemic circulation. Neonates are prone to toxicity due to low serum α-globulin levels and immature metabolic system.

Information for prolonged infusions of local anesthetics in neonates is limited. Studies have shown that the plasma level of bupivacaine continues to rise even after 48 hours of continuous infusion.[2] Most hospital laboratories are able to analyze therapeutic lidocaine but not bupivacaine levels. Monoethylglycinexylidide (MEGX), the metabolite of lidocaine, rises with continuous epidural infusion.[3] MEGX has a convulsant property similar to that of lidocaine, so an additive effect of lidocaine and MEGX can contribute to toxicity. Serum lidocaine levels are checked twice a day in neonates for the first 48 to 72 hours and are maintained at less than 4 µg/mL. If required, the infusion is held for few hours, or if the levels continue to rise, then the dose of local anesthetic is reduced. Bupivacaine is not recommended for prolonged infusions in infants younger than 6 months due to limited information. In older children, bupivacaine continuous infusions should be limited to 0.4 mg/kg/h (0.2 mg/kg/h in infants less than 6 months). The site of epidural catheter is assessed daily to rule out the presence of any erythema or discharge. The dressing is changed every fifth day by the pediatric pain service. If there is any evidence of local or systemic signs of infection such erythema, drainage, or unexplained fevers, the epidural catheter is discontinued, the tip is sent for culture, and the patient is closely observed. If an epidural abscess is suspected, an MRI of the spine must be obtained immediately.

Benzodiazepine

Intravenous diazepam 0.1 to 0.2 mg/kg is administered q4–6 hours as a PRN or scheduled dosing for treatment of bladder spasms and sedation.

Anticholinergic

An oxybutynin patch is used for treatment of bladder spasms. Rule out any urinary tract infections or occlusion of ureteric stent as a contributing factor.

Narcotics

In spite of epidural infusion, some patients do require intravenous opioids. This is administered via a PCA pump (patient/parent/nurse-controlled analgesia). Rarely, a continuous infusion is added to the PCA bolus.

In infants, fentanyl, with a short duration of action, is used with bolus dose of 0.2 to 1 µg/kg/dose with a lockout interval of 10 minutes to a maximum of three to four doses per hour. Following the removal of the tunneled epidural catheter, patients may be transitioned to an intravenous opioid regimen using PCA as described with a basal rate of 0.5 to 1 µg/kg/h. The dose is titrated to effect.

In older children, morphine at a continuous rate of 10 to 30 µg/kg/h and a bolus of 10 to 30 µg/kg, or hydromorphone at 4 to 6 µg/kg/h with an intermittent bolus of 4 to 6 µg/kg every 10 minutes to maximum of five doses per hour can be used.

Once the child tolerates oral intake, a transition is made to oral opioids, generally oxycodone 0.1 to 0.2 mg/kg/dose given every 4 hours. With the start of oral oxycodone, the basal infusion rate of PCA must be turned to zero.

Methadone 0.1 mg/kg/dose may be used in older children q12h. Being a long-acting drug, less frequent dosing is needed, and oral and intravenous doses are interchangeable.

In cases of difficult sedation butorphanol, an opioid agonist-antagonist may be alternated with diazepam for sedation and opioid-induced pruritus at a dose of 0.03 to 0.05 mg/kg/dose q4h on an as-needed basis or scheduled.

Antiinflammatory Agents

Acetaminophen 10 to 15 mg/kg q4–6h to a maximum of 75 mg/kg/day and ibuprofen 4 to 10 mg/kg q6h are also used as an adjuvant.

"Hey, buddy, we are all over with your pain control."

SIDE EFFECTS DUE TO OPIOIDS

1. Nausea/vomiting: Prescribe ondansetron 0.1 to 0.15 mg/kg IV, diphenhydramine 1 mg/kg IV, or metoclopramide 0.1 to 0.2 mg/kg IV.
2. Constipation: Laxative or stimulant from day one such as Colace and senna.
3. Pruritus: Naloxone infusion 1 µg/kg/h or diphenhydramine 1 mg/kg IV,
4. Respiratory depression: Stop PCA, call for help. Check for ABCs; if required, provide supplemental oxygen or bag-mask ventilate the patient, and prescribe IV naloxone (opioid antagonist) 1 to 2 µg/kg/dose to a maximum dose of 10 µg/kg.

After approximately 4 to 6 weeks an x-ray of the pelvis is performed to ensure proper callus formation after osteotomies, so that immobilization in traction can be discontinued. The patient is then prepared for discharge within next few days.

"It's time for us to say goodbye."

WITHDRAWAL

Any patient who has received benzodiazepine or narcotics for a period of 10 to 14 days must be weaned gradually. Weaning is done typically every alternate day with a reduction of the total dose by 10% to 20% each time. These patients also need to be monitored for any withdrawal symptoms. At Johns Hopkins, we have an opioid weaning flow sheet that is used both in the intensive care and the inpatient units. The scoring includes three broad categories:

1. Central nervous system: excessive crying, sleeping, Moro reflex, tremors, increased muscle tone
2. Metabolic: temperature, respiratory rate, sweating, yawning, sneezing, nasal stuffiness, increased secretions (suctioning)
3. Gastrointestinal: emesis, loose or watery stools

The symptom from each category is scored on a 0 to 3 or 1 to 2 point scale. A score >8 to 12 would indicate withdrawal; change back to the opioid dose with which no withdrawal symptoms were noted and maintain for 48 hours and reassess.

Many of these patients are also sent home on a weaning schedule. To improve parental compliance intervals between individual dose should be at least 8 hours. Detailed instructions, with dosing for each day and information regarding any signs of withdrawal, are given. A contact number in case of any questions or concerns should be provided.

CONCLUSION

Managing a patient with bladder exstrophy requires a multidisciplinary approach with close cooperation with members of the team for a successful outcome.

"Hurray, finally it's over. I am going home."

REFERENCES

1. Meldrum KK, Baird AD, Gearhart JP. Pelvic and extremity immobilization after bladder exstrophy closure: complications and impact on success. *Urology* 2003;62(6).
2. Larsson BA, Lonquist PA, Olsson GL. Plasma concentrations of bupivacaine in neonates after continuous epidural infusion. *Anesth Analg* 1997;84(3):62.
3. Miyabe M, Kakiuchi Y, Kihara S, et al. The plasma concentration of lidocaine's principal metabolite increases during continuous epidural anesthesia in infants and children. *Anesth Analg* 1998;87:1056–1057.

SUGGESTED READING

Bailey AG, McNaull PP, Jooste E, Tuchman JB. Perioperative crystalloid and colloid fluid management in children: Where were we and how did we get here? *Anesth Analg* 2010;110(2):375.

Kost-Byerly S, Jackson EV, Yaster M, Kozlowski LJ, Mathews R, Gearhart JP. Perioperative anesthetic and analgesic management of newborn bladder exstrophy repair. *J Pediatr Urol* 2008;4:280–285.

Miller RD. Anesthesia. 5th ed. The Curtis Center, Independence Square West, Philadelphia, Pennsylvania, 19106: Churchill Livingstone, a Harcourt Health Sciences Company.

Yaster M, Krane EJ, Kaplan RF, Cote CJ, Lappe DG. Pediatric Pain Management and Sedation Handbook. Copyright 1997 by Mosby-Year Book Inc, 11830 Westline Industrial Drive, St. Louis, Missouri 63146.

PART V
REGIONAL

CHAPTER 30

REGIONAL BLOCK OF THE UPPER EXTREMITY

GEZA K. KISS
AHDEV KUPPASAMY
SARAH LASALLE

Mortal arm and nerve must feel.
     Sir Walter Scott, *Harold the Dauntless* (1817)

INTRODUCTION

I won't try to resolve the ongoing question as to whether patient outcomes are improved with peripheral regional versus general anesthesia. Many anesthesiologists believe that it is the catabolic stress response to surgery and underlying comorbidities that ultimately determine postoperative morbidity and mortality. Our job as anesthesiologists is to attenuate that stress response. Patients do well with both types of anesthetics in the hands of competent physicians.

So I ask again, why regional? (Pardon the perseveration. If something is repeated here, it's probably important to remember.)

- Sometimes patients request ABG (anything but general) for whatever reason, and patient choice is a good thing.
- Sometimes it makes OUR lives easier. Take the 86-year-old patient from the nursing home with hypertension, diabetes mellitus, Alzheimer's disease, and tsutsugamushi fever with an ejection fraction (EF) of 10% for a repair of an open wrist fracture. Sure, prope/sux/tube will work. But there is sick and then there is our demented octogenarian. Can't use OK anesthesia here. It would be great to have an alternative.
- Occasionally the surgeon will request that we do a regional (WHHHHHAAATTTT?). It's true; more surgeons are requesting regionals these days.
- Other reasons include faster discharge to the floor or home, decreased postoperative nausea and vomiting (PONV), excellent postoperative analgesia while sparing opioids and their side effects.

I'm probably preaching to the choir and won't win any converts from the "I know the best regional, the polyvinylchloride tube block" school, so let's just discuss the where's and how's of upper extremity regional anesthesia.

This chapter discusses the details of the brachial plexus blocks:
- Supraclavicular
- Interscalene
- Infraclavicular
- Axillary

If you can perform these four, you'll be able to anesthetize any part of the upper extremity, except for maybe the proximal axilla. These will all be one-shot techniques; placing catheters is a whole other ballgame.
- Got ultrasound? You can do these blocks.
- Got a nerve stimulator? You can do these blocks.
- No ultrasound or nerve stimulator? You can still do these blocks, via a paresthesia technique, maybe not as elegantly or as comfortably for the patient, but ultimately all you need are a regional block needle and a syringe filled with local anesthetic.

- When relief doctors went to Haiti after the earthquake, they had to "rediscover old ways of doing blocks" as there were no ultrasound or nerve stimulator devices. The day may come when you have to do these "the old-fashioned way" as well.

THE ANATOMY OF THE BRACHIAL PLEXUS OR WHY ROBERT TAYLOR DRINKS COFFEE BLACK

Who in the name of Gray's Anatomy is Robert Taylor? He was a huge movie idol from the 1930s through the 1950s who always got the girl and who is persistently part of a mnemonic for the organization of the brachial plexus:
- Roots
- Trunks
- Divisions
- Cords
- Branches

We have all managed to memorize the brachial plexus (BP) anatomy at least 100 times, but unfortunately, if you want to know how to do the upper extremity blocks, you HAVE TO, HAVE TO, HAVE TO, HAVE TO memorize it again.
- Despite the fact that the plexus looks like the track arrangement at Penn Station, it does like to hang around the subclavian/axillary artery conduit.
- Ultrasound-guided techniques are facilitated by the neural structures' perivascular location.

Did I mention that you have to KNOW YOUR ANATOMY? (Figure 30-1)

I did.
- Don't just memorize it for the 100th time without really visualizing the three-dimensional relationship among the vessels, the nerves, and the "Ssssssssss" (lungs and pleura).
- Also, know which nerves innervate which muscles and know the actions of those muscles. Try to get to the anatomy lab and look at the structures in situ.

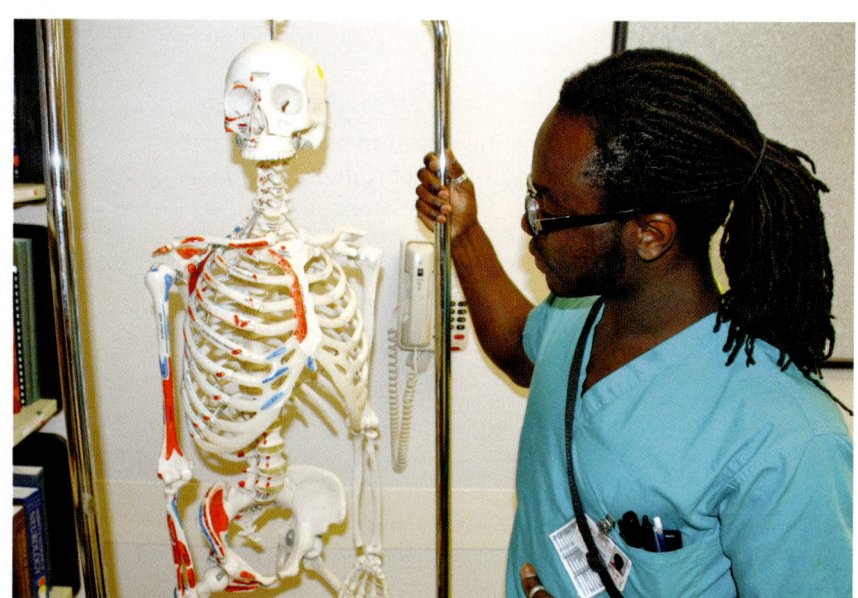

FIGURE 30-1 "Hey, how ya doin? Want to study some anatomy?"

MAYBE I SHOULDN'T DO THIS BLOCK

Contraindications

- Patient refusal: No brainer. It's also a no brainer for the jury if you violate this one. (This is an absolute contraindication. The others are relative.)
- Infection at the site of injection: Why make it easier for the microbe to move to better digs? Let it get a job and a mortgage like the rest of us.
- Coagulopathy: As hematoma is the potential result, you must realize that not all hematomas are created equal. If you can compress the area, the patient will usually do OK. The interscalene and axillary areas are easily compressible, even the supraclavicular area. Not so for a vessel in the infraclavicular area.

"I DON'T WANT TO HEAR THE HAMMERING"

Who does? I can't blame you. The anesthetic experience is about amnesia as much as anything else, so we usually accede to the patients' requests for this. Sedation is an important part of regional anesthesia, both during the block and during the surgery.

- A little midazolam and fentanyl go a long way, but it's important not to snow patients to the point where they will be unable to communicate the symptoms of an intraneural injection (big screaming radicular-like ouchie).
- During the procedure, a propofol or remifentanil infusion can help with anxiolysis, patient comfort, and even analgesia if there is inadequate tourniquet coverage.
- Taken too far, however, you end up with GANA (not the country, silly) an acronym for "general anesthesia, no airway," resulting from a larger than average dose of mu and γ-aminobutyric acid (GABA) agonists (also known as RAG: "room air general").

If the surgical position makes the patient's airway inaccessible to us, we will often intubate and use the block for postoperative analgesia. Try avoiding the following scenario:

- The block goes south.
- The patient gets all squirrelly.
- The surgeon is questioning your parentage, and you have to try to induce and maintain the airway while the patient is prone.
- It makes for an interesting day that had, up to that point, been very boring.

LOCAL ANESTHETICS

Tailor your locals to type and duration of surgery:

- Short cases (1 to 2 hours) where postoperative pain is minimal call for intermediate-duration anesthetics such as lidocaine or mepivacaine (1.5% to 2%). Onset is about 15 to 20 minutes and duration between 2 and 4 hours. Epinephrine (1:200,000 or 5 μg/cc) adds about 10% to 20% to your duration while allowing you to test for intravascular injection.
- For cases longer than 3 hours or where you are concerned about postoperative pain, bupivacaine and ropivacaine (0.5%) are commonly used. (Bupi is a little more potent than ropi.) Expect surgical block of about 6 hours, and postoperative analgesia of about 12 to 24 hours. These drugs take a longer time to work, usually upward of 30 minutes. Take that into account when timing your blocks.
- Estimation of surgical duration is between you and the operating physician. Remember to factor in your STC (surgeon's time coefficient, the value by which you multiply the surgeon's stated time to completion to get your actual surgical time).

LOCAL ANESTHETIC TOXICITY

Local anesthetics block impulse conduction along cell membranes that utilize sodium channels as the primary means of action potential transmission. They do that in a reversible fashion.

- That's a good thing if you are injecting the local perineurally.
- If one injects the species intravascularly in a large enough dose, action potentials are blocked in unintended places, such as the central nervous system (CNS), where the result is a seizure, or the myocardium (which also utilizes sodium channel–based action potentials), where the result can be a life-threatening arrhythmia or asystole.
- How much local is bad? It depends on where you inject. If you inject 1 cc of 2% lidocaine into the vertebral artery in a 70-kg patient, you may get a seizure in a flash, while an intravenous injection of 5 cc will probably be well tolerated.
- How bad is bad? A lido-induced seizure isn't something to strive for, but if you give propofol and manage the airway, you can often escape unscathed.

- On the other hand, bupivacaine (ropi less so) likes to check in but not check out of myocardial sodium channels.
- Always be careful of your long-acting anesthetic volumes and concentrations (never >0.5%).

Always keep airway management equipment and 20% lipid emulsion in your regional cart (Figure 30-2).
- The lipid emulsion (1.5 cc/kg bolus over 1 minute and then 0.25 cc/kg/min) has been shown to be successful as part of a regimen to treat bupivacaine-induced cardiovascular collapse.

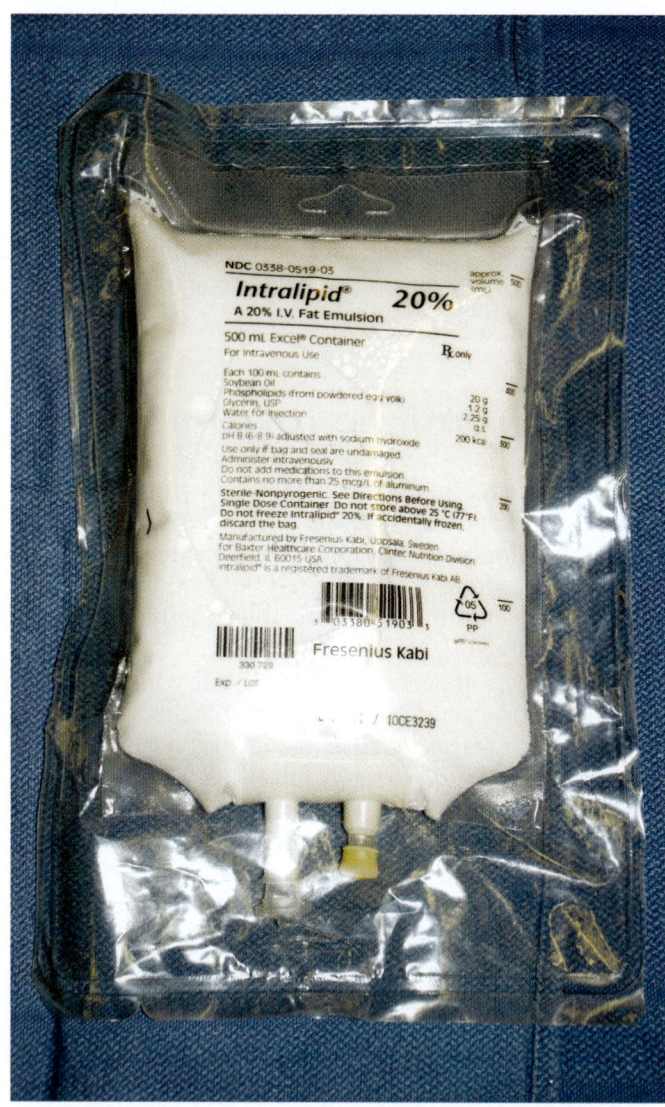

FIGURE 30-2 "20% Intralipid. Don't leave home without it."

TIME OUT

Avoid doing a block on the wrong extremity and/or the wrong patient; it's really bad form.
- Perform a TIME OUT to confirm patient identity, surgical procedure, and laterality in the presence of a nonsedated patient (or patient representative), yourself, and a preoperative or circulating nurse.
- Classic setup for a wrong-sided surgery happens when a patient comes to the OR with both arms bandaged. Make sure of site and side!

MAXIMIZING DATA: THE PROGRESSION OF BLOCK TECHNIQUE OR HOW TO AVOID THE *SPACE OF HALL*

The *Space of Hall* is the eponymous abstract anatomical area into which one injects inordinately large amounts of local anesthetic without visible clinical effect. No backboard, no net, no basket, no nuthin'.

Let's set the WAYBAC machine for the early 1960s and listen in on our attending, our resident, and our patient:
- Attending: "When you feel an electric shock go down your arm let me know."
- *{Manipulation of 22-gauge (G) 3.5-inch regional block needle in the patient's interscalene space}*
- Patient: "YYYYEEEEEEEEEEEOOOOOOOOOO WWWW!!!!!!!!!!!! *#%%$^# $&#&@*$!"
- Attending to resident: "Inject!"

An abridged but succinct summary of the paresthesia technique for nerve localization:
- Believe it or not, the technique was not associated with frequent nerve injuries when used with a short bevel needle, providing you didn't inject into resistance or get radiating pain on injection.
- It didn't have a bad success rate either. In the hands of an experienced operator, the technique works well, especially if you are in a bare-bones practice. (The other technology-free technique, the transarterial axillary block, will be discussed later.)

We need more data to know when we are close to the nerve, don't cha think? Someone took an idea from the clinical electrophysiologists to use electrical nerve stimulation.
- As you get close to a nerve with an insulated stimulating needle (the tip gives off current, the shaft of the needle does not), motor fibers fire and the end-organ muscle contracts.
- If you're in another county, no muscle stimulation.

- If you are intraneural (a bad thing), you can get contraction with infinitesimal amounts of current. It's an excellent nerve localization technique.

Sometimes, however, it seems impossible to find Mr. Nerve. Body habitus, a dearth of landmarks, and the bane of the regionalist's existence—anatomic variation—make for a challenging day. You've also got those pesky structures, the pleura and lungs, which hang like the Sword of Damocles over the supraclavicular and infraclavicular blocks.

"One ping only, Vasily."

Sean Connery to Sam Neill in *The Hunt for Red October* (1989)

I know another obscure movie reference. The "ping" as in sonar, as in ultrasound, as in "How do we find the nerve we want to block?" Ultrasound imaging is just another part of our information armamentarium (Figure 30-3).

Most anesthesiologists have been using it to find vascular structures for years.
- The pulsating thingy is the artery and the compressible thingy next to it is the vein.
- (If you're using Doppler, one is a red thingy, the other a blue thingy.)
- Close to the vessels are hyperechoic (whitish) or hypoechoic (darkish) tubular or honeycombed structures.
- With a little bit of practice, experience, and imagination, you will this as recognize as neural tissue.

ULTRASOUND PHYSICS FOR THE REGIONALIST IN 135 WORDS OR LESS

- The ultrasound generator produces sound waves at a frequency of between 2 and 15 MHz.
- Higher frequencies are great for spatial resolution but so-so for penetration.
- Lower frequencies give you depth of penetration with a trade-off on resolution.
- For brachial plexus (BP) blocks, we use frequencies between 6 and 13 MHz.
- Body tissues, depending on their composition, reflect or absorb sound waves to varying degrees. This property is known as their acoustic impedance.
- The software compiles these relative differences in absorption and transmission and generates a black and white image. It is essentially a tomogram using the ultrasound as your cutting tool.
- The image can be transverse, sagittal, or coronal, or any combination thereof.

WHICH WAY DO I POINT THIS THING?

Your needle will reflect most of the sound back and appear hyperechoic (white).
- If you go across the ultrasound beam at 90 degrees (out-of-plane), the needle will appear as a white dot (better for catheter insertion) (Figure 30-4).
- If the needle is placed along the long axis of the transducer at 0 degrees (in-plane), you will see the needle shaft in its entirety (Figure 30-5).
- Remember that the beam is ultrathin, so needle positioning under the transducer must be exact. For the one-shot techniques described here, the in-plane technique will be used.

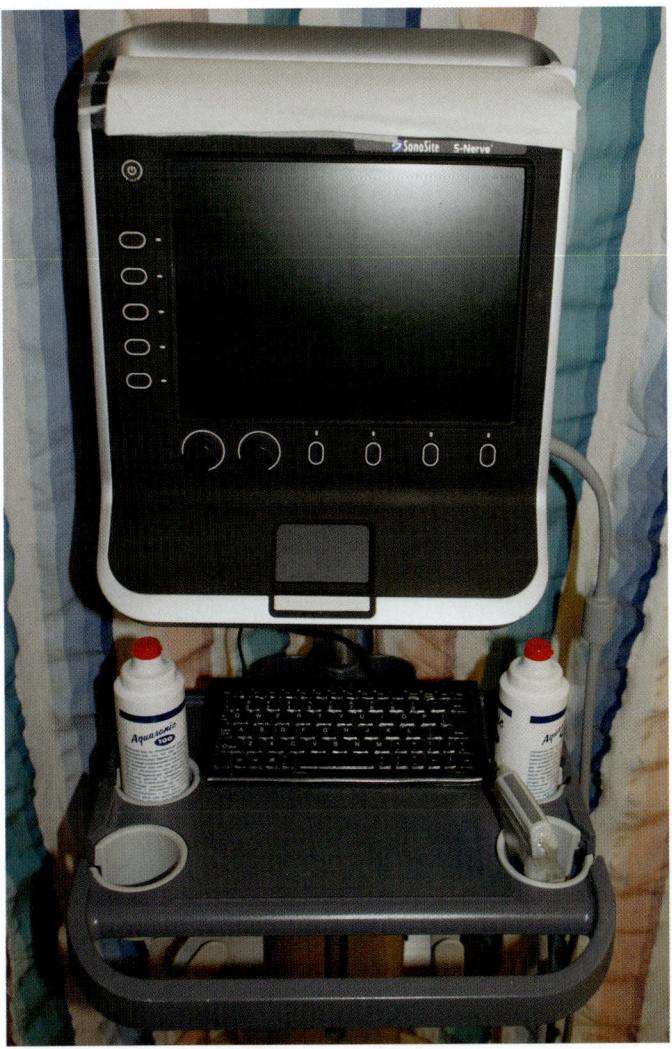

FIGURE 30-3 "Ultrasound good for patient."

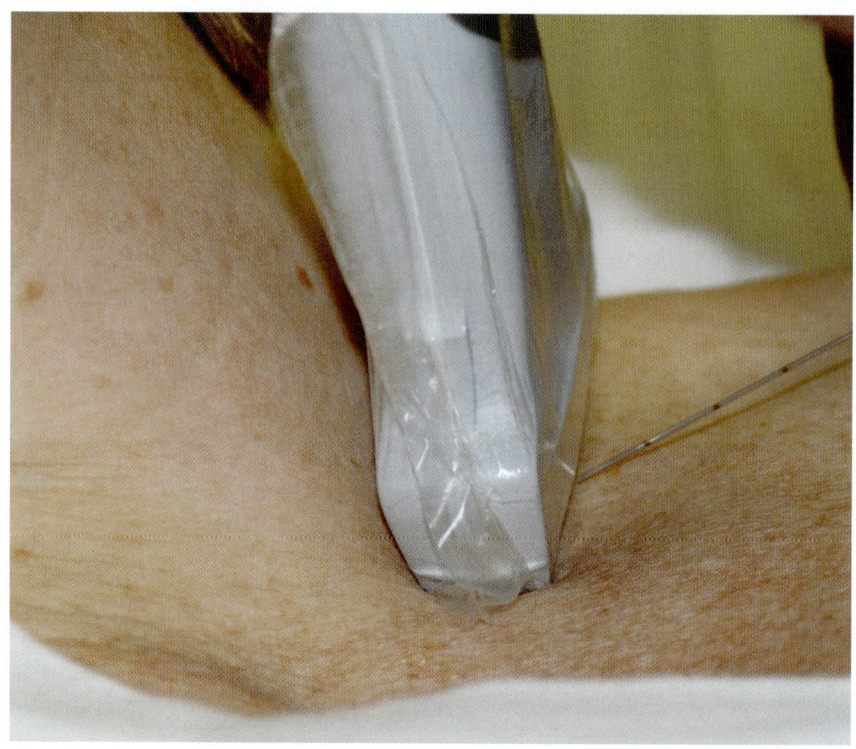

FIGURE 30-4 Out-of-plane needle/transducer orientation.

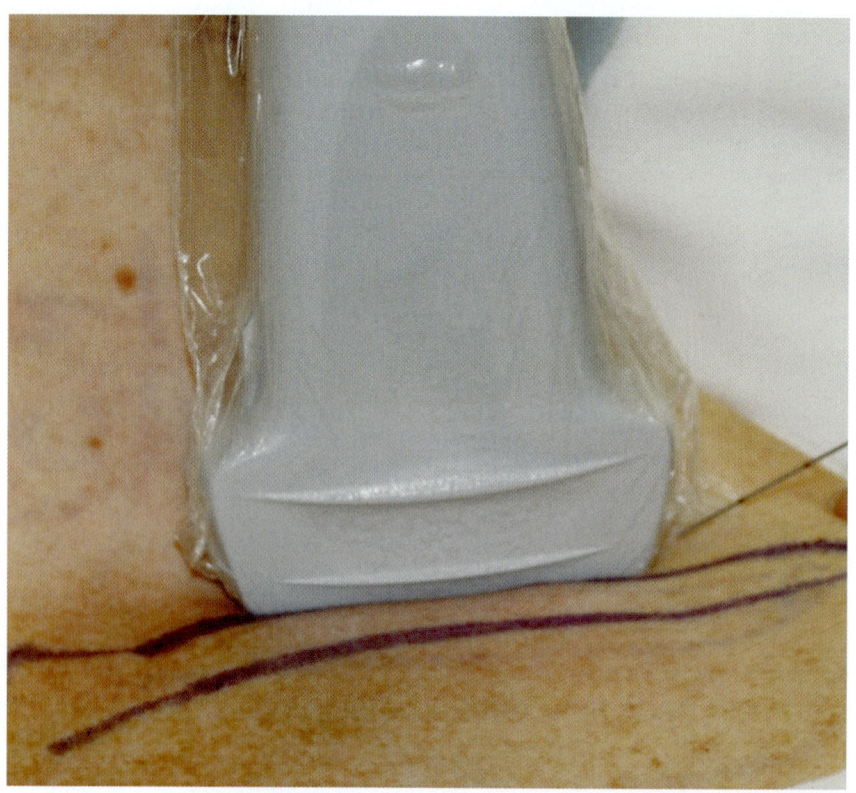

FIGURE 30-5 In-plane needle/transducer orientation.

- You'll get the big picture in no time. Remember to KNOW YOUR ANATOMY and try to visualize everything in 3-D (without the glasses). Practice needle insertion on a Blue Phantom™, a piece of raw chicken, or your in-laws.

MORE DATA, PLEASE!

What if the ultrasound image is less than stellar? Once again, it might be because of body habitus, anatomical variation, sunspots, bad hangover, etc. How about combining the use of ultrasound with a nerve stimulator? What a great idea, wish I would have thought of it.
- Actually, it's pretty intuitive to use multiple sampling techniques, and many docs have used it for a while.
- Use the ultrasound to visualize the anatomy and to "show me the needle."
- Once you're in the ballpark, assure yourself with the nerve stimulator that the structure you're about to inject is not the belly of the coracobrachialis muscle or its ilk in the *Space of Hall*.
- The more data you can obtain for needle localization, the better and safer your block technique will be.

POINTS TO AVOID GENERAL BADNESS

- Don't inject into resistance: Try using a two-syringe technique (a 10-cc syringe on a three-way stopcock with a 30- or 60-cc syringe). You get a much better feel using the smaller syringe when you inject. DON'T FORCE.
- Use epinephrine (1:200,000) in your local to help detect and prevent intravascular injection.
- Inject 5 cc of local, aspirate, inject, aspirate, inject, etc., for the same reason.
- Don't oversedate your patient. You need some feedback to avoid intraneural injection, which would be manifest as searing radicular pain. You'll learn to differentiate between the patient's sensation of pressure at the injection site and genuine discomfort.
- Maintain sterility.
- Always follow up with your patient either at home or on the ward. Paresthesias and hypoesthesias may last for a few days, and patients need to be reassured.
- Always document your procedure. Write a narrative or use a comprehensive check-off list, but just make sure you document.

SETUP

Efficient equipment setup facilitates your block procedure. In fact, it often takes longer to do the setup than the actual block. For those of us without indentured servants, it makes sense to take the time to prepare the equipment well in advance. A checklist is helpful. Some centers will have trays prepared in advance.

Every patient gets a pulse ox, blood pressure cuff, and supplemental oxygen (Figure 30-6).

Have an airway setup available (laryngoscopes, ET tubes, drugs, etc.) The picture below is worth a thousand, well, many words (Figure 30-7).
- Sterile gloves
- Sterile prep sponges
- Local anesthetic for skin infiltration in a small syringe with a 25-G needle
- Syringe setup (30- or 60-cc syringe on three-way stopcock, with a 10-cc syringe, extension tubing)
- Local anesthetic for nerve block
- Epinephrine ampule, 1 cc, 1:1000
- Nerve block needle, either 21-G, 10-cm or 22-G, 5-cm insulated nerve stimulating needle or some variant (short bevel good, long bevel not as good, can act as a blade)
- Nerve stimulator
- Electrocardiogram pad for nerve stimulator
- Ultrasound imaging device
- Transducer cover, either long sterile sleeve or Tegaderm
- Sterile ultrasound conduction gel

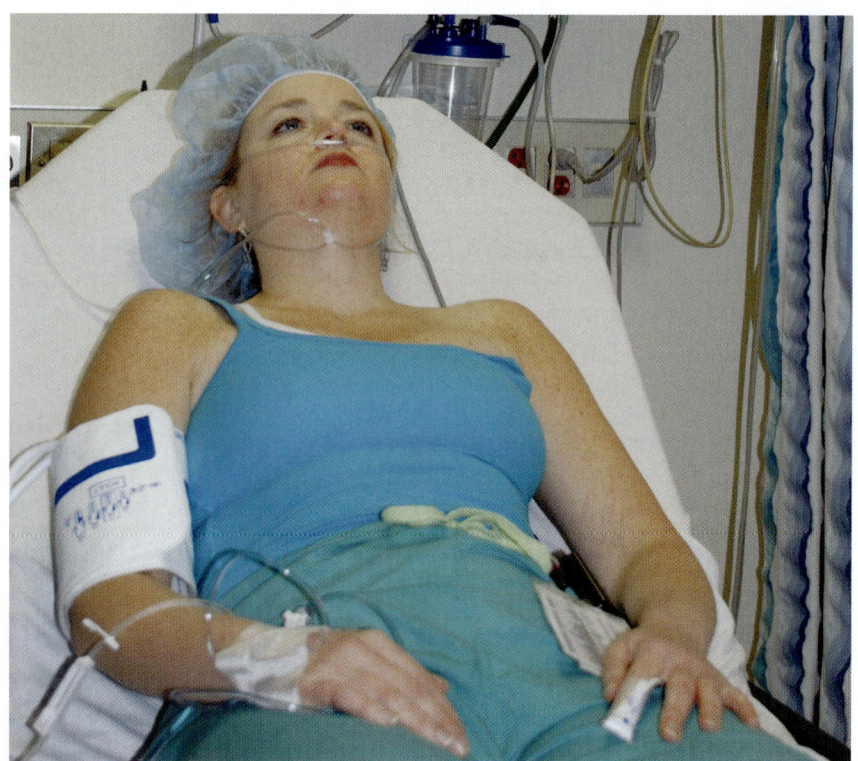

FIGURE 30-6 Everyone gets a pulse oximeter, supplemental O₂, and blood pressure cuff.

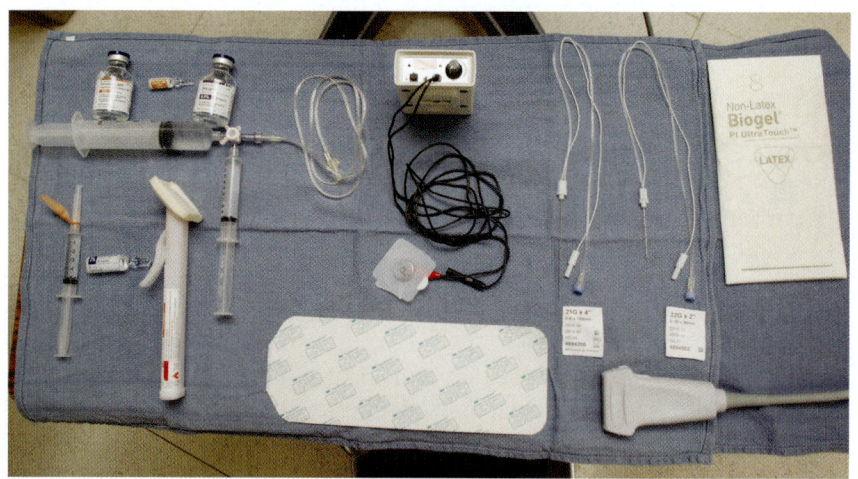

FIGURE 30-7 A standard nerve block setup. Notice the three-way stopcock. "He said three-way."

SUPRACLAVICULAR BRACHIAL PLEXUS BLOCK

This block is affectionately termed the "spinal of the arm" because it can anesthetize almost the entire upper extremity, although it can often miss the proximal shoulder and proximal axilla (C5 and T2).

Indications

- If you want to do surgery on the arm distal to the shoulder, then this block should cover it. It gives good tourniquet coverage, usually without any supplementation. I wouldn't try this one for shoulder surgery; the interscalene is a better pure shoulder block.

Cautions

- If your patient has bad chronic obstructive pulmonary disease (COPD) or significant contralateral lung pathology, you might find him or her intubated for a while as diaphragmatic paralysis may occur from phrenic nerve block. If you really

Chapter 30 REGIONAL BLOCK OF THE UPPER EXTREMITY

- need to do a regional for these patients, then the more distal infraclavicular or axillary approaches might be a better idea.
- This block has experienced a resurgence with the use of ultrasound guidance.
- Pneumothorax rates aren't astronomical with those approaches (between 0.6% and 5.0%), but they do occur more frequently than other blocks.
- Once again, infraclavicular and axillary techniques are less risky alternatives if you don't have ultrasound to keep you away from the pleura.

Technique

- Let's concentrate on the ultrasound-guided placement of this block for the reasons just mentioned.
- After sterile prep and appropriate sedation (keep the patient happy but maintain meaningful contact, as they say), apply your sterile ultrasound gel (hereafter referred to as "goop") in the supraclavicular fossa.
- The patient should be either supine or head up about 30 degrees. The arm can be at the patient's side.
- Adjust the depth of penetration on the ultrasound and slide your transducer parallel to and adjacent to the clavicle to be able to view the subclavian artery (SA), the pleura and lungs, and the brachial plexus (BP), which will appear as a honeycomb along the lateral margin of the SA (Figures 30-8 and 30-9).
- After giving a few cc of skin local, insert the block needle, (either 22-G, 5-cm or 21-G, 10-cm insulated tip attached to your syringe setup) and slowly advance it medially so as to visualize your needle on the screen.
- Your angle of approach will be between 10 and 30 degrees. Remember that the ultrasound beam is narrow.
- Try to keep your needle centered under the transducer. This is an in-plane technique so the long axes of the needle and transducer will be parallel (Figure 30-10).
- If you can't see your needle after a few centimeters of advancement, come back out and reassess your position.
- Your target will be just short of the SA, at the inferior edge of the BP (seen as the 7 o'clock position in the accompanying figure) (Figure 30-11).
- Try to distribute the injection of local anesthetic evenly throughout the plexus. The goal is to inject the local within the fascial sheath while avoiding nerve shish kebab; i.e., don't violate the epineurium.
- If you are concerned about needle position or your visualization is generally funky, use the nerve stimulator.
- Your goal is to get some sort of distal stimulation like wrist or finger contraction. Start at 1.0 mA and decrease to no less than 0.3 mA.
- The beauty of the supraclavicular block is that it is reasonably forgiving.
- There is an anatomic confluence of the nerves here so the local gets where it's supposed to pretty easily.
- Once you're happy with your needle position, inject 1 cc to confirm your location on the screen and continue 5 cc at a time, with frequent aspirations, to a total of about 30 cc. You will see your injectate expand in the perivascular area.
- Piece of cake, right?

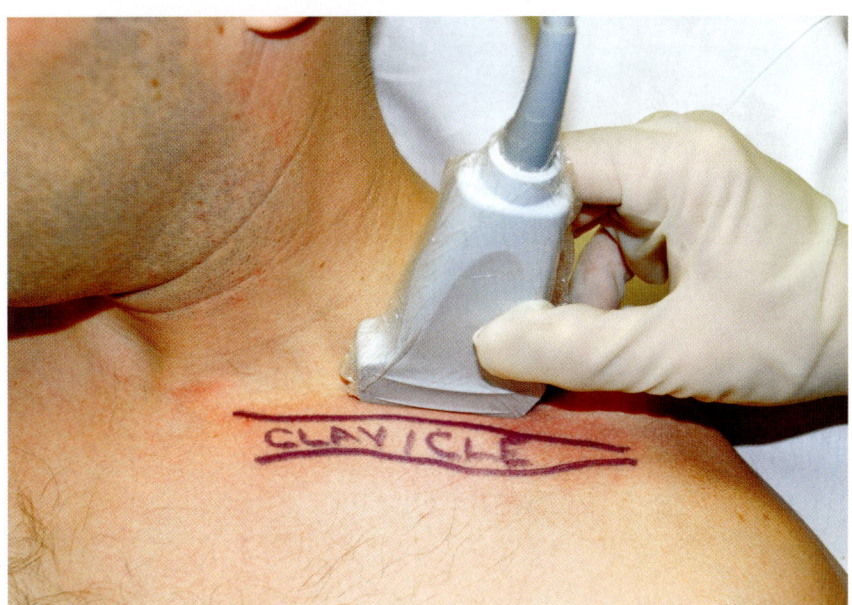

FIGURE 30-8 "Nice clavicle, why is it so red?"

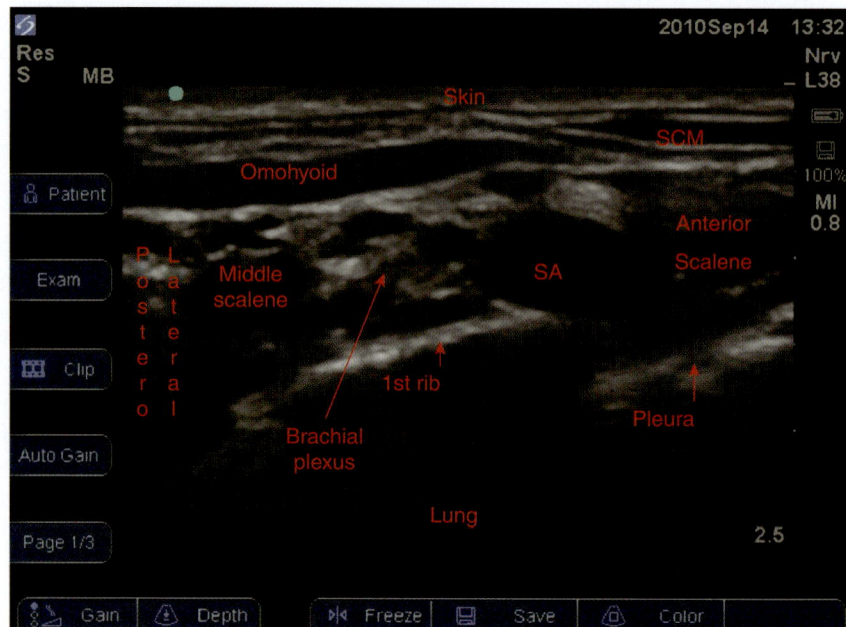

FIGURE 30-9 Ultrasound anatomy of the supraclavicular area.

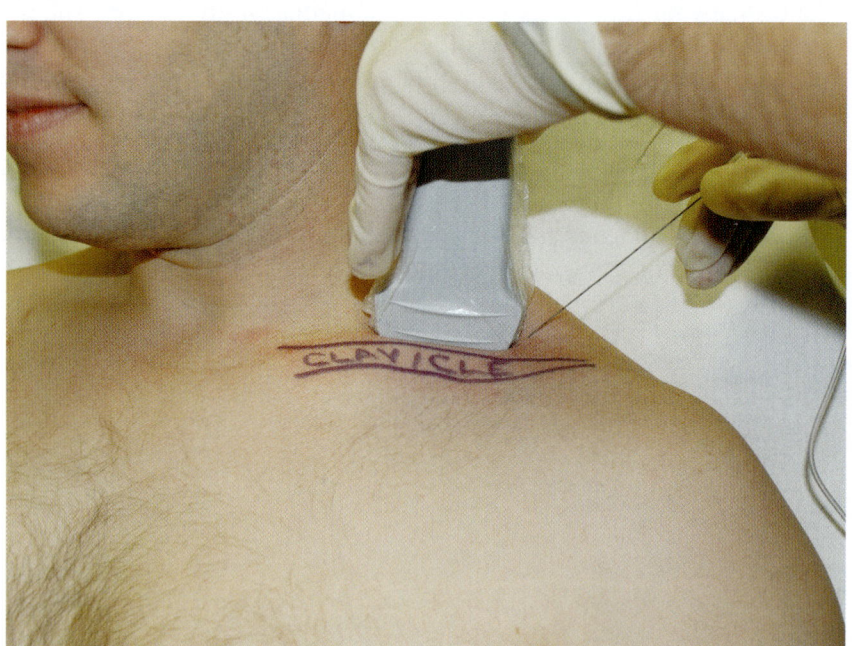

FIGURE 30-10 In-plane approach to the supraclavicular block.

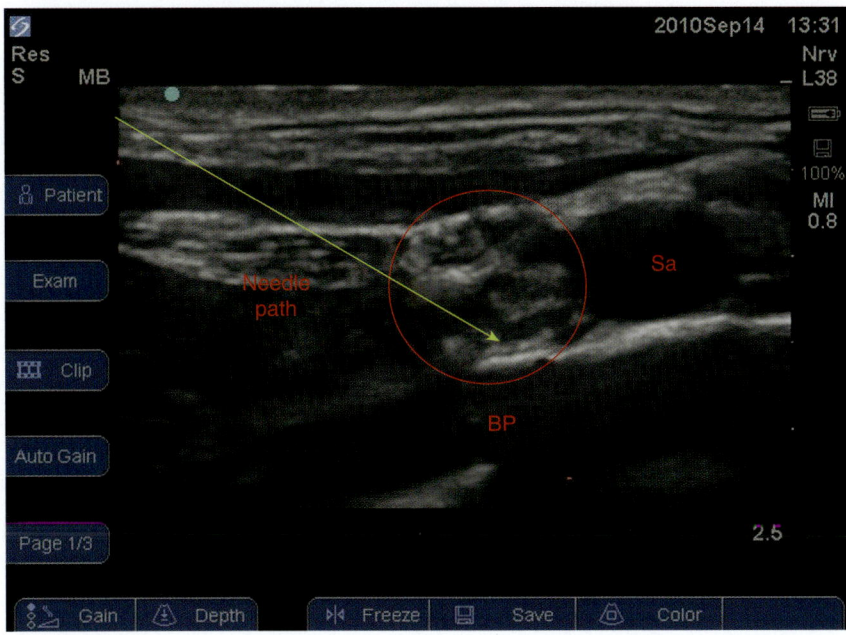

FIGURE 30-11 "Get into the fascial sheath, but not into the nerve."

Complications and Side Effects

- Infection: Be meticulous with sterile technique.
- Hematoma: Visualize the anatomy (in your head and on the screen). Visualize the needle on ultrasound. Don't use a huge needle (like an 18 G). If you do get a hematoma, hold compression.
- Nerve injury: Don't inject into resistance. Use the two-syringe technique to get a better feel. Don't inject at less than 0.3 mA. Make sure to use a short bevel needle.
- Neurotoxicity/vascular injection: Use epinephrine in your block juice. Inject in 5-cc aliquots with frequent aspirations. Use Doppler on your ultrasound if you're not sure if that dark thing you see is a vessel. Patients with pulmonary hypertension or increased filling pressures can be hypervascular with an ultrasound image that looks like a map of the Finger Lakes. Stay away from that minefield. Use a pulse oximeter to monitor for tachycardia after injection.
- Diaphragmatic paralysis: Good chance you'll get this but it's not 100% like the interscalene. Smaller injectate volumes may spare you this side effect.
- Pneumothorax: That's why we're using ultrasound. Don't advance the needle unless you can visualize the pleura and the needle. "SHOW ME THE NEEDLE!!!"

INTERSCALENE BRACHIAL PLEXUS BLOCK

The interscalene block is an upper trunk block, i.e., C5 and C6, with maybe a tinge of C7. You're going to miss the distal and medial upper extremity with this one, i.e., the middle and lower trunks.

Indications

- Shoulder surgery, surgery of the lateral arm

Cautions

- Phrenic nerve paralysis occurs about 100% of the time with this one, so the same caveats with COPDers and contralateral lung pathology apply as with the supraclavicular block.
- You can do this block by landmarks alone, but it is sometimes difficult because of the patient's body habitus. Ultrasound is a great backup. The plexus is pretty superficial in this area. Don't go drilling for oil here.

Technique

- Mark out or find your anatomy (Figure 30-12).
- The goal is to place a 22-G, 5-cm nerve-stimulating needle into the interscalene groove at or slightly below the level of the cricoid cartilage.

- Finding that magic space between the anterior and middle scalene muscles is the key, and since there are lots of sinews in the neck, it ain't always easy.
- The neck is a busy place!
- Identifying the sternocleidomastoid muscle (SCM) is easy, so do that first. Sit the patient up at about 45 degrees with the neck turned away from you, against the resistance of your hand. A taut SCM is now apparent.
- With your fingers palpating the posterior edge of the clavicular head of the SCM, have the patient sniff forcefully. The scalenes are accessory muscles of respiration, so you should feel them contract under your fingers just superior to the clavicle.
- The groove will be more prominent inferiorly. If you push hard enough and you're in the sweet spot, the patient will complain of neck and proximal arm discomfort. Mr. Spock used to do this block on a regular basis.

Whenever you do a relatively blind technique KNOW YOUR ANATOMY!!! (Figure 30-13).

- The brachial plexus passes in a latero-inferior-anterior direction from the neck to the upper extremity.
- Point your needle in a slightly medial-inferior-anterior direction. Remember the bad, evil structures that live there, namely the pleura (inferior and deep), the carotid/internal jugular (IJ) complex (way medial), and the intervertebral foramen, spinal cord, vertebral artery housing project (posterior) (Figure 30-14).
- Don't oversedate since you need patient communication, but have a heart as well.
- Give a small amount of local (about 1 cc) as a true skin wheal since the plexus may be as superficial as 1 cm. You can actually dampen or extinguish the nerve stimulation response if that injection is too deep.

This technique may be performed using paresthesia as an end point. The paresthesia you're looking for is anything in the upper extremity. It's not subtle and the patient will communicate this in no uncertain terms.

If using the nerve stimulator, begin at 1.0 mA until you get upper extremity stimulation, i.e., deltoid, biceps, triceps, or pectoralis.

- Contraction of the diaphragm means you are too anterior; trapezius, too posterior. Scapular contraction means you are too deep and stimulating the thoracodorsal nerve.
- If you trigger the cremaster muscle, you are in the wrong specialty.
- Decrease the current to about 0.4 to 0.3 mA. Greater than 0.5 mA, the needle may be too far from the nerve; less than 0.3 it may be intraneural.
- Inject when you are happy with your needle placement. Make sure the needle is immobilized against the skin and inject 40 cc of local (in the usual 5-cc aspirate-inject pattern).
- You don't want to let the needle hang loosely, as it is disconcerting to all parties involved when it pops out of the patient like the space shuttle and flies around the room.

What's that? Your patient has a body mass index (BMI) of 45 and you can't feel jack? Time for the ultrasound, I think. Prep out the neck and supraclavicular areas.

- Cover the transducer with the megacondom or Tegaderm. Squirt some sterile goop on the prepped area.
- Visualize the SA and BP as you did for the supraclavicular block.
- Slowly move the transducer in a superior direction toward the interscalene groove (or where you think it should be.)
- Keep the BP in the center of the screen. As you move upward, the hypoechoic nerves will appear between the anterior and middle scalene muscles (Figure 30-15).
- Once you get to slightly below the level of the cricoid cartilage, you're probably in good position.
- Pass the needle in an in-plane fashion under the transducer and aim for the plexus. Do this with or without a nerve stimulator, depending on your expertise or confidence level (Figure 30-16).
- Inject in the usual fashion.

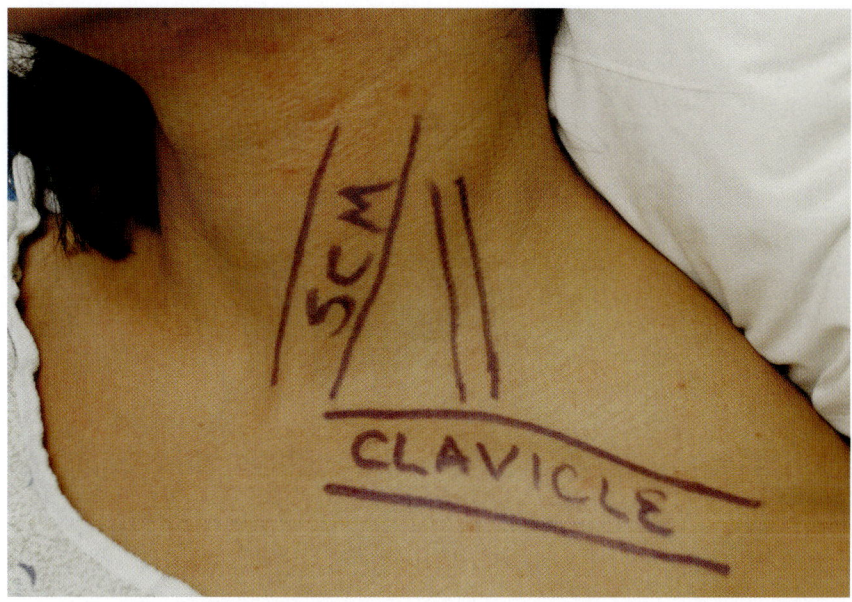

FIGURE 30-12 Landmarks for the interscalene block.

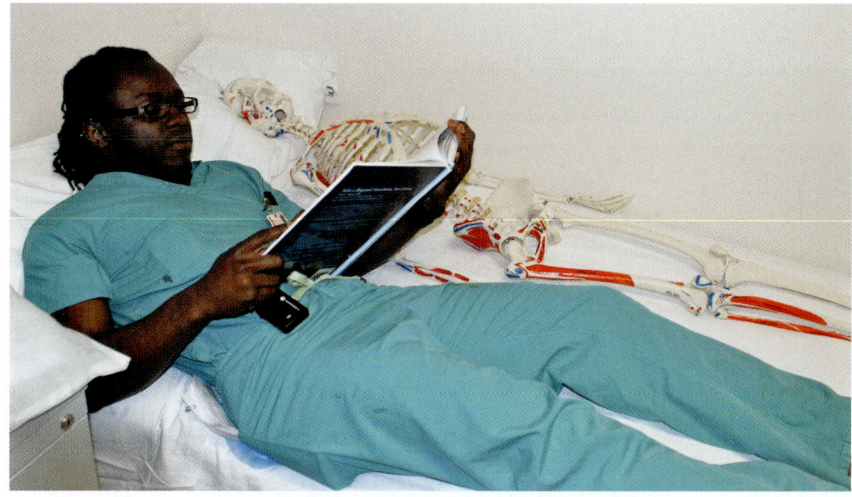

FIGURE 30-13 "I know I said, 'Know your anatomy,' but this is ridiculous...Or is it?"

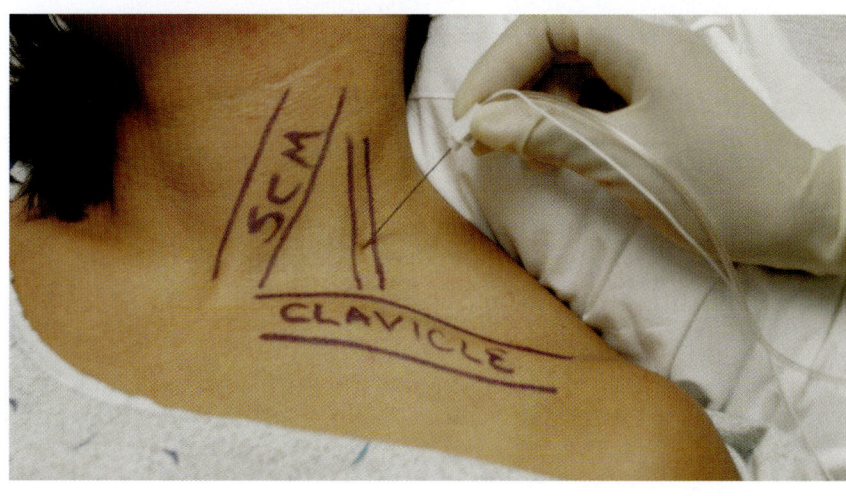

FIGURE 30-14 "Medial, inferior, anterior, and not too deep."

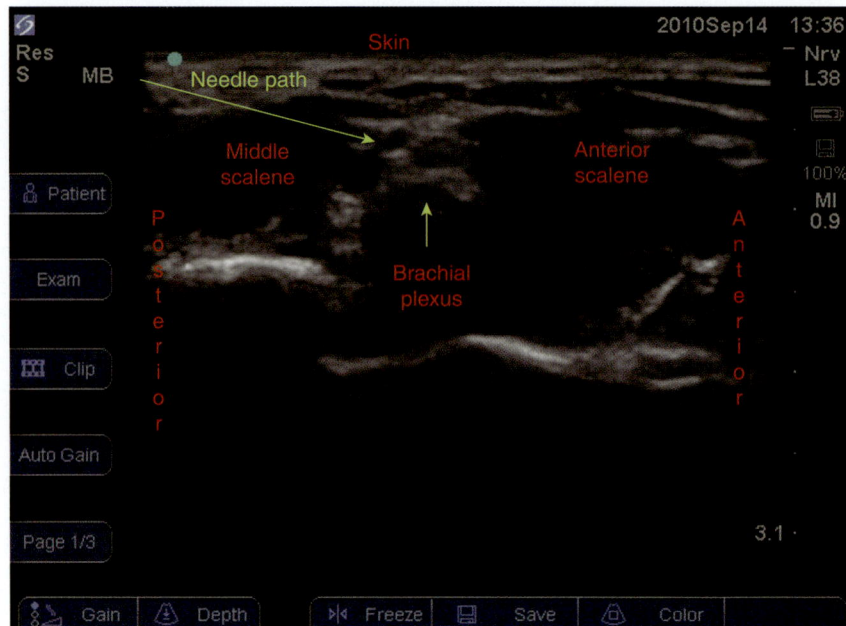

FIGURE 30-15 Ultrasound anatomy of the interscalene area.

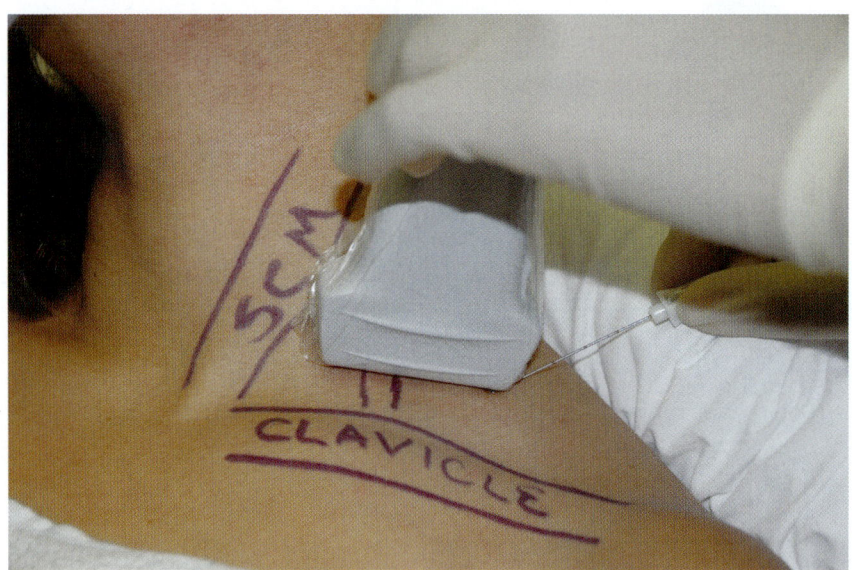

FIGURE 30-16 Ultrasound-guided interscalene approach.

Complications and Side Effects

Same as the supraclavicular with the following additions:
- Vertebral artery injection: DON'T AIM POSTERIORLY!! Always aspirate!
- Total spinal: Whoooaaa!!! If the needle is intraneural and you inject into big-time resistance, the local can backtrack up the dural sleeve and BINGO! Doesn't happen often but.... If the nerve stimulator is still getting a response at less than 0.2 mA, the needle is way deep; back the needle out and start again.
- Carotid artery puncture and injection: Know your anatomy, use Doppler if you're using ultrasound. Hold compression to avoid a hematoma.
- Hoarseness: Recurrent laryngeal nerve block sequelae.
- Diaphragmatic paralysis: If the block is working, expect that the ipsilateral hemidiaphragm isn't.

- Pneumothorax: Don't go deep. Rarely will you need to go more than 2 or 3 cm.
- Horner's syndrome: Good chance of getting some lid lag and pupillary constriction. Let the patient know about it beforehand.

INFRACLAVICULAR BRACHIAL PLEXUS BLOCK

The infraclavicular block hits the brachial plexus at the level of the cords. It's a good alternative to the supraclavicular block when you are concerned about pulmonary issues and phrenic nerve involvement. It is slightly more difficult to do than the supraclavicular and at least two targets must be injected.

Indications

- Infraclavicular blocks are typically good for surgery involving the hand, forearm, elbow, and distal arm. Don't attempt this block for shoulder surgery; the patient will be very disappointed.

Technique

- Avoid doing a paresthesia technique as the needle goes pretty deep into potentially precarious territory.
- Let's concentrate on the nerve stimulator and ultrasound-guided approaches.
- If you wish to use a pure stimulator technique, place the patient supine. The arm may be kept at the patient's side or abducted to 90 degrees.
- After prepping the infraclavicular area, draw a line from the sternoclavicular joint to the coracoid process (CP) and mark the midpoint of the line (Figure 30-17).
- At that point, or slightly caudal to it, infiltrate a little skin local. The angle of the needle (21-G, 10-cm nerve stimulator needle) should be about 45 degrees and aiming toward the axilla (Figure 30-18).
- An alternate insertion point may be 2 cm medial and 2 cm caudal to the coracoid process (CP). The needle angle here will be closer to 90 degrees.
- In either case, know your anatomy, and avoid the thorax.
- Begin stimulating at 1.0 mA and look for twitches in the wrist or hand until you reach 0.4 to 0.3 mA (no lower).
- Volume of local should be 35 to 40 cc, injected in the usual, customary and reasonable manner.

For the ultrasound-guided approach, patient positioning is the same.

- After prepping, place the probe medial to the CP just caudal and nearly perpendicular to the clavicle (Figure 30-19).
- Find the big pulsing thing. This is the axillary artery.
- The three hyperechoic (or white) dots at the 2 o'clock, 6 o'clock, and 10 o'clock positions are the cords and money-shot targets.
- Superior is the lateral cord, inferior is the medial cord, and posterior, well, take a guess: posterior cord (Figure 30-20).
- Take the 21-G, 10-cm stimulating needle and insert it in-plane with your probe.
- Aim for the cords and fire, injecting each cord individually, if possible. Use the nerve stimulator to confirm depending on your experience, confidence, or hubris.

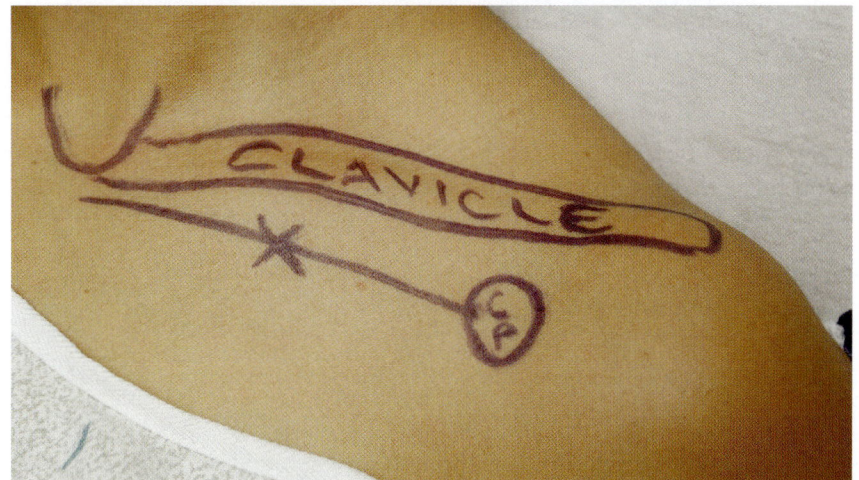

FIGURE 30-17 Infraclavicular landmarks. CP, coracoid process.

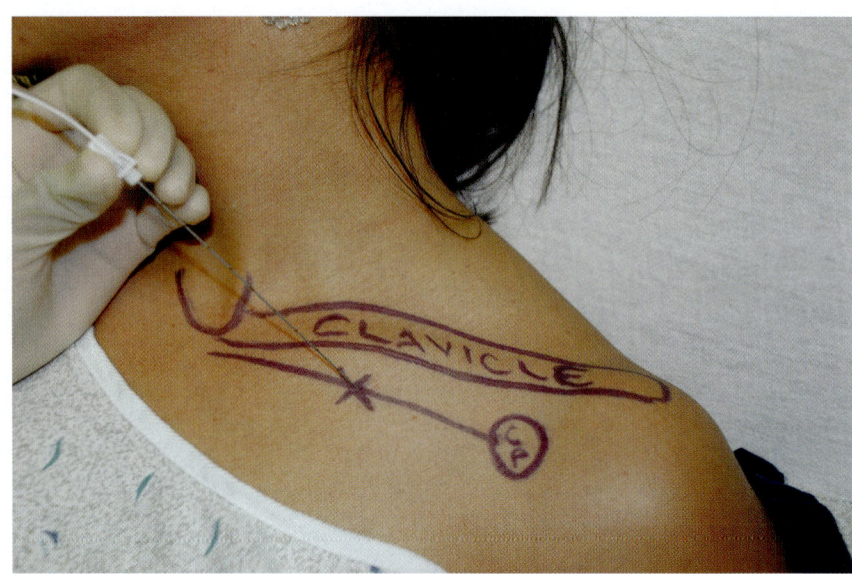

FIGURE 30-18 "Don't forget, the lung is down there, somewhere."

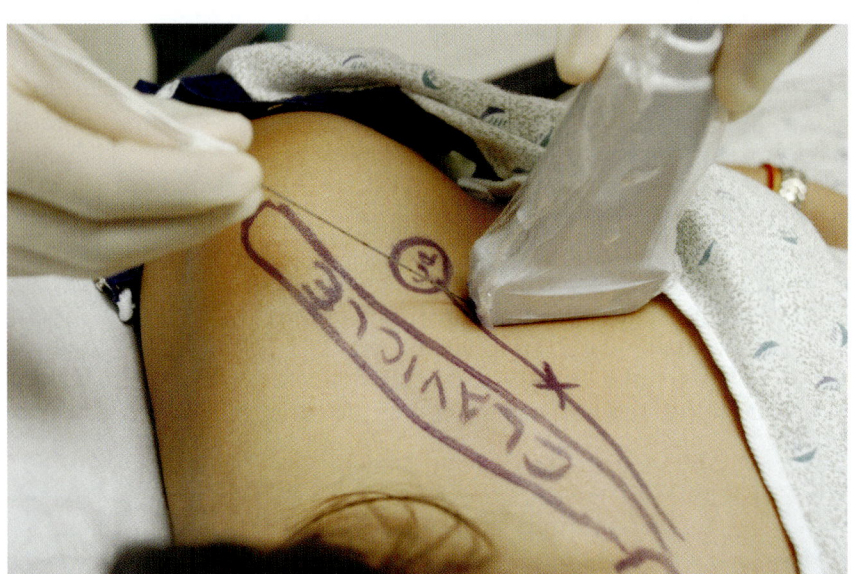

FIGURE 30-19 Infraclavicular ultrasound-guided approach.

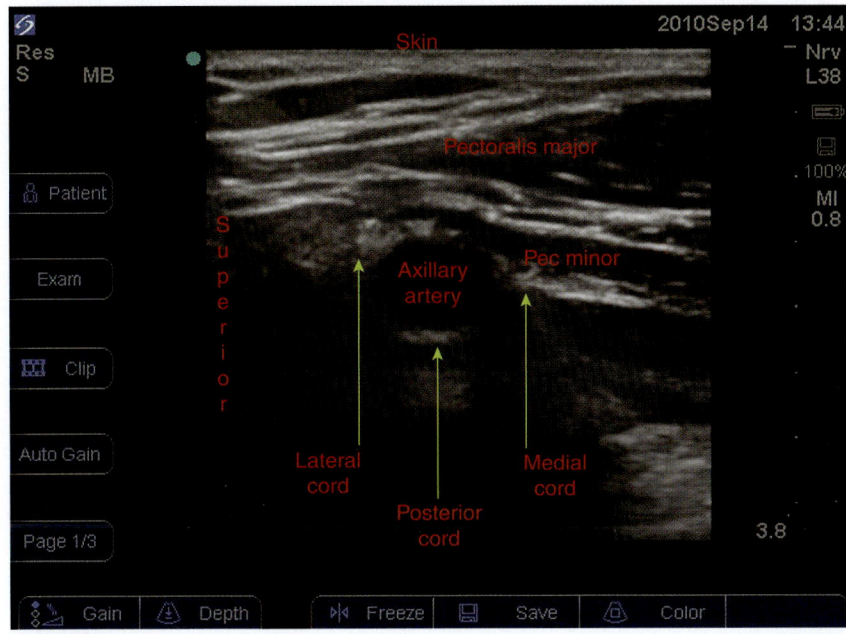

FIGURE 30-20 Infraclavicular ultrasound anatomy.

Complications and Side Effects

- Infection, nerve injury, and vascular injury: You're practically a pro; you know what to do to avoid these.
- Hematoma: Definitely stay away from coagulopaths.
- Pneumothorax, hemothorax, and chylothorax (with a left-sided block): Don't go blindly poking around. Know where your needle is relative to the lungs and pleura.

AXILLARY BRACHIAL PLEXUS BLOCK

This is one of the oldest nerve blocks; it has a reasonably good success rate and can be performed with a minimum of technology.

Indications

- The axillary is good for any procedure below the elbow. The musculocutaneous nerve is often missed with it though (lateral forearm), so that nerve needs to have supplemental blockade (see below).

Technique

The block may be performed using one of the four techniques: transarterial, paresthesia, nerve stimulator, or ultrasound guided. The one commonality for all four is patient positioning. The patient should be supine with the hand behind the head, arm abducted to 90 degrees (Figure 30-21).

For the transarterial approach, feel for the pulse of the axillary artery. Try to find it as high in the armpit as possible.

- Sterilely prep, then grab your 22-G, 5-cm needle and try to get an axillary A-line. (Of course, you infiltrate the skin first.)
- Aim proximally (Figure 30-22).
- Once you aspirate blood, keep aspirating until the perfusionist can go on pump.
- Seriously, once you have aspirated blood, advance the needle a tiny bit until no blood is aspirated (i.e., the far side of the artery) and inject 20 cc of local.
- Withdraw back through the artery until no blood is aspirated and inject another 20 cc. (Aspirate, inject, etc.)
- Old timers were wont to say, "No blood, no block."

Let's say that during the transarterial attempt, you get a paresthesia down the patient's arm.

- Many anesthesiologists will take that as a positive end point and inject 20 cc of local.
- Remember that you need to get to the other side of the artery to increase the probability of successful anesthesia, due to the anatomical relationship between the cords and the vessels. Otherwise, *blockus partialis* may result.

If you'd like to utilize the nerve stimulator modification, perform your transarterial technique with the stimulator set at 1.0 mA.

- Perform as above.
- If muscle twitch is obtained before aspirating blood, take that as an end point and inject local at 0.4 to 0.3 mA.
- Was that the radial, ulnar, or median nerve you just injected?

- You need to get the radial (20 cc) AND either the median or ulnar nerves (the other 20 cc) injected since they are on opposite sides of the artery, often separated by levees and reinforced concrete.
- Otherwise, *surgeon unhappiness magnus* precedes induction and intubation.

If you'd like to use ultrasound, place the transducer in the sterilely prepped axilla perpendicular to the long axis of the humerus (Figure 30-23).

Look for the axillary artery (Figure 30-24).

At this point, you should be able to identify three nerves surrounding the artery: the median (lateral), the ulnar (medial), and the radial (deep to the artery).
- After giving skin local, insert the stimulating needle (22 G, 5 cm) in plane with the ultrasound probe.
- Inject each of the three nerves with about one third of the 40 cc of local.
- Augment your confidence by using the nerve stimulator if you wish.

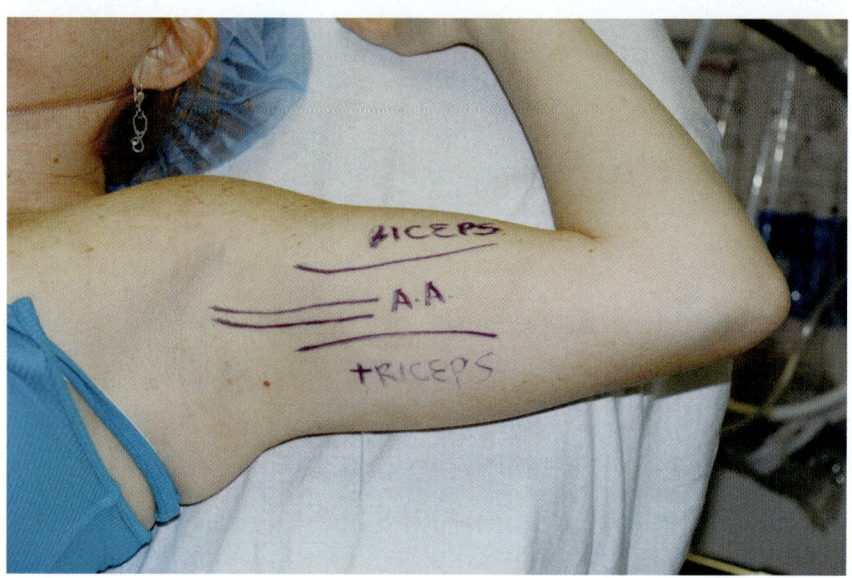

FIGURE 30-21 "Frankie say relax."

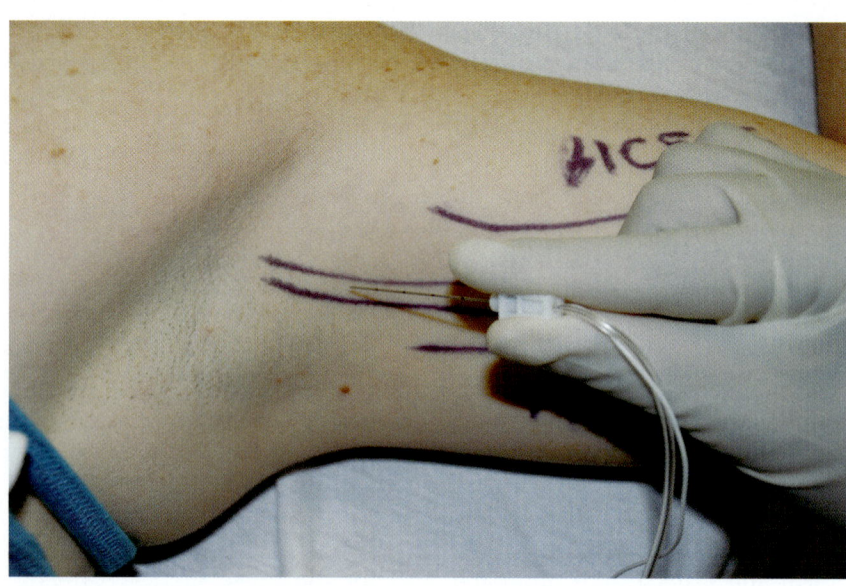

FIGURE 30-22 "Aim high in the axilla and proximally."

Chapter 30 REGIONAL BLOCK OF THE UPPER EXTREMITY

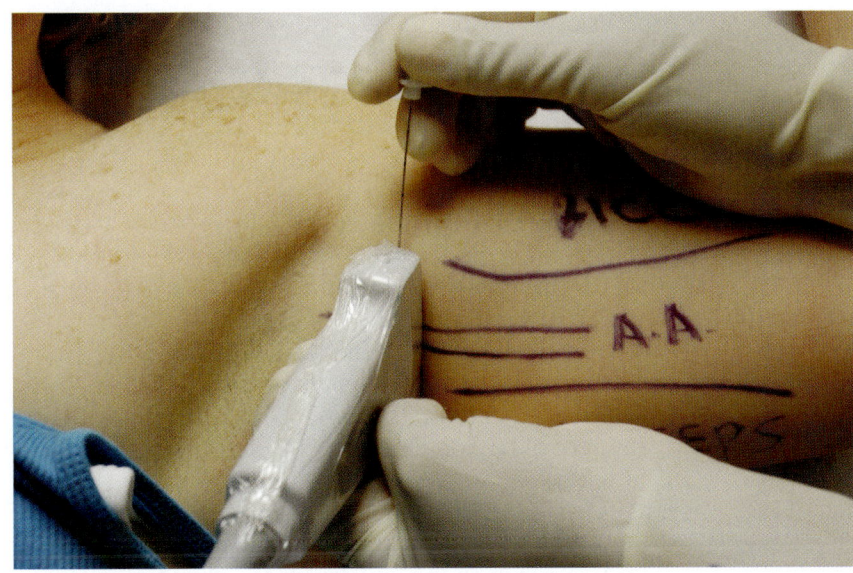

FIGURE 30-23 Ultrasound-guided axillary approach.

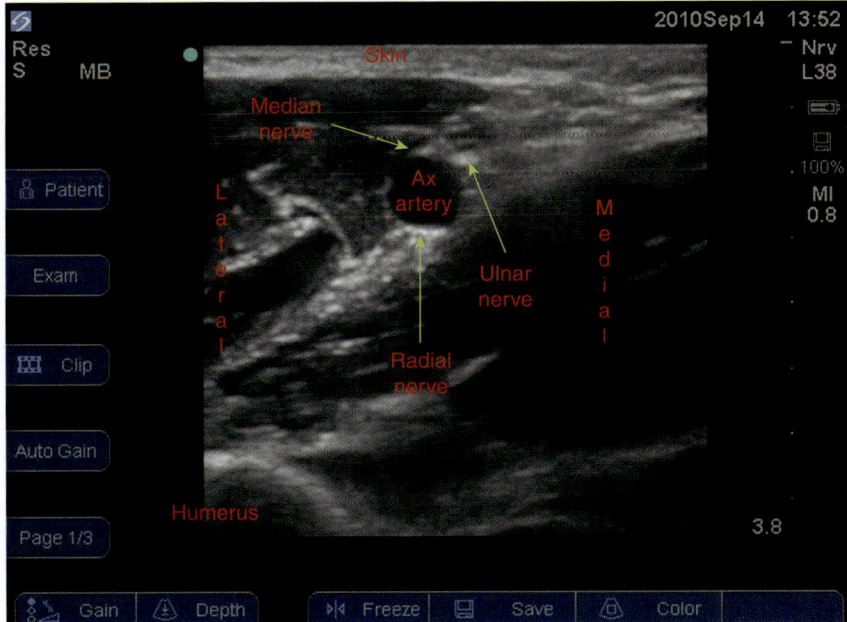

FIGURE 30-24 Axillary ultrasound anatomy.

Complications and Side Effects

- Infection, nerve injury as usual
- Vascular puncture or injection: Use the tried and true aspirate inject mantra along with epi containing local and a pulse oximeter monitor.
- Hematoma: Sure you can compress the axillary hematoma, but avoid the situation by using a small needle and staying away from coagulopaths.
- I know of one person who, yes, dropped a lung doing a transarterial axillary block. There is truly nothing we are incapable of screwing up.

MUSCULOCUTANEOUS BLOCK

The musculocutaneous nerve is a terminal branch of the lateral cord and the most proximal to emerge from the brachial plexus. It innervates the biceps and brachialis muscles and ends as the lateral antebrachial cutaneous nerve of the forearm, which is sensory for the lateral aspect of the forearm and wrist.

Indications

- It is often used to supplement an axillary block to complete the anesthesia for the lateral forearm and wrist.

Technique

- Once you have completed the axillary block, redirect the needle superiorly and proximally.
- Pierce through the coracobrachialis, and perform a field block.
- The nerve may also be blocked at the elbow.
- At this level the nerve runs superficially at the interepicondylar line. Identify the insertion of the biceps tendon and mark the site 1 to 2 cm laterally.
- Perform a field block at this point.
- On ultrasound, the musculocutaneous nerve is seen superior to the axillary artery, near the humerus, between the biceps and coracobrachialis (Figure 30-25).
- Injection volumes are between 5 and 10 cc.

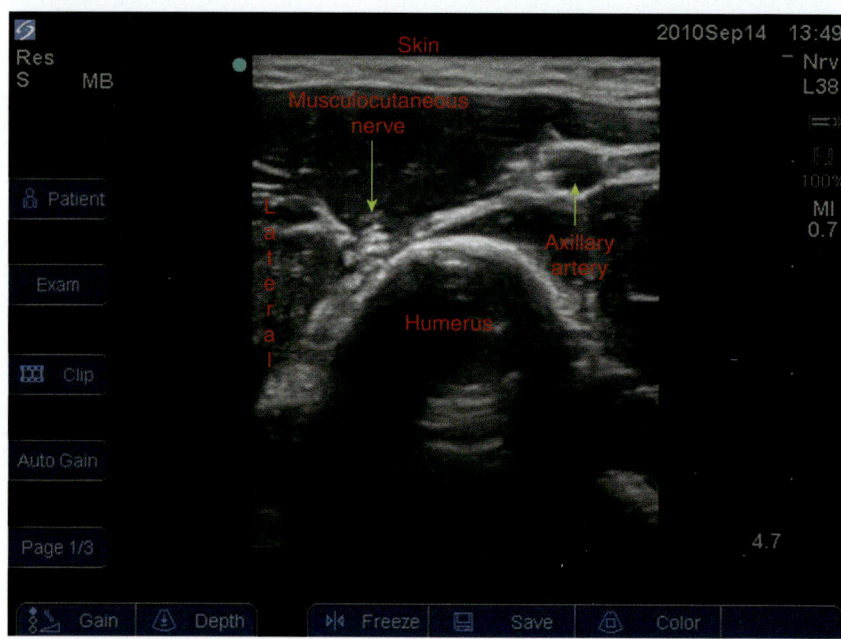

FIGURE 30-25 Musculocutaneous nerve on axillary ultrasound.

SUGGESTED READING

Brown D. *Atlas of regional anesthesia*, 3rd ed. Chapter 4 (37–44), Chapter 5 (45–54), Chapter 6 (55–62), Chapter 7 (63–70). Philadelphia: Elsevier Saunders, 2006.
Great anatomic drawings to help you KNOW YOUR ANATOMY.

Hahn M, McQuillan P, Sheplock G. Regional anesthesia: an atlas of anatomy and technique. Chapter 12 (95–100), Chapter 13 (101–106), Chapter 14 (107–112). St. Louis, Mosby, 1996.
Good source that is heavy on cadaveric pictures and imaging.

Kapral S, Krafft P, Eibenberger K, et al. Ultrasound-guided supraclavicular approach for regional anesthesia of the brachial plexus. *Anesth Analg* 1994;78:507–513.

New York School of Regional Anesthesia. www.nysora.com.
At your fingertips info anywhere you can receive a wi-fi signal.

CHAPTER 31

LOWER EXTREMITY NERVE BLOCKS

ANDRES MISSAIR
CARLOS DE LA HOZ
RALF E. GEBHARD

Once in Africa I lost the corkscrew and we were forced to live off food and water for weeks.
Ernest Hemingway

NERVE BLOCK SELECTION

The innervations of the dermatomes, myotomes, and osteotomes do not always coincide. The surgical site must always be identified along with the surgical approach in order to ensure that all relevant nerves are anesthetized as the incision passes from skin to bone (Table 31-1).

Joints present special situations, whereby multiple nerves are often involved from disparate sites of origin:
- Hip joint:
  - Femoral nerve anteriorly
  - Sciatic nerve posteriorly
  - Obturator nerve (anterior branch) medially
  - Spinal roots of T11-12: skin overlying the hip
- Knee joint:
  - Femoral nerve anteriorly
  - Sciatic nerve posteriorly
  - Obturator nerve (posterior branch) medially
- Ankle joint:
  - Sciatic nerve
  - Saphenous nerve (branch of femoral nerve) medially

ULTRASOUND VS. NERVE STIMULATION

Whereas nerve stimulation provides functional anatomical information regarding what structures the needle is in contact with, ultrasound provides visual guidance of those structures that surround the needle and its intended path. Neither modality has demonstrated (individually) greater patient safety in recent randomized-control studies.[1,2] According to some investigations, ultrasound guidance results in faster block onset and smaller total local anesthetic dose when used by experienced regionalists.[3] We advocate the combined use whenever possible, since each modality yields complementary information.

SINGLE SHOT VS. CONTINUOUS NERVE BLOCK INFUSION

The indications for placement of a lower extremity nerve block catheter are as follows:
- Joint surgery
- Patients who will undergo early physical therapy postoperatively
- Limb amputations
- Sympathectomy for limb salvage following an ischemic insult
- Serial wound débridements

The approaches utilized for catheter placement are the same as for any single-shot nerve block. Special care must be taken, however, to ensure perfect sterility of the catheter site during placement. Some techniques are more amenable to catheter placement: lumbar plexus, femoral, sciatic (Raj and subgluteal), and the lateral popliteal are all recommended for this application.

The infusate for most continuous nerve blocks are:
- Ropivacaine 0.1% to 0.2%
- Bupivacaine 0.125% to 0.25%

TABLE 31-1 Block Selection for Lower Extremity Surgery

Nerve Block	Surgical Indication	Special Considerations
Lumbar plexus	Hip, knee, saphenous vein stripping, patella tendon repair, ACL repair, above the knee amputations	Achieves anesthesia of the lateral femoral cutaneous and obturator nerves; for amputations, combine with sciatic nerve block
Femoral	Knee, saphenous vein stripping, patella tendon repair, ACL repair, above the knee amputations	Will spare the obturator and lateral femoral cutaneous nerve territories; for amputations combine with sciatic nerve block
Sciatic: posterior/parasacral	Posterior knee, tibia and fibula, Achilles tendon repair, foot and ankle procedures, below the knee amputations	Saphenous nerve block required for medial lower leg/ankle; achieves anesthesia of the posterior cutaneous nerve of the thigh also
Sciatic: Raj technique/subgluteal	Posterior knee, tibia and fibula, Achilles tendon repair, foot and ankle procedures, below the knee amputations	Saphenous nerve block required for medial lower leg/ankle; spares the posterior cutaneous nerve of the thigh; well-suited for catheter placement
Sciatic: popliteal	Tibia and fibula, Achilles tendon repair, foot and ankle procedures, below the knee amputations	Saphenous nerve block required for medial lower leg/ankle; tibial nerve stimulation yields better block
Ankle	Procedures of the foot and toes	Can be very painful due to numerous injections required

ACL, anterior cruciate ligament.

We prefer to use ropivacaine for our continuous nerve blocks due to its reduced cardiotoxicity and motor block. As such, ropivacaine provides a safe analgesic that will not interfere with the motor exercises required during a patient's physical therapy (Table 31-2).

TABLE 31-2 Continuous Peripheral Nerve Block (CPNB) Infusion Rates for Lower Extremity Blocks

Nerve Block	Infusate Rate (mL/h)
Lumbar plexus	10–14
Femoral	8–10
Sciatic	10–12

NERVE BLOCK PATIENT SETUP

Prior to starting a nerve block, it is paramount to ensure patient safety by placing monitors and having resuscitation drugs/equipment easily available:
- American Society of Anesthesiologists (ASA) monitors
- Oxygen via face mask
- Suction
- Intubation equipment
- Ambu bag and mask
- Crash cart with defibrillator
- Resuscitation drugs:
  - Advanced cardiac life support (ACLS) medications
  - Phenylephrine
  - Ephedrine
  - Intralipid 20%
- Sedatives
  - Propofol
  - Midazolam

LUMBAR PLEXUS BLOCK

Indications

Hip, anterior thigh, knee

Landmarks

1. Posterior spinous processes
2. Iliac crest
3. L3-L5 interspaces (Figure 31-1)

Technique

- Needle insertion is 4 to 5 cm lateral to the line connecting the posterior processes of L3, L4, and L5, along Tuffier's line running tangential to the iliac crest at the level of L4.
- The needle should be perpendicular to the patient's back.
- Objective: contact L4 transverse process, and walk off caudally onto the lumbar plexus approximately 2 cm deeper (Figure 31-2).

WARNING!! Anticoagulation: Follow American Society of Regional Anesthesia (ASRA) guidelines for neuraxial blockade in the anticoagulated patient.[4]

Complications

- Epidural or intrathecal spread
- Kidney, ureter, or bowel puncture
- Retroperitoneal hematoma

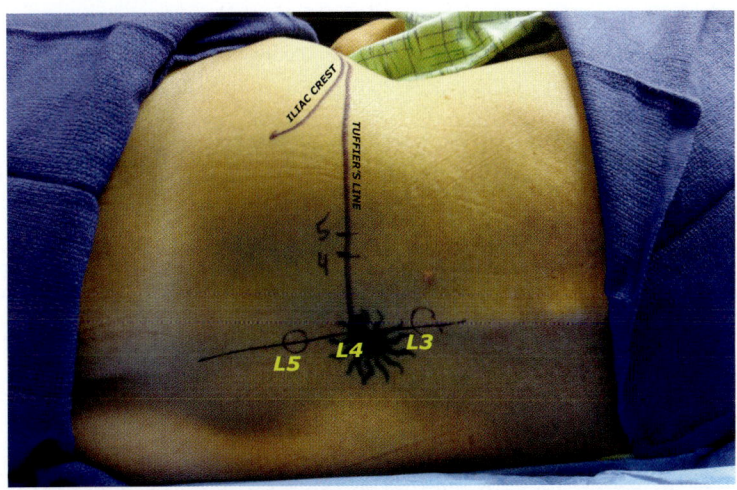

FIGURE 31-1 Lumbar plexus block landmarks.

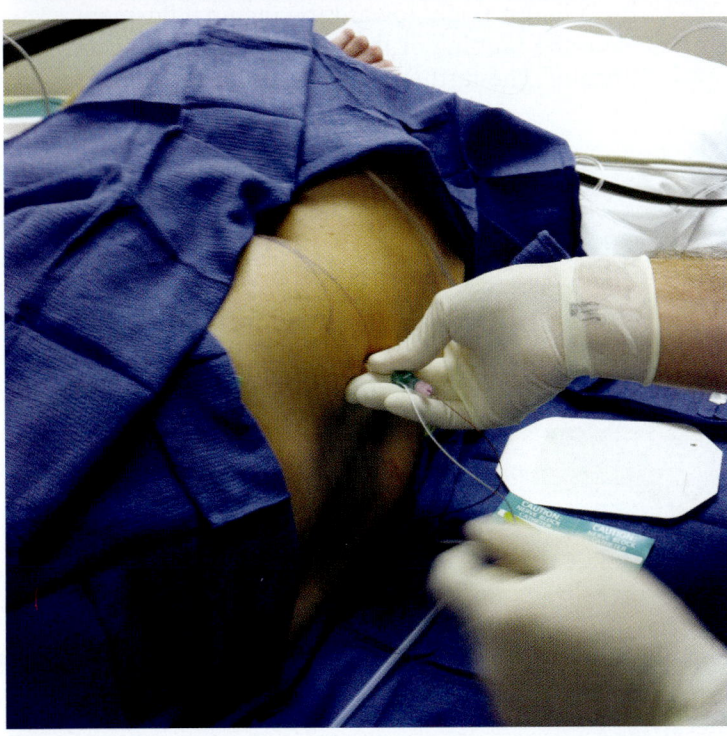

FIGURE 31-2 Lumbar plexus block needle insertion and orientation.

TABLE 31-3 Lumbar Plexus Block Twitch Responses[5]

Motor Response	Anatomical Explanation	Solution
Erector spinae muscle twitch	Isolated stimulation of paraspinal muscles due to shallow needle placement	Advance needle SLOWLY
Hamstring muscle twitch	Sciatic nerve stimulation resulting from caudal needle placement	Redirect needle cranially after withdrawal; confirm lumbar interspace.
Flexion of thigh	Stimulation of psoas muscle due to deep needle placement	Withdraw completely; reinsert following landmarks and technique
Bone contact without twitches	Needle in contact with transverse process	Return to skin and redirect caudally
Needle inserted >10 cm, no twitches and no bone encountered	Needle missed transverse process and lumbar plexus roots	Withdraw completely; reinsert following landmarks and technique

Clinical Pearl

The lumbar plexus block carries a higher risk of local anesthetic toxicity due to its deep location and vicinity to vascularized muscle. We therefore avoid high concentrations of local anesthetics with this block. The sympathectomy resulting from this block and the possible epidural spread can cause significant hypotension (Table 31-3).

FEMORAL BLOCK

Indications

Thigh, knee, medial leg/ankle

Landmarks

1. Femoral artery
2. Inguinal crease

NOTE: If you fail to palpate the femoral artery, draw a line from the anterior superior iliac spine to the pubic tubercle. This line represents the inguinal ligament. The femoral artery should lie beneath the medial third (Figure 31-3).

Technique

- Enter the skin parallel to the artery and 45 degrees to the anterior thigh, toward the inguinal ligament.
- Note the fanning of the femoral nerve as it courses distally. The farther away from the inguinal

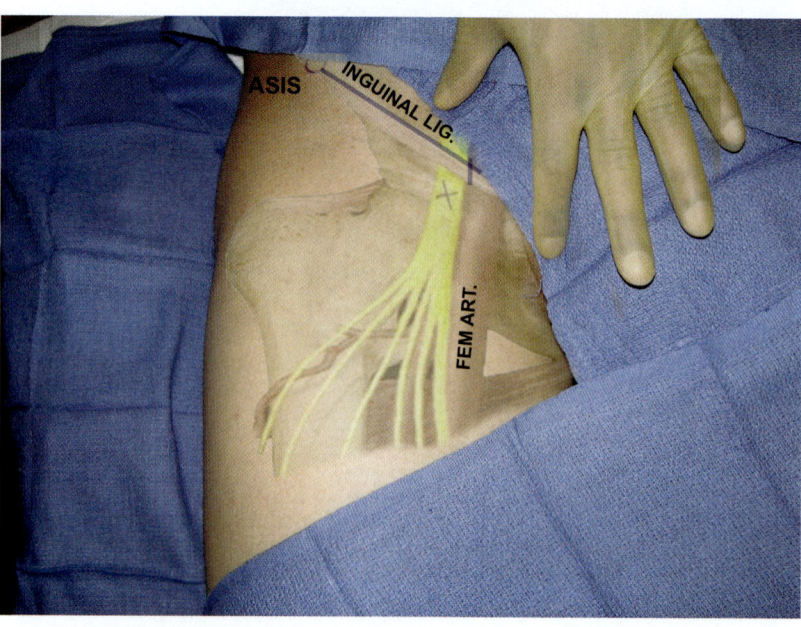

FIGURE 31-3 Femoral nerve block landmarks.

Chapter 31 LOWER EXTREMITY NERVE BLOCKS

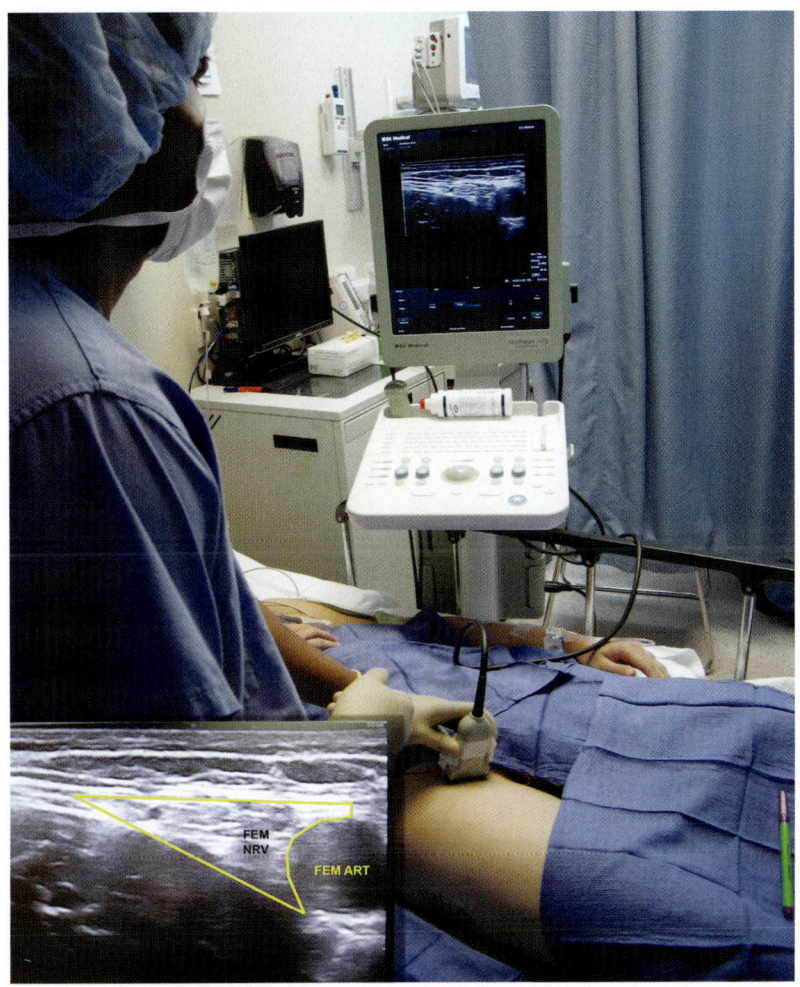

FIGURE 31-4 Ultrasound-guided femoral nerve block.

ligament, the greater the chance of an incomplete block.
- Based on a recent study, the speed of injection during a femoral block should not exceed 10 mL/min in order to avoid generating pressures that can produce nerve barotrauma (Table 31-4).[6]
- Objective: The goal is to stimulate the patella (rectus femoris). Redirect the needle medially if the vastus lateralis is encountered, or laterally if the vastus medialis is stimulated.

Ultrasound

See Figure 31-4.

Complications

- Hematoma due to venous or arterial puncture

TABLE 31-4 Femoral Block Twitch Responses[5]

Motor Response	Anatomical Explanation	Solution
No response	Disconnected nerve stimulator	Check grounding wire, connection to needle, and battery charge
Local twitch	Stimulation of the iliopsoas or pectineus muscle	Needle redirection following reassessment of femoral artery pulsation
Sartorius muscle twitch	Stimulation of the sartorius muscle	Redirect laterally and advance 1–3 mm
Vascular puncture	Needle placement into femoral artery or vein	Hold pressure for 3 minutes then withdraw and redirect laterally

POPLITEAL BLOCK

Indications
Tibia, ankle, foot

Posterior Approach
Landmarks
1. Popliteal fossa crease
2. Biceps femoris tendon
3. Semitendinosus tendon

Technique
- Insert needle 7 cm above the crease, along the bisecting line. The needle should be advanced in a slightly craniolateral direction. Correct placement will not elicit any local muscle twitch until the sciatic nerve is encountered.
- Objective: stimulation of the common peroneal (foot dorsiflexion) or tibial nerves (plantar flexion) (Figure 31-5).

Lateral Approach
Landmarks
1. Vastus lateralis
2. Biceps femoris

Technique
- Insert needle between the vastus lateralis and biceps femoris, 10 cm proximal to the lateral epicondyle. Correct placement will elicit a biceps femoris twitch just before encountering the sciatic nerve.
- Objective: stimulation of the common peroneal (foot dorsiflexion) or tibial nerves (plantar flexion) (Figure 31-6).

NOTE: The common peroneal nerve lies just lateral to the tibial nerve. Therefore, the needle should stimulate plantar dorsiflexion and foot eversion first, at more shallow needle depths. Deeper and more posterior insertion will yield tibial nerve responses.

Ultrasound
See Figure 31-7.

Complications
- Hematoma due to popliteal artery or vein puncture (Table 31-5)

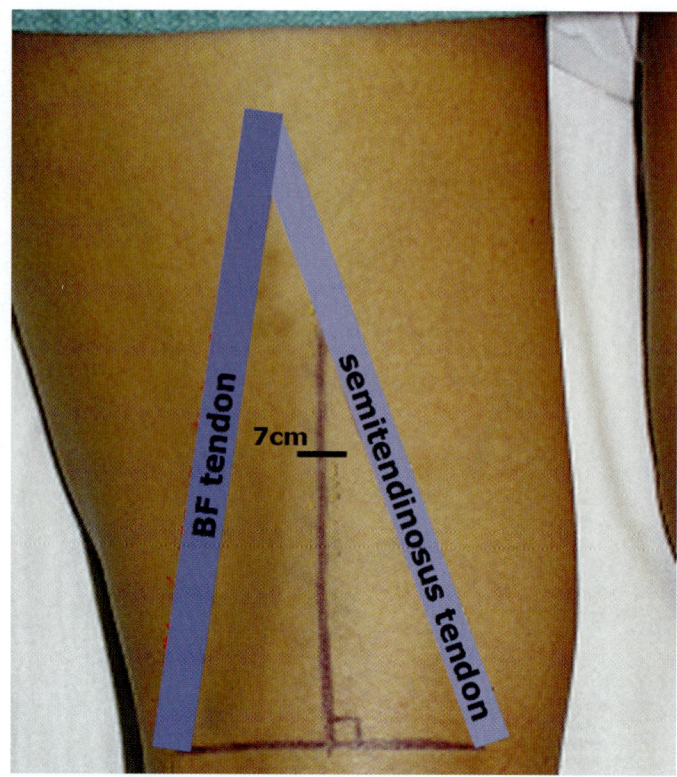

FIGURE 31-5 Posterior popliteal nerve block landmarks.

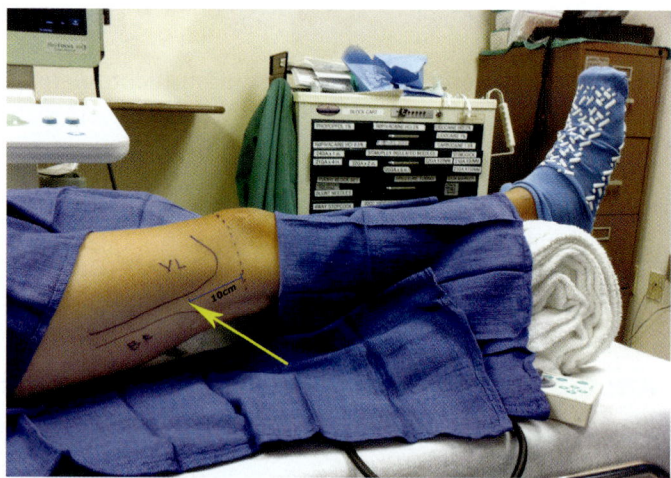

FIGURE 31-6 Lateral popliteal nerve block landmarks. VL = Vastus lateralis; BF = Biceps femoris.

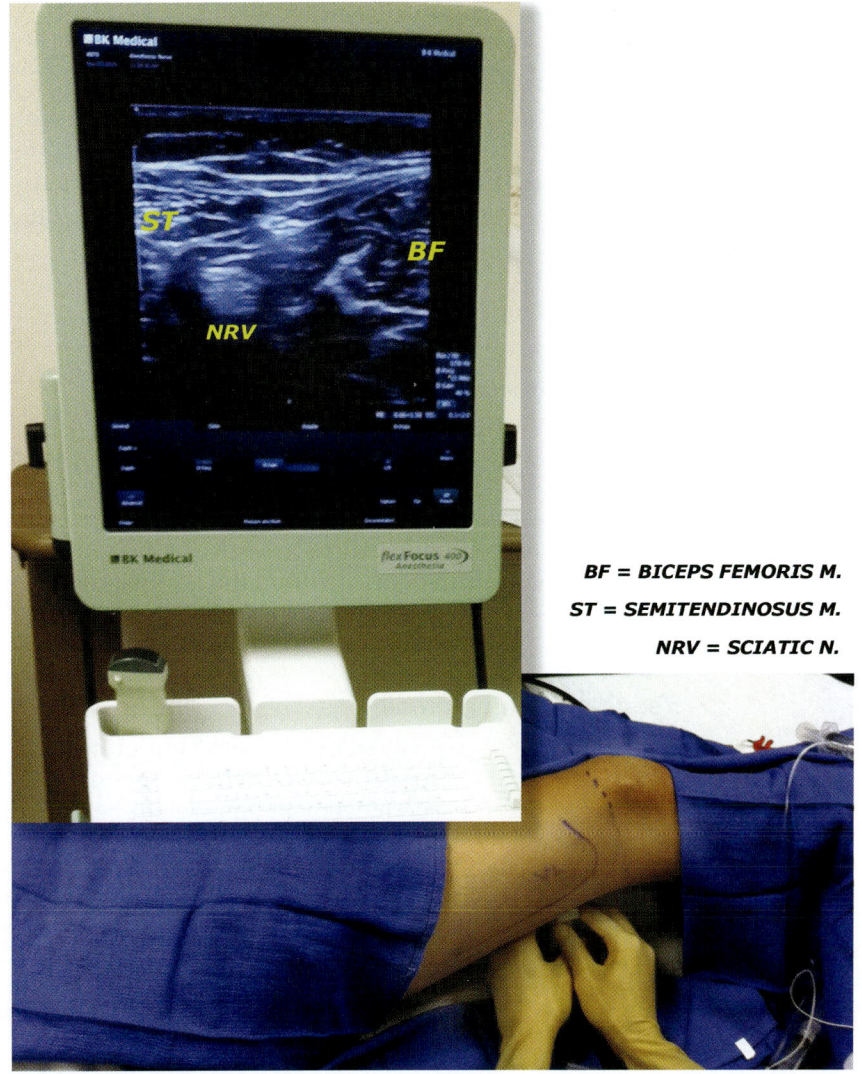

BF = BICEPS FEMORIS M.
ST = SEMITENDINOSUS M.
NRV = SCIATIC N.

FIGURE 31-7 Ultrasound-guided lateral popliteal nerve block.

TABLE 31-5 Lateral Popliteal Block Twitch Responses[5]

Motor Response	Anatomical Explanation	Solution
Biceps femoris muscle twitch	Direct stimulation of biceps femoris muscle	Advance needle 1–2 cm past the muscle
Isolated gastrocnemius muscle twitch	Stimulation of nerve branches outside the sciatic nerve	Advance needle until twitches in the foot/toes are observed
Vascular puncture	Needle advanced into popliteal artery or vein, which lies between the femur and sciatic nerve	Withdraw and redirect needle posteriorly

SCIATIC BLOCKS

Indications

Knee, tibia, ankle, foot (Figure 31-8)

Posterior Classic Approach of Labat

Landmarks

1. Posterior superior iliac spine (PSIS)
2. Greater trochanter (GT)
3. Sacral hiatus (SH)

Technique

- A line is drawn from the GT to the PSIS. At the bisection, a perpendicular line is drawn caudally 4 to 5 cm. The needle can be inserted at this point. Another technique involves inserting the needle at the intersection of the latter with the line drawn from the GT to the SH.
- Objective: common peroneal or tibial nerve twitch (plantar flexion and dorsiflexion of the foot), hamstring twitch is also acceptable (Figure 31-9).

Complication

- Neuropraxia secondary to microvascular hematomas irritating the sciatic nerve

Clinical Pearls

According to studies, the sciatic nerve demonstrates greater block success when higher local anesthetic (LA) concentrations are used versus larger volumes.[7]

Animal studies have demonstrated that epinephrine can reduce blood flow to the sciatic nerve by 40%, and should thus be avoided.[5,8]

Plantar flexion is more reliable than dorsiflexion during the Labat approach to the sciatic nerve block.[9]

Parasacral Approach (Technique of Mansour)

Landmarks

1. Ischial tuberosity (IT)
2. Posterior superior iliac spine (PSIS)

Technique

- Needle insertion is 6 cm caudally, along the PSIS-IT line, perpendicular to all planes.
- Advance the needle in a slight cephalad orientation for 5 to 7 cm until bony contact at the superior aspect of the greater sciatic notch (GSN). Then, redirect caudally to pass into the GSN and advance no further than 2 cm until stimulation of the sciatic nerve is achieved.
- Objective: common peroneal or tibial nerve twitch (plantar flexion and dorsiflexion of the foot), hamstring twitch is also acceptable.
- Caution: needle advancement beyond 2 cm following bony contact increases the risk of complications (Figure 31-10).

Caution: Potential risk for sigmoid colon, iliac vessel, and ureter perforation if needle is passed deep to the sacral plexus. This block is also associated with urinary retention due to the proximity of the pelvic splanchnic nerves, perineal, and pudendal nerves.

Subgluteal and Raj Approach

Landmarks

1. Greater trochanter (GT)
2. Ischial tuberosity (IT)

Technique (Raj)

- Needle insertion occurs at the midpoint of the GT-IT line, perpendicular to the posterior thigh. Needle passage should lie within the sciatic groove between the biceps femoris and semitendinosus muscles.

Technique (Subgluteal)

- Needle insertion 5 cm below the midpoint of the GT-IT line; good for catheter placement due to decreased soft tissue movement and weight-bearing on the catheter site.
- Objective: for either approach, we seek a nerve twitch response from the common peroneal or tibial nerves. A hamstring response should NOT be accepted as these fibers will lie outside the sciatic nerve at this point of needle insertion (Figures 31-11 and 31-12).

Anterior Approach

Landmarks

1. Anterior superior iliac spine (ASIS)
2. Pubic symphysis (PS)
3. Greater trochanter (GT) of femur

Technique

- A line is drawn from the ASIS to the PT. At the midpoint, the perpendicular bisecting line is drawn caudally.
- A third line originating at the GT is drawn parallel to the ASIS-PT line, toward the intersection with the perpendicular bisector of the ASIS-PT line. This point corresponds to the needle insertion site.
- The needle is advanced perpendicular to the skin, toward the lesser trochanter (LT).
- Objective: contact with the LT followed by caudal redirection to contact the sciatic nerve 1 to 2 cm deep (Table 31-6) (Figure 31-13).

TABLE 31-6 Sciatic Nerve Block Twitch Responses[5]

Motor Response	Anatomical Explanation	Solution
Biceps femoris muscle twitch	Direct stimulation of biceps femoris muscle	Advance needle and redirect slightly medially
Hamstring twitch during Labat or Mansour approaches	Sciatic nerve stimulation	Accept and inject
Hamstring twitch during Raj or subgluteal approaches	Stimulation of muscular branches of the sciatic nerve, which lie outside the nerve sciatic nerve sheath	Disregard and continue advancing until foot/toes twitches are obtained
Gluteal twitch	Direct stimulation of the muscle due to shallow needle placement	Advance needle
Foot or toes twitches	Sciatic nerve stimulation	Accept and inject

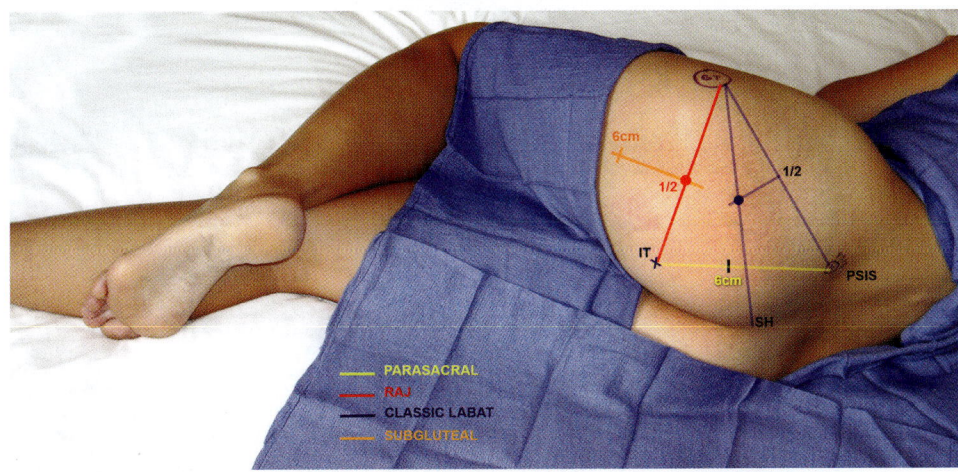

FIGURE 31-8 Overview of landmarks for sciatic nerve block techniques.

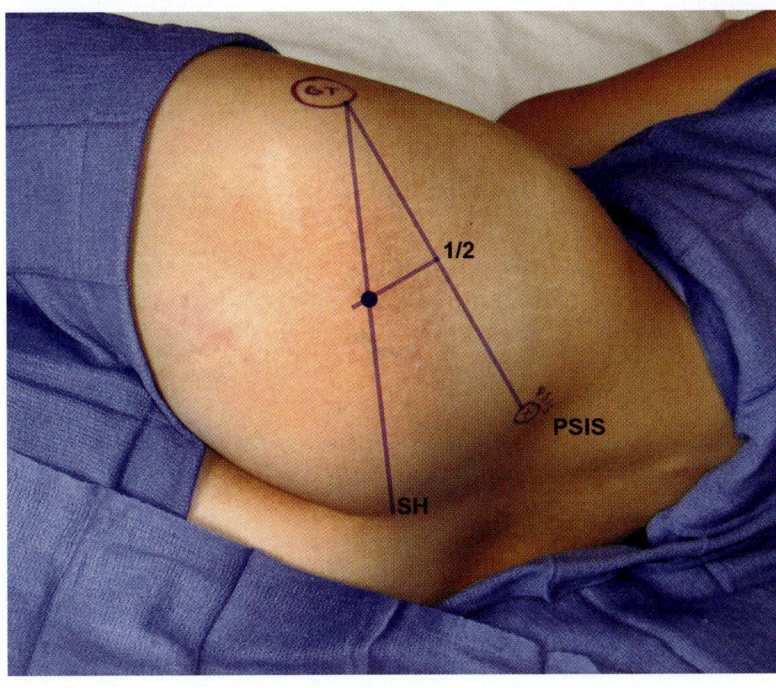

FIGURE 31-9 Sciatic nerve block: classic posterior approach of Labat landmarks.

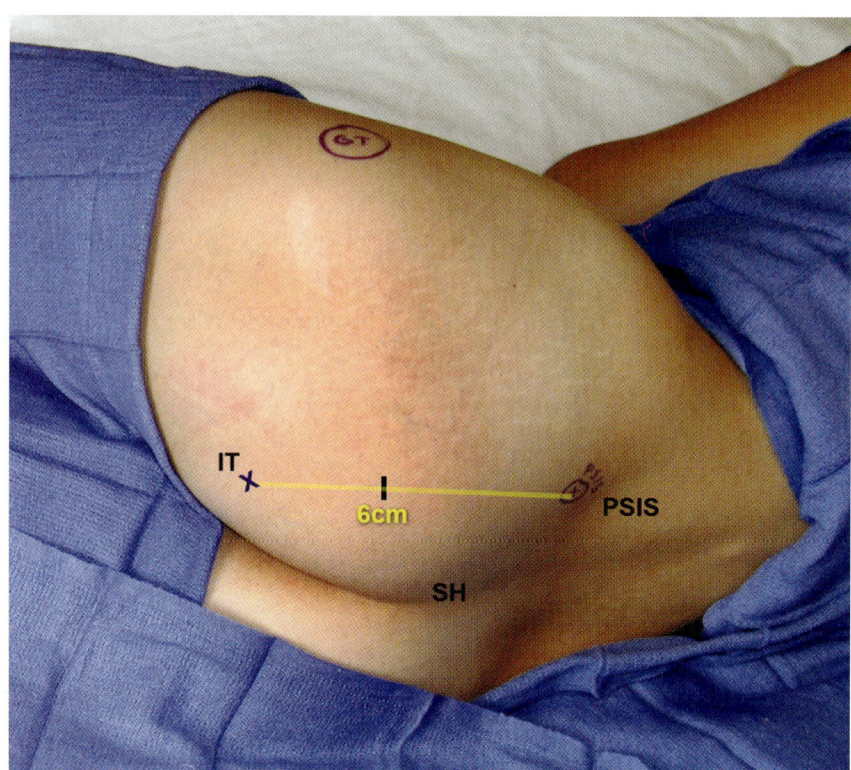

FIGURE 31-10 Sciatic nerve block: parasacral approach landmarks.

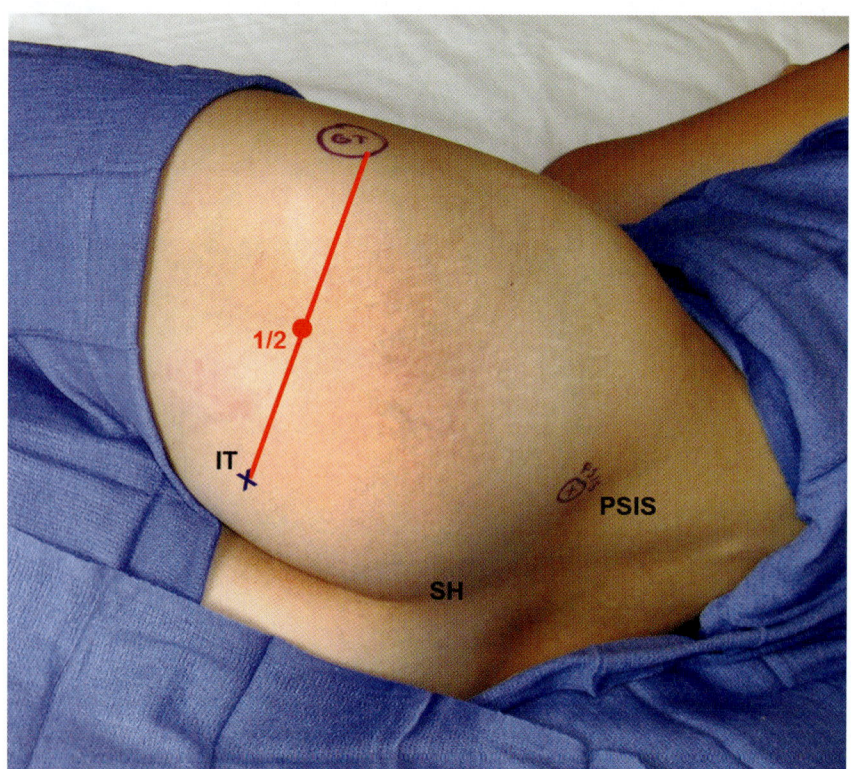

FIGURE 31-11 Sciatic nerve block: Raj approach landmarks.

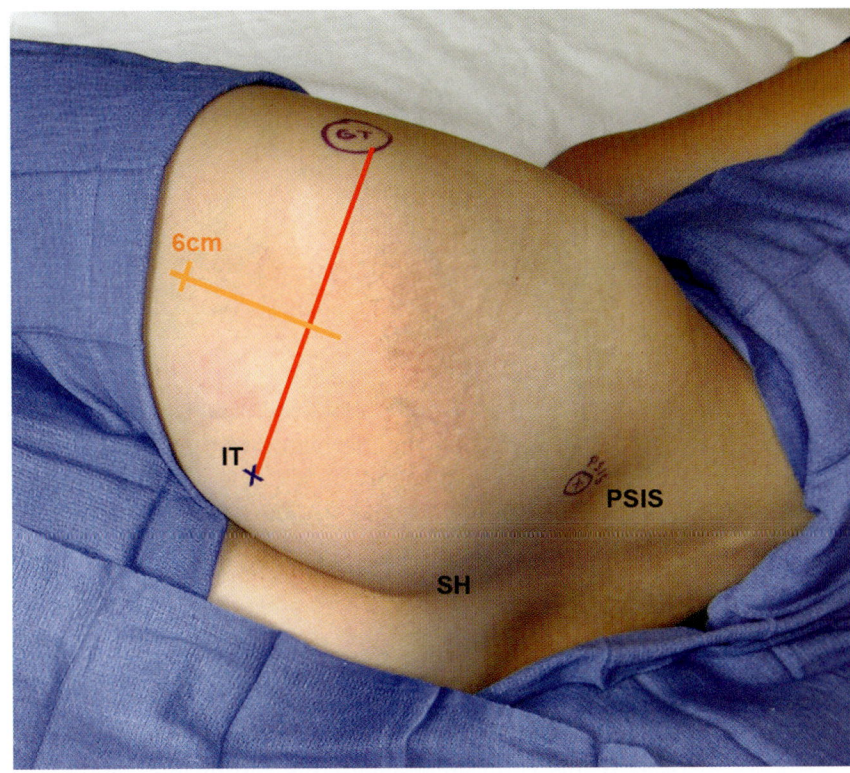

FIGURE 31-12 Sciatic nerve block: subgluteal approach landmarks.

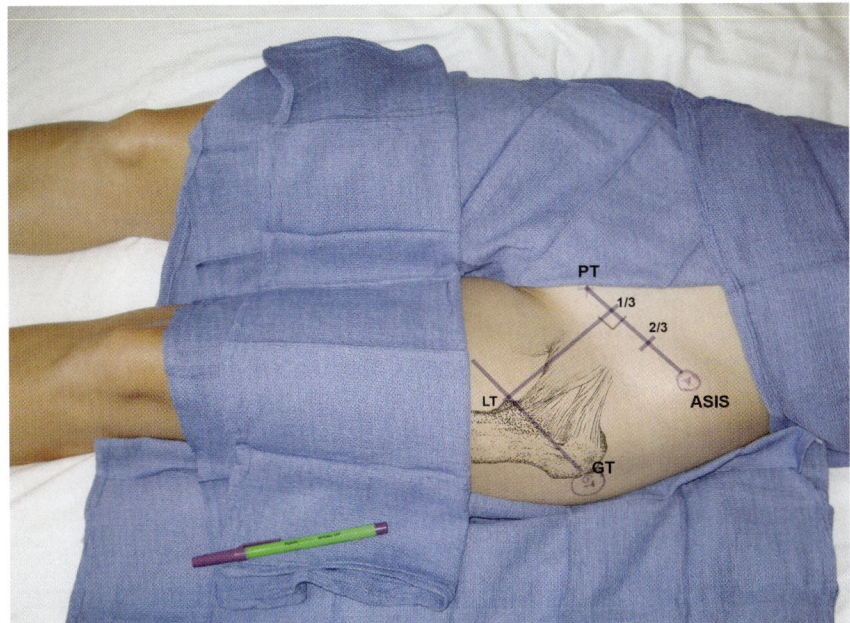

FIGURE 31-13 Sciatic nerve block: anterior sciatic landmarks.

ANKLE BLOCK

Indications

Foot, toes

Landmarks

1. Lateral malleolus (LM)
2. Medial malleolus (MM)
3. Dorsalis pedis artery (DPA)
4. Extensor hallucis longus (EHL)
5. Extensor digitorum longus (EDL)

Technique

- All needle insertions are to occur at the height of the lateral malleolus.
- Deep peroneal nerve: Needle insertion occurs between the tendon of EHL and EDL, just lateral to the DPA. Needle advancement to contact bone, followed by withdrawal 2 to 3 mm and injection of 3 to 5 mL of local anesthetic. The injection should be repeated in a slightly medial and lateral redirection.
- Superficial peroneal nerve: Needle insertion should be in the subcutaneous plane, along the line connecting the EHL and LM.
- Posterior tibial nerve: Needle insertion occurs from posterior to anterior just behind the MM, toward the bony groove where the posterior tibial nerve lies. Upon bony contact, the needle is withdrawn 2 to 3 mm and injection of 3 to 5 mL of local anesthetic. The injection should be repeated in a slightly medial and lateral redirections.
- Sural nerve: Needle insertion should be in the subcutaneous plane, along the line connecting the LM and Achilles tendon.
- Saphenous nerve: Needle insertion should be in the subcutaneous plane, along the line connecting the EHL and MM (Figure 31-14).

CONCLUSION

The innervation of the dermatomes, myotomes, and osteotomes do not always coincide. The surgical site must always be identified along with the surgical approach in order to ensure that all relevant nerves are anesthetized as the incision passes from skin to bone. The ideal block selection is that which ensures adequate coverage of all these disparate innervations. Likewise, it is not necessary to block each individual nerve with the identical local anesthetic. Blocks can be tailored to take advantage of the short- or long-acting properties of each agent. Finally, the ideal block technique (ultrasound vs. nerve-stimulation) depends on the user's level of experience with each modality. Practitioners should always select that technique with which they are most proficient in order to maximize patient safety.

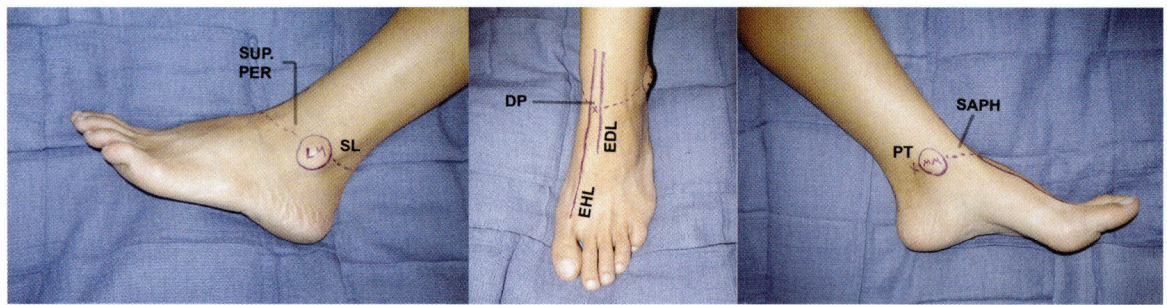

FIGURE 31-14 Landmarks for ankle block.

REFERENCES

1. Liu SS, Zayas VM, Gordon MA, Beathe JC, et al. A prospective randomized, controlled trial comparing ultrasound versus nerve stimulator guidance for interscalene block for ambulatory shoulder surgery for postoperative neurological symptoms. *Anesth Analg.* 2009;109(1):265–271.
2. Barrington MJ, Watts SA, Gledhill SR, et al. Preliminary results of the Australasian Regional Anaesthesia Collaboration: a prospective audit of more than 7000 peripheral nerve and plexus block for neurologic and other complications. *Reg Anesth Pain Med.* 2009;34(6):534–541.
3. Warman P, Nicholls B. Ultrasound-guided nerve blocks: efficacy and safety. *Best Pract Res Clin Anaesthesiol.* 2009;23(3):313–326.
4. Horlocker T, Wedel DJ, Rowlingson JC, et al. Regional anesthesia in the patient receiving antithrombotic or thrombolytic therapy: American Society of Regional Anesthesia and Pain Medicine Evidence-Based Guidelines (Third Edition). *Reg Anesth Pain Med.* 2010;35(1):64–101.
5. Hadzic A, Vloka JD. *Peripheral Nerve Blocks: Principles and Practice.* 1st ed. New York, NY: McGraw-Hill Companies, Inc.; 2004.
6. Missair A, Vale H, Pyram C, et al. Injection pressure during local anesthetic injection at three different velocities for femoral nerve blocks—how slow should we inject? *Reg Anesth Pain Med.* 2009;32:80.
7. Muniz MT, Rodriguez J, Bermndez M, et al. Low volume and high concentration of local anesthetic is more efficacious than high volume and low concentration in Labat's sciatic nerve block: a prospective, randomized comparison. *Anesth Analg.* 2008;107(6):2085–2008.
8. Masuda T, Cairns B, Sadhasivam S, et al. Epinephrine prevents muscle blood flow increases after perineural injection of tetrodotoxin. *Anesthesiology.* 2004;101(6):1428–1434.
9. Taboada M, Atanassoff P, Rodriguez J, et al. Platar flexion seems more reliable than dorsiflexion with Labat's sciatic nerve block: a prospective, randomized comparison. *Anesth Analg.* 2005;100(1):250–254.

CHAPTER 32

ABDOMINAL PAIN BE GONE: THE TAP BLOCK

BRANDON TOGIOKA
JEAN-PIERRE OUANES
RICHARD ELLIOTT

Life is pain and the enjoyment of love is an anesthetic.
Cesare Pavese (1908–1950),
Italian poet, critic, novelist, and translator

Love can be a powerful anesthetic, but in our experience it does not match up to sodium channel blockers.
Brandon Togioka

INTRODUCTION

Did you know that there is a new option for blocking pain in patients who have abdominal surgery? This technique avoids the side effects found with narcotics (sedation, itchiness, constipation, depressed breathing, nausea, etc.) and can be offered to patients who may not tolerate the side effects that go along with epidurals and spinals (hypotension, motor block, etc.). This new technique is the transversus abdominis plane (TAP) block, and it is a relatively new regional anesthetic technique for providing pain relief after lower abdominal surgery.

In contrast to spinals and epidurals, which have been around for over 100 years, the TAP block was described only recently, in 2001. Like most procedures in regional anesthesia, the TAP block was first described as a landmark guided technique, and it later adopted the use of the ultrasound. It is thought that the accuracy and safety of the block are improved by directly watching with the ultrasound as local anesthetic is injected.

Then came the controversy. Physicians performing the block began to argue about what levels the TAP block could affect. Some physicians (most early case reports) stated the block could affect the T7 to L1 levels.[1] However, as more case reports were published, it was found that cephalic spread past T10 was unlikely, making the block pertinent only for lower abdominal surgeries.[2] Thus, the subcostal TAP block was born. In the subcostal technique, local anesthetic is deposited into the same plane as the standard block (between the internal oblique and transversus abdominis muscles); however, it is injected more cephalad immediately under the 12th rib. This approach was shown to affect nerve segments up to T7[3] or the upper abdominal wall.

So now the TAP block, or a variation of it, can be used to provide postoperative analgesia for the entire abdomen (upper and lower). The only problem is that such a block would require at least four needle sticks (OUCH!!!) as each block will only numb one side of the abdominal wall.

ANATOMY

Yikes! I know this isn't a favorite of residents but truly the key to being a good regional anesthetist is understanding your anatomy. So...a brief review:
- The anterior abdominal wall is innervated by the anterior rami of nerves T7 to L1.
  - Nerves from T7 to T11 are known as the intercostals.
  - T12 is the subcostal nerve.
  - The iliohypogastric and ilioinguinal nerves are included in L1.

- Terminal branches of these nerves course through the lateral abdominal wall within a plane bound by the internal oblique and transversus abdominis muscles. This plane is known as the transversus abdominis plane (TAP) (Figure 32-1).
- The peritoneal cavity lies deep to the transversus abdominis muscle layer. Moving from deep to superficial from the peritoneal cavity are the transversus abdominis muscle, the internal oblique muscle, and the external oblique muscle.
- Injection of local anesthetic into the TAP can numb the skin, muscles, and parietal peritoneum of the anterior abdominal wall. Note: The abdominal viscera are not numbed.
- The nerves from T7 to L1 do not cross the midline and so injection of local anesthetic into one side of the abdomen provides only unilateral analgesia.
- As one goes from T6 to L1 the nerves enter the TAP at increasingly more lateral positions, such that T6 enters the TAP just lateral to the linea alba (remember that pale line that runs from the belly button to the pubic bone and gets dark during pregnancy), T7–T9 enter the TAP medial to the anterior axillary line (basically the front of your armpit), and T10–L1 enter the TAP lateral to the anterior axillary line. This anatomical finding has been used to explain why some anesthesiologists have found the TAP block (a block performed quite laterally) to be suitable only for lower abdominal surgery (Figure 32-2).
- The triangle of Petit is an area bound by the latissimus dorsi muscle posteriorly, the external oblique muscle anteriorly, and the iliac crest inferiorly.
  - If you have a hard time feeling the triangle of Petit, and believe me sometimes it just won't seem to exist, you can try needle insertion about 1.5 cm above the iliac crest and 9 to 10 cm working midline from the midaxillary line (the middle of the armpit). Unfortunately, the study that acquired those numbers found a quite variable depth from skin to the TAP (0.5 to 4 cm). Sorry.[4]

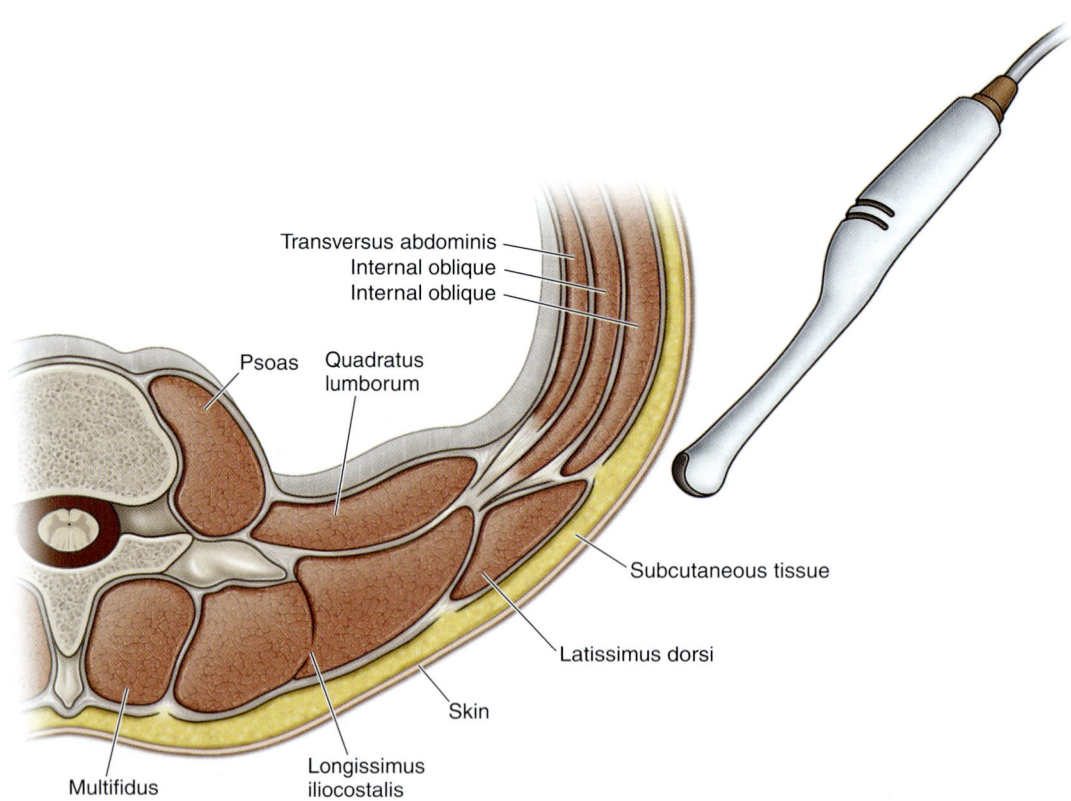

FIGURE 32-1 Transverse section through the abdomen showing the muscle layers pertinent to performing a TAP block.

Chapter 32 ABDOMINAL PAIN BE GONE: THE TAP BLOCK

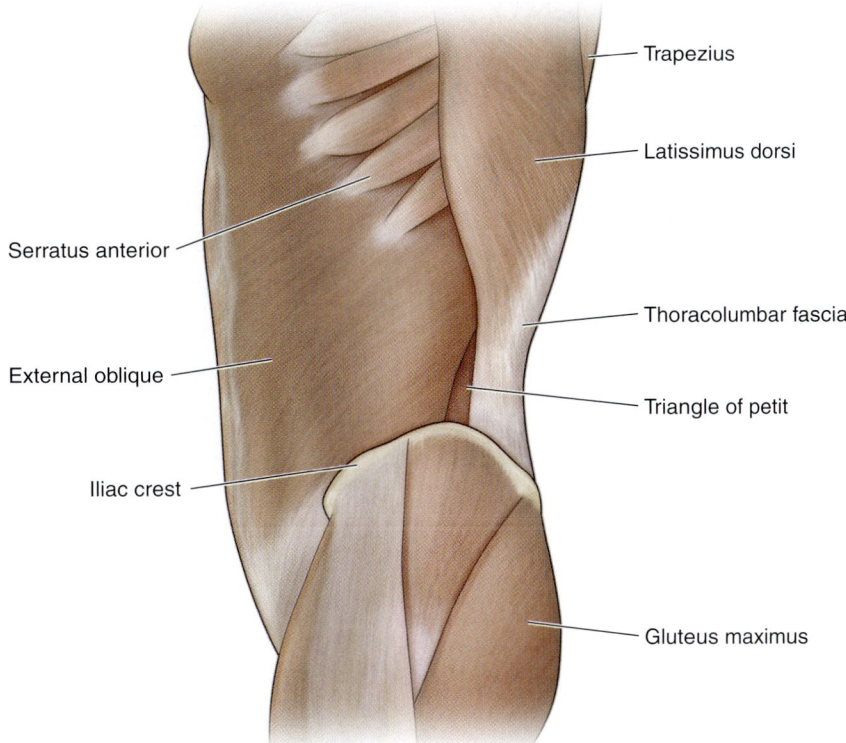

FIGURE 32-2 Side profile of the thoracoabdominal region showing anatomy pertinent to performing a TAP block.

SO WHY PERFORM THE TAP BLOCK?

Well, in addition to the advantages of avoiding narcotics and neuraxial anesthesia (spinals and epidurals), as referred to above, the TAP block has been linked to improved postoperative analgesia and a lessening of the surgical stress response. In fact, some studies have even found that the TAP block is associated with reduced morbidity and an improvement in outcome in selected surgeries.[3,5]

GREAT! NOW WHEN DO I DO IT?

- To be precise, the TAP block has been shown to provide effective postoperative analgesia for the following surgical incisions:[5,6]
  - Inguinal hernia repair
  - Orchiopexy
  - Pfannenstiel cesarean section
  - Open and laparoscopic appendectomy
  - Laparoscopic cholecystectomy
  - Total abdominal hysterectomy
  - Radical retropubic prostatectomy
  - Bowel resections requiring midline laparotomy incisions
- That's a lot to remember! Can you simplify it for me?
  - The TAP block is basically recommended for lower abdominal surgery in cases where neuraxial blockade may be less desirable.
  - This includes patients with spinal abnormalities, coagulopathies, or severe cardiovascular disease who may not tolerate a large sympathectomy.

WHEN CAN I ABSOLUTELY NOT DO IT?

- Patient refusal (as always)
- Anterior abdominal wall infection around the triangle of Petit
- Local anesthetic allergy
- Preexisting neurologic impairment (relative)
- Psychologic instability (relative)
- Peritonitis (relative)

THE SCAVENGER HUNT (EQUIPMENT)

- Sterile towels and 4" × 4" gauze packs
- Two 20-mL syringes filled with the local anesthetic of your choice
- Sterile gloves, mask, cap
- Skin antiseptic, typically chlorhexidine or iodine
- 21- to 22-gauge 50- to 150-mm short beveled block needle
- Ultrasound machine with linear, high-frequency transducer for visualization of shallow anatomic structures (ultrasound-guided technique only)
- Ultrasound probe cover (ultrasound-guided technique only)
- 1.5", 25-G needle and 1% lidocaine to numb skin prior to block (optional)

PHILOSOPHY OF THE TAP BLOCK

The TAP block is great for covering the pain of incision from the skin, muscles, and parietal (outer) peritoneum, but it will not cover any visceral pain (pain from the internal organs). Thus, it can only be used as part of a multimodal approach to pain control.

LOOK, MOM, I CAN DO IT WITH MY EYES CLOSED: THE BLIND/LANDMARK-GUIDED TECHNIQUE

1. Place the patient supine and then drape and prep the abdomen.
2. The needle is inserted into the area of the triangle of Petit.
3. The needle can be inserted either perpendicular to the skin or at a slightly oblique angle, with the advantage of the oblique angle being that the "pops" through the fascial layers are often easier to appreciate. Similarly, using a more blunt tipped needle can help the operator to appreciate the "pops."
4. As the needle is inserted, the operator will first feel one "pop," indicating penetration of the external oblique fascia and entry into the plane lying between the external and internal oblique muscles. The second "pop" indicates penetration of the internal oblique fascia and entry into the TAP.
5. Once the TAP has been entered, the operator aspirates to make sure the needle is not in a blood vessel and then incrementally (5 mL at a time) injects local anesthetic to desired volume (Figure 32-3).

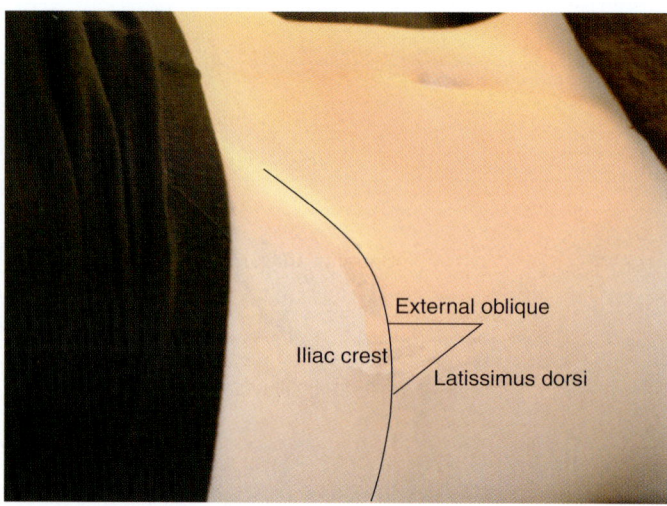

FIGURE 32-3 Live model surface anatomy pertinent to performing a TAP block.

SEEING IS BELIEVING: THE ULTRASOUND-GUIDED TECHNIQUE

1. After placing the patient supine and draping and prepping the triangle of Petit, place the ultrasound transducer above the iliac crest in a transverse plane (i.e. parallel to the ribs).
2. Using the ultrasound probe, identify the three muscular layers of the abdominal wall from superficial to deep: external oblique, internal oblique, and transversus abdominis muscle (Figure 32-4).
   a. Muscles will appear hypoechoic (dark) with the fascial sheaths between muscles appearing bright or hyperechoic.
   b. Please note the internal oblique muscle is usually the most prominent (thickest) muscular layer of the abdominal wall.
   c. Deep to all three muscles will appear a hypoechoic (dark) region, the peritoneal cavity, that is bound by a hyperechoic (bright) line, the peritoneum.
3. Identify the TAP, as this will be your target.
   a. Individual nerves are usually not seen.
4. Insert the needle in-plane (i.e., parallel and under the ultrasound probe) from a medial to lateral direction (Figure 32-5).
5. Visualize needle tip, NOT JUST NEEDLE SHAFT, to avoid entering undesired structures (Figure 32-5).
6. Once the TAP is entered, inject a small amount of local anesthetic (1 to 2 mL) looking for

hydrodissection (i.e., separation of the transversus abdominis and internal oblique muscles) to confirm correct needle placement
   a. Fluid will appear hypoechoic (dark) on the ultrasound image (Figure 32-6).
7. Inject a total of 20 to 30 mL of local anesthetic into this plane in adults (Figure 32-7).
8. Scan the abdomen cephalad and caudad to determine the extent of local anesthetic spread.
9. Repeat these steps on the other side of the abdomen if bilateral pain relief is desired.
10. Remember not to exceed the recommended maximum dose for each local anesthetic (with epinephrine added)
    a. Ropivacaine and bupivacaine 3 mg/kg
    b. Lidocaine and mepivacaine 7 mg/kg

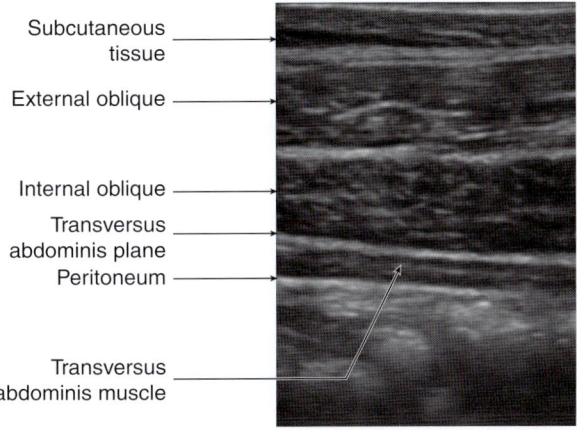

FIGURE 32-4 Ultrasound anatomy of muscles and planes pertinent to the TAP block.

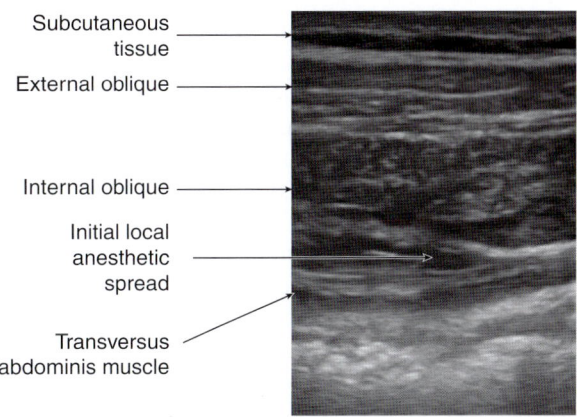

FIGURE 32-6 In-plane ultrasound technique showing hydrodissection of the transversus abdominis and internal oblique muscles.

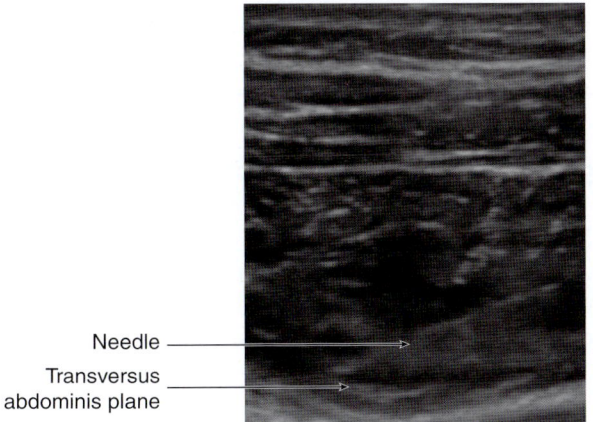

FIGURE 32-5 In-plane ultrasound technique with needle approaching the TAP.

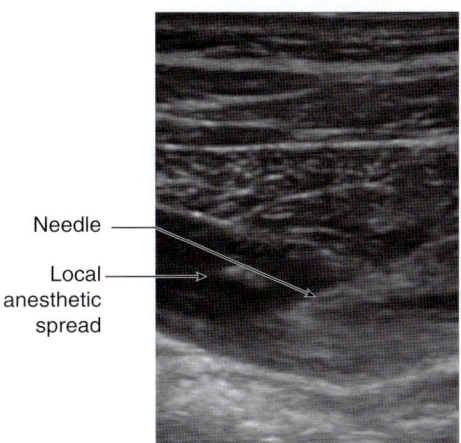

FIGURE 32-7 In-plane ultrasound technique showing local anesthetic injection into the TAP.

BUT WHAT ABOUT THAT BLOCK FOR THE UPPER ABDOMEN—THE SUBCOSTAL TAP BLOCK

The subcostal TAP block is performed very similarly to the above-described approaches, with the notable exception that the ultrasound probe is placed just caudad and parallel to the 12th rib.

PROLONGED POSTOPERATIVE ANALGESIA: CATHETER INSERTION

Catheters are inserted when practitioners desire postoperative analgesia longer than that which can be obtained with a single dose of local anesthetic. The procedure for inserting a catheter into the TAP is described below. Please note that the procedure for finding the TAP must be performed with a Tuohy needle when catheter insertion is desired.

1. After finding the correct plane, as described above, and confirming correct placement with hydrodissection with 1 to 2 mL of local anesthetic, introduce the catheter through the Tuohy needle.
2. The catheter is typically introduced 3 to 5 cm beyond the needle tip.
3. Confirm correct placement of the catheter with a 20- to 30-mL bolus of local anesthetic.
4. After confirming correct placement remove the Tuohy needle while leaving the catheter in place.
5. Secure the catheter in place noting depth at skin.
6. A 7- to 10-mL/h infusion can be started with a dilute solution of local anesthetic such as 0.2% ropivacaine or 0.0625% to 0.125% bupivacaine.

RULES TO STAY OUT OF TROUBLE

It's easier to stay out of trouble then get out of trouble.
H. Jackson Brown Jr., American author

So now you are ready to perform the block for the first time. Not real sure of yourself…that's OK. You can perform the block on an anesthetized patient. In doing this you will ensure that the patient won't move and you don't have to be as embarrassed if it takes you awhile. However, you should know that performing the block on a patient who is asleep masks some of the warning signs of nerve damage, namely paresthesias. Also, when you perform the block, don't forget to include epinephrine in your local anesthetic solution so that intravascular injection can be detected quickly. Lastly, if possible, use the ultrasound. Ultrasound use is associated with a more successful block and the need to use less local anesthetic in experienced hands.[7]

DECISIONS, DECISIONS, DECISIONS: LOCAL ANESTHETIC OPTIONS

- Mepivacaine 1% to 2% with 1:200,000 epinephrine
  - Provides intermediate duration analgesia with quick onset
- Lidocaine 1% to 2% with 1:200,000 epinephrine
  - Provides pretty much the same thing as mepivacaine
- Ropivacaine 0.25% to 0.75% with 1:200,000 epinephrine
  - Provides more prolonged analgesia, but with longer onset
- Bupivacaine 0.25% to 0.75% with 1:200,000 epinephrine
  - Provides pretty much the same thing as ropivacaine with more potential for cardiac toxicity

HOW MUCH TO USE: DOSAGE

The TAP block is a volume-dependent block. In other words, the block depends on local anesthetic spread and not concentration. Thus, it is suggested that you use dilute local anesthetic solutions to stay below toxic dosages. This will allow you to use a high volume to maximize your chances of creating a happy postanesthesia care unit (PACU) patient.

Don't forget: if you are performing this block for a midline incision, you will have to block both sides of the abdomen. If this is the case, be sure your TOTAL dosage stays well below toxic levels.

POTENTIAL MAJOR COMPLICATIONS

- Intrahepatic injection
- Intraperitoneal injection or hemorrhage[6]
- Bowel puncture and hematoma
- Pelvic hematoma
- Transient femoral nerve palsy
- Local anesthetic toxicity

KIDDIE BLOCKS: SPECIAL PEDIATRIC CONSIDERATIONS

Wow, you have advanced quickly! Off to treat the kiddies. If the block is to be performed on children it is recommended that the operator start first on older children and lower the age as experience increases. Children can be more challenging, as their smaller size places nerves closer to critical structures. To this extent, only use sharp needles when doing ultrasound-guided TAP blocks in children. Blunt needles require more pressure and can "pop" through to injure other organs. The ultrasound is almost a necessity in children, as there is no easily identifiable triangle of Petit. When using the ultrasound, look for an area in the flank where the three lateral abdominal muscles can be easily visualized. Once you find the TAP, inject between 0.1 and 0.2 mL/kg of local anesthetic up to a total dose of 20 mL per side (in older children). In one journal article it was recommended that the total dosage of bupivacaine be limited to 2 mg/kg for neonates and 3 mg/kg for children to avoid toxicity.[8]

NOW I AM A PRO: TROUBLESHOOTING PROBLEMS

"Ahhhhhh...I cannot find the three muscle layers of the anterior abdominal wall!"

- If this occurs, it can be helpful to start scanning with the ultrasound probe in the midline over the rectus abdominis muscle. In this area the rectus abdominis muscle is the only muscle. The ultrasound can then be used to scan laterally to a point where all three muscles are identified and these can be traced to the region above the iliac crest where the block can be performed.

"Where is the TAP?"

- If this question occurs to you, you can use Doppler technology to identify small blood vessels within the TAP.[4] You can look for bowel peristalsis to identify the peritoneal cavity.

"All I see is fat:" difficulty in placing the block secondary to patient obesity:[9]

- If this occurs, the operator can ask an assistant to provide manual retraction of the abdomen by standing opposite the side being blocked and pulling soft tissues toward him- or herself.
- Another technique that has been described is to have the patient lift his or her head off of the bed, which will tense the abdomen and make palpating the triangle or Petit easier.
- Using a lower frequency curvilinear ultrasound probe can be helpful, as lower frequency ultrasound waves will have a greater depth of penetration.

"I can see the target; I just can't get there:" difficulty in achieving the shallow needle trajectory required to place the TAP block:

- If this occurs, try inserting the needle further from the transducer.

CONCLUSION

- The TAP block is a relatively new regional technique for providing postoperative pain relief for patients having abdominal surgery.
- Its major advantage is that it avoids some of the disadvantages that go along with spinals and epidurals.
  - There is less worry with anticoagulation with the TAP block.
  - The TAP block should not cause any motor block of the legs.
  - The TAP block avoids sympathectomy mediated hypotension.
- The TAP block is usually performed within the triangle of Petit, which is an area bound by the latissimus dorsi (posteriorly), the external oblique muscle (anteriorly), and the iliac crest (inferiorly).
- The TAP block will cover pain due to an incisional injury to the skin, muscles, and parietal (outer) peritoneum.
  - It will not cover any pain due to injury/manipulation of the internal organs.
  - The TAP block should be used only as a multimodal approach to pain control.
- The TAP block is commonly performed either by feel, using landmarks to guide placement, or via ultrasound guidance.
- If prolonged pain control is desired, a catheter can be inserted into the TAP.
- Potential complications of the TAP block include intrahepatic injection, intraperitoneal injection, bowel puncture, femoral nerve injury, and local anesthetic toxicity.

REFERENCES

1. McDonnell J, O'Donnell B, Farrell T, et al. Transversus abdominis plane block: a cadaveric and radiological evaluation. *Reg Anesth Pain Med* 2007;32:399-404.
2. Tran TM, Ivanusic JJ, Hebbard P, Barrington MJ. Determination of spread of injectate after ultrasound-guided transversus abdominis plane block: a cadaveric block. *Br J Anaesth* 2009;102(1):123-127.
3. Lee TH, Barrington M, Tran TM, Wong D, Hebbard PD. Comparison of extent of sensory block following posterior and subcostal approaches to ultrasound-guided transversus abdominis plane block. *Anaesth Intensive Care* 2010; 38(3):452-460.
4. Jankovic ZB, Du Feu FM, McConnell P. An anatomical study of the transversus abdominis plane block: location of the lumbar triangle of Petit and adjacent nerves. *Anesth Analg* 2009;109:981-985.

5. Petersen PL, Mathiesen O, Torup H, Dahl JB. The transversus abdominis plane block: a valuable option for postoperative analgesia? A topical review. *Acta Anaesthesiol Scand* 2010;54:529–535.
6. Finnerty O, Carney J, McDonnell JG. Trunk blocks for abdominal surgery. *J Assoc Anaesthetists Great Britain Ireland* 2010;65:76–83.
7. Willschke H, Marhofer P, Bosenberg A, et al. Ultrasonography for ilioinguinal/iliohypogastric nerve blocks in children. *Br J Anaesth* 2005;95(2):226–230.
8. Suresh S, Chan V. Ultrasound guided transversus abdominis plane block in infants, children and adolescents: a simple procedural guidance for their performance. *Pediatr Anesth* 2009;19:296–299.
9. Gravante G, Castri F, Araco F, Araco A. A comparative study of the transversus abdominis plane (TAP) block efficacy on post-bariatric vs aesthetic abdominoplasty with flank liposuction. *Obes Surg* 2010; published online ahead of print.

CHAPTER 33

NERVE BLOCKS FOR ABDOMINAL SURGERY

JONI MAGA
LUIS NARCISO

"Ouch, my stomach hurts like never before!"
Surgical Patient

INTRODUCTION

There's good news! We can prevent these kinds of complaints. In this chapter we will discuss certain techniques that will allow us to do so. Blocks are fun...and easy (don't tell anyone; let people think you are a superstar). Many of the blocks in this chapter are limited to providing analgesia only since the viscera cannot be blocked. They are great for postoperative pain relief and, if done preoperatively, can decrease opioid usage and the associated risks (nausea, vomiting, itching, confusion) during and after the anesthetic.

ANATOMY

Abdominal Wall Innervation[1,2]

- Anterolateral abdominal wall neurovascular plane
  - The plane between the inferior oblique and the transverse abdominis muscles where all the abdominal cutaneous nerves along with the ilioinguinal and iliohypogastric nerves run (see Table 33-1 and Figure 33-1).

Abdominal Visceral-Sensory Innervation[2]

Visceral sensation is carried via the afferent nerve fibers of the thoracic and abdominal sympathetic nerves. There is a significant overlap in the vertebral level of origin among the spinal nerves innervating individual abdominal organs. The spinal nerves consist of the presynaptic nerve axons. These nerves form junctions with bundles of nerve bodies that form the postsynaptic ganglia, which then go on to innervate the organs individually. This network of postsynaptic nerves form elaborate nerve plexi. The autonomic nervous innervation of any particular abdominal organ is described by the specific spinal nerves from which they originate. The sympathetic and visceral sensory innervations consists of spinal nerves T5–L2.

- Greater splanchnic nerve
  - T5–T9
  - Synapses with the celiac ganglia
    - Innervates upper abdominal organs
- Lesser splanchnic nerve
  - T10–T11
  - Synapses with the superior mesenteric ganglia
    - Innervates lower abdominal organs
- Least splanchnic nerve
  - T12
  - Synapses with the aorticorenal ganglia
    - Innervates lower abdominal organs
- Lumbar splanchnic nerves
  - L1–L2
  - Synapses with the inferior mesenteric ganglia and hypogastric plexus
    - Innervates lower abdominal and pelvic organs

TABLE 33-1 Abdominal Wall Innervation

Nerve	Source	Sensory	Motor
Intercostal nerves	T7-T11 (ventral primary rami of spinal nerves)	Skin, anterolateral abdomen	Intercostal muscles and abdominal wall muscles
Subcostal nerve	T12 (ventral primary ramus of T12)	Skin, anterolateral abdomen	Abdominal wall muscles
Iliohypogastric nerve	T12, L1 (ventral primary rami of T12 and L1)	Skin, lower abdominal wall, upper hip, and upper thigh	Lower abdominal wall muscles
Ilioinguinal nerve	L1 (ventral primary ramus of L1)	Skin lower abdominal wall, anterior scrotum, labia majora	Lower abdominal wall muscles

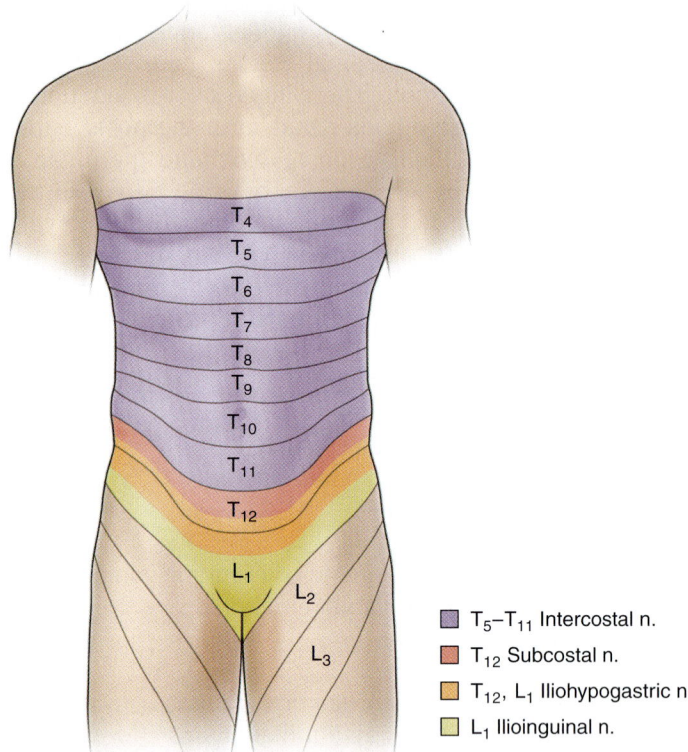

FIGURE 33-1 Dermatomes.

REGIONAL ANESTHESIA TECHNIQUES

Neuraxial Anesthesia

- Is the most commonly used technique that provides analgesia, continuous analgesia, and intraoperative anesthesia for abdominal, pelvic, and lower extremity procedures
- These techniques include epidural, spinal, and combined spinal-epidural anesthesia.
- Please refer to the individual chapters of the techniques mentioned above for detailed explanations on these procedures.

Transversus Abdominis Plane Block

- A technique used as an anesthetic adjunct for abdominal surgery, cesarean sections, and pediatric abdominal surgery
- Provides postoperative analgesia
- See Chapter 32 for a detailed explanation of this procedure.

Thoracolumbar Paravertebral Nerve Blocks[3,4]

- Description
  - Technique where local anesthesia is introduced into the triangular paravertebral area where the spinal nerve exits the vertebral column. It provides segmental analgesia and can also provide surgical anesthesia to the area. It works like a one-sided epidural with the added benefit of less hypotension and urinary retention.
- Indications
  - Analgesia for abdominal procedures and inguinal procedures, surgical anesthesia for inguinal herniorrhaphy. It can also be used to decrease pain from herpes zoster outbreaks.

- Technique
  - Can be performed with the patient in the sitting, lateral, or prone position
  - Palpate and mark the spinous process, then measure 2.5 cm lateral and mark it. This designates the transverse process. Repeat for each level (Figure 33-2).
  - Note: C7 is the most prominent; T7 corresponds to the inferior tip of scapula, and the iliac crest corresponds to the L3–4 interspace.
  - Prepare and drape the area sterilely.
  - Inject a small amount of local anesthetic superficially to make a skin wheal at each level.
  - A 22-gauge (G) needle with depth markings is introduced perpendicular to the skin, until the transverse process is felt (3 to 5 cm deep in T-spine, 4 to 7 cm deep in the L-spine). Note the depth of the process, withdraw the needle to the skin, and reposition your hold on the needle to 1 cm more than the depth that the transverse process was encountered. Maintain hand contact on the body for stabilization (Figure 33-3: 1st needle position).
  - Redirect 20 to 30 degrees caudally. It is inserted 1 cm deeper than where the transverse process was felt. Since you are holding the needle at this point, just insert the needle to the point where your fingers are in contact with the skin. A "pop" will not be felt unless a larger gauge needle is used. Paresthesias are unlikely. This is a fixed depth technique (Figure 33-3: 2nd needle position).
  - When in the thoracic region: After redirecting caudally, a more shallow bone may be encountered. If so, this bone is actually the transverse process. The first bone that was encountered is the rib and not the transverse process. Remove needle and begin the procedure caudad to the original needle insertion point to encounter transverse process (Figure 33-3).
  - Note: Redirecting cranially could be potentially hazardous if the first point you encounter is the rib and you assume it is the transverse process. Advancing 1 cm deeper could land you in the pleura (see Figure 33-3).
  - Aspirate to check for blood or cerebrospinal fluid (CSF)
  - Inject 3 to 5 mL of the local anesthetic of your choice. (We recommend 0.5% ropivacaine for maximal postoperative pain relief.)
  - It is recommended that at least three segments be blocked in order to provide reliable results.
  - Medial to lateral scanning with an ultrasound to map out structures prior to procedure can be utilized. Using the ultrasound to guide the needle during the actual procedure is challenging and is a more advanced technique.

- Risks
  - Pneumothorax
  - Infection
  - Bleeding
    - Note: use the same anticoagulation guidelines here as you do for neuraxial anesthesia due to its proximity to the epidural space.
  - Anaphylactic reaction
  - Larger volumes of local anesthetic will increase the likelihood of epidural spread and ipsilateral sympathetic blockade, resulting in bradycardia and hypotension. Avoid directing the needle medially.
  - Subarachnoid injection with total spinal anesthesia, especially in the thoracic spine area. Avoid directing the needle medially.
  - There is a high risk of intravascular injection in this area, so make sure you aspirate.

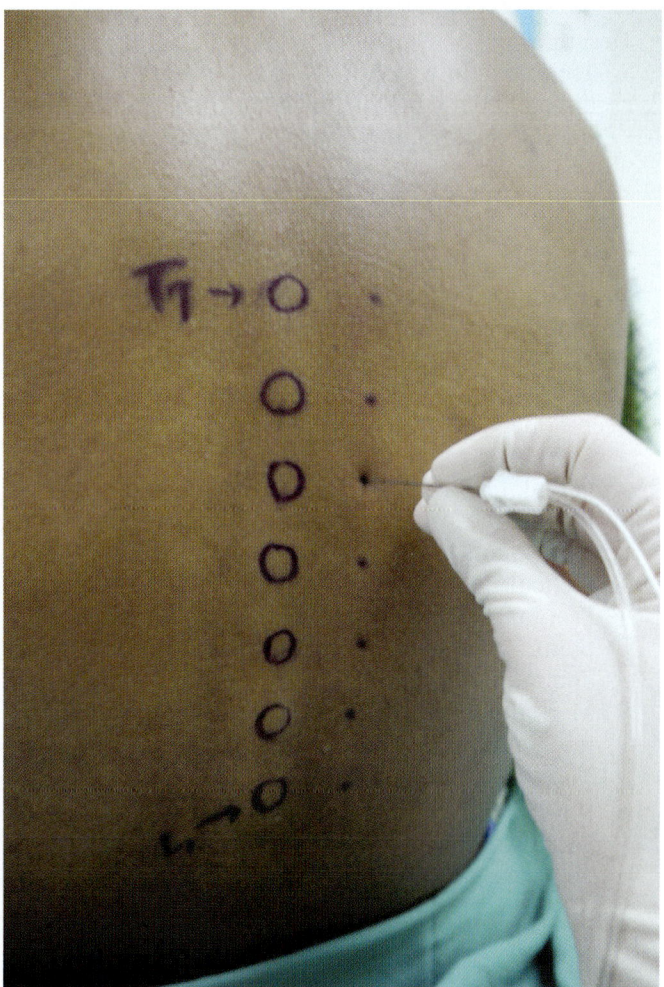

FIGURE 33-2 Paravertebral block.

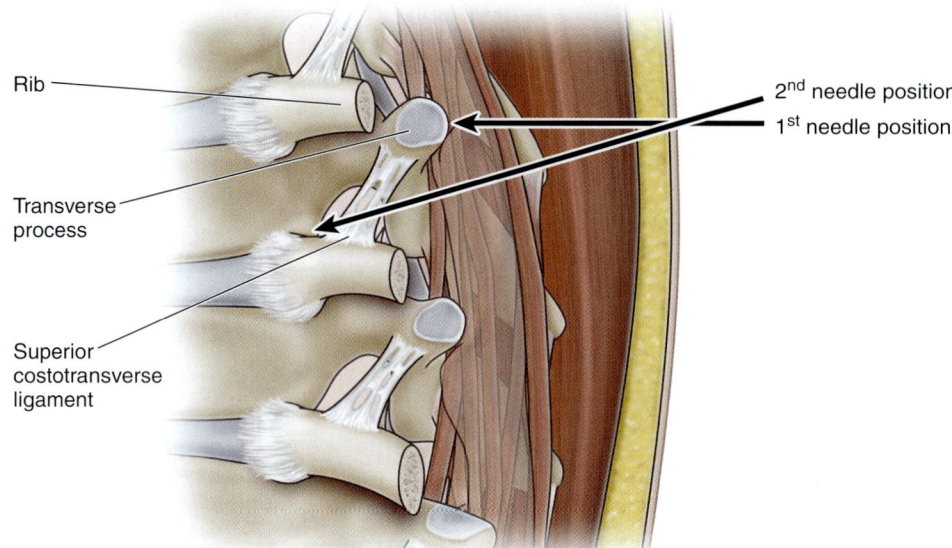

FIGURE 33-3 Paravertebral space.

Intercostal Nerve Block[3]
- Description
  - Technique in which local anesthetic is introduced directly below the rib adjacent to the underlying neurovascular bundle, which supplies the motor and sensory innervation of the abdominal wall and the thoracic wall. It can be used for intraoperative and postoperative analgesia.
- Indications
  - Upper abdominal procedures, more commonly thoracic procedures and broken ribs, and can also be used to decrease pain from herpes zoster outbreaks.
- Technique
  - Can be performed with the patient in the sitting, lateral, or prone position
  - Palpate the spinous processes of T7–T12 and mark them.
  - Difficult to perform above T7 due to the scapula
  - Feel for the inferior border of the most angulated point (6 to 8 cm lateral from the spinous process) and mark it.
  - Mark the rest of the ribs' inferior borders along this parasagittal line (Figure 33-4).
  - The area is then prepared and draped sterilely.
  - Inject a small amount of local anesthetic superficially to make a skin wheal.
  - A 22-G needle with depth markings is then introduced into skin at the lower border until it comes in contact with the rib.
  - The needle is then "walked" down below the rib.
  - The needle should be pointing slightly toward the head the entire time (20 degrees cephalad) (Figure 33-5).
  - It is then advanced about 3 to 4 mm below the rib.
  - Aspirate your needle.
  - Inject about 5 mL of the local anesthetic of your choice. We suggest 0.5% ropivacaine for a long-lasting block.
  - Several segments must be blocked in order to provide reliable analgesia to the area.
  - Ultrasound guidance may be used to help better localize the ribs initially for marking. The technique remains otherwise the same.
- Risks
  - Pneumothorax
  - Infection
  - Bleeding
  - Anaphylactic reaction
  - Intravascular injection
  - Large quantities of local anesthetic can be absorbed quickly with potential overdose.
  - Careful consideration should be given to patients who depend on accessory muscle use for breathing.

Chapter 33 NERVE BLOCKS FOR ABDOMINAL SURGERY

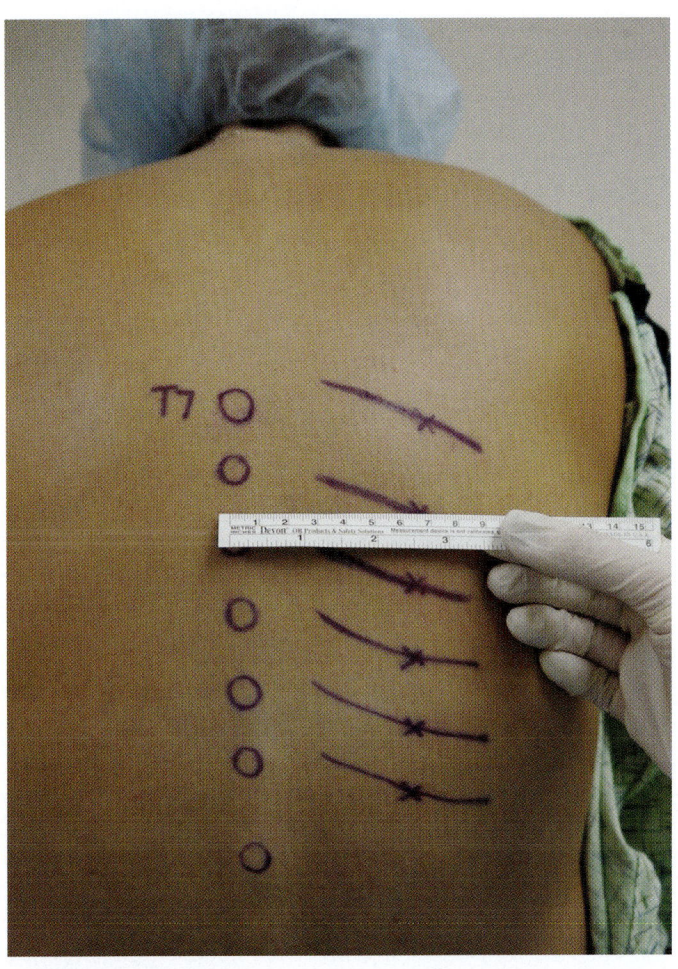

FIGURE 33-4 Intercostal block.

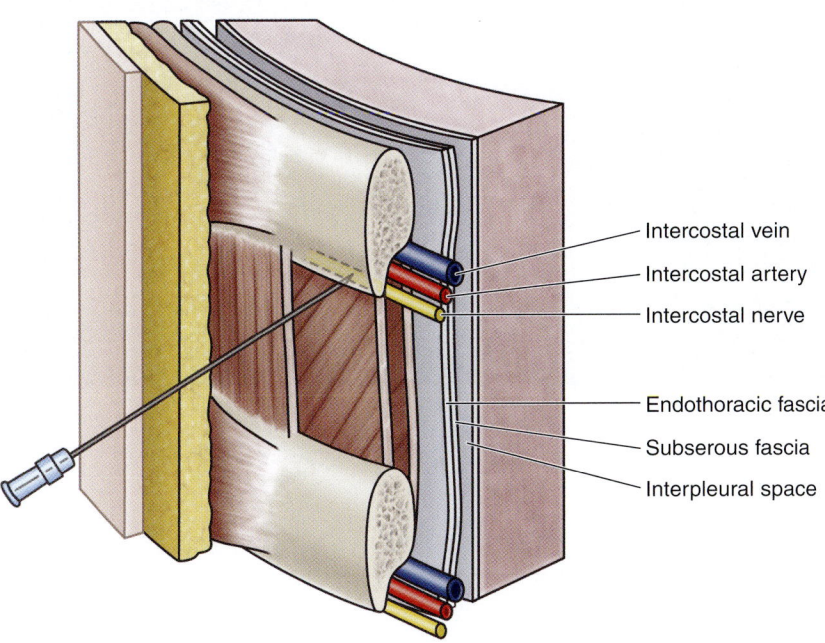

FIGURE 33-5 Intercostal space.

Ilioinguinal and Iliohypogastric Nerve Blocks[4]

- Description
  - L1 (ventral primary ramus)
  - Course
    - Superomedial to anterior superior iliac spine (ASIS): Lies between transversus abdominis and internal oblique muscles, courses inferomedially, and pierces the internal oblique and cutaneous branches, and then pierces the external oblique. Iliohypogastric continues to run anteroinferiorly to the superficial inguinal ring.
  - Iliohypogastric: innervates skin over inguinal region
  - Ilioinguinal: innervates skin over superomedial aspect of thigh
- Indications
  - For postoperative pain relief, will not be enough for surgical anesthesia as it does not cover viscera. Can be performed pre- or postoperatively.
  - Analgesia from incisions: Pfannenstiel, inguinal herniorrhaphy, and other lower abdominal wall procedures and inguinal area incision sites
  - Note: To block entire lower abdominal wall, you need to block T11, T12, iliohypogastric and ilioinguinal.
  - Note: If combined with injection of the peritoneum (from surgeon), it may be used for surgical anesthesia.
- Technique
  - Loss of resistance technique using a blunt needle. Deposition of local anesthetic between the external oblique and the internal oblique. Feel for a "pop."
  - Find ASIS.
  - The needle insertion point lies 2 cm medial and 2 cm superior to the ASIS (Figure 33-6).
  - Direct a blunt-tip needle perpendicular to skin; after "pop." inject 3 cc (recommend 0.5% ropivacaine); remove needle.
  - Repeat at 45 degrees lateral and 45 degrees medial for a total of 9 cc.
- Risks
  - Infection
  - Bleeding
  - Anaphylactic reaction
  - Intravascular injection: local anesthetic toxicity
  - Injury to abdominal organs

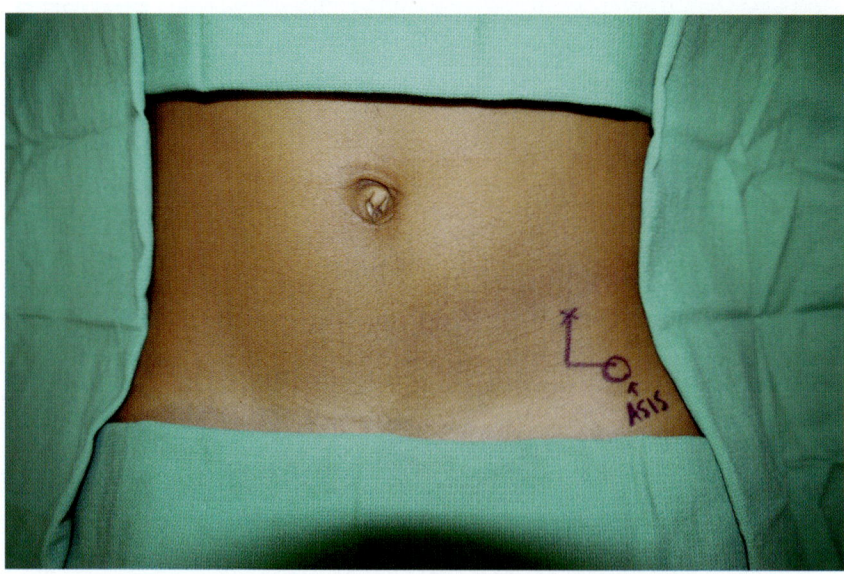

FIGURE 33-6 Ilioinguinal block.

Other Techniques

- Intraabdominal local anesthetic irrigation
  - This is a technique in which the abdominal organs affected by the surgery are irrigated with small amounts of local anesthetic, usually lidocaine or bupivacaine.
  - It is usually applied by the surgeon on the operative field.
  - It has been shown to have some benefit in providing postoperative analgesia by decreasing visceral discomfort following cholecystectomies, hysterectomies, and cesarean sections.
- Field blocks
  - Technique in which local anesthetic, usually lidocaine or bupivacaine, is injected either directly into the site of incision or in a square pattern around the area of incision to provide intraoperative and postoperative analgesia.
  - Typically performed by the surgeon prior to incision for abdominal procedures that involve small surgical and incision sites.

CONCLUSION

There are many different anesthetic adjuncts that may be used during abdominal surgery for a well-balanced multimodal approach to perioperative pain control. Remember that practice makes perfect. The more you practice, the more comfortable and more efficient you will become, and, best of all, the happier your patients will be.

REFERENCES

1. Anatomy tables—abdominal wall. *Medical gross anatomy—home*. http://anatomy.med.umich.edu/gastrointestinal_system/abdo_wall_tables.html#nerves.
2. Moore KL, Dalley AF, Agur AMR. *Clinically oriented anatomy.* Philadelphia: Lippincott Williams & Wilkins, 2009.
3. Barash PG, Cullen BF, Stoelting RK. *Clinical anesthesia.* Philadelphia: Lippincott Williams & Wilkins, 2006.
4. Hadzic A. *Textbook of regional anesthesia and acute pain management.* New York: McGraw-Hill, Medical Publishing Division, 2007.

CHAPTER 34
PERIPHERAL NERVE CATHETERS— COMFORTABLY NUMB

JOSEPH C. HUNG
MARIE HANNA

When I was a child
I caught a fleeting glimpse
Out of the corner of my eye.
I turned to look but it was gone.
I cannot put my finger on it now.
The child is grown,
The dream is gone.
But I have become comfortably numb.

Pink Floyd

INTRODUCTION

Sometimes being numb can be a good thing. Like performing under pressure. Or during a painful procedure. Or in the few days after someone cuts you open in a surgery. Being numb is great in all of these situations.

We had a patient once who was getting bone marrow harvested from her hip. They were using a big needle. She was okay with it, though, because she was numb from her waist down. Why? Because we had given her a single shot of spinal anesthesia. Things were going well.

But as they say, "All good things must come to an end." Pain control is a good thing. In this particular bone marrow harvest case, it came to an end. The patient's cell counts were not great. The oncologists took a long time to harvest the needed amount of marrow. The spinal wore off in about 90 minutes. The patient began complaining. She was face down to allow the team to gain access to her hip. She would periodically look up to call us names. She called the harvesting team names. They were not nice names.

In this particular case, pain control did not necessarily have to come to an end. We could have left in a catheter to redose the anesthetic in the form of an epidural catheter. However, hindsight is always 20/20. Peripheral nerve catheters follow a similar principle. Single-shot peripheral nerve blocks wear off. People with pain are upset when this occurs (both during surgery and after surgery). If you don't like being called names, put in a peripheral nerve catheter.

INDICATIONS

Other chapters in this book offer indications to consider when weighing regional anesthesia techniques versus general anesthesia; see especially Part V.
- Compared to neuraxial blockade, peripheral nerve catheters offer the following:
    - No need for Foley placement (reducing the risk of urinary tract infection)
    - Easier use of anticoagulation postoperatively
    - Less risk of epidural infection, meningitis, or hematoma
    - Improved side-effect profile (compared to opiate only regimens), including greater hemodynamic stability, less pruritus, less nausea, less

constipation, less sedation, and less urinary retention
- What is a good thing to have in yoga, karate, and perioperative analgesia?
  - Answer: Mobility and flexibility
  - Continuous local anesthetic infusions through a peripheral nerve catheter (PNC) allow for prolonged infusions of more dilute concentrations.
  - Patients can be exercising yet comfortable after joint replacement.

Other Things That Patients Don't Like
- Other than pain, people also tend not to like falling because of a very numb leg.
- Because dense nerve blocks are avoided through dilute anesthetic infusions, fewer people tend to fall secondary to sensory loss. There is also less theoretical risk of limb injury secondary to neglect.
- Patients also tend to be happier when they are able to feel their extremities.
- Side effects such as respiratory insufficiency following single-shot interscalene block have also been mitigated by using lower concentrations of local anesthetic through a PNC.[1]
- Show me the money!
  - There have been significant cost savings associated with a reduced need for hospitalization for pain control made possible through PNC analgesia.[2]
- Patients with significant trauma require multiple surgeries. Leave a catheter in!
- Along the same lines, PNCs can be used for prolonged diagnostic/treatment options for painful pain syndromes. Treatment of complex regional pain syndrome (CRPS) is a common example.
- Love and pain tolerance are key. Leaving in a PNC can be useful for more effective postoperative rehabilitation and physical therapy.

Contraindications
- Similar to contraindications for single-shot peripheral nerve blocks. They are very few and far between, and include:
  - Patient refusal or mental incompetence for informed consent: "No means no!!"
  - Bacteremia
  - Infection at PNC insertion site
  - Significant allergies to local anesthetic or other drugs you are planning on administering through the peripheral nerve catheter
  - Per the American Society of Regional Anesthesia (ASRA) guidelines, anticoagulation should not factor into peripheral nerve blockade or peripheral nerve catheter placement except with deeper blocks such as a paravertebral block or lumbar plexus block.[3]

Equipment (Not Optional)
- Placement needle (may or may not be stimulating needle, i.e., have ability to attach to a nerve stimulator to confirm location)
  - Some use the Tuohy needle with the standard epidural catheter (see below).
  - If not using a stimulating needle, then you will have to use ultrasound technique to confirm correct location of needle tip.
- Infusion catheter (may or may not be stimulating catheter, i.e., have ability to attach to a nerve stimulator to confirm location). Some use a standard epidural catheter.
- Chlorhexidine antiseptic solution
- Sterile drape
- Sterile gown and gloves
- Mask and cap (so the patient can't recognize you in case of a failed block)
- Sterile syringe for nerve block local anesthetic
- Sterile syringe for superficial anesthesia local anesthetic
- Surgical adhesive strips or one of many commercially available fixation devices
- Tegaderm or other transparent dressing
- Infusion pump and tubing (to infuse your local anesthetic solution through the PNC)
- Standard monitoring equipment
  - Pulse oximeter
  - Blood pressure cuff
  - Electrocardiogram (ECG) leads
  - Oxygen by nasal cannula or facemask
- Resuscitation equipment
  - Ambu bag
  - Suction
  - Emergency drugs (phenylephrine, atropine, ephedrine, and epinephrine)
- Sedation drugs (midazolam and/or fentanyl)
  - For patients with low pain tolerance and high sedation requirements, consider the use of propofol, ketamine and/or dexmedetomidine.

Equipment (Optional, Depending on Technique)
- Sterile marking pen
- Nerve stimulator (to stimulate some lucky nerve out there, if using nerve stimulator technique for nerve localization)
- Ultrasound machine (if using ultrasound-guided technique for nerve localization)
- Sterile ultrasound sleeve with ultrasound gel
- 18-gauge AngioCath or other non-safety IV catheter (if you want to tunnel your nerve catheter; see below)

Peripheral Nerve Catheter History and Physical Examination (Checklist)

- Is this the correct patient, and am I doing the procedure at the correct side/location?
- Is there any evidence of infection at the PNC site?
  - Pain (dolor)
  - Erythema (rubor)
  - Edema, induration (tumor)
  - Heat (calor)
- Does this patient have frank bacteremia?
- Is this patient allergic to anything I plan on infusing through this catheter?

Technique (Broadly Divided Into Nerve Stimulator Techniques and Ultrasound Techniques)

- Pick an appropriate nerve block technique given the indication.
- Given relevant surface anatomy for block, pick a site for needle insertion.
- Make sure patient is appropriately monitored (ECG, pulse oximetry probe, blood pressure) and well oxygenated.
- Make sure the patient is appropriately positioned given the nerve block technique.
- Confirm adequacy of resuscitation equipment.
- Time-out and confirm patient identity, procedure, correct procedure site, allergies, and informed consent.
- Use IV sedation if needed.
- Sterilely prep and drape the anatomical area involved.
- After opening supplies in a sterile environment, put on gown and gloves.
- Make a 2- to 3-cm skin local anesthetic wheal (1% lidocaine) at needle insertion site with subcutaneous infiltration.
- Flush catheter and placement needle/cannula with 3 to 5 cc of sterile normal saline or local anesthetic to confirm patency and no leaks (Figure 34-1).
- With a nerve stimulator
  - Reasonable initial stimulator settings: 1.2 to 1.5 mA, 2 Hz, and impulse duration of 0.1 ms
  - Connect placement needle/catheter needle to stimulator
  - Advance placement needle toward target nerve.
    - Monitor for motor response in muscles innervated by target nerve.
    - Reduce the nerve stimulation current incrementally until motor response is maintained at less than 0.5 mA.
  - If inadequate motor response is elicited with reasonable needle advancement, withdraw needle to skin and redirect in a systematic fashion (e.g., fan-shaped distribution) to isolate the desired nerve.
  - After you are happy with your motor response, deposit the desired amount of local anesthetic around the target nerve through the placement needle (always with incremental injection after negative aspiration). Inject local anesthetic only if you are not planning on using a stimulating catheter (see below).
  - Thread the peripheral nerve catheter through the placement needle 3 to 5 cm beyond the cannula tip.
- With ultrasound
  - The many possible ultrasound techniques used to identify target nerves for peripheral nerve blockade are beyond the scope of this chapter.
  - The idea is to use an in-plane approach for placement of the needle/cannula to visually confirm the proximity of the needle tip to the target nerves (as opposed to confirming location by using a motor response and nerve stimulator).
  - Deposit desired amount of local anesthetic around target nerves with ultrasound confirmation of injection (always with incremental injection after negative aspiration). Inject local anesthetic only if you are not planning on using a stimulating catheter (see below).
  - Thread the peripheral nerve catheter 3 to 5 cm beyond the placement needle/cannula tip (Figures 34-2 to 34-4).
- If using a stimulating catheter
  - Use of a stimulating catheter allows confirmation of the placement of the peripheral nerve catheter (either with ultrasound or nerve stimulator technique).
  - It is very possible to isolate a great motor response using a stimulating insertion needle/cannula, only to have a poorly working catheter after placement.
  - If using a stimulating catheter, remember not to deposit local anesthetic through the placement needle, as this will make isolating a motor response through subsequent placement of the stimulating catheter difficult.
    - Some kits have a stimulating wire to manipulate through the peripheral nerve catheter for stimulation, while others have wires integrated within the catheter itself.
  - Transfer the stimulating lead to the stimulating catheter.
  - Use similar stimulator settings (1.2 to 1.5 mA, 2 Hz, and impulse duration of 0.1 ms) to isolate motor response from the target nerves.
    - Maintain motor response while decreasing current to ≤1 mA.
    - Note that higher currents may be needed to elicit a motor response with the catheter as compared with the stimulating introducer needle/cannula.[4]
    - There is no magic current threshold to isolate motor response using a nerve stimulator. Using

a stimulating catheter, a higher threshold (up to 1 mA) may be needed.
- If an appropriate motor response cannot be elicited using the stimulating catheter, try to withdraw the stimulating catheter incrementally.
  - If you are still not happy with the motor response, then withdraw the stimulating catheter completely.
  - Reattempt rethreading through the placement catheter or consider a new needle entry point with the placement needle/cannula.
- Once you are satisfied with the isolated motor response, deposit the desired amount of local anesthetic around the target nerve through the stimulating catheter (always with incremental injection after negative aspiration).
- With all techniques, withdraw the placement needle/cannula while feeding the peripheral nerve catheter through to maintain the position of the catheter tip, similar to withdrawing the epidural placement needle after placing an epidural catheter.
- To maximize the accuracy of catheter placement, the distance threaded beyond the insertion needle/cannula tip should be minimized (3 to 5 cm). Do not feed the catheter more than 5 cm to avoid coiling and knotting around nerves.
- Sterilely secure the peripheral nerve catheter using one of many commercially prepared kits, sutures, and/or adhesive strips (Figure 34-5).
- To Tunnel or not to Tunnel?
  - Some initial studies have shown an extremely low rate of infection with subcutaneous tunneling of peripheral nerve catheters. Further randomized and controlled studies are needed to confirm decreased rates of infection as compared with nontunneling techniques for securing nerve catheters.[5]
  - A commonly used technique for tunneling catheters:
    - Using 1% to 2% lidocaine, provide superficial anesthesia to the skin 3 cm lateral to the insertion site of your peripheral nerve catheter.
    - Using an 18-gauge (G) AngioCath or other non-safety IV catheter, insert 3 cm lateral to the insertion site of the peripheral nerve catheter or simply away from the surgical site.
    - Aim the IV catheter (and needle) to come out 3 to 4 mm cephalad to the insertion site of the peripheral nerve catheter.
    - Remove the needle from the IV catheter and dispose off safely.
    - Run the peripheral nerve catheter retrograde through the IV catheter (and through the subcutaneous tunnel you just created).
    - Withdraw the IV catheter through the skin while holding the now tunneled peripheral nerve catheter.
  - Of course, if you are tunneling, you cannot connect the injection port to the proximal end of the peripheral nerve catheter to inject anesthetic before this step.
  - Secure with one of many commercially available kits, sterile adhesive strips, and/or sutures.

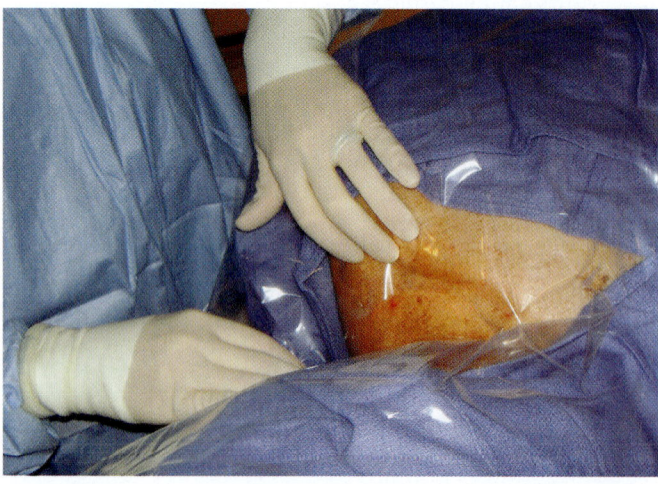

FIGURE 34-1 Sterile prep and drape for placement of posterior interscalene catheter.

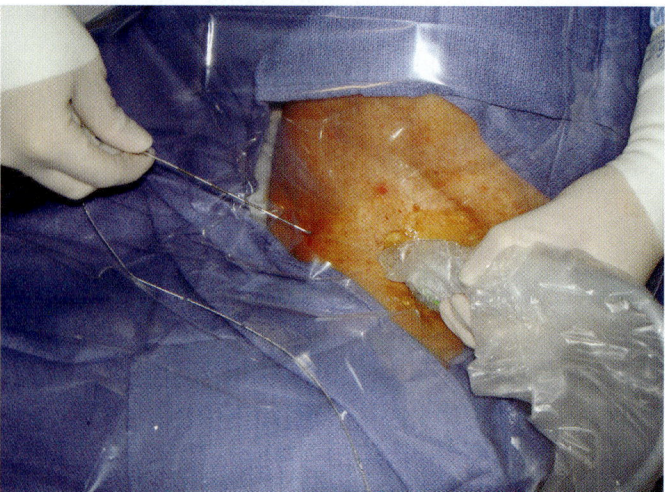

FIGURE 34-2 In-plane ultrasound technique to visualize brachial plexus for placement of posterior interscalene peripheral nerve catheter.

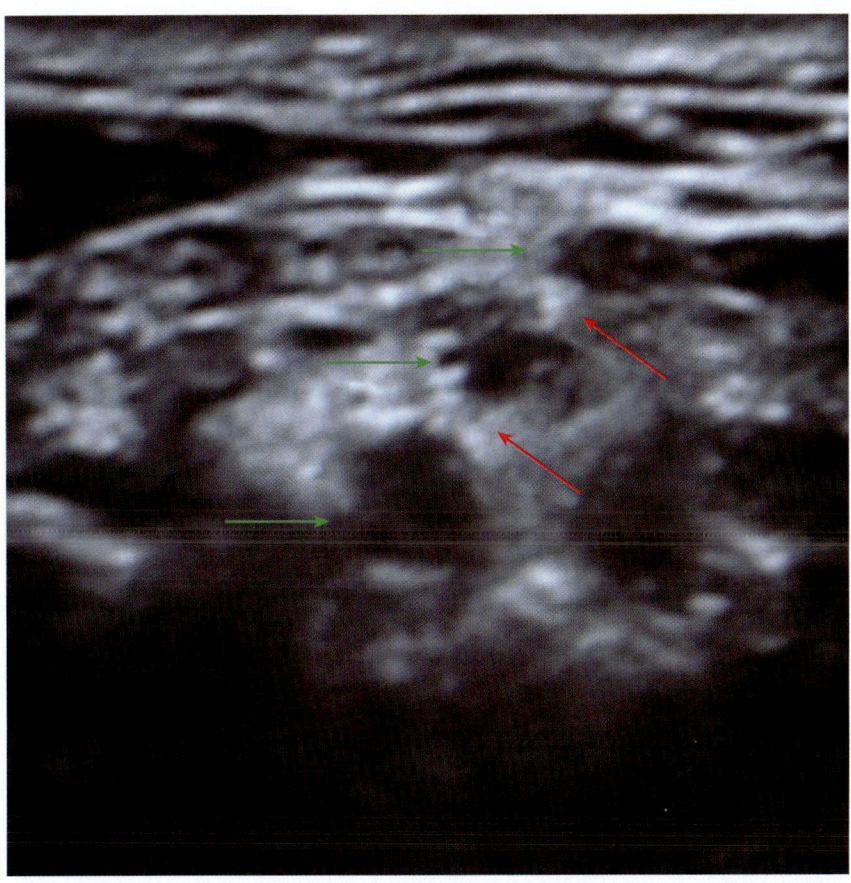

FIGURE 34-3 Ultrasound view of C5-C7 nerve roots (green arrows). Note the transverse processes of C5 and C6 (red arrows) underlying their respective nerve roots. Also note that the C7 transverse process is less prominent.

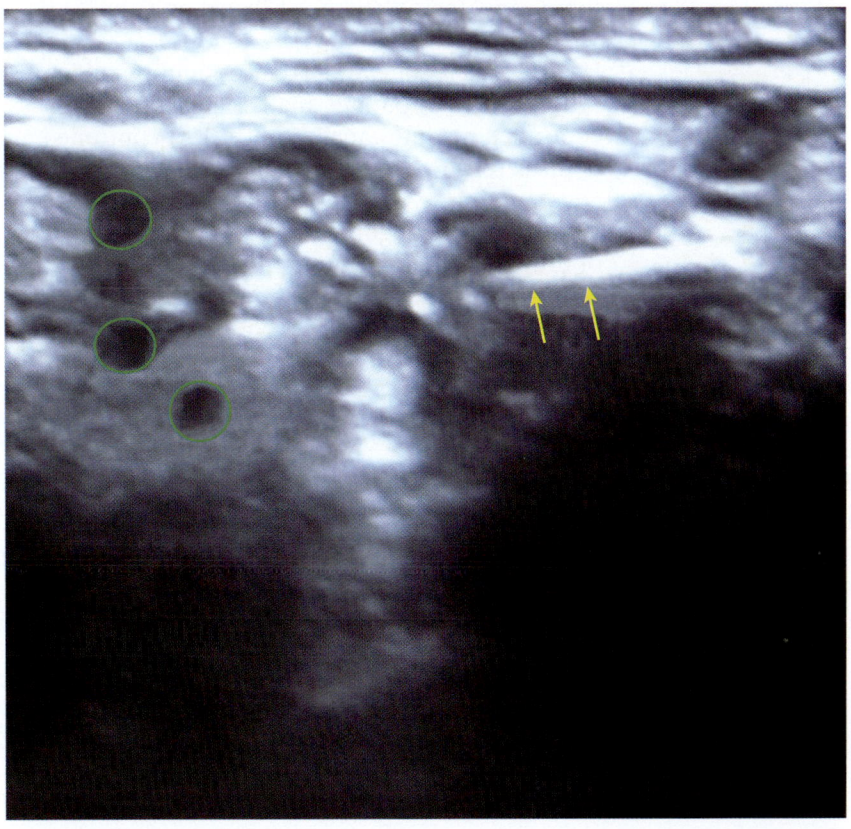

FIGURE 34-4 Ultrasound in-plane view of advancing the Tuohy needle (yellow arrows) toward targeted nerve roots (highlighted in green).

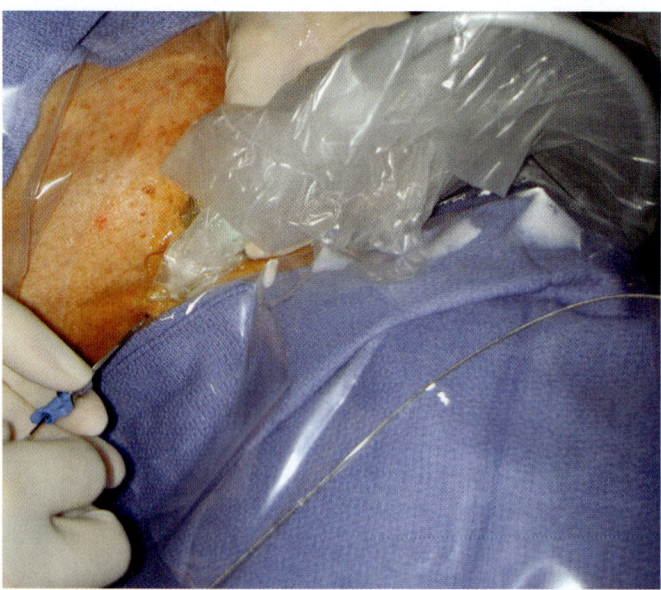

FIGURE 34-5 Feeding the peripheral nerve catheter through the placement needle after correct placement using ultrasound.

TABLE 34-1 American Society of Regional Anesthesia Pain Resource Center[8] Recommended Dosing for Patient Controlled Analgesia (Using 0.2% Ropivacaine)

Catheter Site	Basal Rate	Bolus Dose	Lockout Interval
Brachial plexus	6–8 mL/h	4 mL	30 min
Femoral nerve	4–6 mL/h	2–4 mL	30–60 min
Lumbar plexus	4–6 mL/h	2–4 mL	30–60 min
Sciatic nerve	6–8 mL/h	4 mL	30–60 min

Choice of Drugs

- Bupivacaine and ropivacaine are most commonly used for continuous infusion in peripheral nerve catheters.
- Studies suggest that ropivacaine is less cardiotoxic while providing less motor block with equal analgesia (as compared with bupivacaine).[6]
- Addition of epinephrine (5 µg/cc) increases the duration of single-injection nerve blocks by up to 100% to 200% and also decreases blood levels of local anesthetic 20% to 30% via vasoconstriction.[6] Potentiation of ropivacaine may be less compared with other local anesthetics.[6]
  - Most importantly, the use of epinephrine with local anesthetics allows early detection of intravascular injection.
  - However, epinephrine also has the potential to cause ischemic neuropathy via concentration-dependent reductions in neural blood flow by 20% to 35%.[6]
- The addition of clonidine (0.1 µg/kg) to single-shot local anesthetic bolus also provides a 50% to 100% increase in analgesic duration.[6]
  - Clonidine acts to further decrease nerve transmission through pain fibers (with local anesthetic).
  - There is no evidence of increased hypotension or sedation with the use of (1 µg/cc) clonidine in continuous local anesthetic infusions.
- Theoretically, there is no role for adjuvant opiate therapy in local anesthetic solutions for peripheral nerve blockade.
  - There is a paucity of opiate receptors located at sites for continuous plexus analgesia.
- In comparing dosing regimens (basal only, bolus only, versus basal and bolus):
  - Having a basal rate allows for optimum patient satisfaction and patient analgesia, while patient controlled epidural analgesia (PCEA) controlled boluses result in lower overall local anesthetic consumption.[7]
  - While there is no gold-standard for the choice of drugs used for peripheral nerve catheters, ropivacaine 0.2% is a very common choice.
- Remember to test the catheter with Epinephrine/local anesthetics before starting the infusion (Table 34-1).

COMPLICATIONS

- Using dilute solutions of local anesthetic with hourly infusion rates of 5 to 10 cc virtually eliminates any risk of local anesthetic toxicity (see drug selection, above).
- Learn to recognize signs of local anesthetic toxicity: metallic taste, perioral numbness, tinnitus, drowsiness, dizziness, restlessness, respiratory depression, seizure, cardiovascular system depression, and coma.

- Infection
  - Studies show that for inpatients, incidence of catheter infection ranges from 0% to 3.2%.[9]
  - Outpatient infection rates are usually less than 1%.[9]
  - ASRA guidelines recommend maximum sterile precautions for peripheral nerve catheter insertion, including sterile hand washing, sterile prep and drape with alcohol-based chlorhexidine solutions, sterile gloves, and use of surgical hats/masks.
  - Sterile precautions should also be used for filling infusion pumps.
- Neurologic complications and injury
  - Studies show incidence of neurologic injury ranging from 0.3% to 2%.[9]
  - Neurologic symptoms are often transient.
  - Injury can occur both during the block and in the postoperative period.
  - Case reports have also shown postdischarge injuries in patients with peripheral nerve catheters, most often from neglect injuries in extremities with little or no sensation.
    - Proper positioning is key!!
    - Must always balance the level of analgesia while maintaining some degree of motor function, sensation, and proprioception.
  - With lower extremity catheters, always instruct patients not to bear weight on the affected extremity to minimize the risk of falls.
- When sending patients home with peripheral nerve catheters, patient education on the specific delivery system being used and on potential complications from nerve catheters is key!
  - Last word of wisdom: you cannot have a successful PNC service unless you have a dedicated acute pain service that makes rounds on the patients daily and is available for consultations 24/7.

CONCLUSION

- Continuous peripheral nerve blockade provides flexibility and mobility.
  - Selective nerve blockade allows for earlier ambulation (compared to general anesthesia) and avoids hospital admission for certain patient populations.
  - Catheters allow for a prolonged infusion of a more dilute local anesthetic solution (compared to single-shot nerve blockade techniques), possibly providing an increased safety margin.
- There are few contraindications to placement of peripheral nerve catheters.
  - Infection at the desired site for catheter placement is one of the few contraindications for this procedure.
  - Clean the site properly and use sterile technique (cap, gown, gloves, drape).
- Double-check patient monitors and resuscitation equipment before proceeding.
- If planning on confirming placement using a stimulating catheter (as opposed to a stimulating placement needle), do NOT first inject local anesthetic through the placement needle before catheter placement/stimulation.
- Advance the catheter only 3 to 5 cm beyond the tip of the placement needle to avoid coiling.
- Higher currents may be needed to elicit a motor response with a stimulating catheter as compared with a stimulating introducer needle/cannula.
- When discharging patients with peripheral nerve catheters, education on proper care and recognition of complications are key!
  - There must be a dedicated acute pain service for support 24/7.

REFERENCES

1. Al-Kaisy AA, Chan VWS, Perlas A. Respiratory effects of low dose bupivacaine interscalene block. *Br J Anaesth* 1999;82:217–220.
2. Ilfield BM, Mariano ER, Williams BA, Woodard JN, Macario A. Hospitalization costs of total knee arthroplasty with a continuous femoral nerve block. *Reg Anesth Pain Med* 2007;32:46–54.
3. Horlocker TT, Wedel DJ, Rowlingson JC, et al. Regional anesthesia in the patient receiving antithrombotic or thrombolytic therapy. *Reg Anesth Pain Med* 2010;35:64–101.
4. Phamdang C, Kick O, Collet T, Gouin F, Pinaud M. Continuous peripheral nerve blocks with stimulating catheters. *Reg Anesth Pain Med* 2003;28:83–88.
5. Compère V, Legrand JF, Guitard PG, et al. Bacterial colonization after tunneling in 402 perineural catheters: a prospective study. *Anesth Analg* 2009;108:1326–1330.
6. Liu SS, Salinas FV. Continuous plexus and peripehral nerve blocks for postoperative analgesia. *Anesth Analg* 2003;63:263–272.
7. Ilfeld BM, Thannikary LJ, Morey TE, Griend V, Enneking FK. Popliteal sciatic perineural local anesthetic infusion: a comparison of three dosing regimens for postoperative analgesia. *Anesthesiology* 2004;101:970–977.
8. Continuous peripheral nerve blocks, 2010. http://www.asra.com/pain-resource-center-acute-pain-continuous-peripheral-nerve-blocks.php.
9. Swenson JD, Cheng GS, Axelrod DA, Davis JJ. Ambulatory anesthesia and regional catheters: when and how. *Anesthesiology Clin* 2010;28:267–280.

CHAPTER 35
KIDDIE NERVE BLOCKS

J. GABRIEL TSANG
RICHARD ELLIOTT

"Hold still!"

Many a parent

INTRODUCTION

The benefits of regional anesthesia apply to the pediatric population as much as they do to the adult population (adults are really just kids with years of psychological baggage). These benefits include, but are not limited to, decreased use of opioid analgesia, decreased requirement of intraoperative general anesthetics, and a decreased stress response.

The use of ultrasound for regional anesthesia has become more common in recent years and appears poised to dominate the practice of regional anesthesia for the near future. As such, the majority of the blocks described in this chapter are ultrasound-guided techniques. For the beginner, ultrasound images may look like you're hunting for a polar bear in a snow storm, but don't despair! With persistence and practice you'll find your target through the blizzard. For all procedures, follow your practice's guidelines for maintaining a sterile field.

SPECIAL CONSIDERATIONS FOR THE PEDIATRIC POPULATION

As you may have been told many times before, we cannot think of the pediatric patient simply as a small adult. But it is true that some things are miniaturized: smaller nerves, less space between anatomical structures, and immature neural structures. Such issues can frustrate our ability to get a good block. Read on for more details and helpful hints.

When comparing kids to adults, there are marked differences in physiology, anatomy, pharmacology, and psychology that we must know. Here's a quick list:

- Anatomy
  - Incomplete myelination of nerves (up to age 3): better penetration of local anesthetics to the nerve, but different appearance (the myelin sheath tends to be hyperechoic, **i.e. brighter**)
  - Loose perineurovascular sheath: facilitates greater spread of local anesthetic
  - Structures within the epidural space are more gelatinous and less fibrous than in adults: may affect the spread of local anesthetics and facilitate the threading of the epidural catheter
  - The spinal cord ends at L3 for neonates, rising to L1 by 1 year of age
- Physiology
  - Reduced hypotensive response to sympathectomy caused by neuraxial anesthesia: less likely to need preprocedure fluid bolus
  - Relatively higher cardiac output and regional blood flow: rapid systemic uptake may increase risk of toxicity
  - At less than 2 months of age infants have immature hepatic metabolism; dose amides carefully!
- Pharmacology
  - Children >6 months old have a larger volume of distribution; should tolerate relatively larger doses of local anesthetics
  - At less than 2 months there is a decrease in plasma proteins, such as α-1 acid glycoprotein. This results in higher amide local anesthetic concentrations; max amide dose lowered by 50%
- Psychology
  - It is very rare to find a child calm enough to tolerate a block while conscious (heck, it's hard to

get some to sit still for a haircut). Therefore, most of our blocks must be performed under general anesthesia.

A Few Words on Safety

- Use epinephrine where possible to detect intravascular injection. Do not use for end-arterioles (e.g., digital blocks and penile blocks); "No epi to nose, toes or hose."
- An increase of as little as 10 beats per minute may indicate a positive test dose with epinephrine (an inadvertent intravascular injection).
- Watch for changes in the electrocardiogram; 25% increase in T-wave amplitude may indicate an intravascular injection.
- Always aspirate before you inject!

NOW ON TO THE BLOCKS!

Block of Arnold (or Block the Auricular Branch of the Vagus) (Fig. 35-1)

- Commonly used for: myringotomy tube placement; some evidence to indicate that it is equivalent to intranasal fentanyl[1]
- Anatomy: This nerve provides sensory innervation to the external acoustic canal and the inferior tympanic membrane. The superficial portion of this nerve passes between mastoid process and the tympanic portion of the temporal bone.
- Equipment needed:
  - 30-gauge (G), ½-inch needle
  - 0.2 mL of 0.25% bupivacaine c 1:200,000 epi
- Technique:
  - Turn the head to the contralateral direction of the side to be blocked.
  - Pull the tragus away from the block.
  - Insert the needle just posterior to the tragus, piercing the cartilage.
  - Confirm placement with negative aspiration, then inject 0. 2 mL of 0.25% bupivacaine.

Trigeminal Nerve Blocks:
V1: Ophthalmic Division (Fig. 35-2)

- Commonly used for: procedures that involve incision to the forehead region, e.g., nevus excisions, frontal craniotomies
- Anatomy: The supraorbital and supratrochlear nerves exit the skull from the supraorbital foramen. These two nerves are the terminal branches of V1. They provided sensory information to the forehead and anterior scalp.

- Equipment:
  - 27-G, 1-inch needle
  - 1 to 2 mL of 0.25% bupivacaine with 1:200,000 epinephrine
- Technique:
  - Locate the supraorbital notch.
  - Insert the needle perpendicular to face.
  - Hit bone, withdraw slightly, then inject.
  - Direct the needle medially to ensure block of the supratrochlear nerve.
  - Withdraw needle and hold pressure on procedure site to minimize hematoma formation.

V2: Maxillary Division (Fig. 35-3)

- Commonly used for: cleft lip and various nasal surgeries
- Anatomy: The infraorbital nerve is the terminal branch of V2 and our target here. It exits the skull from the infraorbital foramen (think: around cheek bone, just below eye).
- Equipment:
  - 27-G, 1- to 1½-inch beveled needle
  - 0.5 to 2 mL (depending on size/age of child) 0.25% bupivacaine with 1:200,000 epinephrine
- Technique: intraoral approach
  - Identify the infraorbital groove via palpation.
  - Fold the patient's lip back.
  - Guide the needle through the subsulcal groove, staying parallel to the canine tooth or first maxillary premolar on the ipsilateral side.
  - Hit bone, then inject (after negative aspiration).

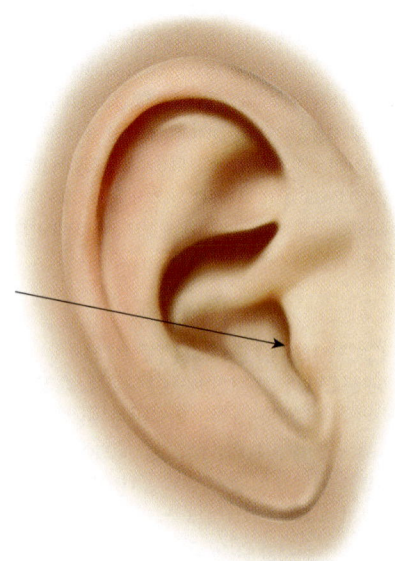

FIGURE 35-1 Block of Arnold. *Arrow* denotes direction of needle. Remember to head behind the tragus.

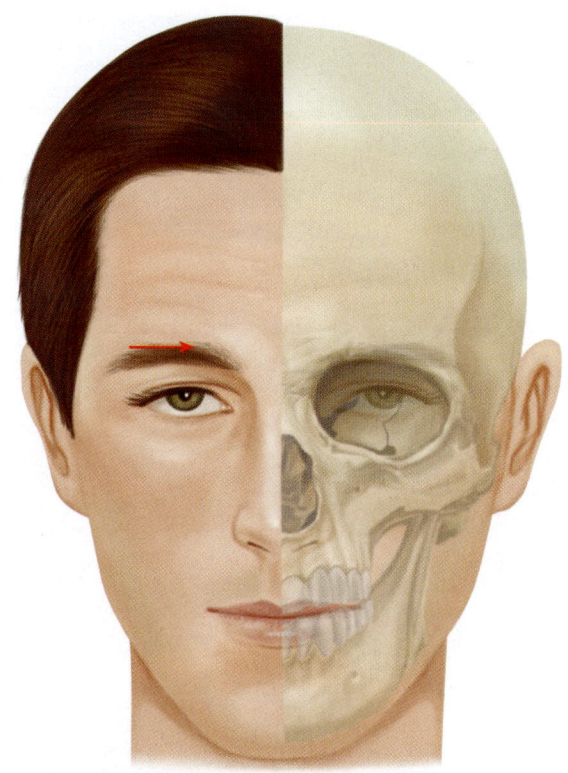

FIGURE 35-2 V1 block. This image shows an "older child" (he's had a hard life). The landmarks remain the same regardless of age. *Arrow* denotes direction of needle.

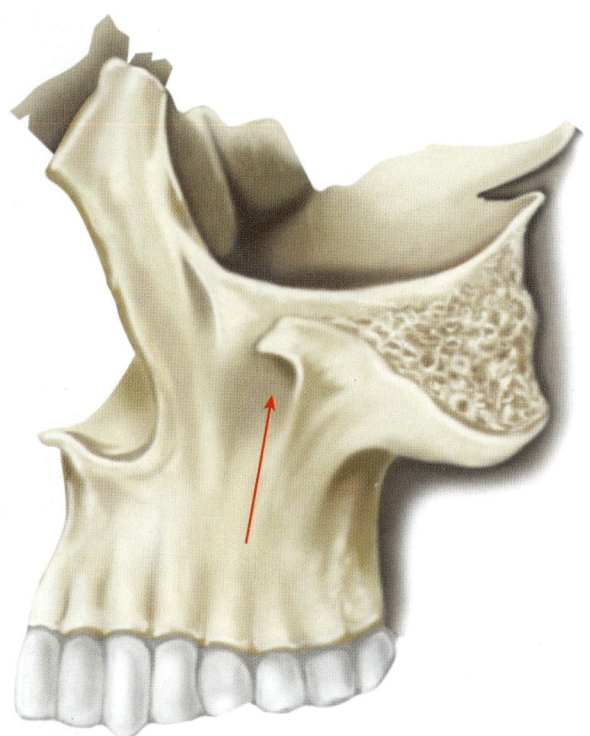

FIGURE 35-3 V2 block. A view of the underlying skeletal anatomy. *Arrow* denotes direction of needle, pointing toward the infraorbital foramen.

Upper Extremity Blocks

- Standard equipment recommendations:
  - Ultrasound (US) with 7- to 13-MHz linear probe; use the lower frequencies for deeper structures (for older or just chubbier kids)
  - Short beveled, 22- to 25-G, 35- to 50-mm needles
  - 0.2 to 0.5% ropivacaine or 0.5% bupivacaine; avoid using >0.5 mL/kg

Typically, the larger the probe, the lower the frequency. Remember, with lower frequencies you gain depth, but you lose definition in your image. Luckily, in pediatrics we can usually get away with the smaller, 7- to 13-MHz linear probe for all blocks. But for those kids who've had one too many French fries, the 4- to 8-MHz curvilinear probe may be more appropriate for the deeper blocks, e.g., subgluteal sciatic nerve block.

Axillary Block (Fig. 35-4)

- Commonly used for: hand and arm surgery (below shoulder); appropriate for syndactyly repair
- Anatomy: The brachial plexus branches should lie just inferior to the axillary artery.
- Ultrasound road map:
  - Median nerve: relatively superficial, sandwiched between the axillary artery and the biceps brachii
  - Ulnar nerve: lies medial and superficial to axillary artery
  - Radial nerve: lies just deep to the artery
  - Musculocutaneous nerve: This one may not be easy to find in young children. If detectable, it should be between the biceps brachii and coracobrachialis.
- Technique:
  - Place the patient supine with the shoulder externally rotated and abducted to 90 degrees. Flex the patient's arm at the elbow to 90 degrees (think: waving "hi," or throwing a ball).
  - Align the US probe so that it lies transverse to the humerus.
  - Direct the needle in plane to the US probe (i.e., parallel to beam).
  - Identify structures: trace the nerves distal and proximal if there is any doubt.
  - Block the deep nerves first, and move superficial, to minimize distortion of the anatomy.
  - The musculocutaneous nerve may lie above the biceps muscle.

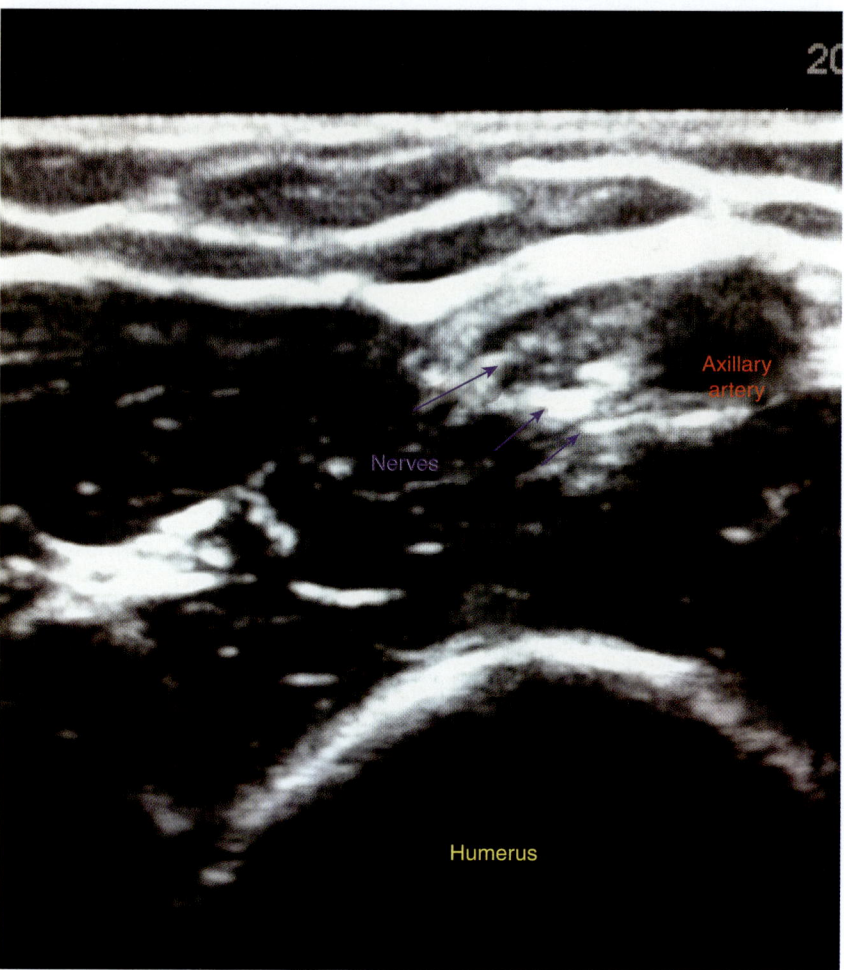

FIGURE 35-4 Axillary nerve block. This is the ultrasound image you should try to obtain. The labels indicate where the nerves (*blue arrows*), the humerus, and the axillary artery are.

Supraclavicular Block (Fig. 35-5)

- Commonly used for: Upper arm (mid-humerus) to hand
- Anatomy: Trunk level of brachial plexus, superior to subclavian artery
- Ultrasound road map:
  - The brachial plexus appears as a hypoechoic "cluster of grapes."
  - Subclavian artery is deep and medial to the plexus.
  - Scalenus anterior muscle is medial to the plexus.
- Technique:
  - Align the US probe in the coronal oblique plane (think: parallel to clavicle) at the upper border of the clavicle.
  - Move lateral to medial to find the subclavian artery.
  - Identify structures.
  - Insert needle from lateral to medial toward the plexus; keep the needle in plane to the US probe.
  - "Pop" through the nerve sheath and inject deep to superficial. Look for the "donut sign" (hypoechoic halo around nerves) as a sign of success.

Note: be vigilant regarding the potential of a pneumothorax. Even if you swear it was the easiest block you've ever placed, bad things do happen.

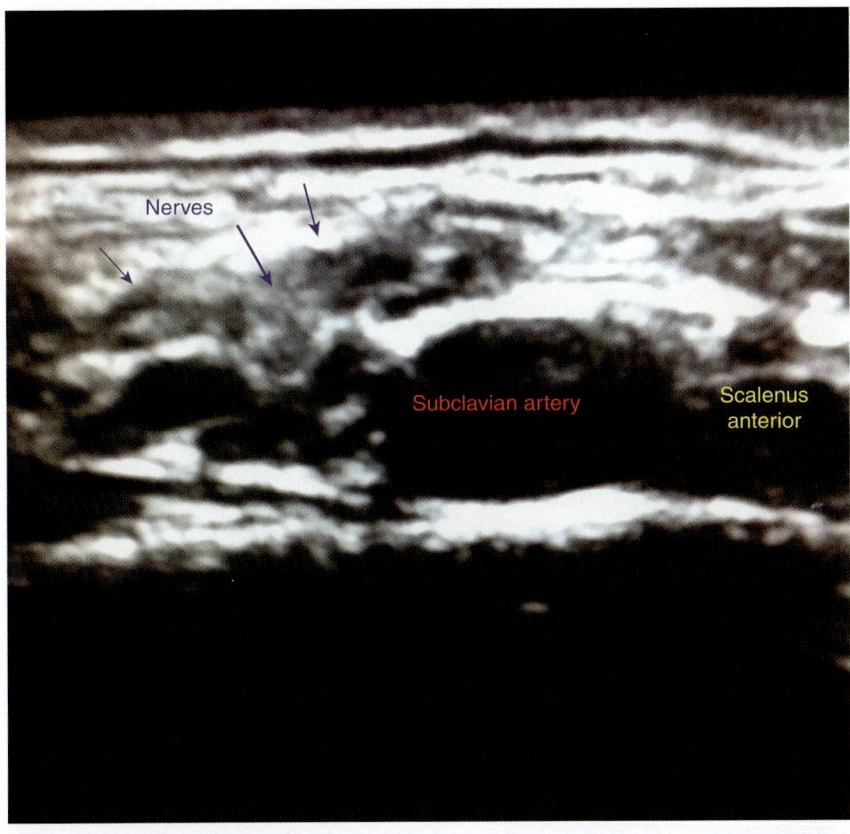

FIGURE 35-5 Supraclavicular nerve block. This is the ultrasound image you should try to obtain. The labels indicate where the nerves (*blue arrows*), subclavian artery, and scalenus anterior muscle are. Remember, try to aim the needle "below" the nerves.

Infraclavicular Block (Fig. 35-6)

- Commonly used for: arm/hand procedures
- Anatomy: Cord level of the brachial plexus; medial and inferior to coracoid process
- Ultrasound road map: The plexus lies deep and medial to the pectoralis muscles. The medial cord lies near the axillary artery and vein. The posterior cord is deep to the axillary vessels. The lateral cord is cephalad to the axillary artery.
- Technique:
  - Align the ultrasound probe in the parasagittal plane (perpendicular to clavicle) just medial and inferior to coracoid process.
  - Identify the structures.
  - Drive the needle cephalad to caudad, in plane to the US beam.
  - Aim the needle to the posterior cord.
  - After negative aspiration, inject around the nerves.

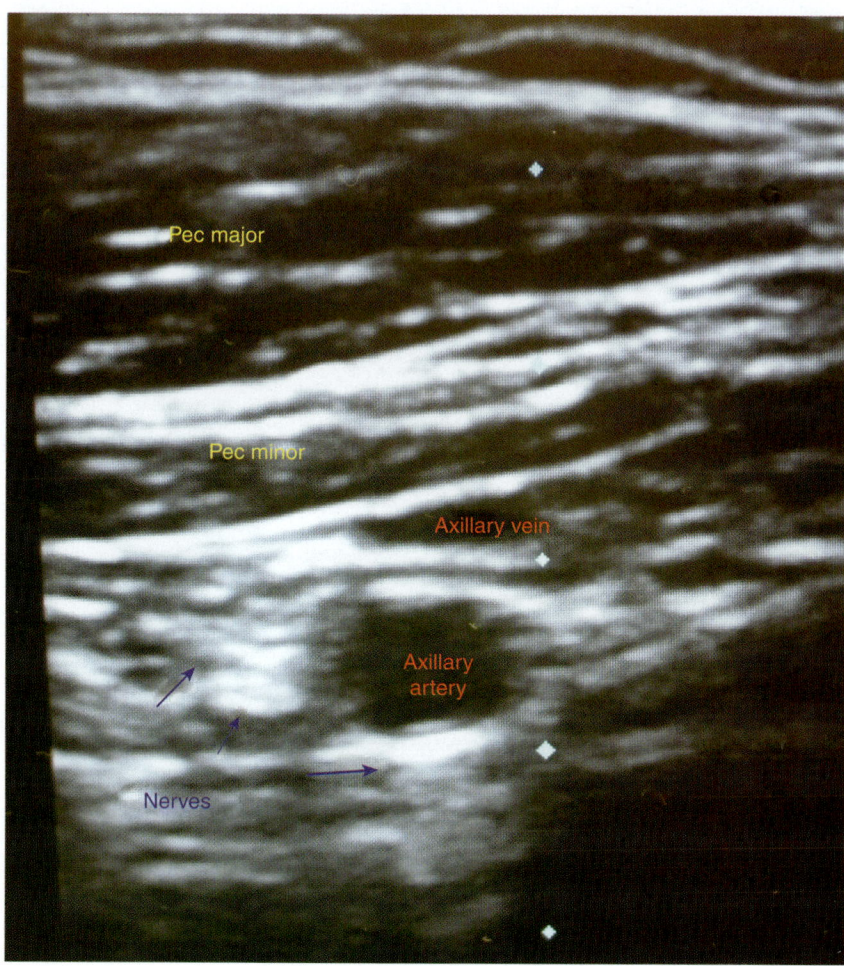

FIGURE 35-6 Infraclavicular nerve block. This is the ultrasound image you should try to obtain. The labels indicate where the nerves *(blue arrows),* axillary vein, axillary artery, and pectoralis muscles are.

Lower Extremity Blocks
- Standard equipment recommendations:
  - Same as above

Femoral Nerve Block
- Commonly used for: anterior thigh, knee procedures
- Anatomy: The femoral artery is the key landmark. It lies medial to the nerve and lateral to the vein.
- Ultrasound road map:
  - Vein and artery are medial to the nerve as described above.
  - The fascia lata is a linear hyperechoic structures that lies superficial to the femoral nerves and vessels.
  - The fascia iliaca lies just on top of the femoral nerve.
  - The femoral nerve appears as a hyperechoic bundle.
- Technique:
  - After identifying the location of the femoral artery via palpation, place the US probe over the area, parallel and inferior to the inguinal ligament.
  - With the needle, approach the nerve laterally, in-plane to the probe.
  - As the needle punctures the fascia, there may be a slight "popping" sensation.
  - With the needle at the deep margin of the nerve, inject the local anesthetic, looking for medial and lateral spread.

Sciatic Nerve Block: Subgluteal Approach
- Commonly used for: surgery on lateral aspect of lower leg and ankle, tibia/fibula and foot
- Anatomy: deep to gluteus maximus, lateral to the origin of the biceps femoris, lateral to ischial tuberosity
- Ultrasound road map:
  - The cortex of the greater trochanter appears as a hyperechoic structure lateral and deep to the nerve.
  - The nerve itself appears as an elliptical, hyperechoic structure.
- Technique:
  - Place the child in the lateral decubitus position, procedure side up.

- Flex the operative hip and knee (aka Sims' position).
- Place the US probe parallel to the gluteal crease; a lower frequency may offer a better view due to depth.
- Insert needle in-plane to US probe; inject local anesthetic so that it surrounds the nerve.

Popliteal Nerve Block (Fig. 35-7)

- Commonly used for: ankle/foot procedures
- Anatomy: The sciatic nerve in this position is bordered by the hamstring muscles. The semimembranosus and semitendinosus lay superomedially, and the biceps femoris superolaterally. The branch point of the nerve, into the tibial and peroneal nerves, is variable.
- Ultrasound road map:
  - The popliteal artery is deep and medial to the nerve.
  - Trace the sciatic nerve cephalad and caudad to identify the location of the bifurcation into tibial and peroneal nerves. The nerves appear as round, relatively hyperechoic structures.
  - The femoral condyles may not be readily visible (i.e., as hyperechoic structures), as they are mostly cartilaginous in young children (1 to 3 years old).
- Technique:
  - Place the patient the supine or in Sims' position.
  - Place the US probe at the superior border of the popliteal crease.
  - Scan cephalad and caudad until the bifurcation of the sciatic nerve is noted.
  - Position the probe just proximal to the bifurcation.
  - Approach the sciatic nerve with the in-plane to the probe.
  - Start injection at the deep border of the nerve; aim to get the donut sign.

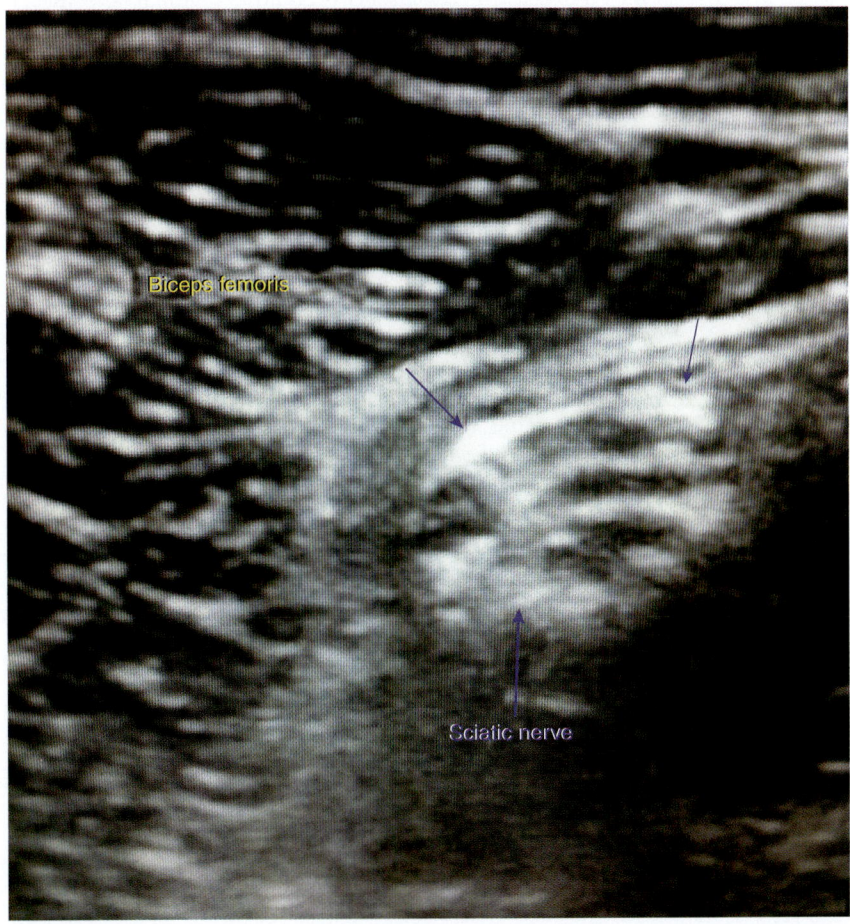

FIGURE 35-7 Popliteal/sciatic nerve block. This is the ultrasound image you should try to obtain. The *blue arrows* surround the nerve, with the biceps femoris labeled superolaterally.

Ilioinguinal (and Iliohypogastric) Nerve Block

- Commonly used for: inguinal hernia repair, orchidopexy
- Anatomy: a branch of the first lumbar nerve; lies lateral to the psoas major; passes through the transverse abdominus near the anterior portion of the iliac crest
- Ultrasound road map:
  - The anterior superior iliac spine appears as a large hypoechoic structure lateral to the nerve.
  - The ilioinguinal nerve is medial to the iliohypogastric nerve.
  - Both of the nerves are on the same plane, and appear as round hyperechoic structures.
  - The nerves are sandwiched between the hypoechoic layers of the internal oblique (superficially) and transverse abdominis (deep) muscle.
- Equipment: See above.
- Technique:
  - Place the US probe along the anterior superior iliac spine (ASIS), in horizontal alignment with the umbilicus.
  - Identify the muscle layers and the nerves.
  - Direct the needle, in-plane, with the tip pointed medially.
  - Hydrodissect the muscle layers from the nerves with a dextrose solution (just push enough fluid to get decent separation of the tissue planes).
  - Inject local anesthetic so that it surrounds the nerves.

Dorsal Penile Nerve Block

- Commonly used for: circumcisions/penile procedures
- Anatomy: This is a branch of the pudendal nerve. It is lateral to and paired with the dorsal arteries of the penis.
- Equipment:
  - 27-G, short beveled needle
  - 2 to 5 mL of 0.25% bupivacaine (no epinephrine; yes, this is the "hose")
- Technique:
  - Insert needle into infrapubic space/base of penis, until a pop is felt.
  - Aspirate, then inject ~1 mL of local.
  - Then withdraw needle slightly and direct it laterally to the each side of the shaft, depositing a couple of milliliters of local on either side.

ACKNOWLEDGMENT

Special thanks to Triska (triska@drawingblank.com) for providing the original illustrations for Figures 35-1 to 35-3.

REFERENCE

1. Voronov P, Tobin MJ, Billings K, Coté CJ, Iyer A, Suresh S. Postoperative pain relief in infants undergoing myringotomy and tube placement: comparison of a novel regional anesthetic block to intranasal fentanyl—a pilot analysis. *Pediatr Anesth* 2008;18(12):1196–1201.

SUGGESTED READING

Ross AK, Eck JB, Tobias JD. Pediatric regional anesthesia: beyond the caudal. *Anesth Analg* 2000;91:16–26.

Good review with excellent pictures. Good "how-to" guide for neurostimulator techniques, for those without access to an ultrasound.

Tsui BCH, Suresh S. Ultrasound imaging for regional anesthesia in infants, children and adolescents—a review of current literature and its application in the practice of extremity and trunk blocks. *Anesthesiology* 2010;112(2): 473–492.

An excellent review of ultrasound for regional anesthesia in the pediatric population. Excellent images.

Tsui BCH, Suresh S. Ultrasound imaging for regional anesthesia in infants, children and adolescents—a review of current literature and its application in the practice of neuraxial blocks. *Anesthesiology* 2010;112(3):719–728.

Part two of the review above.

Voronov P, Suresh S. Head and neck blocks in children. *Curr Opin Anaesthesiol* 2008;21(3):317–322.

Great review with excellent pictures. Doubles as a "how-to" guide on pediatric regional anesthesia for the head and neck.

CHAPTER 36
CHRONIC PAIN BLOCKS

BRIAN DURKIN

EPIDURAL STEROID INJECTION

Background

Epidural steroid injections (ESIs) are a common treatment option for many forms of low back pain and leg pain secondary to spinal stenosis, spondylolysis, or disk herniation. ESIs may also be performed in the cervical and thoracic regions to treat corresponding pain caused by irritated nerves. The steroid injected reduces the inflammation or swelling of nerves in the epidural space. This may in turn reduce pain, tingling, and numbness and other symptoms caused by nerve inflammation, irritation, or swelling. The effects of ESI tend to be temporary. Pain relief may last for several days or even years. The goal is to reduce pain so that the patient may resume normal activities and a physical therapy program.

Indications

Patients with pain in the neck, arm, low back, or leg (sciatica) may benefit from ESI. Specifically, those with the following conditions may benefit:
- Spinal stenosis
- Spondylolysis
- Herniated disks
- Degenerative disks
- Sciatica

Contraindications (Relative or Otherwise)

- Active infection
- Very high blood pressure
- Patients on anticoagulant therapy
- Hemorrhagic disorder
- Allergies to medications injected
- Local neoplasm
- Local vascular anomalies
- Elevated intracranial pressure

The Procedure

- Patients usually remain awake for the procedure. Sedatives can be given to help anxiety. If IV sedation is used, blood pressure, heart rate, and breathing are monitored during the procedure.
- The appropriate vertebral levels are selected based on clinical history, physical examination, and radiographic evidence (most commonly MRI).
- The patient is placed in a prone position on the table, and a fluoroscope is then used to identify the correct vertebrae.
- The patient is prepped and draped in an aseptic fashion and given a local anesthetic, which will numb the skin before the injection is given (Figure 36-1).
- The physician directs a Tuohy needle through the skin and between the spinous processes into the epidural space or spinal needle toward the neural (Figure 36-2).
- Fluoroscopy allows the clinician to watch the needle in real time on the fluoroscope monitor, thus ensuring that the steroid medication is delivered as close to the inflamed nerve root as possible. Some discomfort occurs, but patients typically feel more pressure than pain.
- Contrast is then injected through the needle to confirm epidural placement prior to injection of the corticosteroid (Figure 36-3).
- The needle is then withdrawn.

There are three ways to deliver steroids into the epidural space: interlaminarly, transforaminally, or caudally. The best method depends on the location and source of pain.

- The interlaminar approach places the needle between the lamina of two vertebrae directly

from the middle of the back. Medication is able to be delivered to the nerve roots on both the right and left sides of the inflamed area at the same time.
- The needle is placed to the side of the vertebra in the neural foramen, just above the opening for the nerve root and outside the epidural space for the transforaminal approach.
- Use of a contrast dye helps to confirm where the medication will flow when injected (Figures 36-4 and 36-5).
- This method treats one side at a time. It is preferred for patients who have undergone a previous spine surgery because it avoids any residual scars, bone grafts, metal rods, and screws.

Complications
- Spinal headache from a dural puncture
- Bleeding
- Infection
- Allergic reaction
- Nerve damage/paralysis (rare)
- Corticosteroid side effects may cause weight gain, water retention, flushing (hot flashes), mood swings, or insomnia, and elevated blood sugar levels in people with diabetes.

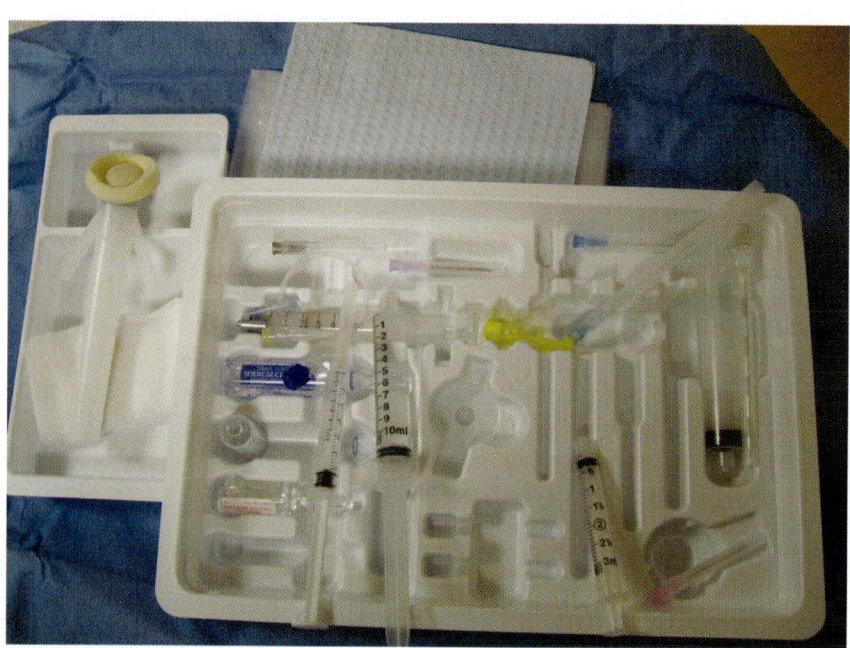

FIGURE 36-1 Basic disposable epidural kit.

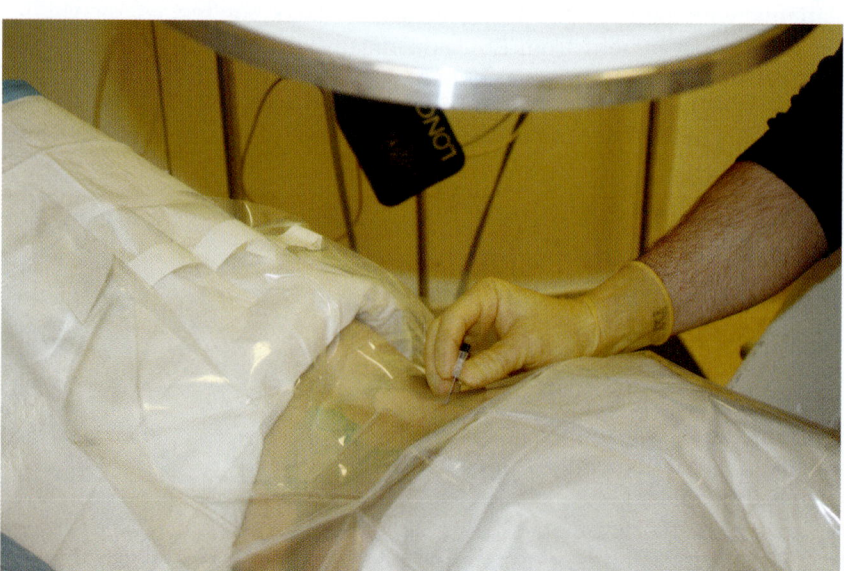

FIGURE 36-2 Fluoroscopically guided lumbar foraminal injection.

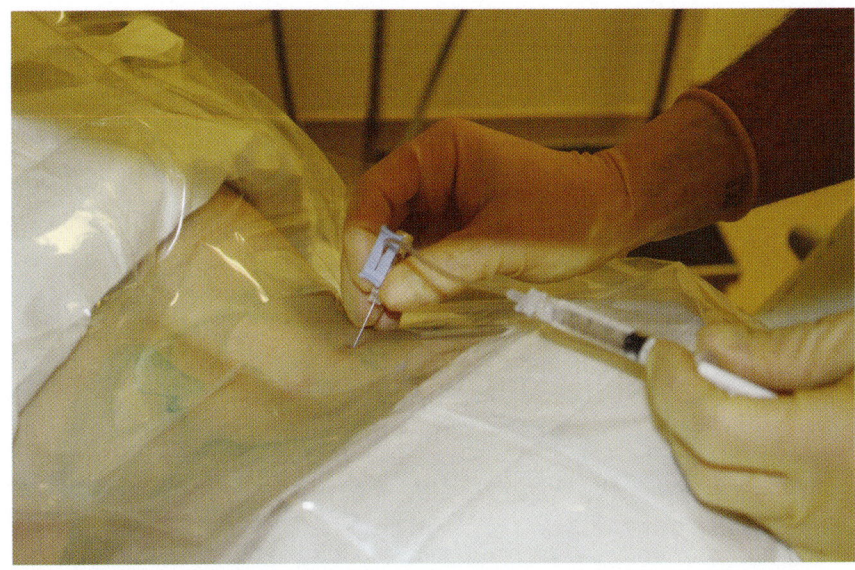

FIGURE 36-3 Injection of radiographic contrast.

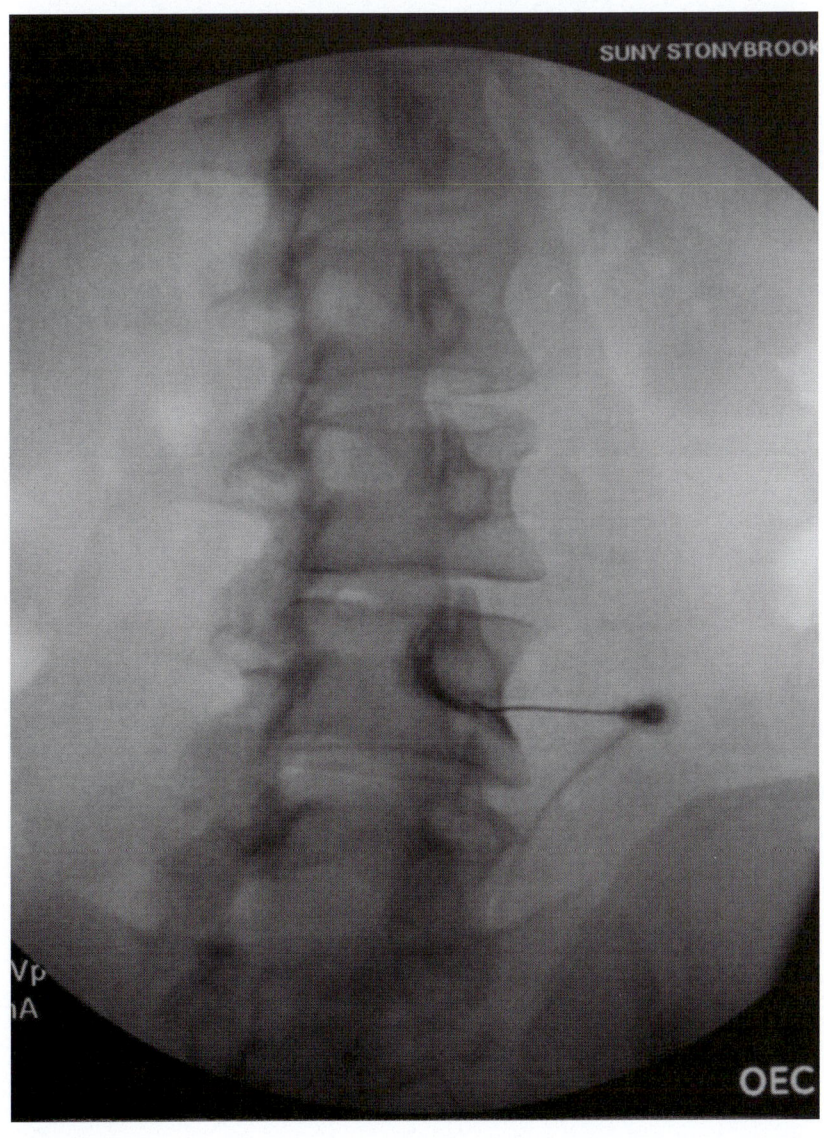

FIGURE 36-4 Oblique fluoroscopic view of contrast around the right L4 root.

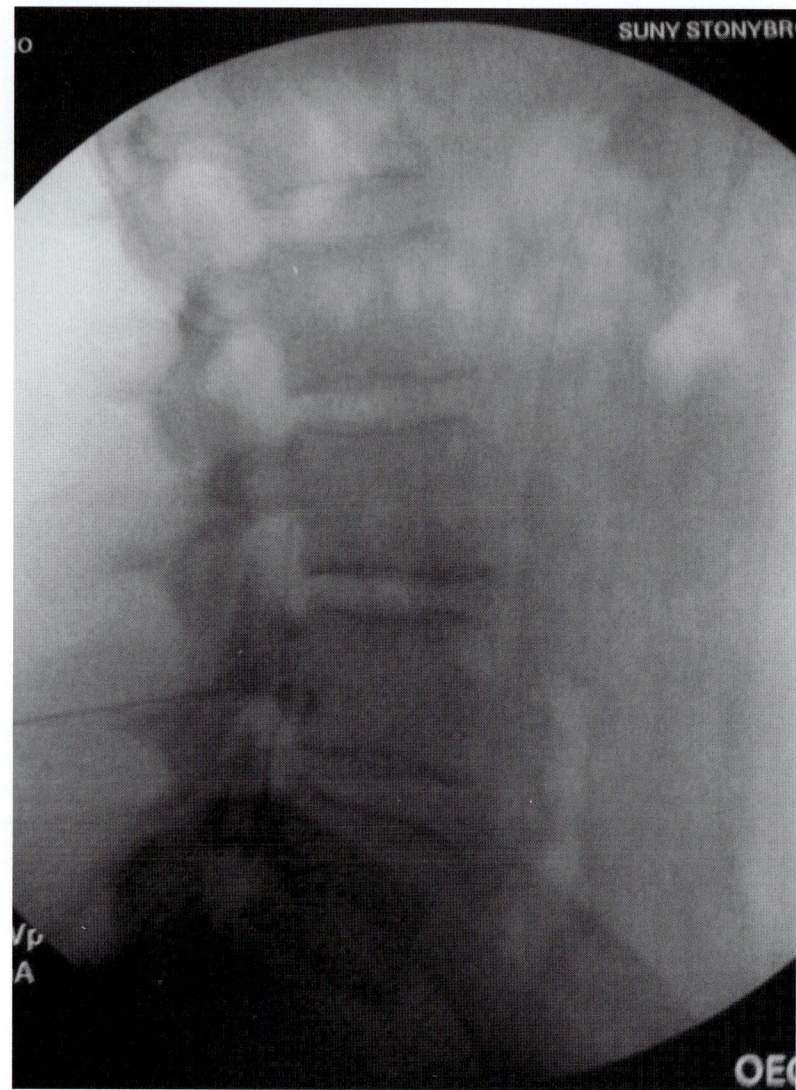

FIGURE 36-5 Lateral fluoroscopic view of contrast in the anterior lumbar epidural space.

STELLATE GANGLION BLOCK

Background

Sympathetic innervation of the head, neck, upper chest, and most of the arm is supplied by the cervical sympathetic chain, which is composed of superior, middle, intermediate, and inferior cervical ganglia. However, the inferior cervical ganglia and the first thoracic ganglia often fuse to form the stellate ganglion. Stellate ganglion blocks use an injection of local anesthetic into the anterior neck in order to diagnose or treat pain located in the head, neck, chest, or arm caused by sympathetically maintained pain. Stellate ganglion blocks may also be used to see if blood flow can be improved in disorders of circulation. Following the performance of a sympathetic block, the pain may not go away despite evidence of a sympathetic block, i.e., the pain is not responsive to sympathetic blocks, which is of diagnostic value; the pain does not go away, and there is no evidence of a sympathetic block, i.e., the block is a technical failure; or the pain goes away after the injection and stays away longer than the life of the local anesthetic, i.e., the block was of therapeutic value. The procedure will likely need to be repeated to achieve long-lasting benefit.

Indications

- Diagnosis and treatment of head, neck, arm, and upper chest pain syndromes
  - Sympathetically mediated pain syndromes (complex regional pain syndromes [CRPS] types I and II)

- Angina
- Postherpetic neuralgia/herpes zoster
- Neoplastic related pain
- Phantom limb pain
- Vascular headaches
- Vasospastic disease or vasculopathies of head, neck, and upper extremity
  - Raynaud's syndrome
  - CREST syndrome
- Treatment of circulatory insufficiency
  - Peripheral vascular disease
  - Revascularization after limb reimplantation

Contraindications (Relative or Otherwise)

- Active infection
- Very high blood pressure
- Patients on anticoagulant therapy
- Hemorrhagic disorder
- Allergies to medications injected
- Local neoplasm
- Local vascular anomalies

The Procedure

- The stellate ganglion is located medially to the scalene muscles, lateral to the longus coli muscle, esophagus, trachea, and recurrent laryngeal nerve, anterior to the transverse processes and prevertebral fascia, superior to the subclavian artery and posterior aspect of the plura, and posterior to the vertebral vessels at the seventh cervical level.
- Stellate ganglion blocks have traditionally been performed blindly by palpation using a paratracheal technique (Figure 36-6).
- With the patient's head extended, a 5-cm, 22-gauge needle is inserted at the medial edge of the sternocleidomastoid muscle just below the level of the cricoid cartilage, which corresponds to Chassaignac's tubercle (anterior tubercle of the C6 level). The needle is advanced to the tubercle and withdrawn 1 to 2 cm prior to injection.
- Careful aspiration must be done prior to injection to exclude unintentional intravascular injection (vertebral or subclavian arteries) or subarachnoid injection into a dural sleeve.
- The block is dependent on enough volume reaching the stellate ganglion to result in an effective block. This method also has a relatively high rate of inadequate block and adverse effects.
- Image-guided stellate ganglion blocks have the advantages of increased safety and accuracy compared with blind injections because the needle can be accurately placed close to the ganglion itself.
- A smaller amount of local anesthetic can be used, because of the close proximity of the needle to the ganglion, resulting in a decrease in adverse effects.
- The patient is placed in the supine position monitors are placed and the neck is prepped and draped in a sterile fashion (Figure 36-7).
- The stellate ganglion is identified using landmarks and fluoroscopic or ultrasound guidance.
- After injection of subcutaneous local anesthetic, a 5-cm, 25-gauge needle is inserted onto the anterior tubercle of the transverse process of C6 or C7 under direct visualization with fluoroscopy or ultrasound.
- Confirm negative aspiration of blood and cerebrospinal fluid (CSF).
- If using fluoroscopy, radiographic contrast medium is injected to confirm proper placement (Figures 36-8 and 36-9).
- A dilute volume of local anesthetic solution is injected to a total of 10 to 15 mL.
- The patient is then observed for signs of a successful block.
- Following successful placement of local, the skin temperature of the ipsilateral arm promptly increases along with the onset of Horner's syndrome.

Complications

- Vascular injury of internal jugular vein or carotid artery resulting in hematoma or hemothorax
- Traumatic neural injury of vagus nerve or the brachial plexus secondary to needle or intraneural injection
- Pneumothorax
- Chylothorax secondary to injury of thoracic duct
- Mediastinitis after inadvertent esophageal puncture
- Infectious process resulting in abscess, meningitis, and osteitis or osteomyelitis
- Accidental epidural or intrathecal injection of local anesthetic
- Brachial plexus block
- Hoarseness secondary to recurrent laryngeal nerve blockade
- Phrenic nerve block with loss of ipsilateral hemidiaphragm innervation and subsequent respiratory distress
- Intravascular injection with resultant seizure or cardiac arrest

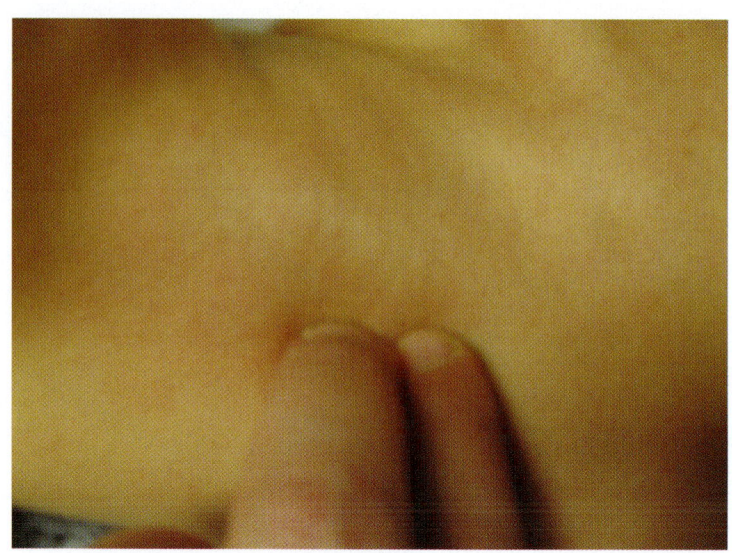

FIGURE 36-6 Palpating the left carotid artery.

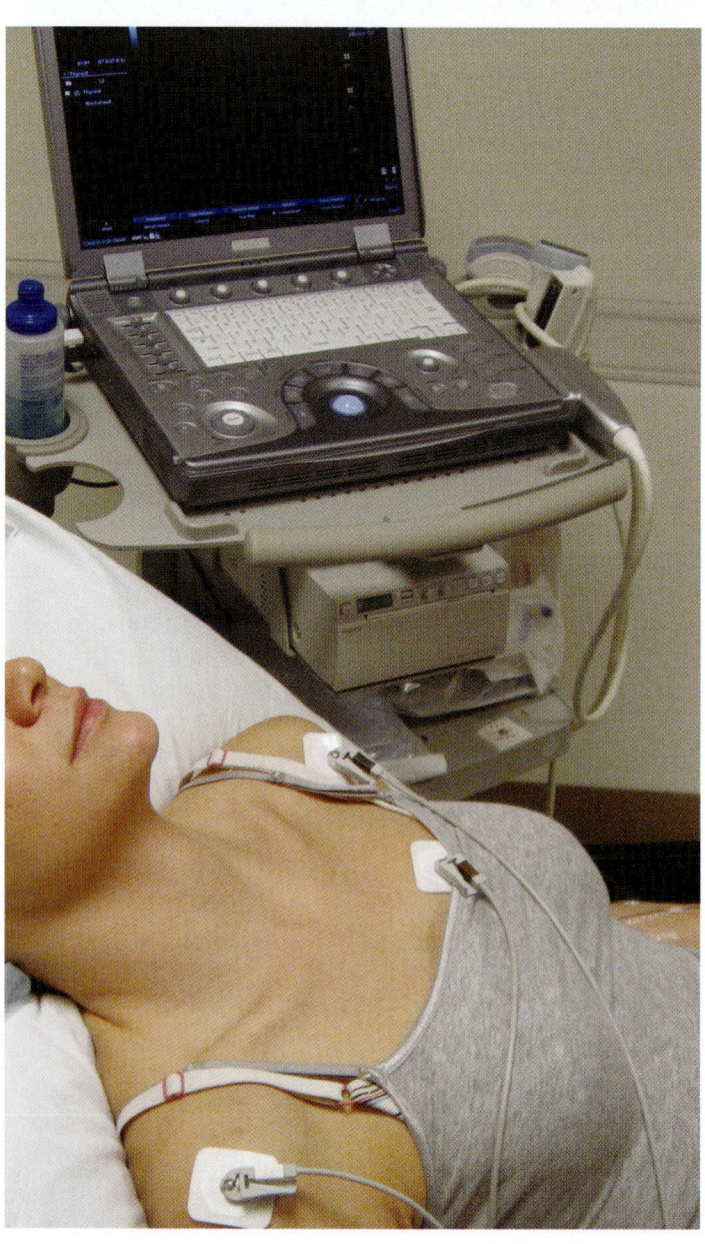

FIGURE 36-7 Getting ready for an ultrasound-guided stellate ganglion block.

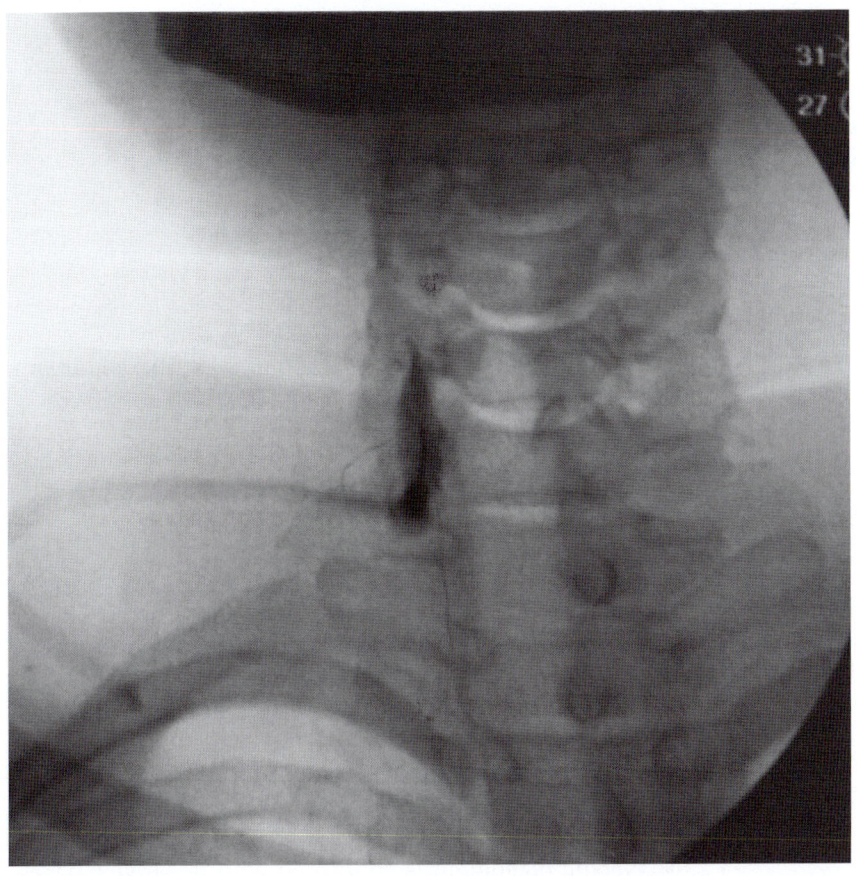

FIGURE 36-8 Anterior fluoroscopic view of contrast injection for right stellate ganglion block.

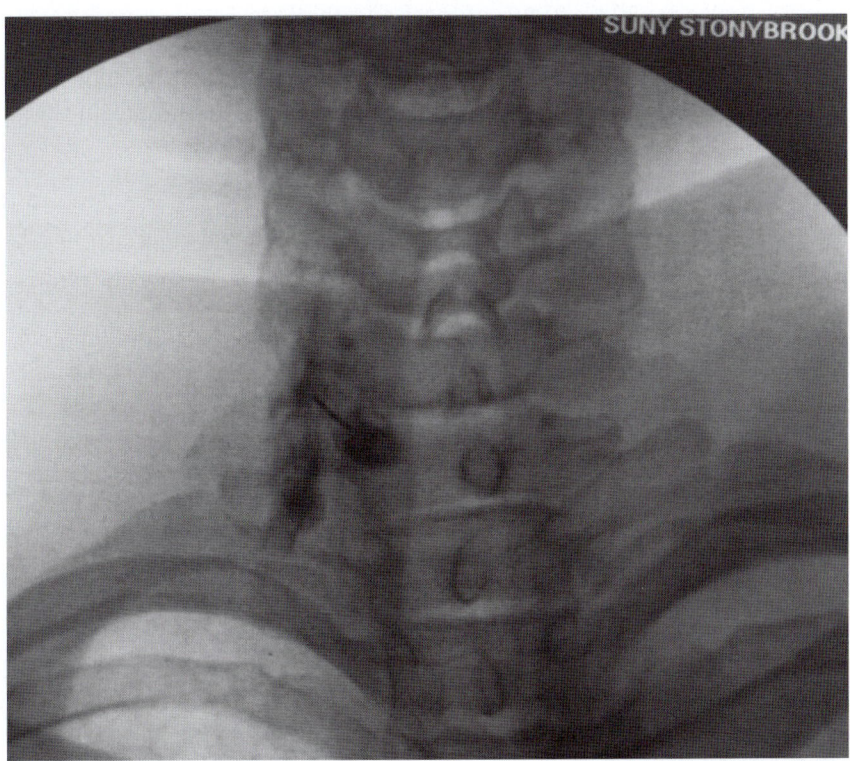

FIGURE 36-9 Fluoroscopic image of injectate spreading to C7–T1 level indicating probable right stellate ganglion block.

LUMBAR SYMPATHETIC BLOCK

Background

The lumbar sympathetic plexus is a collection of preganglionic and postganglionic efferent nerve fibers that provide sympathetic innervation the lower extremities. The paired lumbar sympathetic chains enter the retroperitoneal space under the right and left crura and travel inferiorly in the groove between the anterolateral vertebral bodies and the psoas muscle. The ganglia are usually posterior to the vena cava on the right and anterolateral to the aorta on the left. The white and gray rami communicans pass to their associated ganglia under the fibrous attachments of the psoas to the vertebral bodies, usually along the middle of the vertebral body. The ganglia of the lumbar sympathetic chain can be variable in position and number. Frequently there is a fusion of the L1 and L2 ganglia; rarely are five ganglia found on each side of an individual.

Evidence indicates the postganglionic sympathetic fibers may act at the effector terminal in addition to primary afferent sites in certain pathological states. The exact mechanism of the interaction remains unclear; however, blockade of the sympathetic efferent fibers may interrupt the function of the primary afferent neuron. Blockade of the lumbar sympathetic plexus may also block visceral afferent fibers from the lower extremities that travel with the sympathetic nerves.

Indications

Diagnosis and treatment of:
- Sympathetically maintained perineal pain
- Complex regional pain syndromes types I and II
- Postherpetic neuralgia
- Visceral pelvic pain
- Cancer pain
- Inoperable peripheral vascular disease and vasospastic disease of the lower extremities
- Phantom limb pain

Contraindications (Relative or Otherwise)

- Active infection
- Very high blood pressure
- Patients on anticoagulant therapy
- Hemorrhagic disorder
- Allergies to medications injected
- Local neoplasm
- Local vascular anomalies abdominal aortic aneurysm (AAA).

The Procedure

- The patient is placed in the prone position and the anterolateral border of the L2, L3, or L4 vertebral body is visualized using fluoroscopy (Figure 36-10).
- Once the chosen vertebral body is identified and after aligning the inferior end plate, the fluoroscope is rotated in order to place the superior articular process at one third of the inferior end plate.
- The patient is then prepped and draped in an aseptic fashion and a 22-gauge, 15-cm needle is advanced under fluoroscopy to the anterolateral aspect of the target vertebral body (Figure 36-11).
- Needle placement is confirmed with negative aspiration and contrast placement (Figures 36-12 and 36-13).
- After confirmation of the correct needle location, 20 to 40 mL of local anesthetic is administered.
- Upon completion of the block, the patient must be assessed for sympathectomy. Increasing skin temperature, decreasing pain, and anhidrosis in the distal extremity indicate a sympathectomy.

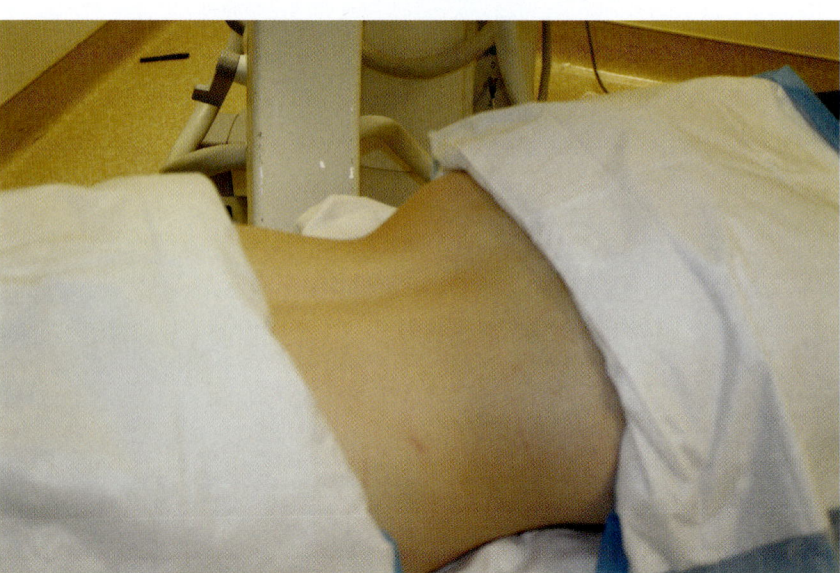

FIGURE 36-10 Positioning a patient for a lumbar sympathetic block.

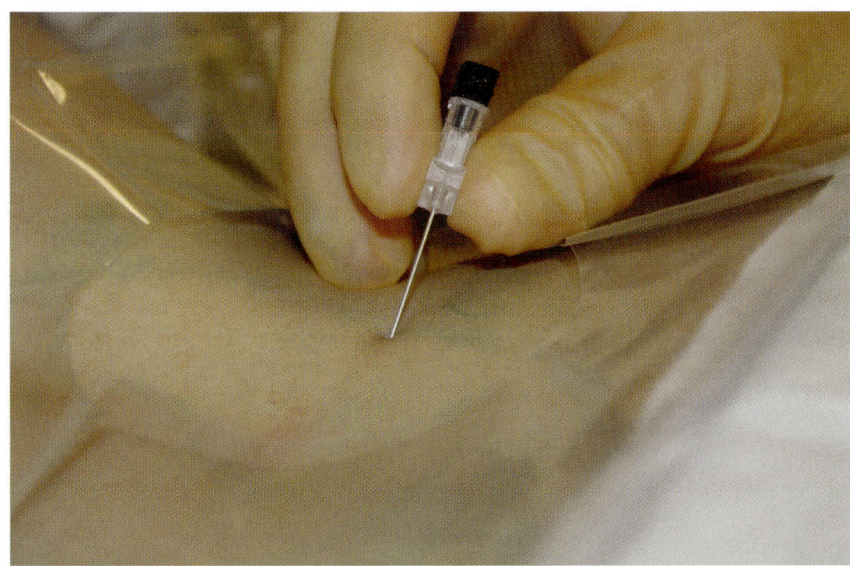

FIGURE 36-11 Placing the needle for a lumbar sympathetic block at L4.

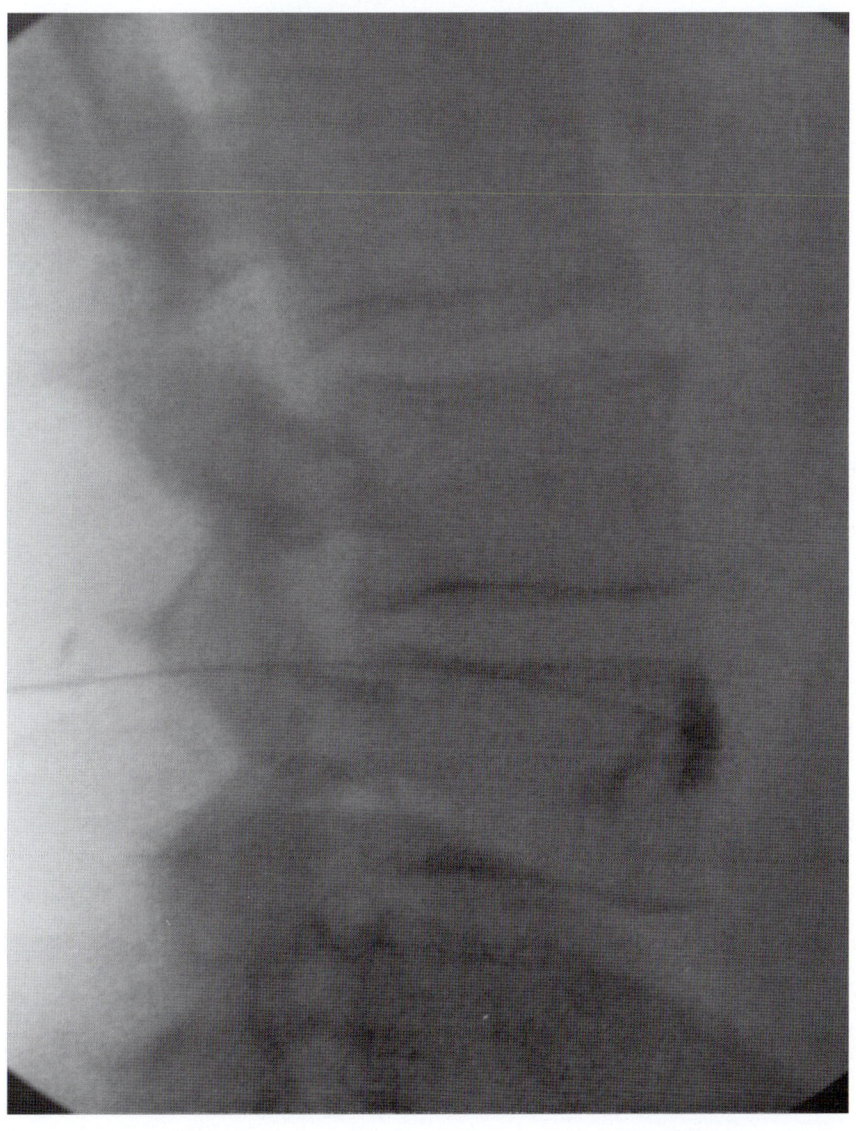

FIGURE 36-12 Lateral fluoroscopic view of right lumbar sympathetic block at L4.

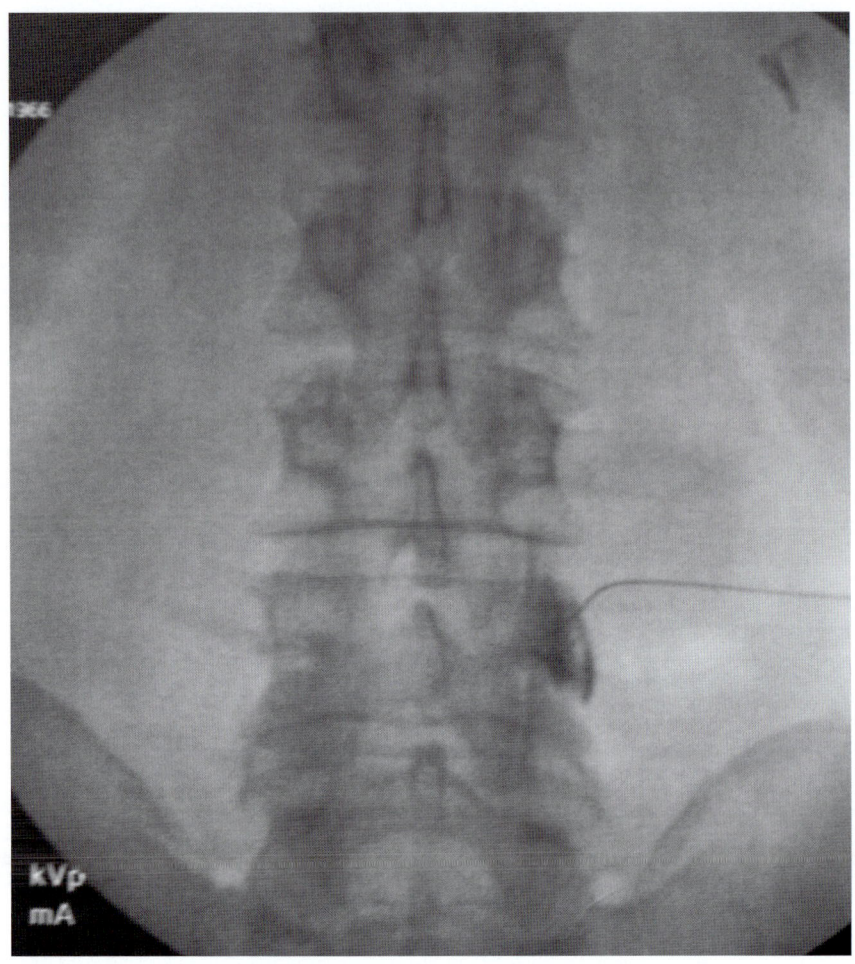

FIGURE 36-13 Anterior fluoroscopic view of right lumbar sympathetic block at L4.

Complications

- The most troublesome and frequent complication is simultaneous blockade of the L2 somatic nerve root.
- Inadvertent injection into the subarachnoid space, epidural space, intravascular (vena cava, aorta, lumbar vessels)
- Damage by needle or neurolytic solution to the kidneys, renal pelvis, ureters, and intervertebral disks
- Infection
- Mild backache
- Neuropathic pain
- Retroperitoneal hematoma
- Sympathalgia

- Destruction of sympathetic fibers produces cramping or burning pain in the anterior thigh.
- Sympathectomy-mediated hypotension
- Intravascular steal may occur in arteriosclerotic patients
- Failure of ejaculation: real risk after bilateral block. The risk must be explained to male patients.

SUGGESTED READING

Raj PP, Lou L, Erdine S, Staats PS, eds. *Interventional pain management: image-guided procedures,* 2nd ed. Philadelphia: Saunders/Elsevier, 2008.

Rathmell JP. *Atlas of image-guided intervention in regional anesthesia and pain medicine.* Philadelphia: Lippincott Williams & Wilkins, 2006.

CHAPTER 37
INSIGHTS ON OPHTHALMIC ANESTHESIA

STEVEN GAYER

"Aye yai yai, I have to block an eye, eye, eye!"
*Anonymous Anesthesiologist,
first day in private practice*

INTRODUCTION

- Ophthalmic anesthesia is mostly eye block + monitored anesthesia care (MAC). MAC is important because angina, arrhythmias, hypertension, apnea, hypoxia, hypercarbia, confusion, seizures, and more can occur (Figure 37-1). Personnel with airway and resuscitation skills must be immediately available.
- Most anesthesiologists skip the block and default to the ophthalmologist, claiming anesthetizing eyes is too risky. When was the last time you went to do an urgent C-section and told the obstetrician, "This patient's too risky, you do the block"?
- Real anesthesiologists know how to block eyes.

Philosophy

- Surgeons do retrobulbar blocks (RBBs) because (a) that's what they were taught way back when in residency, and (b) onset of anesthesia is almost immediate.
- Anesthesiologists perform peribulbar blocks (PBBs) because they are generally safer since (a) brainstem anesthesia is much less likely, (b) the odds of skewering the back of the eye are far less, and (c) damage to other key orbital structures is rare.
- The fact that more volume and time are needed is immaterial to the anesthesiologist who blocks patients awaiting surgery ahead of time in a holding area.

Indications

- Ophthalmologist's need for an akinetic, anesthetized eye. Corneal transplant, retina surgery, glaucoma surgery, enucleation, any procedure of long duration.
- Patient's need or desire for an akinetic, anesthetized eye. Hypernervousness, painful eye, etc.
- Anesthesiologist's need for a good day in the OR in the face of 10 to 20 eye surgery patients or a patient with difficult airway, crippled ventilatory status, or feeble cardiovascular function that would otherwise need an awake intubation or postoperative ventilation or an ICU bed after general anesthesia.

Contraindications

- Most are relative contraindications.
- Severe bleeding diathesis, ultra-gross infection, marked bony orbit deformation, actual honest-truth allergy to local anesthetics.
- If a patient will not be able to lie relatively still during surgery, the best option may be general anesthesia or postponing elective surgery until such time as the patient can repose tranquilly, allowing surgery via regional anesthesia and MAC.

Let's take a moment to reflect:
- Patients with longer than normal or deeply recessed eyes are at greater risk of having their globes skewered by a needle. Some patients have abnormal outpouched areas (staphylomata) in the side or back of the eye.
- Recessed eyes are noted by looking at the patient (interesting notion). Near-sighted people and those who had prior scleral buckle surgery have longer eyes. Eye length and shape are determined by ultrasound.

The most important preoperative test for eye patients is...?
- The CBC → No.
- The ECG → No.
- The U/A? → No.
- The serum porcelain level? → 'Fraid not.
- The ultrasound of the eye → Bingo! An ultrasound is a prerequisite for the ophthalmologist in order to determine the appropriate lens implant to insert and is done on every patient scheduled for *cataract* surgery (Figure 37-2). Due to the outpatient nature of cataract surgery, this information rarely is placed in patients' surgical charts (Figure 37-3). Be aware: it exists. If one intends to perform an eye block, ask the ophthalmologist for the ultrasound data. Confirm that the eye length is normal (<26 mm) and that the shape of the eye is normal (Figure 37-4). Write this down on the chart somewhere. Even if you just scrawl, "US OK per Ophth" or "US wnl," it indicates that you took eye length and shape into account before blocking the eye.

Equipment
- Standard stuff: pulse oximeter, rhythm monitor, blood pressure cuff, and O_2 by nasal cannula
- Clearly marked indicator of side-of-anesthesia and surgery on the patient
- Cap shouldn't be pulled down, obscuring that clearly marked indicator of side-of-anesthesia and surgery.
- RN or other assistant to confirm patient ID, consent, side-of-anesthesia, and to hold the patient's hand, eyelid open as needed, etc.
- Precautionary materials nearby: ampule of atropine and syringe (just in case of severe oculocardiac reflex). Narcotic and benzodiazepine reversal agents.
- Resuscitation equipment.
- Syringe of local anesthetic. A few units of hyaluronidase is always nice. Some prefer their hyaluronidase derived from sheep testicles rather than the bovine stuff. We don't think it matters. We don't bother adding epi since tachycardia from absorbed epi isn't always a good thing for elderly patients.
- Label on the syringe. We know of one poor soul who accidentally injected a syringe of unlabeled pentothal. Bad day.
- Needle. Long or short? The once commonly used 1.5" (38-mm) needle can reach the apex of the orbit in 20% of patients, so a shorter needle, ≤1.25" (31 mm), is more prudent. Sharp or dull? Controversial. More difficult to puncture an eye with a dull needle, but it causes more damage if the globe is penetrated. Sharp needles are less painful.
- Topical drops: optional prior to block
- Antiseptic prep
- Some gauze to wipe the shmutz away and keep the eye shut if needed
- An oculo-occlusive device to encourage the local to diffuse posteriorly; we usually just use digital pressure and skip the oculo-occluder

Technique
- Confirm you have the correct patient in front of you.
- Check the ultrasound data, if available.
- Make sure that you are about to block the proper side.
- Provide appropriate sedation.
- Alcohol wipe the lower eye lid if that makes you happy.
- Apologize to the patient for making his/her eye sting from the alcohol wipe.

Next time consider giving a few anesthetic drops before searing someone's eye with alcohol (Figure 37-5).
- Style point: tetracaine drops sting, proparacaine drops do not. If one is using anesthetic drops to prevent stinging from the prep, use one that doesn't sting!
- Examine the surface anatomy to assess if there is significant recession of the eye (increases risk of puncture!).
- With the patient's eyes in neutral gaze, draw a plumb line down from the lateral border of the pupil to the bony ridge of the orbit (Figures 37-6 and 37-7). Alternatively, identify the same spot at the junction of the lateral third and medial two thirds of the orbital rim. This is the traditional injection point (Figure 37-8).
- We are not traditionalists, so we shift our needle entry point further laterally toward the inferotemporal corner of the orbit. The further lateral you move the injection point, the less likely you are to have postoperative strabismus from trauma to the inferior rectus or inferior oblique muscle (Figure 37-9).
- Place a finger on the orbital rim and ballot the globe, creating a space between bone and globe. This is where the needle will go (Figure 37-10). Remember that the eye's equatorial margin may extend into that space somewhere below your fingertip. Be careful! Don't puncture the eye!
- Orient the needle bevel toward the globe. This maneuver lessens the chance of globe puncture by creating another millimeter or so of distance from the eye (Figures 37-11 to 37-13).
- Angle the needle essentially parallel with the globe (Figures 37-14 and 37-15). Enter the orbit close to the rim while encouraging the eye cephalad and away from the oncoming needle. A few things to avoid:

the floor of the orbit (pain, bleeding), the eye (duh), the apex of the orbit (nerve and muscle trauma, brainstem anesthesia), and intravascular injection (seizures).

- Fix the needle hub between two fingers while abutting the back of your hand against the patient's cheek. This provides stability and helps ensure that the needle will not impale the patient's brain should the patient decide he/she no longer wants to participate in today's activities (Figures 37-16 to 37-21).
- Look for evidence of blood in the needle hub prior to injecting local anesthetic. Alternatively, consider aspirating the syringe to determine if the needle tip is in a blood vessel.
- Consider wiggling the needle 2 to 3 mm in a plane parallel to the eye or ask the patient to gaze outward in order to ensure that the needle is not in the eye. The only thing worse than puncturing the eye is penetrating the eye and injecting local anesthetic (Figure 37-22).

Inject slowly. Watch the eye. Look for *the Good, the Bad, and the Ugly*:

- *The Good:* Observe the lid droop slightly (sign of sympathetic block), the globe shift forward, and/or the pupil to begin to dilate (Figures 37-23 and 37-24).
- *The Bad:* Arterial hemorrhage. Soft, mushy eye = punctured eye. Milky floaters in the pupil—this is local anesthetic precipitating in an eye that has been punctured and injected. Usually associated with a terrible postoperative visual outcome. A rock-hard eye may have excessive intrinsic or extrinsic pressure on it that may compromise perfusion and jeopardize vision (Figure 37-25).
- *The Ugly:* Local anesthetic can dissect under the conjunctiva. This is self-resolving and usually meaningless (Figure 37-26). A small bleed may result in a lower lid shiner. This too is self-resolving, although it may take a few weeks. It is usually not otherwise significant (Figure 37-27).
- Remove the needle, examine the eye for evidence of bleeding, close the lid, and assess globe pressure while gently encouraging backward flow of local anesthetic by intermittent digital pressure.
- Ask the patient to gaze left, right, up, down. Assess that onset of akinesia is occurring (Figure 37-28). Place a drop of anesthetic or betadine on the eye to confirm that analgesia is present (Figure 37-29).
- Betadine needs to be in place for at least 3 minutes (Figure 37-30). Many times it seems as though an OR prep is placed and rinsed off in under 60 seconds; therefore, we are in the habit of dripping and/or swabbing betadine on/around the eye after a block and letting it sit until later when it gets rinsed off with the prep in the OR. Note: Patients will not like you if you reverse the order and place the betadine before the block.
- Proprioception of the eyelid is lost with a good block, so manually close the patient's eye (Figure 37-31). Tape a gauze pad over the eye to keep the lid shut if it insists on remaining open (Figure 37-32).

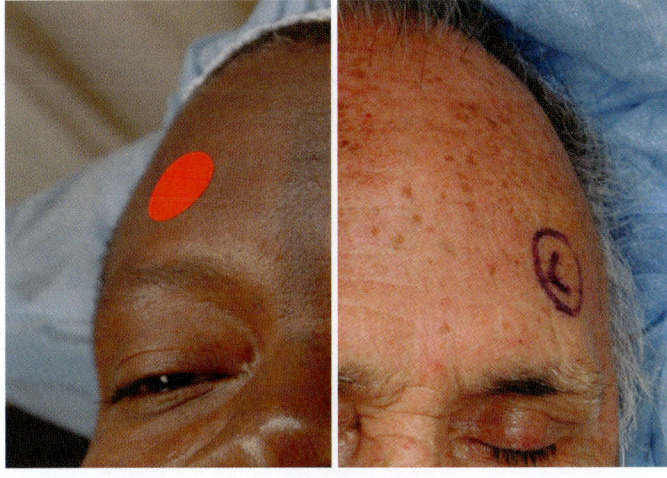

FIGURE 37-1 Always confirm patient, procedure, and side-of-surgery prior to performing regional anesthesia. The side to be operated should be clearly marked. Patient's cap should not obscure the label.

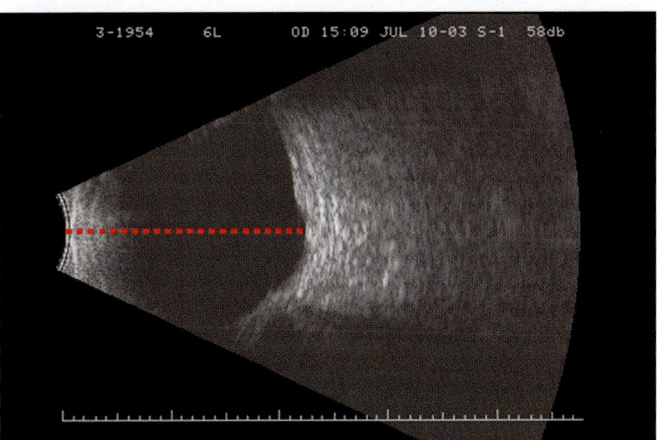

FIGURE 37-2 The ultrasound reveals the length and shape of the globe.

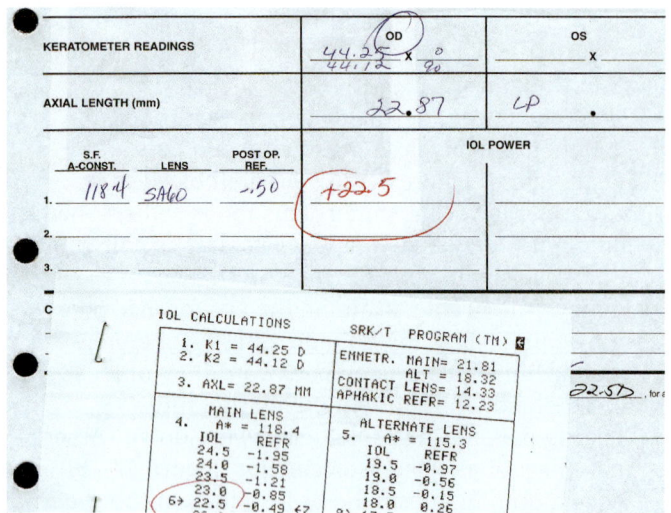

FIGURE 37-3 The ultrasound report may be handwritten or computerized. Make note of the length of the eye. Note that this patient's axial length is 22.87 mm, not 22.5!

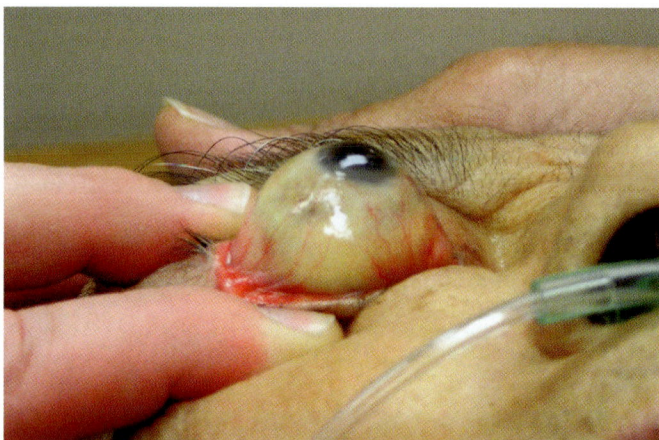

FIGURE 37-4 Examine the surface anatomy. Deeper set eyes are more likely to be punctured.

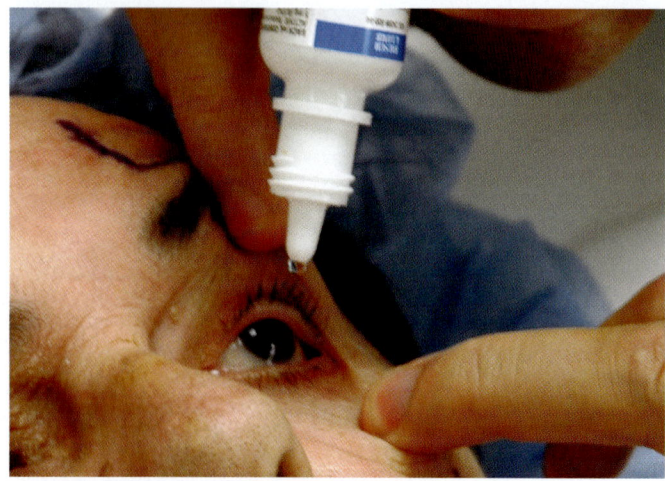

FIGURE 37-5 Consider placing a drop or two of local anesthetic.

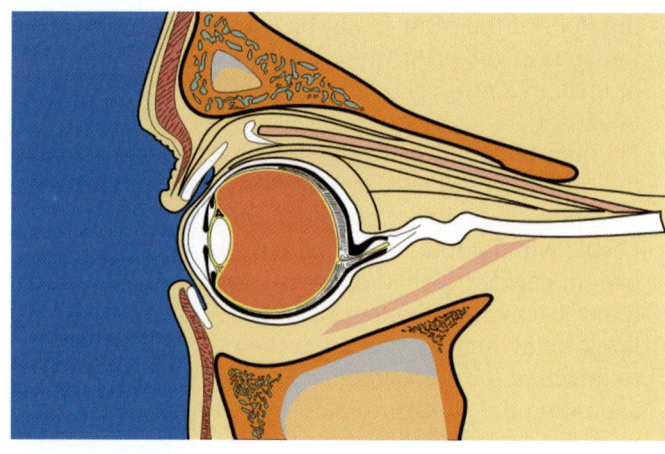

FIGURE 37-6 This allows the optic nerve to rest loosely in the posterior orbit. A taut optic nerve is easily damaged by an oncoming block needle…

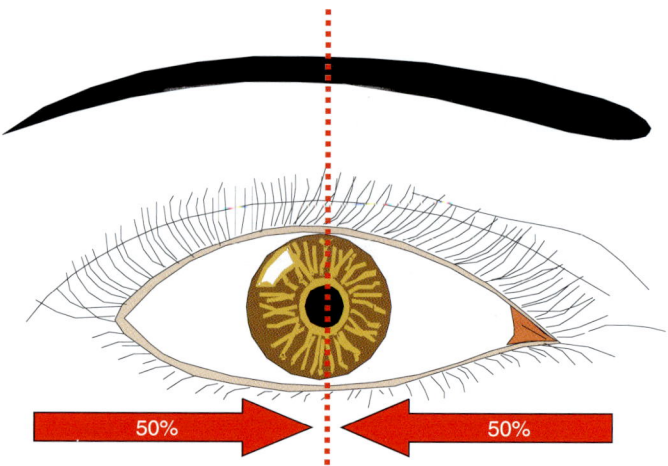

FIGURE 37-7 …Ask the patient to gaze forward, placing the globe in a midline, neutral position.

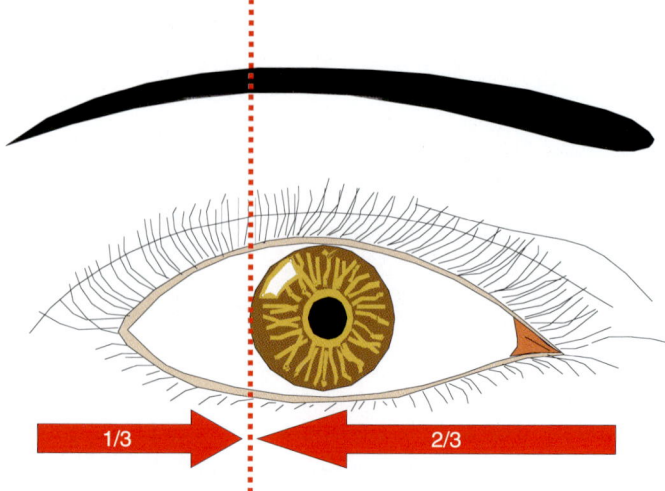

FIGURE 37-8 The traditional entry point is located at the one-third to two-thirds margin under the eye.

Chapter 37 INSIGHTS ON OPHTHALMIC ANESTHESIA

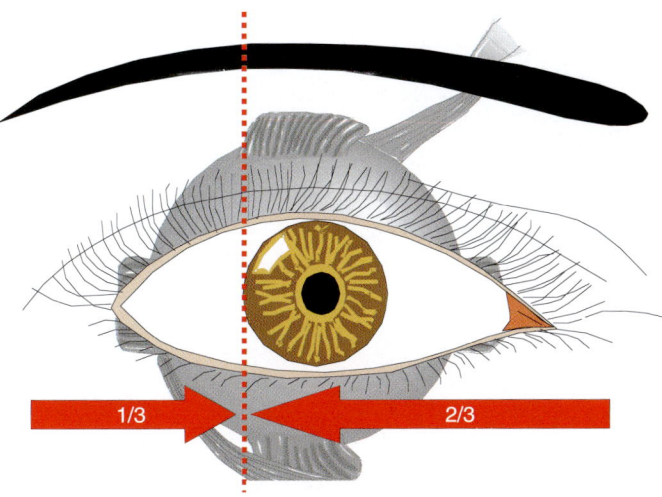

FIGURE 37-9 The needle may encounter the inferior rectus muscle or the inferior oblique muscle.

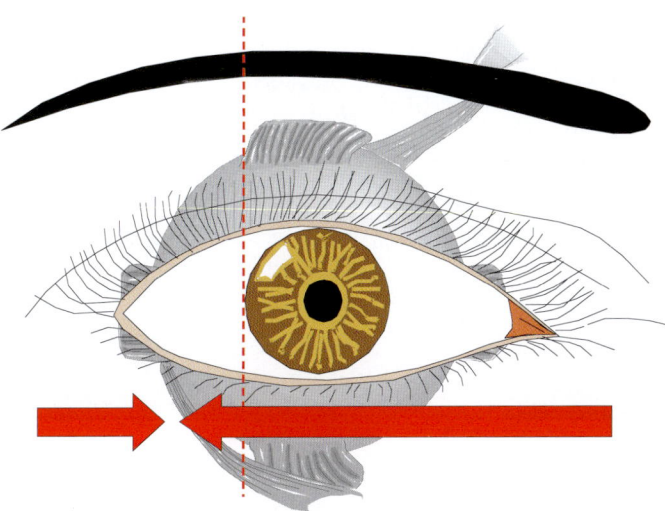

FIGURE 37-10 Moving the needle insertion point more laterally than the traditional entry point is recommended.

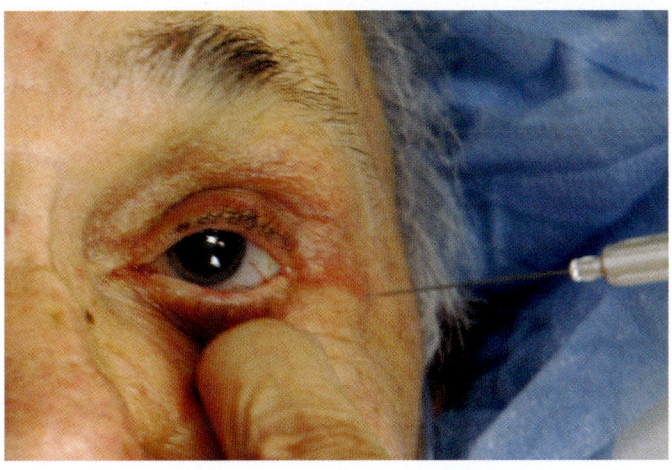

FIGURE 37-11 Ballot the globe away, creating space between inferior orbital rim and the eye.

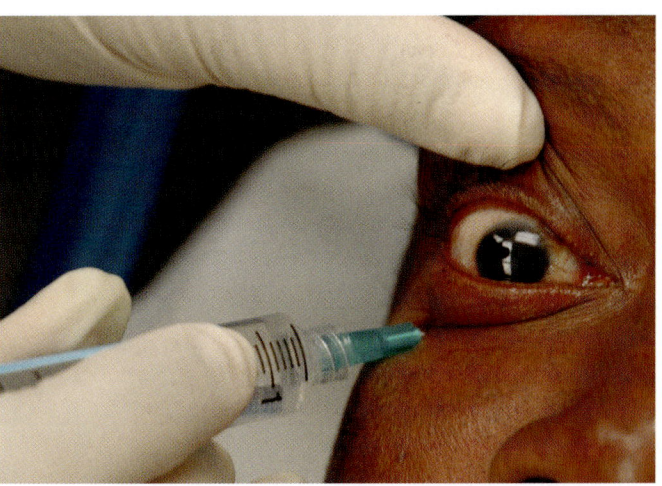

FIGURE 37-12 Decide if you will go through skin…

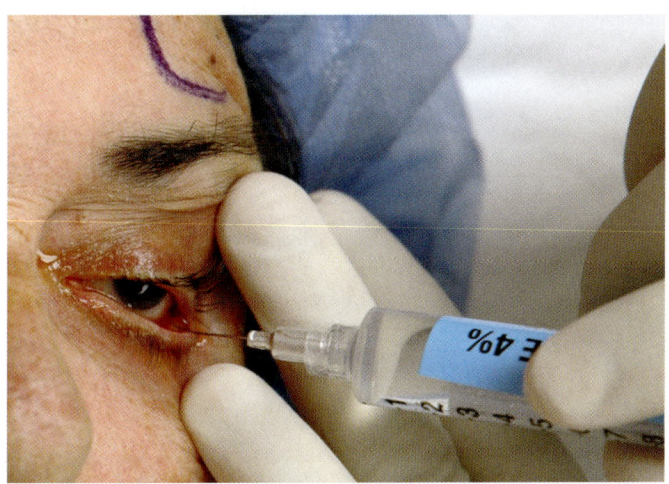

FIGURE 37-13 …or across conjunctiva

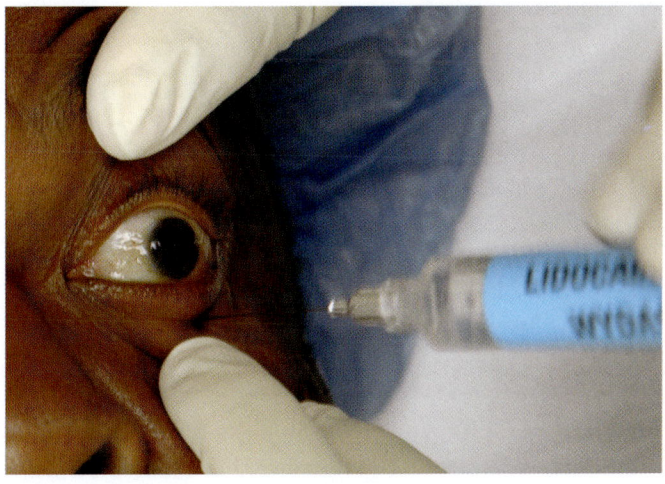

FIGURE 37-14 Angle the needle parallel to the axis of the eye…

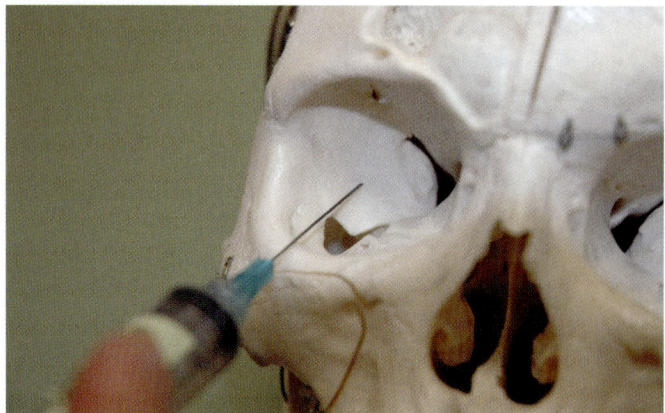

FIGURE 37-15 ...such that the needle tip avoids the apex of the orbit. (Dangerous structures lurk there—optic nerve, cranial nerves, veins, and arteries). This is the proper direction for a peribulbar block.

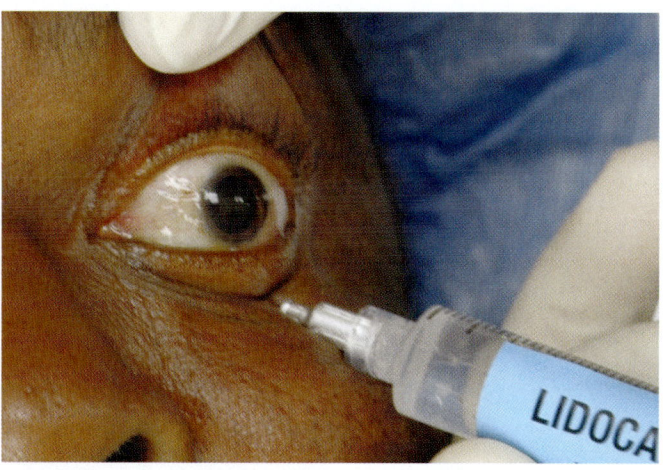

FIGURE 37-16 Alternatively, the traditional angulation of a needle...

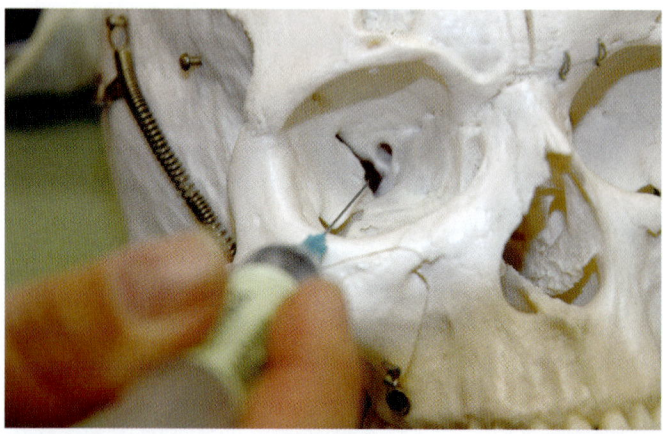

FIGURE 37-17 ...has been along the axis of the orbit. This is a retrobulbar block and is associated with more complications; therefore, it is not recommended for the novitiate.

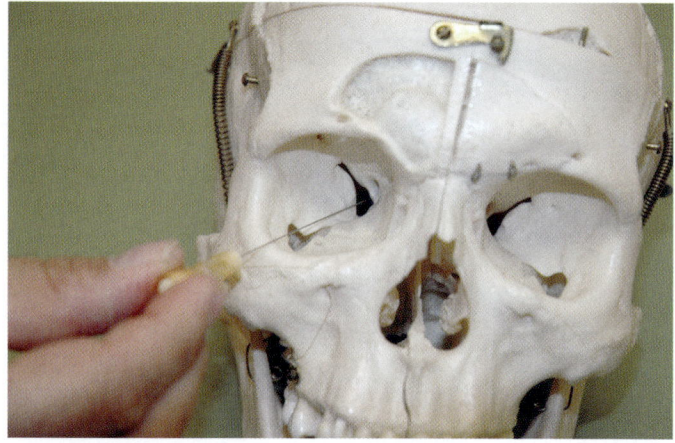

FIGURE 37-18 If you perform a retrobulbar block using a long needle, this may happen.

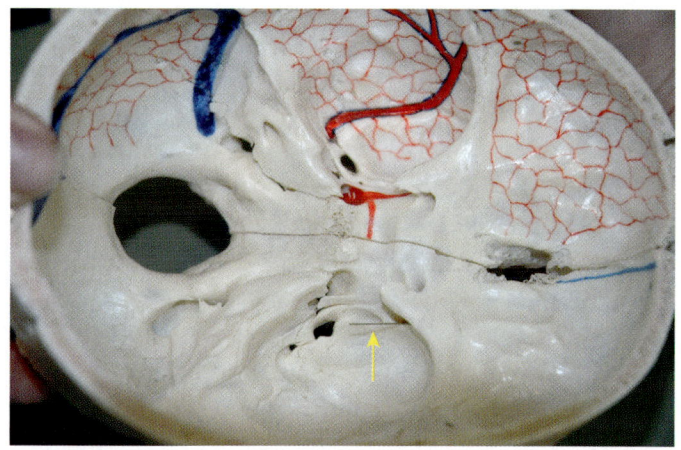

FIGURE 37-19 Another view. Note the position of the needle tip.

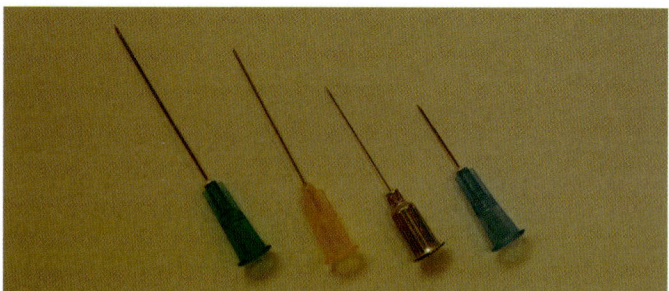

FIGURE 37-20 Use a proper-length needle: 5/8" to 1.25".

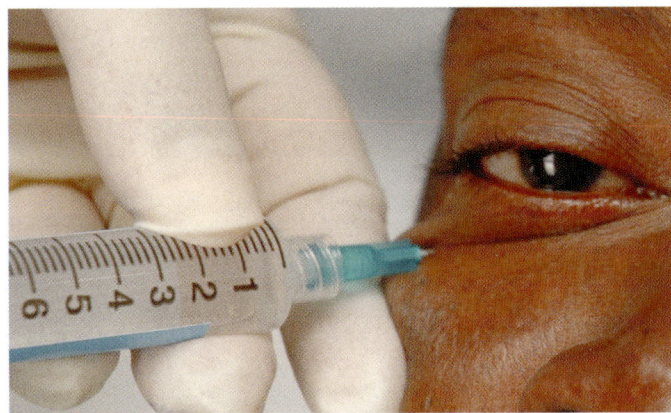

FIGURE 37-21 When the needle has been placed to suitable depth, fix the position such that it will remain in place as anesthetic is injected or if the patient should move.

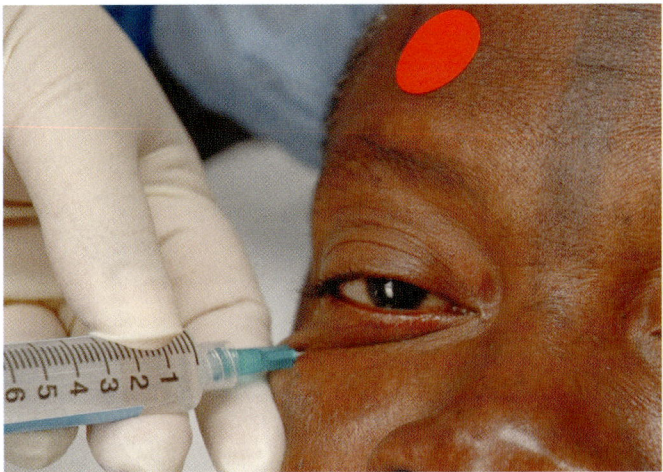

FIGURE 37-23 Sympathetic blockade of Muller's muscle...

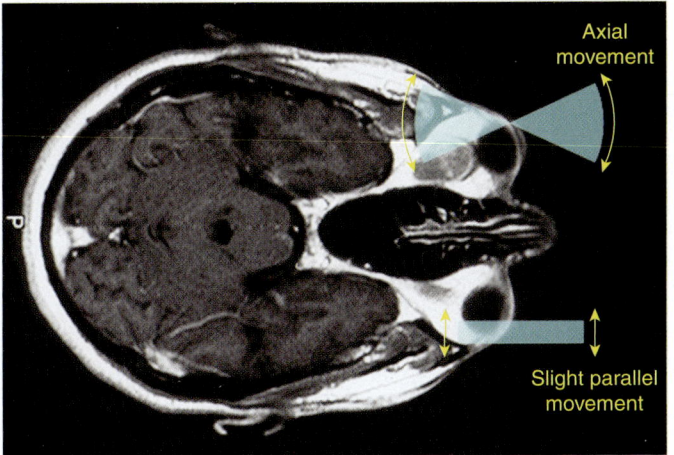

FIGURE 37-22 Prior to injecting, ensure that the needle has not penetrated the globe by asking the patient to gaze to one side and then back into neutral position. Alternatively, consider gently wiggling the needle from side to side with a slight parallel motion. Do not pivot the needle about an axial point, as this creates too much motion of the needle tip in the orbit.

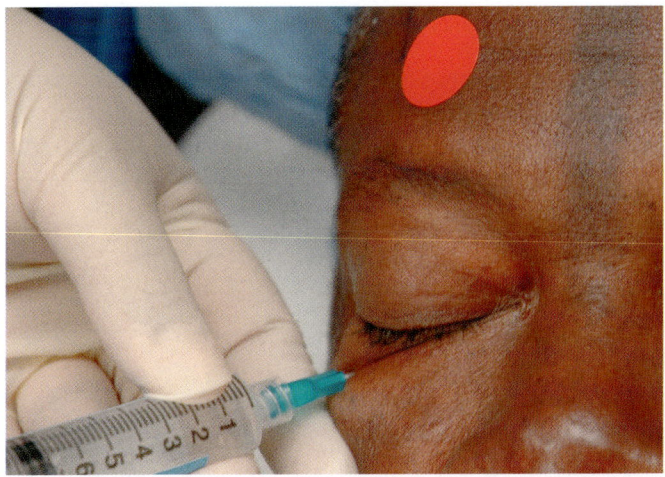

FIGURE 37-24 ...should cause the upper lid should begin to droop as one injects local anesthetic.

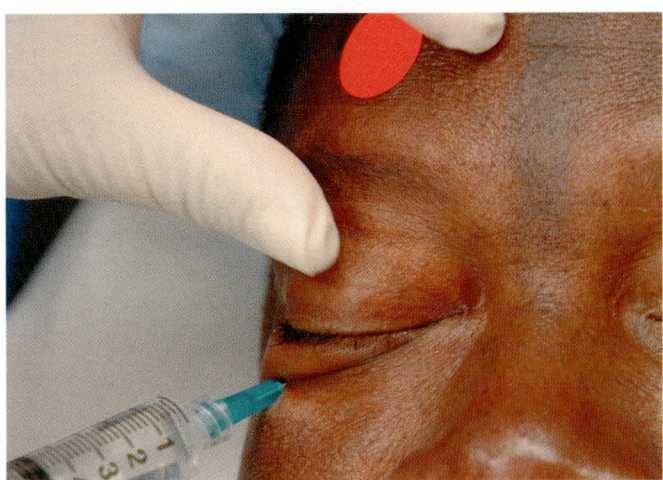

FIGURE 37-25 Assess orbital pressure as the local anesthetic is injected.

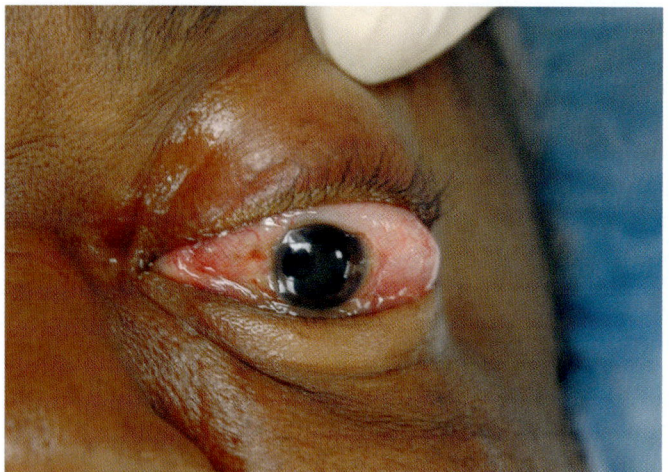

FIGURE 37-26 Chemosis may occur when local anesthetic dissects underneath the conjunctiva. This is normal.

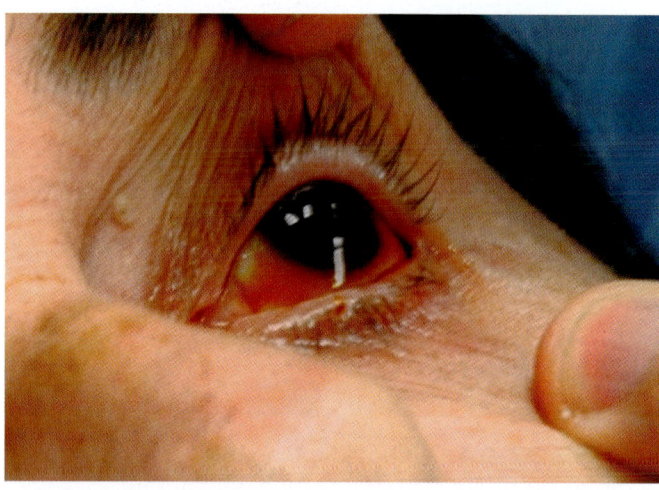

FIGURE 37-27 Minor subconjunctival hemorrhage is not uncommon. This should not be a problem.

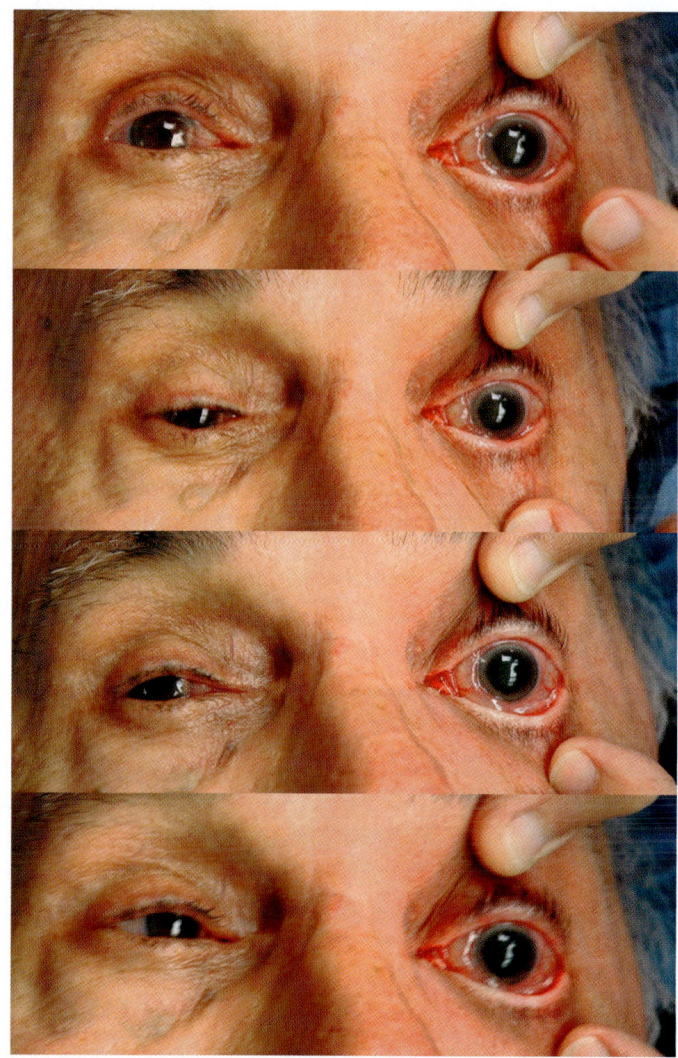

FIGURE 37-28 Assess the extent of akinesia by asking the patient to gaze up, down, right, and left.

Chapter 37 INSIGHTS ON OPHTHALMIC ANESTHESIA

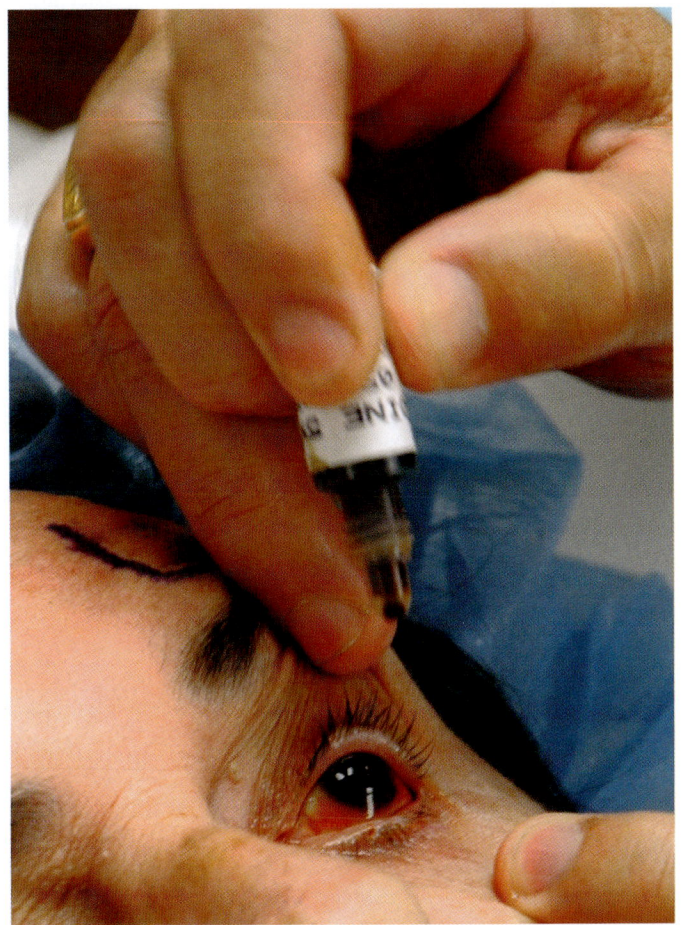

FIGURE 37-29 Consider instilling a drop of 5% povidone-iodine solution.

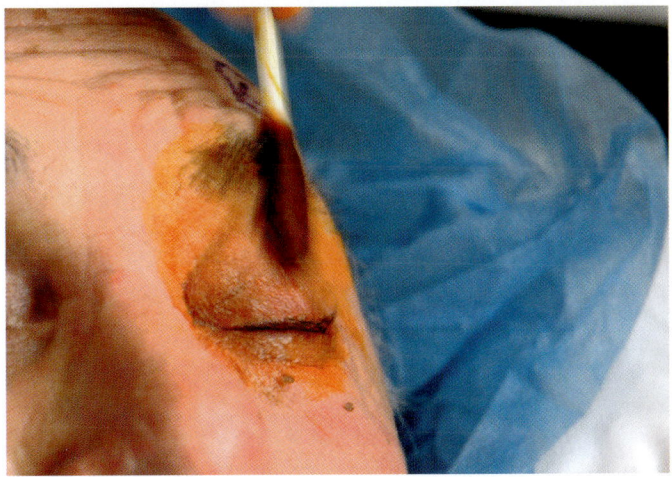

FIGURE 37-30 Consider swabbing the eyelids with povidone-iodine solution.

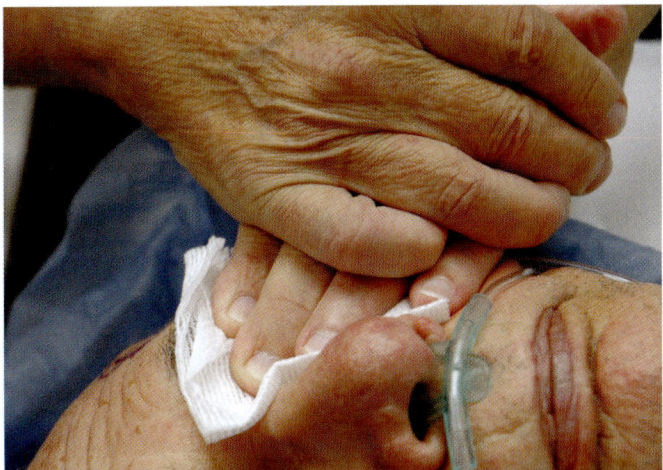

FIGURE 37-31 Close the eyelids and protect them.

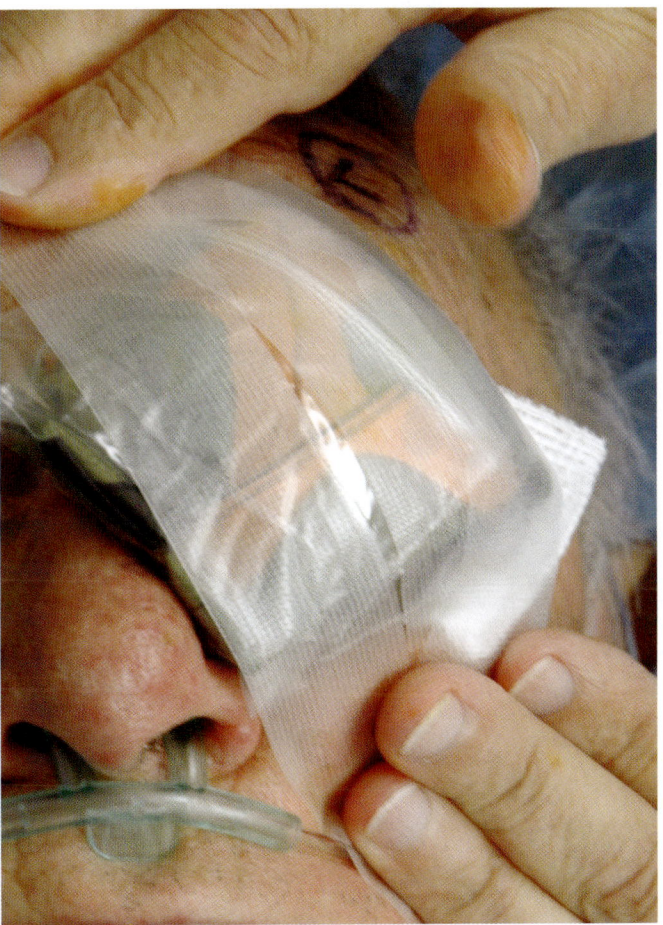

FIGURE 37-32 Consider an oculo-compression device to help spread the local anesthetic and dissipate tension. Avoid prolonged use of such a device, particularly with glaucoma patients.

SUGGESTED READING

Fanning GL. Orbital regional anesthesia. Ophthalmol Clin North Am 2006;19(2):221–232.

Gayer S, Kumar CM. Ophthalmic regional anesthesia techniques. *Minerva Anesthesiol* 2008;74(1–2):23–33.

Schwartz AJ. Ophthalmic anesthesia: more than meets the eye. In: Schwartz AJ, ed. American Society of Anesthesiologists Refresher Courses in Anesthesiology, vol. 34. Philadelphia: Lippincott Williams & Wilkins, 2006, pp 55–63.

PART VI
CHEST

CHAPTER 38

"THE LUNG'S NOT DOWN, YOU IDIOT!"—LUNG ISOLATION

LEBRON COOPER
ADAM SEWELL

Humanity with all its fears,
With all the hopes of future years,
Is hanging breathless on thy fate."
Henry Wadsworth Longfellow,
The Building of the Ship (1849)

INTRODUCTION

One-lung ventilation cases take your breath away, that's for sure. And while you're struggling with that lung that keeps coming up, you'll be taking your patient's breath away, too.

Lung isolation is the most consistent pain in the neck in anesthesia. Just when you think you've finally got the lung down, a patient comes along who didn't read the book. You'll do everything right, and that lung WILL NOT GO DOWN! It won't deflate for love or money. Then the next day a patient comes whose lung goes down, and in close concert with the lung, the saturation goes down, never to rise again.

Ay caramba, what a challenge!

What's the flip side of this often headache-plagued procedure? If you can learn lung isolation, really learn it well, you will be a valuable addition to whatever group (academic or private practice) that you join. You'll even be one of the most sought-after persons when everyone else has floundered in one-lung cases. What a deal, huh?

Isolating the lung is hard.

If you can do the hard stuff, you will always have a job.

ABSOLUTE INDICATIONS

- Here's a mnemonic for absolute indications (better know this mnemonic cold; it has been the salvation on many oral board exams! We promise you will never forget the indications for lung isolation again!):
  - BPOW—blood, pus, oxygen (separate mnemonic for this), and water.
    - Blood: you don't want blood from one lung contaminating the other side.
    - Pus: you don't want pus from one side of one lung contaminating the other side.
    - Oxygen: you don't want an oxygen leak or loss from one side making it impossible to ventilate the other side.
      - ▲ This one has another mnemonic: SUB T.
        - △ Surgical
          - ○ If the surgeons have sectioned a bronchus and you don't have the lung isolated, you will lose all your ventilation.
        - △ *U*nilateral lung cyst
          - ○ This rare beastie is just a giant alveolus, which doesn't contribute any meaningful oxygen exchange, you need to isolate it.

- △ *Bronchopleural/cutaneous fistula*
  - ○ The air leaking out of this will impair ventilation.
- △ *Trauma*
  - ○ A sectioned bronchus from trauma (call it an "amateur surgical sectioning") can also lead to "lost ventilation.
- Water: you don't want irrigating fluid (used to treat alveolar proteinosis) from one lung to contaminate the other side.

RELATIVE INDICATIONS

All these indications are variants of absolute indications.
- A better view (surgical exposure)
  - Lung biopsy
  - Lobectomy
  - Pneumonectomy
  - Esophageal surgery
  - Thoracic aortic aneurysm repair/resection
  - Thoracic spine surgery
    - If the lungs are in the way, and the surgeon wants them out of the way, you have a relative indication for lung isolation!
- Caveats to this:
  - Beware the surgeons who yell loud enough; they feel that they can convert a *relative* to an *absolute* indication.
  - Keep in mind, that the day will come when you won't be able to isolate the lung, and the surgeon, no matter how much he or she screams, "This is impossible. Are you incompetent?" will be forced to deal with it.
  - Guess what? The lung is really soft and squishy, so it is easy to retract. It's not like the surgeon is being asked to retract the acetabulum.
    - With that in mind, learn how to do lung isolation well each and every time…don't rely on a soft and squishy lung!
    - Doing that will make your one-lung ventilation life a perpetual nightmare!

ABSOLUTE CONTRAINDICATIONS

- There are no absolute contraindications to lung isolation, but there are plenty of *precautions*:
  - If a patient is absolutely near death on two lungs (such poor function that he or she can barely oxygenate with both lungs, attempting one-lung ventilation may just be the coup de grace.)
    - Caveat: Don't kill someone to isolate a lung!

- A tracheal tear is a near damnable thing.
  - Big tubes: If you shove a big double-lumen tube (DLT) down blindly (as is typical of the procedure), you can convert a partial rent into a complete section and then it's "Good night Irene."
    - ▲ Beware the large esophageal cancer that can eat into the back of the trachea. Big tubes in such cases have been known to tear the trachea.
    - ▲ There are better ways to place DLTs, by the way. Check later on in this chapter.
  - Big tumors: An obstructing tumor in the upper airway or the trachea may make placement of a DLT problematic.
    - ▲ Beware the obstructing tumor that eats away at the trachea; you'll tear it for sure!
      - △ Heck, even a single-lumen or Univent® might not be able to make that trip.
      - △ Even if you place a small endotracheal tube (ETT) to get past the tumor, blocking the lung through it may still be problematic.
- Remember that in a difficult airway, a DLT will be extra difficult to place. You need such a good view with a big enough airway to place a double lumen, that you should consider alternatives (a Univent or a regular ETT) to at least get the procedure started.
  - Although not impossible to place a double-lumen via fiberoptic scope, it ain't that easy. Just because you're really good at fiberoptic bronchoscopy, don't go all ape and pretend you're King Kong here!

STUFF YOU'LL NEED TO GET STARTED

Equipment

- Stethoscope (yep, if you've gotten used to life without a stethoscope, it's time to steal one, because this is one chest you will probably need to listen to). Then again, if it's your only method of verification that the lung is isolated, you'll probably be about as successful as swimming across the English Channel.
- Fiberoptic bronchoscope (no matter what you hear with the stethoscope, you still need to check with the scope and make sure you're in the right place. Plus, if things go awry in the procedure, you'll need the fiberoptic to reposition things.)
  - What size bronchoscope, you ask? A 37-French (F), or smaller, double-lumen ETT will not admit an adult-sized (8.0 mm) fiberoptic bronchoscope without a fight. Make sure whatever tube you use will admit whatever fiberoptic scope you have.

- Best way? Test it out ahead of time. Place the bronchoscope through the lumen of the ETT BEFORE the tube is in the patient.
- Rules of thumb:
  ▲ Adult-size (8.0 mm) bronchoscope for single-lumen ETTs or Univents larger than 8.0 mm inner diameter (ID) and double-lumen ETTs larger than 37F (you can view things much easier with this scope instead of an intubating scope!).
  ▲ Fiberoptic intubating-size (5.0 mm) bronchoscope for ETTs smaller than 8.0 mm ID and double-lumen ETTs smaller than 37F.
  ▲ Pediatric-size (3.4 mm) bronchoscope for single-lumen ETTs smaller than 4.5 mm ID. (You need some space for a small endobronchial blocker and the scope. The smallest endobronchial blocker available is 5F, but should fit into a 4.5-mm ETT well.)
- Laryngoscope: you must get everything out of the way for the *perfect* view of the cords!
  - A Mac (curved blade) just plain does a better job (according to many of our colleagues) than does a Miller (straight blade) at moving aside the tongue.
  - That said, a Miller blade is much better than a Mac (according to our other colleagues) for intubating difficult airways and placing large things in the trachea.
  - What does all this mean?
    - Use whatever blade makes you happy, but be able to use both kinds of all sizes!
    - You have no idea what you'll see and how you'll get that darned big double-lumen in, so be ready for anything!
- Videolaryngoscope (GlideScope, McGrath, or similar)
  - You may wish to have one of these fancy devices around. While this isn't the place to discuss the different types of videolaryngoscopes, suffice it to say that they are literally lifesavers in certain situations.
  - They tend to take up more space in the mouth than you wish, but you may have a much better chance of seeing where you need to go. Of course, seeing where you need to go is only part of it; you've gotta get that darned big double-lumen there!
- Endotracheal tubes (notice, that's plural)
  - Double-lumen
    - Have a couple of sizes available. The airway may look okay on the examination, but we've all been surprised before. Have different sizes available (just like when you do pediatric cases; you're never sure what you'll run into).
    - In general, use a 35F or 37F for most women (depending on their height) and a 37F or 39F for most men (depending on their height).
    - You may need to go one size larger than suggested if you have a really tall patient (or someone whose tracheal anatomy didn't follow textbooks).
    - We know this is pretty vague advice, but frankly, since there are only five sizes of DLTs (35F, 37F, 39F, 41F, 43F), and the smaller ones are for smaller and shorter people, while the larger ones are for larger and taller people, it's not too hard to have a couple of tubes available.
- Univent ETT, the Fugi Uniblocker®, the Arndt endobronchial blocker, or the Cohen tip-deflecting endobronchial blocker, depending on what you want to do and how you want to drop the lung. (The EZ blocker is available in Europe.)
  - Prejudices abound ("I never use a double-lumen anymore! They're just too big and dangerous! Or "The Univent stinks! It never works right!")
  - Like everything else in medicine, learn to use all of them and you have more tools in your airway toolbox.
  - When using a Univent or Uniblocker, don't forget the swivel adapter. This is the gizmo that connects to your regular, old ETT, allowing you to ventilate, bronch, and slide down your blocker all at the same time. Cool beans!
- A regular, single-lumen ETT.
  - Just in case you can't get the fancy ones in, make sure that you can secure the airway with a plain, old, regular tube. Don't kill a patient because you are hell-bent on isolating the lung!
  - If you are in trouble, go back to the ABCs, and that means secure the airway first and foremost, even if it's not with the exact tube you originally envisioned.
  - Don't forget to call for help! Just because you're trying to prove you can absolutely get that lung out of the way yourself, don't put the patient at risk. Get help early and often!
- Clamp (a Kelley clamp, if you need to be specific, but any clamp will actually work), that is, if you do the double-lumen tube. You don't need a clamp for the Univent or endobronchial blockers.
  - Make sure, when you place the clamp, that you clamp the *connector*, not the *ETT itself*. If you clamp on the ETT, the lung won't deflate, plus you won't be able to put a fiberoptic bronchoscope down the appropriate lumen.
  - Worst of all, if you tear the ETT with the clamp, you'll have to reintubate. (If you tear the connector, you just have to get another connector.)

BEWARE THE DIFFICULT AIRWAY!!!

- If someone comes to your OR with a genuinely difficult airway, you will have a heck of a time placing a double-lumen ETT. The tube is big, clunky, hard to move, and it's easy to tear the tracheal cuff on the teeth.
- If someone looks like he might be a tough intubation, consider intubating him awake with a Univent or regular ETT. (Same rules apply to topicalization; just make sure it's good).
- Once you have the regular ETT in, using a tube exchanger, you can then place a double-lumen or a Univent over it using a Seldinger technique.
- If someone is already intubated and the airway looks really bad (you know, like the patient who has been intubated for 3 weeks, has full-body anasarca, or weighs 400 pounds, etc.):
  - Either place a bronchial blocker down that ETT or use a tube exchanger.
  - Don't just pull a tube out blindly in the belief that you will be able to reintubate easily. That might not happen, and then your day just got really bad!
    - Caveat:
      ▲ Difficult airway plus lung isolation is a supreme challenge! Make sure you're ready for anything!

PHILOSOPHY OF LUNG ISOLATION

- The key in any one-lung case is keeping an open mind.
- When you initiate one-lung ventilation, the saturation can be a real problem.
  - Don't be afraid to reinflate the lungs, stabilize the patient, and then reassess.
  - Just remember, if you keep reinflating the lung, it will be in the way of the surgeon. Your 2-hour procedure just became 6 hours. The better anesthesiologist can do many different maneuvers to improve oxygenation without inflating the lung; see One-Lung Oxygenation Tips and Maneuvers, later in the chapter, for sure-fire ways to make this happen.
  - Don't "suffer in silence" while the patient crashes and dies. The surgeon is in this with you, and you need to work with him or her to make sure the patient does OK. Ego has no place in a one-lung case.
- Keep in mind all the options, including such exotic ones as cardiopulmonary bypass and extracorporeal membrane oxygenation (ECMO). If, due to some wild circumstance, the patient's lungs just absolutely cannot do it alone, you sometimes have to let a machine do it.
- Be quick to get help if you are in trouble.
  - When you are tangling with a cantankerous double-lumen ETT, Univent, or endobronchial blocker, it is easier than easy to take your eye off the patient.
  - Don't let the patient become unstable while you are peering through the fiberoptic!
- If your partner or colleague is doing a double-lumen case, go in there and help out. You will win big brownie points, plus, it's an easy way to get more lung isolation exposure.
  - You will get to look down the fiberoptic and help troubleshoot positioning.
  - Every time you do that, you learn a little. And as we all know, the more we know, the more we know we don't know!

HISTORY AND PHYSICAL EXAMINATION

The H&P is even more critical in a one-lung ventilation case than in other cases.

- Airway, airway, airway. Is this person easy to intubate or just easy enough to intubate with a regular ETT? Yes, there is a difference.
- Lungs: Will they be able to tolerate one-lung ventilation? Check pulmonary function tests (preferably split-lung) for a total pneumonectomy. If it's just a lobectomy but you need one-lung ventilation during the procedure, you may get away without pulmonary function tests, remembering, of course, that you may have issues with oxygenation and ventilation during the procedure.
- Heart: A bad heart with right heart failure, plus the hypoxemia of one-lung ventilation, can lead to some bad news. (Ever hear of hypoxic pulmonary vasoconstriction? Bad news for the failing right ventricle!)
- Pathology
  - Is this an enormous mass wrapped around the pulmonary artery? Be prepared for anything.
  - Is this a little peripheral mass easily gotten at and removed? Different story.
  - Just as the surgeon has to know about your problems in a lung case, you have to know about the surgical problems in a lung case.
    - Caveat: You can't do good anesthesia unless you know the surgical procedure!

OPTIONS FOR ACHIEVING LUNG ISOLATION

(Well, options, at least, for keeping the operative lung down and out of the surgeon's way.)

- Double-lumen endotracheal tube:
  - A Left-sided tube is the most common, while a right-sided tube is less common.
  - Right-sided tubes are more difficult to position correctly because of the difficulty of positioning the right upper lobe port of the tube exactly over the right upper lobe bronchial lumen.
- Univent endotracheal tube:
  - Just like a regular single-lumen ETT with an endobronchial blocker incorporated in the lumen
  - May be more difficult to place than a single-lumen ETT due to its lack of pliability (more on this later)
- Arndt endobronchial blocker or Cohen "tip-deflecting" endobronchial blocker:
  - All of these devices work similarly by placing them through a single-lumen ETT and directing the blocker to the bronchus you intend to block.
  - The Arndt blocker is wire-guided by fiberoptic bronchoscopy. If the wire is removed after placement, however, it may be challenging to reposition, if the need arises.
  - The Cohen tip-deflecting blocker may have an advantage for directing the tip into a not-so-normal anatomical situation and for the inevitable need for replacing/repositioning if the blocker is inadvertently dislodged during the procedure.
- Fugi Uniblocker®
  - This is the Univent blocker that "stands alone," without being attached to an ETT.
  - It seems that a lot of folks like the blocker of the Univent, but they aren't too hip on its tube. So Fugi decided to give them what they wanted—a blocker without a tube.
  - It is placed and managed just like the other blockers, once it's in (Figure 38-1).
- EZ Blocker®
  - This blocker is currently available only in Europe.
  - It has a cool design, with dual blocker cuffs, bifurcated, to sit directly on the carina.
  - This blocker enables the clinician to drop either lung with only one blocker! (Figures 38-2 and 38-3)
- Fogarty catheter:
  - Jury-rigged to be a bronchial blocker through a single-lumen ETT.
  - Unless you have some kind of connector you've previously planned to use and are familiar with, this may not be the wisest choice, but it may be one of your only choices.
- Regular, single-lumen ETT—"Mainstemmed":
  - You can use a regular, single-lumen ETT and "mainstem" it by pushing it into the *opposite* mainstem bronchus you intend to block and inflating the cuff.
  - By selectively placing the tube in the mainstem bronchus of the lung you actually wish to ventilate and inflating the cuff, you effectively have achieved one-lung ventilation, thus passively deflating the operative lung in the process.
- Faking It:
  - By placing a regular, single-lumen ETT in the trachea, you may plan *intermittent apnea*.
    - This technique really works well when your blocker gets inadvertently dislodged and you're trying to replace it. If you do it just right, the surgeon will never know!
  - You may also use very small tidal volumes.
    - You may have to tell the surgeon to deal with it.
  - You may have to keep using regular tidal volumes.
    - You may have to tell the surgeon to deal with it.
    - Using regular or small tidal volumes as methods of lung isolation are called "Not lung isolation," and your surgeon will probably hate you. (Of course, she probably already hates you anyway!)
- Cardiopulmonary bypass:
  - Guess what? Both lungs come down, that is, if you stop the ventilator.
  - Don't forget to restart the ventilator when you wean from cardiopulmonary bypass (CPB); it's probably the number one preventable cause of not separating from CPB!
- Extracorporeal membrane oxygenation (ECMO)
  - As with CPB, both lungs come down.
  - When faced with this option, consider your day as really, really, really bad! You'll have something to tell your grandkids.
    - Caveat: These last two, CPB and ECMO, may seem a little extreme, but hey, if the lungs can't do the job, *something* has to oxygenate the patient, and these "extrapulmonic" lungs are preferable to a hypoxemic death!

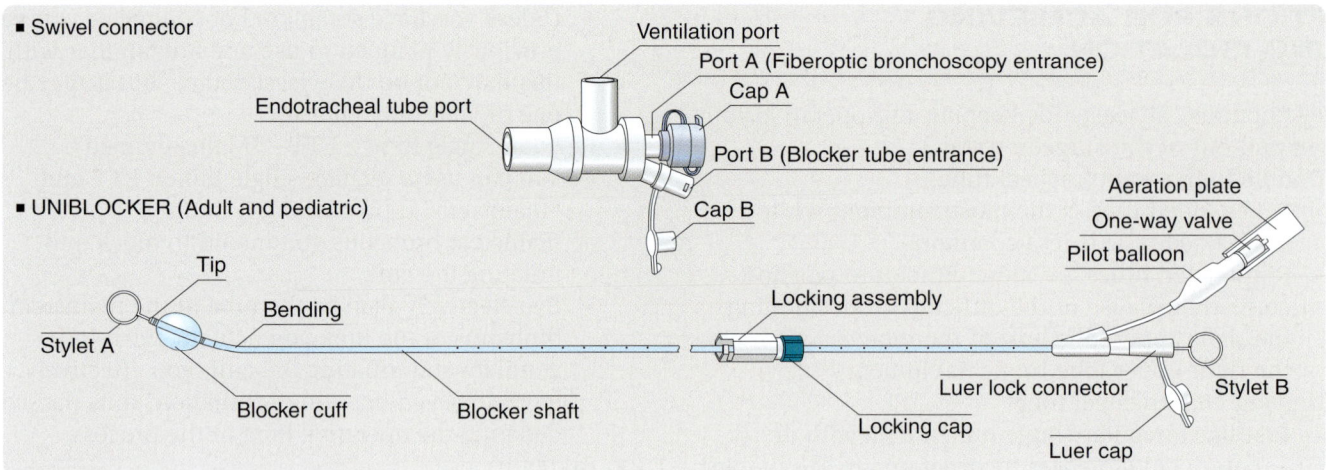

FIGURE 38-1 Fugi Uniblocker.

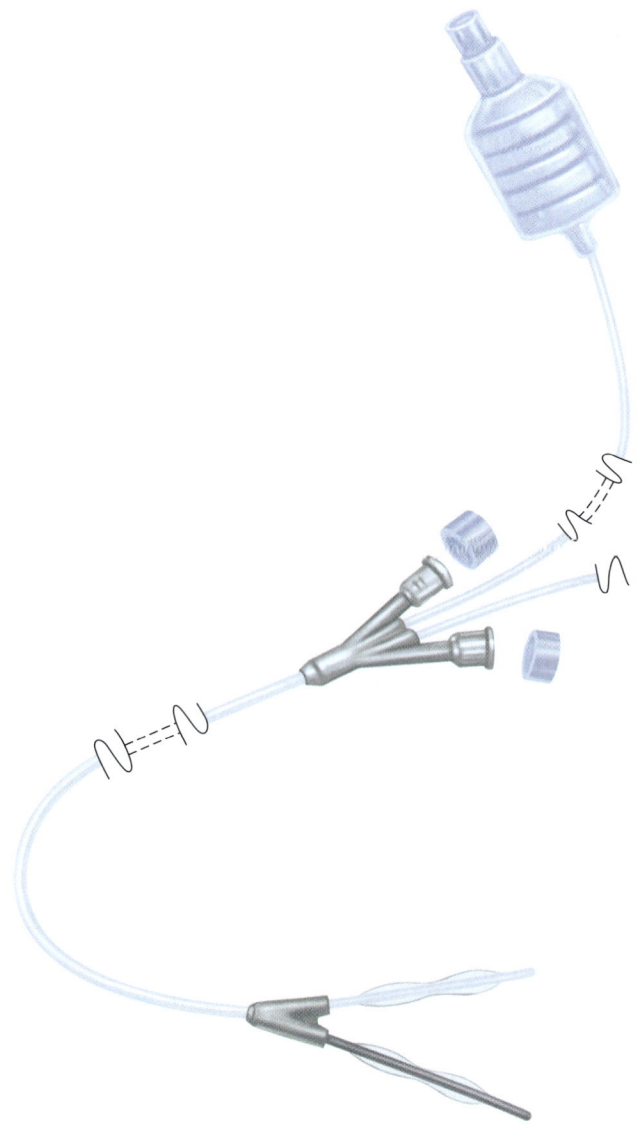

FIGURE 38-2 EZ-Blocker.

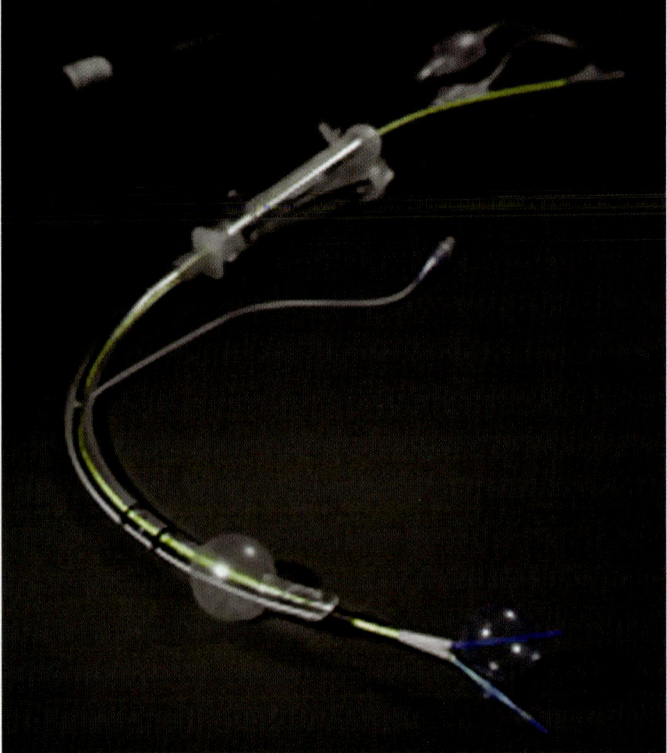

FIGURE 38-3 EZ-Blocker with multiport adapter via regular ETT.

THE CARINA: KNOW IT, LOVE IT, AND BY ALL MEANS RECOGNIZE IT!

- Identifying the carina is the be-all and end-all of lung isolation cases.
- If you can see the carina, you can navigate the treacherous shoals of lung isolation.
- If you can't see the carina, or if you get faked out by a "non-carina" (a division one step further down the bronchial tree from the carina), then you are doomed. You are condemned to flounder about in Nowheresville for the duration of the case. You have a one-way ticket to Unhappy City and that train is leaving the station right now with you on board.
- How do enterprising anesthetists make sure they can recognize the carina?
- If you are a resident or student, get thee to the lung room every time you get a chance and ask if you can sneak a peek through the fiberoptic bronchoscope. The more carinas (carinae?) you see, the better you will be when you are ready to recognize the real deal.
- Ideally, a video camera screen monitor should be used to display an enhanced clear image so others can observe and learn.
- How do you tell the real deal?
  - The carina is sharp.
  - The tracheal rings (cartilages) are *organized* along the anterior aspect of the trachea (kind of like a C-shape).
  - Smooth, longitudinal, muscular, road-like folds framed by dense collections of elastic fibers define the posterior portion of the trachea.
  - The anatomical distance from the tracheal carina to the bifurcation of the left-sided bronchus is approximately 4 to 5 cm.
  - In contrast, the distance from the tracheal carina to the take-off of the right upper lob bronchus is approximately 1.5 to 2 cm.
  - If you are looking at a pseudo-carina, you won't see the organized C's and smooth band along the posterior wall. You may see C's, but they won't necessarily be organized.
- If the surgeon does a bronchoscopy first (often through a single-lumen tube before you place a DLT, or directly through a Univent if that's what you've placed), take a peek through the scope and get a good look at the carina. Then later, when you're looking through the double-lumen or trying to position your blocker, you'll be looking at familiar turf.
- This is a lot of perseveration on "carina ID'ing," but believe me, that carina really and truly is the difference between a good case with nice lung isolation and a miserable case with you suffering all seven circles of Dante's purgatory at once.

CONSIDERATIONS

Double-Lumen ETT

- Good in a lot of ways. This is the "traditional" lung isolator, so most surgeons and anesthesiologists are familiar with it.
- Although it can be a pain to get in (it's so big and clunky), and it's a pain to position just right (if you get faked by a non-carina, you'll be sunk), once you get it in, it tends to stay that way. Note: this is a major plus!
- The double-lumen allows easy deflating of the lung, so the lung comes down quickly without delay.
- The relatively large bronchial lumen allows for suctioning, looking around with the fiberoptic scope, and switching back and forth between lungs (very handy and many times necessary if you do lung transplants. Just because you can do a double-lung transplant with a bronchial blocker, doesn't mean you should).
- But the double-lumen has its dark side. The damn thing is so big, it can be awfully hard to place by direct laryngoscopy.
- A small mouth, big teeth, small chin, fat jowls, etc.— all the things that make plain, old intubation tough— make navigating that DLT damned near impossible to place at times.
- Add to that the size of the laryngoscope or videolaryngoscope in the mouth simultaneously.
- Coupled with that is the human's inability to focus on more than one thing at a time. You look at the cords, and your focal point leaves the tracheal cuff (which by now is hooking on a tooth). You advance the DLT and tear the tracheal cuff at the same time! What a nightmare!
- Now, the next time you attempt intubation, you focus on the tracheal cuff, hoping not to tear it again, but your focal point goes off the cords and now you miss the intubation altogether. Absurd, huh? Just try it. (If you haven't yet torn a tracheal cuff while placing a DLT, you haven't placed enough of them.)
- One more headache with this big bastard: you can tear hell out of the trachea itself (see Relative Contraindications, above). Oh, wouldn't that be just ducky? Think about it, you do a case where the patient has esophageal cancer. That cancer may very well be eating into the trachea, which is just in front of it. In goes your DLT, RRRRRRRRRRRRRIIIIP! Now you have disrupted tracheal tree, which has been known to significantly shorten one's social calendar, may significantly shorten one's day at work, or significantly shorten your patient's life span, among other tragedies. You'll definitely have a story to add to your Facebook page!

Univent®

- The groovy thing about the Univent is that you put it in like a regular ETT.
- If you secure it at about 21 to 22 cm, you know that when you place the fiberoptic bronchoscope, you are probably looking at the carina.
- There is a lot less confusion about which thing is the carina with a Univent.
- Also, the Univent can be placed with the patient awake. (Try that with a double-lumen! Doable, but damned tough, and I personally dare you to try!)
- So for the difficult-intubation-lung-isolation-combo-pack, the Univent is the "bomb."

However:

- The Univent is thick and stiff, and sometimes it's difficult to get it through the cords. It may take a little "elbow grease" and a lot of creativity, but once in, it is a cinch to use.
- The bronchial blocker sticks out the top of the tube a long way so you can hit yourself right in the face!

So:

- Intubating with the Univent is not necessarily a walk in the park. It's easier than a double-lumen, yes, but not as easy as a regular ETT.

Arndt® Bronchial Blocker, Cohen® Tip-Deflecting Blocker, the Fugi Uniblocker®, and the EZ Blocker®

- Whereas the Univent has a built-in bronchial blocker in its own special tube, the Arndt, Cohen, Uniblocker, and EZ blocker gizmos go through a regular ETT.
- Of note, if you try this with an ETT smaller than an 8.0 mm ID, you're going to work extra hard, as there is not enough room for everything (blocker and bronchoscope) in the smaller diameter tubes.
- That said, the Arndt has an option of two smaller size blockers. It comes in a 5F, 7F, and 9F. The smaller the patient, the smaller the tube, and the smaller the blocker.
- These four blockers all have a real advantage when you already have an intubated patient, and you don't want to mess around and take the risk of changing tubes. You use what you already have, only modified.
- We know a lot of people who use the Arndt, some who use the Cohen, and fewer who use the Uniblocker (well, it is fairly new on the market), but in general, we find the Univent much easier to work with. However, with an already-intubated patient, other blockers are probably better.
- When faced with a choice, a lot of people would place a tube exchanger, use that to place a Univent, then work with the "easier" piece of equipment. The Arndt and Cohen take more skill than a Univent. The Uniblocker is just as easy to place as the Univent, so it may get some more press in the future.
- The EZ blocker is available currently only in Europe. Only time will tell whether or not the U.S. will get its turn using it!

TECHNIQUES

Double-Lumen Endotracheal Tube

- Do a good, and we mean a good, airway examination. Look for things that will specifically gum up the works with a DLT: a jagged tooth that can tear the tracheal cuff, a small mouth that won't let you place the monster-sized DLT.
- Review the medical record for things that may bring the double-lumen to grief once past the cords: an invasive esophageal cancer, an obstructive lesion in the left mainstem bronchus that won't allow passage of the double-lumen, the enormous aortic aneurysm that may rupture as the double-lumen pushes past it (that would be a lot of fun, that is, if you're into torture and masochism. Remember, lung isolation shouldn't necessarily require emergency cardiopulmonary bypass!).
- If your case involves first a single-lumen ETT (for bronchoscopy), followed by placement of a double-lumen ETT, then view that first intubation as a preview of "coming attractions."
- If you don't get a good view of the cords but still are able to pass the single-lumen ETT fairly easily, then trust us, there is still no way in the world you will be able to pass a DLT. A single-lumen placement has to be *super-easy* for a DLT to be just *regular easy*.
- Left- or right-sided tube?
  - The traditional argument *against* the right-sided DLT is that the take-off of the right upper lobe bronchus is so close to the carina that you may occlude the right upper lobe. Then, when you try to isolate the lung, you will end up in an imperfect world.
  - But if you look at a right-sided DLT, the bronchial cuff is manufactured on a slant, which allows you to ventilate the right upper lobe with no problem! Hey, what do you know? Somebody actually thought of things like this before they marketed this thing! So, the absolute dictum, "Thou shalt not ever use a right-sided DLT," isn't really so absolute a dictum after all.
  - But, to tell the truth, most folks use the left-sided DLT anyway. It's just plain easier to use.
  - So, unless you have a penchant for pain, left-sided will probably be your choice.
  - Just a little hint: the left-sided tube always goes in the left mainstem bronchus. Just because you

are dropping the right lung, you don't have to put the lumen in the right side. Left-sided means left! You drop the respective lungs by clamping the appropriate size, not by intubating the appropriate side (that is, at least with a DLT).

Placing the Double-Lumen Endotracheal Tube

- Do your usual good induction, do your usual good laryngoscopy. Use whatever laryngoscope blade makes you a superhero in really bad situations, and go for the gold.
- Place the tube in the mouth (carefully watching the bronchial cuff as it passes the teeth), go through the cords, and then keep on going. Turn the tube until the two openings at the top of the DLT are looking you square in the eyes. This is called the "blind technique."
- If you turn the tube so those two openings are 90 degrees to your eyes, you've turned it around sideways, and you'll have to do the whole case lying in the lateral decubitus position.
- Push the ETT in until it stops; don't force it, jam it, ram it, pound it, or jump on top of it to get it in. Just slide 'til the slide's done slidin'. Then pull out the stylet, hook up the connectors, and make sure you're in.
- An alternate technique is the bronchoscopy-guided technique. Place the fiberoptic scope through the endobronchial lumen. The endobronchial tip is passed beyond the vocal cords and guided through the trachea with the aid of the fiberoptic bronchoscope until the entrance of the left mainstem bronchus is identified. The tube is then introduced into the left bronchus. This might be a little overkill, but it may prevent a "real kill." It's just plain safer than the blind technique. You can see where you're going.
- Inflate the tracheal cuff, and then inflate the bronchial cuff.
- Clamp off the each lumen, in turn (on the connector that you had set up previously, remember), and listen with your newly acquired stethoscope to get your initial impression of whether you're in the right place or not.
- Caveat:
  - Be sure to use your clamp on the connector, not the lumen itself. If you accidentally tear the connector, you get to go and get another connector; if you accidentally tear the actual ventilating DLT lumen, you get the enjoyment of reintubation. (Remember that difficult airway we talked about? You don't want to do that again!)
  - Remember, if you clamp on the connector, that allows air to escape from the lung. If you clamp on the endotracheal or endobronchial lumen, the lung cannot deflate.
- If you clamp the tracheal side, you should only hear breath sounds on the bronchial side (obvious, but that means on the left for a left-sided DLT, and on the right for a right-sided DLT).
- Now, go down the tracheal side with the fiberoptic bronchoscope. You should see the carina, that all-important carina, the this-above-all-else-to-thine-own-self-be-true carina.
- Stop here. If you are using a left-sided DLT, you'll see a little rim of blue, just to the left, just beyond the carina in the left mainstem bronchus. If you are using a right-sided DLT, you'll see that little rim of blue on the right, just beyond the carina in the right mainstem bronchus.
- If you don't see the carina, deflate the bronchial cuff…and pray.
  - Make absolutely sure you are in the trachea!
- If you still don't see the carina (but you are definitely in the trachea), and you are starting to get a rising feeling of panic in your heart that this patient is an-carinic or suffers from hypocarinaemia, relax and take a deep breath.
  - That carina is down there somewhere.
- Pull back the entire DLT and reassess; maybe you're just in too far.
  - Caveat:
    - If nothing seems to work, *change gears*.
- Put the fiberoptic scope down the endobronchial lumen, then pull the DLT way, way, way, way, way back until you are so far out that you must be looking at the carina.
- Don't fret that you might extubate the patient; you have a fiberoptic scope in the trachea, after all, so you can almost always slip the tube back in. (This of course, is not an absolute; just mind your P's and Q's.)
- Once you've pulled back a country mile, and you really do see the carina, then slide the scope down into the appropriate bronchus for whichever DLT you are using. (You're basically planning to do a Seldinger technique over the bronchoscope in this bronchoscopy-guided technique.)
- Using the fiberoptic scope as a makeshift guidewire, slide the DLT down over the scope into whichever bronchial lumen the DLT is intended for (that would be the left bronchus for left-sided tubes and the right bronchus for right-sided tubes.)
- Now, remove the fiberoptic scope and place it in the tracheal lumen. Look for the carina (which you just saw, live and in color) and identify the blue cuff just below the carina.
  - Key point:
    - When you're really lost, do this:
      - ▲ Send your bronchoscope down the bronchial lumen and pull the entire DLT way, way back.

▲ This trick is the best problem solver. It beats thrashing around for a month of Sundays in the tracheal lumen while the surgeon screams at you and you wonder why you ever got into this business!

Univent

- Just like the double-lumen ETT, the Univent can be used to ensure one-lung ventilation.
- Many an anesthesia provider has changed his or her practice since the introduction of the Univent a couple of decades ago, especially after using the following seldom-written-about-or-even-spoken-of technique. You'll be hard-pressed to find someone to tell you that it can almost—once again, almost—replace the DLT in achieving lung isolation.
- However, if you follow the suggestions below *in the exact order in which they appear*, you will almost certainly achieve lung isolation as well, if not better than you can with a DLT.

Advantages of the Univent

- The Univent has several advantages over the standard double-lumen:
  - It is smaller, hence, usually easier to place and less traumatic.
  - If you are planning a bronchoscopy before the actual procedure, you can do the bronchoscopy through the Univent (size 8.0 mm ID or above), thus eliminating the step and risk of intubating with a single-lumen and reintubating with a Univent or double-lumen.
  - It is placed exactly like a regular, single-lumen tube.
  - You can even do an awake, fiberoptic intubation with the Univent; try that with a double-lumen!
  - Nothing is *ever* advanced into a bronchus blindly, like it is with a typical "blind technique" DLT placement; you get to see the lumen *before* you invade it with a foreign object.
  - What if you cannot or choose not to extubate at the end of the case? A Univent can be left in place, just like a single-lumen tube; there is NO NEED TO REINTUBATE!!!
- Caveat: This comes in real handy when you have that bad airway, huge fluid shift case where you are terrified of removing the tube and risking losing the airway!

Disadvantages of the Univent

- You know if there are advantages, there must also be disadvantages, so here they are:
  - Know the absolute indications for a DLT (see above); these, necessarily, would be contraindications for placing a Univent.
    - Remember the mnemonic BPOW: Blood, Pus, Oxygen, Water.
    - You cannot use a Univent anytime there may be cross-contamination between the lungs. The Univent does not protect the other lung!
- Anytime you need to isolate both lungs separately at different times during the same procedure (as in a double-lung transplant without cardiopulmonary bypass), the Univent is probably not your best choice. Although it can be done, it really can be a hassle that you do not want to deal with. Trust us on this one; we've done it. You won't like it.
- Occasionally, the right-upper lobe bronchus lumen is so close to the carina that the Univent bronchial blocker cannot adequately occlude the lumen, resulting in inadequate isolation of the right-upper lobe.
- In the rare patient (0.1% to 3% of the population), you'll actually find a "pig bronchus," meaning, of course, that the right-upper lobe bronchus actually comes off the trachea itself, thereby making the Univent useless (if you're trying to block the right side) in these cases.
- All that said, if you follow the procedure below in the exact order in which they appear, you may find that the Univent offers superior lung isolation with much less trauma and grief than does a double-lumen.

Placing the Univent

- Just as with the DLT, do a good airway examination. Just because the Univent is smaller than a DLT doesn't mean it will go in as easily as a regular, single-lumen tube.
  - The Univent is a little stiffer than a regular, single-lumen tube, so sometimes it takes a little creativity to get it through the vocal cords. It may not just slide in, even if you have a good view of the cords.
  - Using a stylet sometimes helps direct the Univent through the treacherous path of the posterior pharynx.
- Also, just like with the DLT, it would probably be a good idea to review the medical record and any studies (such as a CT scan) to rule out any obstructing tumor in either the posterior pharynx or the tracheal/bronchial lumens.
- Choose the correct-size Univent for the patient and procedure. If the surgeons are planning a bronchoscopy, the smallest Univent an adult-size bronchoscopy will pass through is an 8.0 mm ID.
- Getting the blocker down the right side is easy; placing it down the left side can be a challenge.

- Note: Do not remove the bronchial blocker stylet. It improves your ability to direct the blocker into the bronchus you intend to block!
- Although it is not known why the manufacturer suggests removing the stylet prior to intubation, it is assumed to be to prevent tracheal or bronchial damage; however, recent reports have shown this not to be the case, and your chances of successful placement are much greater with the stylet left in place.
- You may have to twist the blocker, or you may even have to twist the entire Univent tube to successfully direct the blocker to the bronchus you intend to block. Don't be shy.
- Before intubating, check both the tracheal AND the bronchial cuffs to make sure they are intact.
- Note: The connector to the bronchial cuff does not adequately fit a Luer-lock syringe!
  - You must use a syringe with a slip lock or place a T-piece with a slip lock on the connector, and then use a Luer-lock syringe to inflate the cuff.
- The bronchial cuff almost always requires between 5 and 7 mL of air to completely occlude the bronchial lumen, not 3 or 4 mL as the manufacturer suggests.
- Intubate as you normally would (you know, videolaryngoscope or laryngoscope blade of your choosing).
- Remember, these ETTs are a bit stiffer than a regular tube, so sometimes it takes a little creativity getting it through the vocal cords.
- Once you've determined you are actually in the trachea, follow these steps *in this exact order*, and you will achieve lung isolation:
  - Place the blocker in the bronchus you intend to block, using the fiberoptic bronchoscope to guide your efforts.
    - Remember, leaving the blocker stylet in place will improve your chances of success.
    - Don't be afraid to twist the blocker or the entire Univent to direct your blocker where you want it to go.
  - Push the blocker all the way in until you get mild resistance.
    - (That's way too far in, I know, but trust me; we'll get to that later.)
  - Place the patient in the lateral decubitus position with an axillary roll, beanbags, pillows, etc. Don't forget about safe patient positioning just because you're worried that the Univent may not work.
  - Once positioned safely, disconnect the ventilator circuit.
    - This will allow the lungs to deflate passively.
    - Give them a couple of minutes or so to deflate, because if these were normal lungs and had normal recoil, you probably wouldn't be doing the surgery you're about to do!
  - Using your bronchoscope, *with the ventilator circuit still disconnected*, position the blocker cuff just past the carina (remember the carina?), so you can just see the edge of the blue cuff.
  - Now, with the ventilator circuit still disconnected, inflate the blocker cuff with 5 to 7 mL of air.
  - Reconnect the ventilator circuit. You should now be ventilating only one lung, the one you didn't block. What a cool trick, huh?

The quick reference guide in Table 38-1 is included for your use in the operating room. Unless you just hate this book, I wouldn't suggest cutting out the page; just photocopy it, or visit the University of Miami Department of Anesthesiology Web site at www.anesthesiology.med.miami.edu, click on "Department," click on "Cardiothoracic," and then click on "Protocols" to access this Univent quick reference guide.

Why, you ask, do I disconnect the circuit and stop ventilation all together?
- Because if you inflate the bronchial cuff while you are ventilating, you will trap air inside the lung, and the lung will never deflate.

Why, you ask, do I place the blocker before I position the patient?
- Because once the patient is positioned, it is almost impossible to get the blocker in the bronchus you intend to block (unless the stars are with you and you are incredibly lucky!)

Why, you ask, do I push the blocker all the way in?
- Because if you place the blocker where it really should be before you position the patient, the blocker will almost always, inevitably, migrate out of the bronchus when you turn the patient.
- This ensures the blocker stays in the bronchus you are planning to block.

Troubleshooting the Univent

- Can't ventilate, high-peak airway pressures:
  - Chances are your blocker has migrated out of the bronchus and the cuff has herniated over the carina, thus blocking both lungs.
  - Simply deflate the blocker cuff, reposition the blocker so the cuff is just past the carina, disconnect the ventilator circuit again to drop both lungs, wait, reinflate the blocker cuff with 5 to 7 mL of air, and then reconnect the ventilator circuit to ventilate the other lung.
- Lung begins inflating, even after you've blocked the bronchus:
  - First and foremost, look into the surgical field, or at least on the video screen! Sometimes surgeons like to whine. Make sure the lung is actually

TABLE 38-1 Univent® Placement Quick Reference Guide

1. Place blocker in the correct bronchus and push all the way in.
2. Position the patient safely.
3. Using a bronchoscope, pull back on the blocker until you see the cuff just past the carina.
4. Disconnect the ventilator circuit to drop BOTH lungs.
5. WAIT, really... WAIT!
6. Inflate the blocker cuff with 5 to 7 mL of air to occlude the bronchial lumen.
7. Reconnect the ventilator circuit to ventilate the other lung.

inflating and you don't just have a whining surgeon.
- And make sure the lung is inflating, not just going up and down with the ventilation of the other lung and resultant movement of the mediastinum. How can you tell the difference? Look at the lung tissue itself. Do you see alveoli opening?
- Keep in mind; the surgeons are working on the lung in question, so they may have intentionally or inadvertently moved the bronchus, thus dislodging the blocker.
- Just disconnect the circuit again, deflate the blocker cuff, wait, reposition the blocker just past the carina, reinflate the cuff, and then reconnect the ventilator circuit to ventilate the other lung.
- This will work about 99% of the time.

Arndt® Bronchial Blocker and the Cohen® Tip-Deflecting Blocker

- Intubate with a regular ETT (preferably size 8.0 mm ID or above), or leave the ETT in place in a patient who is already intubated.
- Place the connector (which comes in the kit) on the ETT, place the fiberoptic scope through the *middle port* of the connector, slide the blocker through the *angled port*, hook up your circuit and ventilate through the *side port*.
- Such a clever design! (Trust us, we know George Arndt. George is scary-smart!)
- For the Arndt blocker, slide the tip of the fiberoptic scope through the loop at the end of the blocker. Now you're using the bronchoscope as a guide for a Seldinger technique.
- Advance the bronchoscope into the target bronchus (you know, the one you intend to block).
- Slide the blocker down the scope into the bronchus. You should slide the blocker all the way in, just like you do with a Univent. Yes, this is too far in, but remember, we have a reason for that.
- Now, position the patient in the appropriate lateral decubitus position, remembering, of course, to use an axillary roll and appropriate padding.
- Once the patient is positioned safely, disconnect the circuit and wait! You must drop both lungs so air can escape. Once the blocker cuff is inflated, you will never be able to deflate the lung!
- Once both lungs have had adequate time to deflate, pull back on the blocker, just to the point where you see the edge of the blue cuff. STOP! Unlike the Univent, if you pull these blockers out of the bronchus you intend to block, you may not be able to replace them. You must get another blocker and start all over.
- Now that your blocker is positioned with the edge of the bronchial cuff just barely visible, inflate the bronchial cuff with 5 to 7 mL of air.
- You should now have successfully blocked the lung you wish to block.
- Don't forget: reconnect the circuit to the side port and resume ventilation of the other lung.
- For the Cohen blocker, place the fiberoptic scope through the middle port of the connector and the blocker through the angled port. Deflect the tip, using the incorporated screw control, toward the bronchus you intend to block. Push the blocker into the intended bronchus under direct fiberoptic guidance.

Differences Between the Arndt and Cohen Tip-Deflecting Blockers

- As the name suggests, the Cohen blocker has the ability to deflect the tip to the direction you wish the blocker to go. Although this is an advantage over the Arndt design, you may still have some difficulty directing the tip into the bronchus you are trying to block.
- The Arndt blocker has a loop at the end of the blocker that is designed to slide over the bronchoscope in a Seldinger manner. Once this loop is removed, the blocker itself essentially becomes unmaneuverable. If indeed you can leave the loop in place during the surgery, you may have more success replacing the blocker in the event of inadvertent dislodgment.

Advantages of the Arndt and Cohen Blockers

- The main advantage of either of these blockers is that you do not have to reintubate a patient who is already intubated just to achieve lung isolation.

- You also do not have to reintubate at the end of the case if, indeed, you plan to leave the patient intubated and mechanically ventilated.

Disadvantages of the Arndt and Cohen Blockers

- The bottom line with either of these blockers is that they're just plain harder to use.
- The Arndt is very difficult to replace in the bronchus if it inadvertently becomes dislodged during the procedure.
- The Cohen, although easier to replace than the Arndt because of its tip-deflecting feature, is still more difficult to save than is a Univent.

Fugi Uniblocker®

- Remove the blocker from the packaging, check the cuff, and make sure the blocker is not damaged.
- Use only a clean syringe when inflating the cuff (lint sticking to a syringe may get mixed into the valve). A trick here is to use a T-piece with a slip lock (or a slip lock syringe), then use a Luer-lock syringe to inflate the cuff.
- As with the Arndt and Cohen blockers, intubate with a regular ETT (preferably size 8.0 mm ID or above), or leave the ETT in place in a patient who is already intubated.
- Place the connector (which comes in the kit) on the ETT, place the fiberoptic scope through the connector, slide the blocker in, hook up your circuit, and ventilate through the ventilating port.
- Leave the stylet in place. Advance the blocker into the intended bronchus (the one you want to block) under direct fiberoptic guidance.
- Disconnect the ventilator circuit.
- Wait.
- Inflate the bronchial cuff.
- Reconnect the circuit.
- This is the same procedure as the Univent. The Uniblocker is simply easier to place than many blockers, but you don't have to worry about using the pre-fashioned ETT that comes with the Univent.

Advantages of the Fugi Uniblocker

- Works with preexisting ETTs
- No need to reintubate the patient at the end of the case
- Because the Uniblocker is separate from the ETT, it is easier to position than the Univent.

Disadvantages of the Fugi Uniblocker

- Can dislodge during patient movement
- Tracheal anatomy that is unusual may make placement difficult.
- The endobronchial blocker contains a wire mesh that can interfere with MRI and CT scans.

EZ Blocker®

- As with the Arndt, Cohen, and Uniblocker blockers, intubate with a regular ETT (preferably size 8.0 mm ID or above), or leave the ETT in place in a patient who is already intubated.
- The EZ Blocker has two cuffs. Check both for leaks prior to placing the blocker.
- The EZ multiport adapter (in the kit) should be placed on the ETT and the patient should be ventilated.
- Deflate both cuffs of the EZ blocker completely.
- Lubricate the distal part of the EZ blocker and the bronchoscope.
- During introduction of the blocking device, the ETT should be positioned 4 cm above the carina to ensure proper functioning of the EZ blocker.
- Introduce the EZ blocker through the port (after removal of the closing plug of port) of the EZ multiport adapter and advance into the ETT.
- Introduce the fiberoptic bronchoscope through the other port of the EZ multiport adapter (after removing the plug of the closing cap) in order to visualize the airway and the EZ blocker.
- By checking and adjusting the EZ blocker position under direct visual guidance, advance the device until both distal extensions have been introduced in both (bilateral) mainstem bronchi.
- Following correct placement under direct fiberoptic guidance, disconnect the ventilator circuit, and drop both lungs.
- Inflate the appropriate distal cuff by inflating the corresponding balloon; the distal cuff on blue extension corresponds with the blue striped proximal balloon.
- Make sure that the balloon cuff is not overinflated, as it can cause damage to the bronchus or trachea.
- Following repositioning the patient or the patient's head, check the cuff position with the fiberoptic bronchoscope again to verify correct blocker position on the carina.
- Once the EZ blocker is in the correct position, the cap, mounted on the shaft of the EZ blocker, can be tightened on the port of the EZ multiport adapter until an airtight seal is created.
- In case of repositioning the patient, the closing cap needs to be unscrewed to the extent that the EZ blocker can move freely through the closing cap to avoid damage to the patient.

Advantages of the EZ Blocker

- The EZ blocker may be easier to place, as the bifurcation fits into the bifurcation of the trachea at the carina.
- The EZ blocker also stays in place better while moving the patient and during repositioning, as the shape of the blocker keeps it from being dislodged.

- Perhaps the biggest advantage of this blocker is that in bilateral procedures that require lung isolation, the blocker does not need to be repositioned and you can use either part of the bifurcation for lung isolation.

Disadvantages of the EZ Blocker
- It has two extensions, straddling the carina, which can potentially injure the airway.
- If the anatomy of the airway doesn't match the shape of the blocker, then it becomes very difficult to place.
- It is not yet available in the United States.

Take-Home Points About Blockers
- With the Univent, the Arndt bronchial blocker, the Cohen tip-deflecting blocker, the EZ blocker, or the Fugi Uniblocker, the blocker is on the end of a long skinny stick. Thus, with a little surgical tugging and pushing, the blocker can easily pop out. No problem when using a Univent or Uniblocker. Just put the fiberoptic scope back down, and push the blocker back in again.
- With the Arndt, however, this probably will not work. Take extra care not to displace the blocker from the bronchus. You may not be successful replacing it. You may have more success with the Cohen because of its tip-deflecting feature, but be careful; it may not work.
- The Univent is like those chronically dislocating shoulders some people have. They pop out easily, but they're easy enough to pop back in. The Arndt, on the other hand, is akin to an amputation; once it's gone, it is almost impossible to save.

LUNG ISOLATION GLITCHES

- Almost every placement glitch ends up being one of two things: you can't intubate or you can't see the carina.
- If you can't intubate, you didn't really consider how clunky and hard to maneuver the DLT is. Maybe you'd better reconsider and use the Univent, Arndt, Cohen, Uniblocker, or EZ blocker.
- If you can't see the carina—well, this boils down to your experience. Try pulling way back on the entire ETT, just in case you're in too far.
  - Do everything in your power to see as many carinas as humanly possible. Go into the lung room on your break and just take a peek.
  - There's no magic to it: the more you see, the better you'll be able to recognize it.
- When the lung doesn't deflate, look with the fiberoptic bronchoscope, after you look in the surgical field to ensure the lung isn't deflated. Look, reposition, look, and look again.

- If the patient has a lot of adhesions, then the lungs will sometimes not come down because they are held up. The surgeon will just have to deal with it. And this time, he will just have to deal with it. You have no control over this one.

One-Lung Oxygenation Tips and Maneuvers
These tips are almost sure to work, every time!
- If the oxygen saturation begins to drop, there are several things you must do to improve oxygenation.
- If you follow these simple maneuvers, you may never have to inflate both lungs and interfere with the surgical field.
- There is only one key point to remember: recruit more alveoli!
- Caveat: If things aren't working, by all means inflate both lungs and take a, pardon the pun, breather. Killing the patient to keep the surgeon happy is not an option.
  - First and foremost, make sure you are ventilating with 100% FiO_2!
  - Make sure the ventilator is working, turned on, and the circuit is connected.
  - Make sure the ETT (doesn't matter which one you're using) is free of kinks, mucus, or other obstruction.
  - Make the ventilation match the patient! What does that mean?
    - Check your inspiratory/expiratory (I:E) ratio. A long I:E ratio (where the inspiratory time is greater than the expiratory time) is used for *restrictive* lung diseases, and a short I:E ratio (expiratory time is greater than inspiratory time) is used for *obstructive* lung diseases.
    - Keep in mind, most of these types of patients have *obstructive* lung disease due to their probable smoking history. However, remember, you just positioned the patient in the lateral decubitus position.
      ▲ The patient is now lying on the lung you are trying to ventilate.
      ▲ To move the chest and ventilate with an adequate tidal volume, you may need to increase your inspiratory pressures.
      ▲ You have, in essence, created an iatrogenic *restrictive* lung disease.
      ▲ Now you have an *obstructive component* and a *restrictive component*!
    - Check the tidal volume and respiratory rate.
      ▲ We know the trend is to use lower tidal volumes, but you have to recruit some alveoli here. You may indeed need a higher tidal volume than you wish to use on one lung, because all the alveoli you can use are in this lung!

- ▲ Make sure your respiratory (ventilation) rate is not too high. Remember, these patients almost always have an obstructive component, and they need time to exhale all the CO_2 before you can replace it with oxygen at the alveolar level. A slower respiratory rate will give you that.
- ▲ Combine a higher tidal volume with a lower rate, and you recruit more alveoli for each individual breath.
  - If you have a newer model of anesthesia machine with the newer model ventilators, try adding an *inspiratory pause*.
    - ▲ This maneuver is based on the same concept as positive end-expiratory pressure (PEEP): you recruit more alveoli.
    - ▲ Remember, your respiratory and lung physiology: alveoli have an *opening pressure*, which is actually an opening pressure *over time*.
    - ▲ If, at the end of the inspiratory phase of the ventilation cycle you add a pause, you are essentially recruiting more alveoli at the same peak airway pressure that only took a couple of extra seconds to open.
    - ▲ This can markedly improve gas exchange!
- Add PEEP to the "dependent" lung.
  - Some people call this the "down" lung, since it is in the inferior position to the other lung. However, this terminology is somewhat confusing, since the other lung, the operative lung, is "down," meaning in this case, "deflated." Get in the habit now of referring to the "dependent" and "nondependent" lungs.
  - How much PEEP should you add? Try starting at 5 cm H_2O. If that doesn't work, increase to 10 cm H_2O.
    - ▲ What if the O_2 saturation goes down? You have just increased the alveolar pressure more than the capillary closing pressure, and you have now effectively caused a huge ventilation-perfusion (VQ) mismatch.
    - ▲ In other words, you have shunted blood *away from* the alveoli you wish to ventilate.
- Add continuous positive airway pressure (CPAP) to the nondependent lung.
  - Make sure you know how to do this. You'll need to know this, not only for your patient's survival, but also for the oral boards.
  - Use a CPAP device that is commercially available. Know where they are located in your facility, and know how to set up and use them.
  - The idea is simply to connect the commercially available CPAP device to the bronchial lumen of the double-lumen ETT and the other end to an additional oxygen source (flowmeter). You can dial an amount of pressure you would like to deliver to that bronchus.
    - ▲ What if you are using a Univent, Arndt, Cohen, or Uniblocker device?
    - ▲ The commercially available CPAP delivery device does not fit the port of the blocker. What to do?
    - ▲ Hint: Get a piece of oxygen tubing, connect it to an oxygen source (flowmeter at 2 L/min), and *intermittently* hold the tubing to the port opening. Do not continuously connect this to the port; you will inadvertently inflate the lung, since there is no way for the oxygen/gases to escape. However, if you hold it only for a few seconds, you just may recruit enough alveoli to improve oxygenation.
- If none of the above steps work, discuss this with the surgeon. You may consider *intermittent* ventilation of the operative (nondependent) lung, as long as the surgeon will work with you on this.
  - When can you not bring up the "nondependent" lung? Only when you are in a crisis situation, such as when you're doing a dissecting thoracic aortic aneurysm and the surgeon just lost the proximal aortic cannula, leaving a big hole in the aorta. You cannot bring up the lung or the patient will bleed to death.
  - This is an example of a really bad day.
- When all of this fails to improve oxygenation, it's time to really discuss with the surgeon (be forceful if you have to) the need to ventilate both lungs.
- There are times when, even though you are now ventilating both lungs again, that the insult caused will result in inability to oxygenate with both lungs.
  - And you just thought your day was bad so far.
  - Don't forget…there is always cardiopulmonary bypass and extracorporeal membrane oxygenation.
  - We don't wish this on anyone, but, hey, we've been there, so don't think you will never have the opportunity!

Intercostal Block

- I know, this, strictly speaking, belongs in the regional chapter, but you will most often do intercostal blocks after thoracotomies, so the technique to this block is included here.
- Intercostal blocks do not provide the same pain relief as a thoracic epidural, no matter how much you love them nor how easier they are to perform.

- Intercostal blocks have a high rate of absorption of local anesthetics, so be careful with the amount of local anesthetic you give here. You really should get in the habit of calculating the toxic dose in mg/kg of your local anesthetics, and do not exceed this amount, especially in intercostal nerve blocks.
- Localize the ribs in the dermatomes you want to block.
- Do yourself a favor. If you perform the blocks *after* a chest tube is already in place (as it will be after a thoracotomy or after a chest tube is placed for multiple rib fractures), you don't have to worry about the No. 1 complication of these blocks: the dreaded pneumothorax.
- Use either a 22-gauge needle or a special regional block needle (these tend to be a little longer and afford you the opportunity to get into the neurovascular bundle, even in people with excess thoracic cage fat pads).
- Insert the needle, hit the rib, then walk the tip of the needle off the bottom edge of the rib.
- Advance the tip of the needle until you are just underneath the rib. (Think "below" the rib "above.")
- You might feel a pop as you enter the neurovascular sheath or you might not.
- Aspirate to ensure you are not in a vein or an artery! (Remember, it only takes about 3 to 5 mL of bupivacaine injected intravascularly to cause complete and total cardiovascular collapse!)
- Inject 3 to 5 mL of local anesthetic per intercostal space (calculating the total toxic dose and dividing it by the number of spaces you intend to block).
- Caveat: You can effectively block only one side of the thorax because of the risk of local anesthetic toxicity.

Setting Up the Nitric Oxide Delivery Device (Inovent® by Ohmeda™)

- This has absolutely nothing to do with lung isolation, except that it may be the only thing that saves you during lung isolation when oxygenation hits the floor.
- This is one special thing you will need to do during some heart, lung, or heart/lung transplants, not to mention a few other selected disaster cases where you can only ventilate one lung.
- Nitric oxide is an inhaled gas delivered by a specially built system. Currently there is only one system, the Inovent System, manufactured and supplied by Ohmeda™. There are other delivery devices currently under investigation awaiting FDA approval, but right now this is the only one you've got, so you may as well know how to set it up and use it.
- The dose of nitric oxide is extremely small, in the 5 to 80 parts per million (ppm) range.
- Nitric oxide is extremely expensive, about $125 per hour of use, up to 96 hours (that's nearly $5000 per day). Of course, it's free for the remainder of the month in use, but the charge recurs at the beginning on the following month if indeed you are still using it.
- Nitric oxide is an attempt to provide a "magic bullet" that can decrease pulmonary artery pressures, yet not affect systemic pressures. In spite of its billing, it does not always work, and it does not always spare the systemic pressures.
- Connect the nitric oxide tank to the Inovent delivery device.
- Open the tank.

Setting Up the System

- Connect the nitric oxide delivery tube to the front of the Inovent (there is only one port on the front of the machine that the delivery tube will fit).
- Connect the other end of the delivery tube to the regulator.
- Connect the electronic cable to the front of the Inovent and to the regulator.
- Place the regulator on the *inspiratory limb* of your circuit, just as it leaves the anesthesia machine.
- Attach the sampling line to the front of the Inovent (once again, there is only one port where it will fit).
- Place the other end of the sampling line in the inspiratory limb of the circuit, at least 6 inches proximal to the "Y". This will allow you to adequately measure inspired nitric oxide concentration without contamination from exhaled nitric oxide.
- You will need to insert an extra bit of corrugated circuit tubing into the inspiratory limb of your circuit so you can connect the sampling line. These extra pieces of circuit are provided by the manufacturer.
- Remember, you will hook each of these devices up on the *inspiratory* limb, since you want to measure the nitric oxide *inspired*.
- Fortunately, each device can only plug into one place on the Inovent, so the device setup is nearly foolproof.
- Dial up the nitric oxide concentration you wish to deliver until you get a response you hope to achieve.
- Keep going until you max out at 80 parts per million.
- Notice the amount of inhaled NO_2 (nitrogen dioxide). This is toxic to humans and causes methemoglobinemia. The Inovent measures the inhaled NO_2 as well as nitric oxide, and any amount of inhaled NO_2 above 3 ppm is unacceptable. You may need to dial back your nitric oxide concentration to reduce the amount of NO_2 you are delivering to the patient.
- Keep an eye on the systemic blood pressure; this "perfect" drug is far from it.

SUGGESTED READING

Campos JH, Hallam EA, Van Natta T, Kernstine KH. Devices for lung isolation used by anesthesiologists with limited thoracic experience: comparison of double-lumen endotracheal tube, Univent torque control blocker, and Arndt wire-guided endobronchial blocker. *Anesthesiology.* 2006;104(2):261–266.

Campos JH. Which device should be considered the best for lung isolation: double-lumen endotracheal tube versus bronchial blockers. *Curr Opin Anaesthesiol.* 2007;20(1):27–31.

Cohen E. Pro: the new bronchial blockers are preferable to double-lumen tubes for lung isolation. *J Cardiothorac Vasc Anesth.* 2008;22(6):920–924.

EZ-Blocker®, IQ Medical Ventures, http://www.iq-medicalventures.com/products/EZ-Blocker. Accessed October, 2011.

Fischer GW, Cohen E. An update on anesthesia for thoracoscopic surgery. *Curr Opin Anaesthesiol.* 2010;23(1):7–11.

Narayanaswamy M. McRae K, Slinger P, Dugas G, Kanellakos GW, Roscoe A, Lacroix M. Choosing a lung isolation device for thoracic surgery: a randomized trial of three bronchial blockers versus double-lumen tubes. *Anesth Analg.* 2009;108(4):1097–1101.

Slinger P. The clinical use of right-sided double-lumen tubes. *Can J Anaesth.* 2010;57(4):293–300.

Ueda K, Goetzinger C, Gauger EH, Hallam EA, Campos JH. Use of bronchial blockers: a retrospective review of 302 cases. *J Anesth.* 2011:16; Epub ahead of print.

CHAPTER 39

PACING: "KEEPING THE PACE"

CHRISTIAN MCDONOUGH
DEEPAK SALUJA
JONATHAN KRAIDIN
ASAD KHAN

Tomorrow and tomorrow and tomorrow
Creeps in this petty pace from day to day.
      Shakespeare, *Macbeth,* Act V

INTRODUCTION

Patients with cardiac electrophysiological disturbances often present a challenge to anesthesiologists in the operating room. Implantable devices are being used more frequently for the treatment of bradyarrhythmia, tachyarrhythmia, and heart failure. When confronted with a pacemaker or cardioverter/defibrillator in the OR, it is incumbent on the anesthesiologist to understand the patient care implications. This chapter presents an overview of device function, its indications, as well as management of patients with temporary and permanent pacemakers.

OVERVIEW/HISTORY

- Currently, 3 million people worldwide have implanted rhythm devices and each year 900,000 new devices are placed, mostly in people over the age of 60. The first battery operated pacing device was developed in 1958 by Dr. Rune Elqvist. Devices have evolved from single-chamber pacemakers to multichamber devices to minicomputers that in some cases have the ability to pace, cardiovert, and defibrillate if needed.
- A pacemaker is an external device that acts to provide a minimal programmable rate; if the intrinsic rate is too slow, the pacemaker speeds it up. Pacemakers cannot slow down rates that are too fast. The sinus node located in the right atrium is the director of the band. It generates an electrical signal that spreads from the atrium to the ventricle, causing it to beat in a synchronous fashion. The pacemaker uses electrical impulses, delivered by electrodes contacting the heart muscles, to regulate the beating of the heart.
- An implantable cardioverter defibrillator (ICD) is a pacemaker that can shock abnormally fast rhythms (such as ventricular fibrillation and ventricular tachycardia) back to normal. All ICDs made today also have pacemaking ability, so that a modern-day ICD has the capability to pace a heart that is going too slow, shock a rhythm that is going too fast, or use antitachycardia-pacing techniques to terminate ventricular tachycardias without resorting to shocks.

PACEMAKER INDICATIONS

- Sick sinus syndrome
- Symptomatic sinus bradycardia
- Tachy-brady syndrome
- Atrial fibrillation with periods significant bradycardia during otherwise controlled rates
- Third-degree atrioventricular (AV) block
- Chronotropic incompetence (inability to increase the heart rate to match a level of exercise)
- Prolonged QT syndrome
- Cardiac resynchronization (biventricular pacing)

PACEMAKER ANATOMY/FUNCTION

Transcutaneous pads are the easiest and most convenient way to achieve rapid application of temporary pacing. Transcutaneous pacing is uncomfortable, since the chest musculature can be activated with every paced beat, and that hurts. Often these patients will require sedation.

- Permanent pacing systems consist of a pulse generator and transvenous pacing leads. In this type of system, leads are inserted transvenously via the cephalic or subclavian vein and advanced to the right ventricle or atrium where they are fixed into the myocardial tissue. They are attached to a pulse generator, which is placed subcutaneously or submuscularly in the chest wall.
- Pulse generators contain a battery as well as sensing, timing, and output circuits. Pulse generators can be set to fixed-rate (asynchronous) or demand (synchronous) modes. In the first, impulses are produced at a set rate independent of intrinsic cardiac activity. Asynchronous pacing carries a small danger of producing lethal dysrhythmias should the impulse coincide with the vulnerable period of the T wave. In the latter, the sensing circuit searches for an intrinsic depolarization potential. If this is absent, a pacing response is generated. This mode mimics intrinsic cardiac electric activity.
- During pacemaker placement, signal amplitude and width are set high enough to reliably achieve myocardial capture, yet low enough to maximize battery life.
- Temporary transvenous leads provide a reliable and comfortable pacing in situations in which a permanent device is not yet indicated or is impractical.
- In these systems, catheters are inserted through a central venous access into the right ventricle. ECG monitoring (specifically V1 and lead II) is used to track catheter positioning. For example, while pacing, the atrium will be captured when the tip of the catheter is in the atrium. As the catheter moves into the ventricle, the morphology in V1 will be left bundle (since the right side of the heart is being paced), and lead II will be upright (since the base of the heart is paced first as the catheter is advanced). As the lead is advanced to its proper place in the RV apex, the morphology in lead II becomes inverted (Figure 39-1).

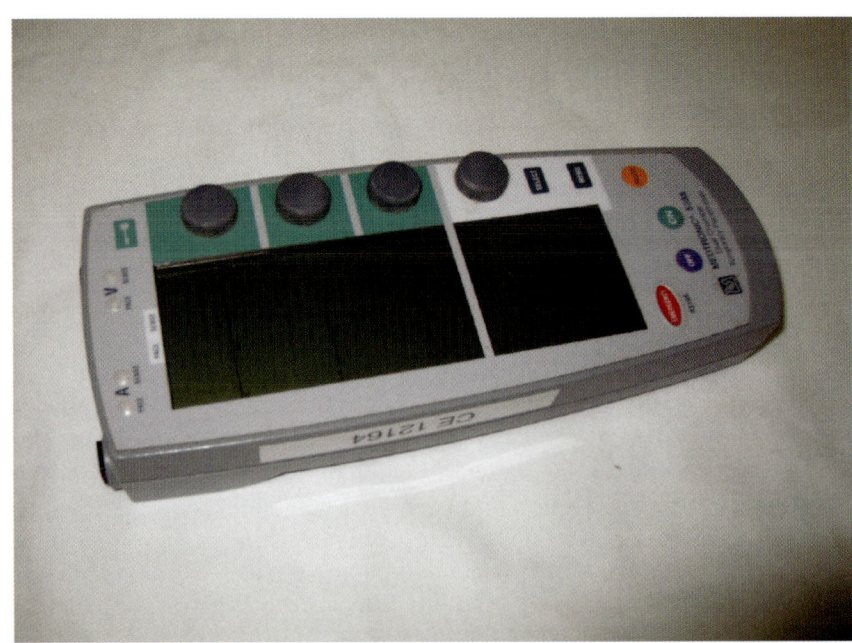

FIGURE 39-1 Common pacemaker found in most operating rooms.

PACING CODES

I know that Rosetta Stone does not yet offer a Pacing Code Language course, but I'm guessing many of you will wish you did after reading the following material. To understand the language of pacing it is necessary to comprehend the coding system for pacemakers (Table 39-1).

Pacing Code Explanation

A typical pacing code consists of three to five letters. The first letter indicates the chamber(s) paced:
- A: Atrial pacing
- V: Ventricular pacing
- D: Dual-chamber (atrial and ventricular) pacing

The second letter indicates the chamber in which electrical activity is sensed:
- A, V, or D
- O is used when pacemaker discharge is not dependent on sensing electrical activity.

The third letter refers to the response to a sensed electric signal:
- T: Triggering of pacing function
- I: Inhibition of pacing function
- D: Dual response (i.e., any spontaneous atrial and ventricular activity will inhibit atrial and ventricular pacing and lone atrial activity will trigger a paced ventricular response)
- O: No response to an underlying electric signal (usually related to the absence of associated sensing function)

The fourth letter represents rate modulation:
- R: Rate-response ("physiologic") pacing
- O: No programmability or rate modulation

The fifth letter represents antitachycardia functions:
- P: Paced
- S: Shocks
- D: Dual (pacing + shock)

- Although the first three letters are used most commonly, a fifth position code is currently in use. The first position denotes the chamber(s) paced; the second position denotes the chamber(s) sensed; the third position denotes the action(s) performed; the fourth position denotes rate response; and finally, the fifth position denotes antitachycardia function. More modern pacemakers have multiple functions. The simplest settings are VVI and AAI.
- The VVI mode senses and paces the ventricle and is inhibited by a sensed ventricular event.
- The AAI mode senses and paces in the atrium, and is inhibited by a sensed atrial event. The most common setting, DDD mode, denotes that both chambers are able to be sensed and paced. This requires two leads, one in the atrium and the other in the ventricle.
- In the ECG, if both atrium and ventricle are being paced, there will be a pacing artifact before the P wave and preceding the QRS.
- The first pacing artifact indicates the atrial depolarization, and the second indicates the initiation of the QRS complex. Given that one of the leads is in the right ventricle, a left bundle-branch pattern may be evident on ECG.
- Rarely, you may encounter specialized single-lead systems that can sense atrial impulses and either sense or pace the ventricle. Thus, this system provides for atrial tracking without the capability for atrial pacing and can be used in patients with AV block and normal sinus node function.

Most pacemaker generators have an x-ray code that can be seen on a chest radiograph; however, the chest radiography may need to be zoomed onto the pacemaker generator for better resolution. The markings, along with the shape of the generator, may assist with deciphering the manufacturer of the generator and pacemaker battery.

TABLE 39-1 Coding System for Pacemakers

1st Position Chamber Paced	2nd Position Chamber Sensed	3rd Position Response to Sensing	4th Position Rate Modulation	5th Position Multisite Pacing
A	A	T	O	O
V	V	I	R	A
D	D	D		V
	O	O		D

Abbreviations: A, atrium; V, ventricle; D, dual (both chambers); O, none; T, triggered; I, inhibited; R, rate adaptive.

Temporary emergency pacing is indicated for therapy of significant and hemodynamically unstable bradydysrhythmias and for prevention of bradycardia-dependent malignant dysrhythmias. Examples include refractory symptomatic sinus node dysfunction, complete heart block (see image below), alternating bundle-branch block, new bifascicular block, and bradycardia-dependent ventricular tachycardia.

MAGNETS

Most of the time we use magnets for things such as sticking our kid's straight-A report card on the fridge, but in the context of this chapter the magnet plays a vital role in managing our device in patients while they are in surgery. There are a couple of issues with surgery:
- If electrocautery is used, electrical interference is sensed during its application as very rapid heartbeats (look at your rhythm strip). Since, as we discussed, devices are stupid, and they cannot tell the difference between electrocautery and actual heartbeats, a device will sense this interference as intrinsic electrical cardiac activity. This means that with pacemakers, pacing will be inhibited (since the pacemaker will think the heart is beating really fast), and with ICDs the patient may get an inappropriate shock (since the ICD will think the heart is beating really fast). More hilarious is that the surgeon, if in close contact with the patient when this happens, may also get a shock.
- When rate-responsive pacing is turned on (i.e., DDDR), the pacemaker will use clues such as the respiratory rate, an accelerometer, or a variety of other things depending on the model to decide what the intrinsic pacing rate should be. Surgery sometimes screws this all up, and pacemakers can get very confused, causing inappropriate rapid pacing and panic in the anesthesiology staff.

PACEMAKER IMPACT ON SURGERY

The proper response to being presented with a patient who is undergoing surgery is to get the device interrogated by someone who knows what he is doing. That way, you will know what kind of device it is (pacemaker? ICD? biventricular ICD?), what the settings are (is rate response on?), and how much the patient is actually using the pacing function (if this device gets inhibited somehow during the surgery, will this patient have heart beats or not?).
- With an ICD, tachycardia settings should always be turned off for the OR.
- With a pacemaker, the right thing to do for the OR depends on the situation. For patients who barely use their pacemaker in real life, chances are they are not going to use it on the table, so you can very likely leave it alone.
- If the rate response is on, you probably want to turn that off. For patients who need their pacemaker to live, you need to do something to ensure it doesn't get inhibited during the procedure.
- All of these things (turning off tachycardia functions and rate response, ensuring pacemaker function in the OR) are most reliably done with the programmer before the procedure (don't forget to have the settings changed back at the end!). Another way to do this is to place a magnet over it.
- In most pacemakers, placing a magnet over the device temporarily "reprograms" the pacer into asynchronous mode. This means that the pacemaker will continue to output regardless of what the heart is doing or if there is any noise present.
- This might be a good choice for a patient who is completely dependent who might have a heart rate of 0 if the pacemaker was inhibited by noise from cautery. In automatic ICDs (AICDs), the magnet will in most cases inhibit the antitachycardia (i.e., shocking) function. It will usually not effect any of the pacemaking functions. This means that the only real option to appropriately prepare patients for surgery who have ICDs but who also require the pacemaking function of the device (i.e., those that are pacemaker dependent) is to interrogate the device. If a patient does not ever use the pacing function, and the device is only there to terminate tachyarrhythmias, putting a magnet over it is usually OK. Just make sure it stays in place.

Major Pacemaker Malfunctions

- Failure to output (i.e., oversensing)
- Failure to capture
- Failure to sense

Other Interesting Pacing Shenanigans

- Pacemaker-mediated tachycardia
- Runaway pacemaker
- Pacemaker Wenckebach phenomenon

Failure to Output

Failure to output occurs when no pacing artifact is present despite an indication to pace (Figure 39-2).
- In most cases in the OR, this is going to be due to the pacemaker sensing noise on the lead and being tricked into thinking that the heart is beating when it actually isn't. The most common cause of this is cautery, as described above, but is can occur for more bizarre reasons such as crosstalk between the leads in a dual chamber device, myopotentials, or from electrical interference from other equipment.

- Other causes of failure to output include a fractured lead (which causes sensed electrical noise), battery depletion, circuit malfunction, or an inadequate connection between the lead and the header, although these are issues that should be identified before the patient hits the OR by doing (you guessed it) an interrogation.
- If output failure occurs in the OR, placing a magnet over the device (if there is not already one in place) will cause the device to switch to asynchronous mode (unless it is completely kaput).
- If your pacemaker problem is caused by the device sensing noise, switching to an asynchronous mode will help you out since the pacemaker no longer looks at what is going on around it and will just start pacing at a fixed rate. If this does not fix the problem and the patient is in need of pacing, the only remedy may be to place a temporary wire.
- Then call the electrophysiologist. The electrophysiology (EP) labs get mad at you when you ask them to come to the OR and help out. Plus they never come in as early as we do, so they are grumpy when they come to the OR. This is a universal law like gravity.

Failure to Capture

Failure to capture occurs when a pacing artifact is not followed by a captured complex.
- This most commonly is due to an inappropriately low programmed output, lead fracture, dislodgment, myocardial infarction at the lead tip, drugs (e.g., flecainide), hyperkalemia, or severe homeostatic abnormalities such as acidosis or alkalosis. There is not much you can do about failure to capture in the OR.
- If there is a programmer handy and someone who knows how to use it, you can try to increase the output. If there is an electrolyte or acid/base abnormality present, you can try to fix it. If all else fails and the patient needs to be paced, you may need to put in a temporary wire. And then call the electrophysiologist.

Undersensing

Undersensing occurs when a pacer incorrectly misses intrinsic depolarization and paces despite intrinsic activity. This is what you intentionally cause when you but a magnet over the device.
- Essentially, a pacemaker that is completely undersensing is a pacemaker operating in asynchronous mode.
- This can occur if the lead dislodges during the procedure, or because of the types of severe homeostatic abnormalities that can result in failure to capture. Since the device is programmed to ignore all voltage that it senses below a certain level, if the sensed voltage goes below that level because of acidosis or hyperkalemia or the like, the device will start ignoring those beats.
- The result may not be as immediately disastrous as failure to capture or output in a pacemaker-dependent patient, but bad things can (and do) still happen. The main danger (this is true during magnet application as well) is that the pacemaker will try to pace the ventricle on the T-wave. Under the right circumstances, this can cause torsades de points, which can be fatal. The disastrous R on T problem!

Pacemaker-Mediated Tachycardia

- A premature ventricular contraction (PVC) in a dual-chamber pacemaker may precipitate pacemaker-mediated tachycardia.
- If a PVC is transmitted in a retrograde manner through the AV node, it may, in turn, depolarize the atria. This atrial depolarization is detected by the atrial sensor, which then stimulates the ventricular leads to fire, hence creating an endless loop.
- Although the maximum rate is limited by the pacemaker's programmed upper limit, the possibility of developing ischemia exists in susceptible patients. This is another opportunity to use a magnet to diagnose and treat the arrhythmia.
- The magnet will place the pacemaker into asynchronous mode and sensing will be deactivated, thus preventing continuation of the dysrhythmia (Figure 39-3).

Runaway Pacemaker

A malfunction of the pacemaker generator resulting in a life-threatening rapid tachycardia (up to 200 bpm) is known as runaway pacemaker (Figure 39-4).
- The most common cause is due to battery failure or external damage. This used to be much more common in the previous generation of devices, but may still occur.
- It is a rare medical emergency that requires immediate action. An external magnet may induce slower pacing, but it is possible that the device will not respond to magnet application, and more aggressive measures may be necessary. If a patient becomes unstable, treatment involves making an incision in the chest wall over the pacemaker and detaching the pacemaker leads from the generator. Note that the patient may require temporary pacing as a result.

Pacemaker Wenckebach Phenomenon

- Let's say you are a dual-chamber pacemaker in a patient with complete heart block. If the patient is in sinus rhythm at 80 beats a minute, you will be sensing that sinus beat and pacing the ventricle at 80 beats a minute in response.
- Let's say the patient goes into atrial fibrillation, with an atrial rate of 400 beats per minute. Are you going to pace the ventricle at 400 beats per minute? Of course not. You will switch to a mode that will essentially ignore the atrium and only focus on how fast the ventricle is going. This *mode switch rate* is usually set to something like 170 beats per minute. So essentially, if the atrium goes over this rate, you will be switching modes.
- Now, let's say this unlucky individual is back in sinus rhythm but now develops atrial tachycardia at a rate of 160 beats per minute. Are you going to switch modes?
- No! That is under the mode switch rate. But are you really going to pace the ventricle at 160 beats per minute? No! That would be way too fast. What you will do is pace as fast as the *upper tracking limit* will allow. This is 130 in the DDD 60–130 setting you may commonly encounter.
- What will happen in this case is that even though the atrium is sensed at 160 beats per minute, the pacemaker will only pace at 130 beats per minute.
- Effectively, the A-V interval will increase in successive beats until one of the atrial beats falls into a period after the ventricular paced beat called the *refractory period*. This is a programmable interval during which atrial events are intentionally not sensed.
- Since the atrial beat falls in the refractory period and is not sensed, no ventricular beat will follow. This looks very much on the ECG like Wenckebach phenomenon, although in this case it is caused by the way the pacemaker is set (Figure 39-5).

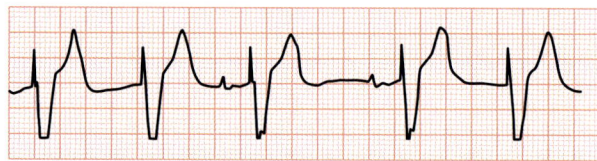

FIGURE 39-2 Failure to output due to oversensing of the T-wave in a patient with complete heart block and a temporary wire.

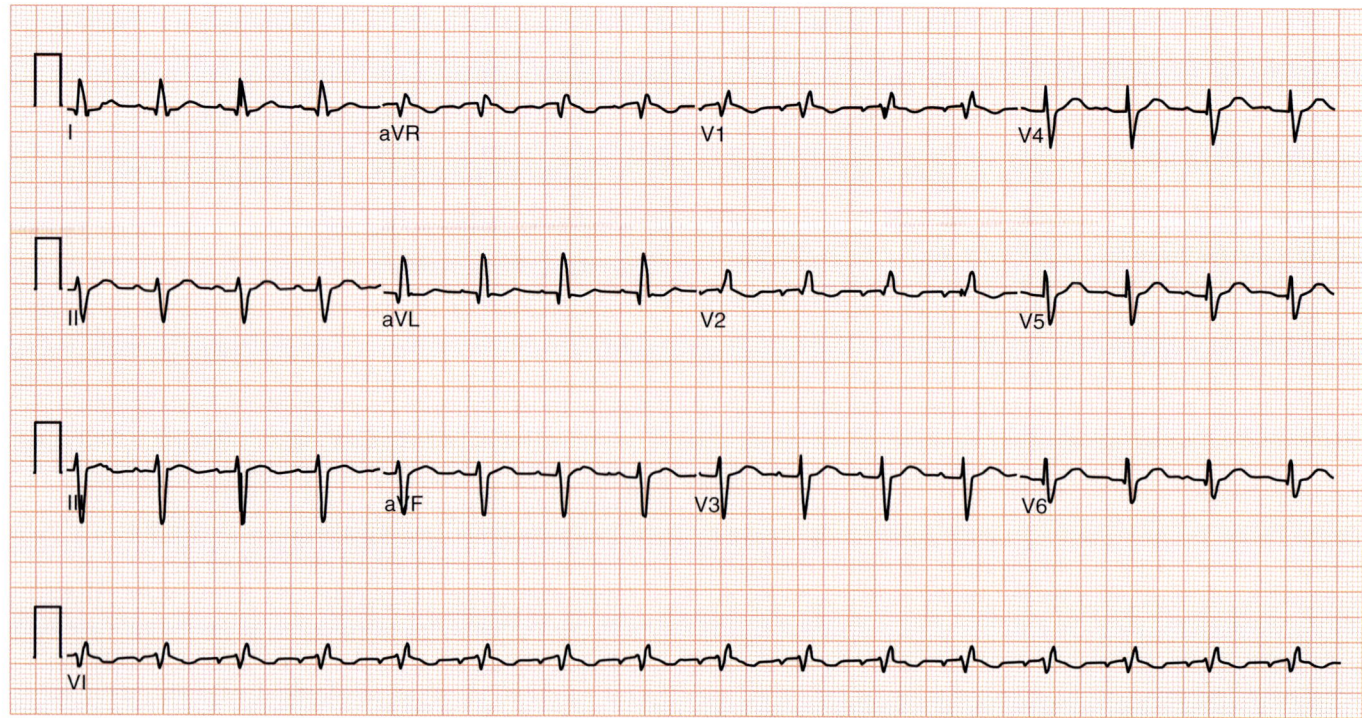

FIGURE 39-3 Pacemaker-mediated tachycardia; note the inappropriate pacing spike in the third QRS.

Chapter 39 PACING: "KEEPING THE PACE"

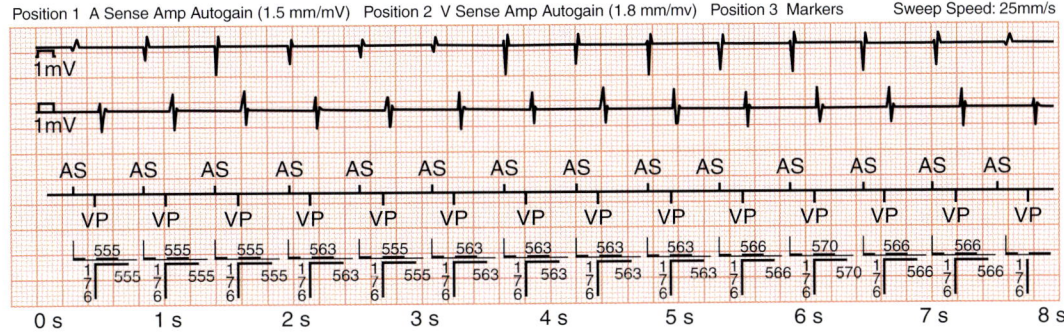

FIGURE 39-4 Runaway pacemaker.

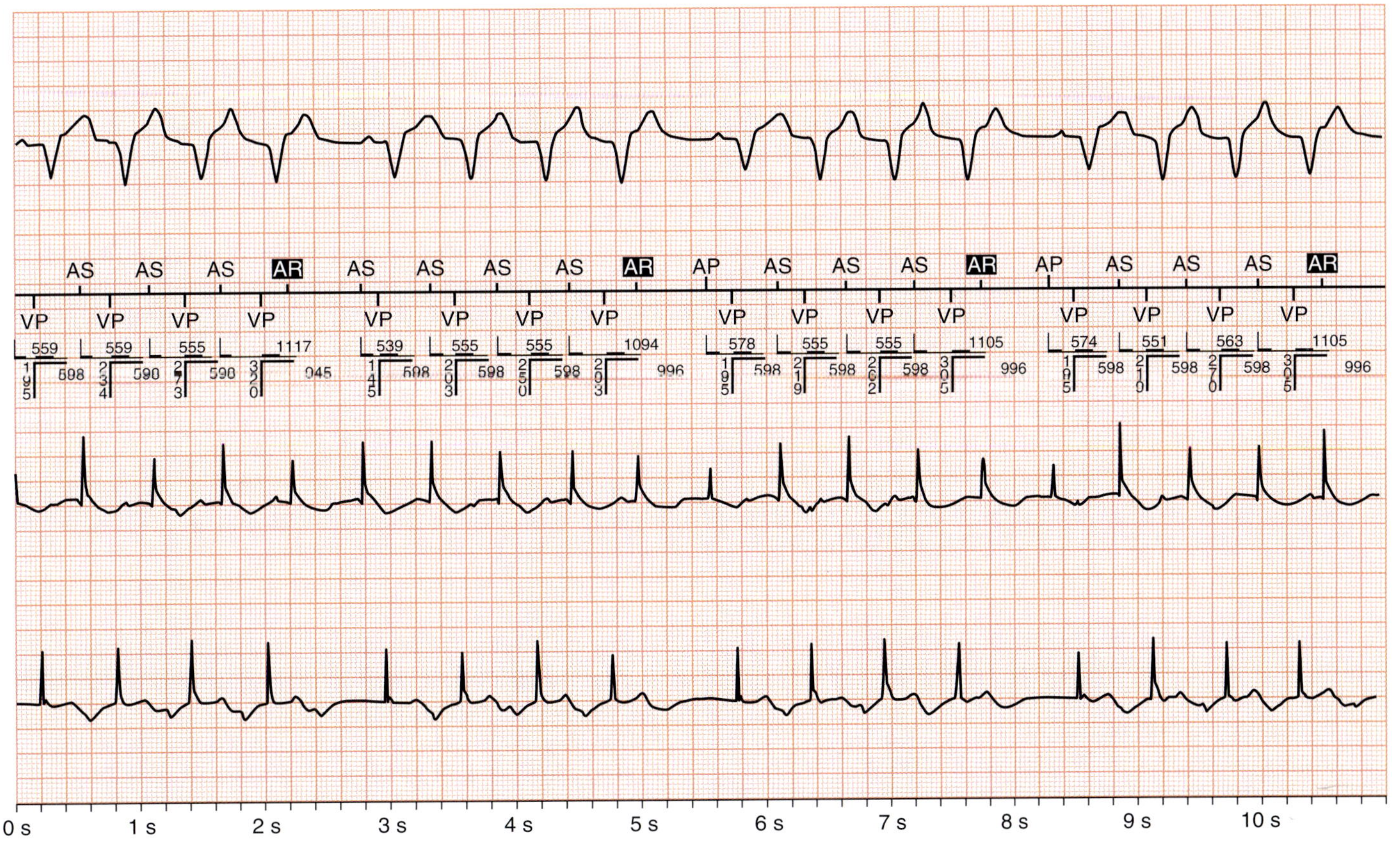

FIGURE 39-5 The channels are (from top to bottom) V1, marker channel, interval channel, atrial channel, and ventricular channel.

PREOPERATIVE MANAGEMENT OF THE PACEMAKER PATIENT

Preoperative evaluation of a patient with a permanent pacemaker should include assessment of both the patient and pacemaker.
- Evaluation and optimization of coexisting diseases in the patient with a pacemaker scheduled for an operating room procedure is of utmost importance.
- Many of these patients have significant comorbidities including severe coronary artery disease (50%), hypertension (20%), and diabetes (10%). It is also important to know the severity of heart disease, the current functional status, and the medications the patient currently takes.
- Asking the patient about the initial indication for pacemaker placement can also help in understanding the patient's underlying conditions. A 12-lead ECG,

chest x-ray for visualization of continuity of leads, and measurement of serum electrolytes (potassium) should be performed.

It is important for the anesthesiologist to review the patient's pacemaker history and follow-up schedule.
- The pacemaker history includes determining the indication for and date of initial pacemaker placement.
- Also determining the last generator test date and battery status is important as it has been reported that 5% of patients presenting for surgery were in need of battery replacement and less than 10% had less than optimal pacing settings.
- Also of importance is determining whether or not the pacing mode should be reprogrammed before surgery in order to avoid intraoperative complications. Reprogramming a device to asynchronous mode at a rate above the patient's normal rate will protect the patient from pacemaker oversensing or undersensing during electromagnetic interference.

In general, pacemaker reprogramming is needed for patients with any rate-responsive device, or patients undergoing major chest or abdominal or thoracic procedures in which monopolar Bovie could cause inappropriate firing of pacemaker. An AICD should also be disabled before anesthesia.
- American College of Cardiology (ACC)/American Heart Association (AHA) guidelines advise that all antitachycardia therapy should be disabled prior to surgery. Alternative cardiac pacing methods should be available if there is a high risk of electromagnetic interference (EMI) in close proximity to pacemaker generator.
- Magnet placement is also an issue that is very important and something that anesthesiologists should be knowledgeable about. Placement of a magnet is advantageous in that it can protect the pacemaker from EMI and inappropriate firing by changing the pacemaker to an asynchronous nonsensing mode.

However, not all pacemakers switch to the asynchronous mode with magnet placement. The response varies with the model and manufacturer.
- Some pacemakers may have a continuous or transient loss of pacing with magnet placement.
- Others may have no change in rate or rhythm or may only have a brief asynchronous pacing period. Also placement of a magnet over a pacemaker is not without risk.
- Switching to an asynchronous mode may trigger ventricular asynchrony in patients with myocardial ischemia, hypoxia, or electrolyte imbalances.
- Constant magnet placement may also alter the pacemaker program causing unexpected or unknown responses to EMI. It is therefore considered safe to use magnets in nonprogrammable pacemakers only.

INTRAOPERATIVE MANAGEMENT

Intraoperative monitoring is dependent on the patient's underlying disease and the type of surgical procedure. Standard American Society of Anesthesiologists (ASA) monitors will suffice, as no special monitoring is needed for patients with pacemakers.
- Pacemaker spikes should be monitored on the ECG strip to ensure proper pacemaker function. Any time there is a pacemaker present, ECG monitoring must be continuous.
- Placement of arterial line, a central line, or a pulmonary artery (PA) catheter again is dependent on the patient's functional status and type of surgery.
- If a PA catheter or central venous line is indicated, careful attention should be focused on not dislodging freshly placed transvenous endocardial electrodes. It is sometimes safer to place these devices on the opposite side or avoid placement if unnecessary.

Any anesthetic technique is appropriate in patients with a pacemaker and should be chosen on a case-to-case basis. Inhalational agents do not alter current or voltage thresholds of the pacemaker, and therefore do not effect pacemaker programming.
- Certain medications such as succinylcholine, ketamine, or etomidate may cause muscle fasciculations or myoclonic movements, which may inappropriately inhibit or trigger stimulation, depending on the pacing modes.
- It is therefore recommended to avoid ketamine and etomidate as well as to use a defasciculating dose of nondepolarizing muscle relaxant before administration of succinylcholine.
- The primary intraoperative issue is the sensitivity of pacemakers to EMI.
- Sources of EMI include nuclear MRI and surgical electrocautery.
- Surgical electrocautery is the most important source of EMI, as it has been associated with fatal arrhythmias and deaths stemming from pacemaker failure.
- Monopolar electrocautery is associated with more EMI than bipolar; therefore, bipolar cautery is the preferred method of cautery.
- If monopolar electrocautery is to be used, then a current return pad should be placed to prevent

the electrocautery current path from crossing the pacemaking system. For head and neck surgery, the pad should be placed on the shoulder contralateral to the device.
- The grounding plate should be as close to the operative site as possible and as far away from the pacemaker as possible. Those patients with unipolar electrode pacemaker configuration have been found to be more sensitive to EMI than those with a bipolar electrode configuration. The pacemaker should be programmed to the asynchronous mode either by magnet placement or by a programmer.
- A programmer should always be present in the OR if cautery is to be used on a patient with a pacemaker. Alternative methods for pacing such as transcutaneous pacing should be readily available in the case of sudden pacemaker malfunction.
- Procedures such as transurethral resection of the prostate (TURP), electroconvulsive therapy, nerve stimulator treatment, lithotripsy, and MRI place pacemaker patients at increased risk of pacemaker failure.
- In general, MRI has been contraindicated in both pacemaker and ICD patients, although in recent years reports have argued that MRI is safe for people with newer devices and who will be totally awake during MRI and in the presence of a cardiologist.

SUGGESTED READING

Hensley F, Martin D, Gravlee G. *A practical approach to cardiac anesthesia,* 4th ed. New York: Lippincott; 2008, pp 410–421.
Gives a clear and concise overview of basic pacemaker function.

Medtronic. Implantable pacemaker and magnet information. www.medtronic.com
Gives information about pacemaker codes and function.

Rastogi S, Goel S, Tempe D. Anesthetic management of patients with cardiac pacemakers and defibrillators for noncardiac surgery. *Ann Cardiac Anesth* 2005;8:21–32.
Gives guidelines on how to manage pacemakers in the perioperative time frame.

CHAPTER 40

TEE
LOOK! IT'S A BIRD...
IT'S A PLANE...
NO, IT'S TEE MAN!

KHURAM KHAN
ENRIQUE PANTIN

> The Bards sublime, whose distant footsteps echo through the corridors of time.
> — *Henry Wadsworth Longfellow*

> Sublimity is the echo of great mind.
> — *Longinus*

INTRODUCTION

Ever wonder what it would be like to have x-ray vision in the OR? Well, transesophageal echocardiography (TEE) is the closest thing we have to that. We are always looking for better ways to assess the hemodynamic status of our patients and TEE has become the best way to do this. You might be asking, "What's the big fuss about TEE?" Well, it's the most direct and accurate way of assessing the cardiovascular and hemodynamic status of our patients. Sometimes staring at a Foley catheter to monitor urine output or trending central venous pressures (CVPs) just doesn't cut it. With TEE, we see (almost) everything! For example, let's say your patient becomes hypotensive in the OR and you're not really sure why. Wouldn't it be amazing to be able to *see* the ventricles and determine whether or not they are sluggish or vigorous, full or empty? (Figure 40-1)

Well, Superman, get a hold of your fancy TEE probe and get ready to save the day. Now, these "super powers" are not just going to come in handy during open heart cases; in fact, there are all kinds of situations that arise in general cases that need your TEE skills. As exciting as all of this sounds, remember you are learning a completely new language, and this takes time, practice, and effort. Initially you should focus on learning what is "normal" and then moving on to identifying basic pathology: severe valvular pathology, pericardial/pleural effusions, aortic disease, and ventricular function assessment (mild, moderate, and severely depressed). We are not going to bore you by repeating stuff you can easily find on the Internet or in books, but there is a must-see Internet site if you are really interested in echocardiography, so take a few minutes and check out http://pie.med.utoronto.ca/TEE/TEE_content/TEE_standardViews_intro.html.

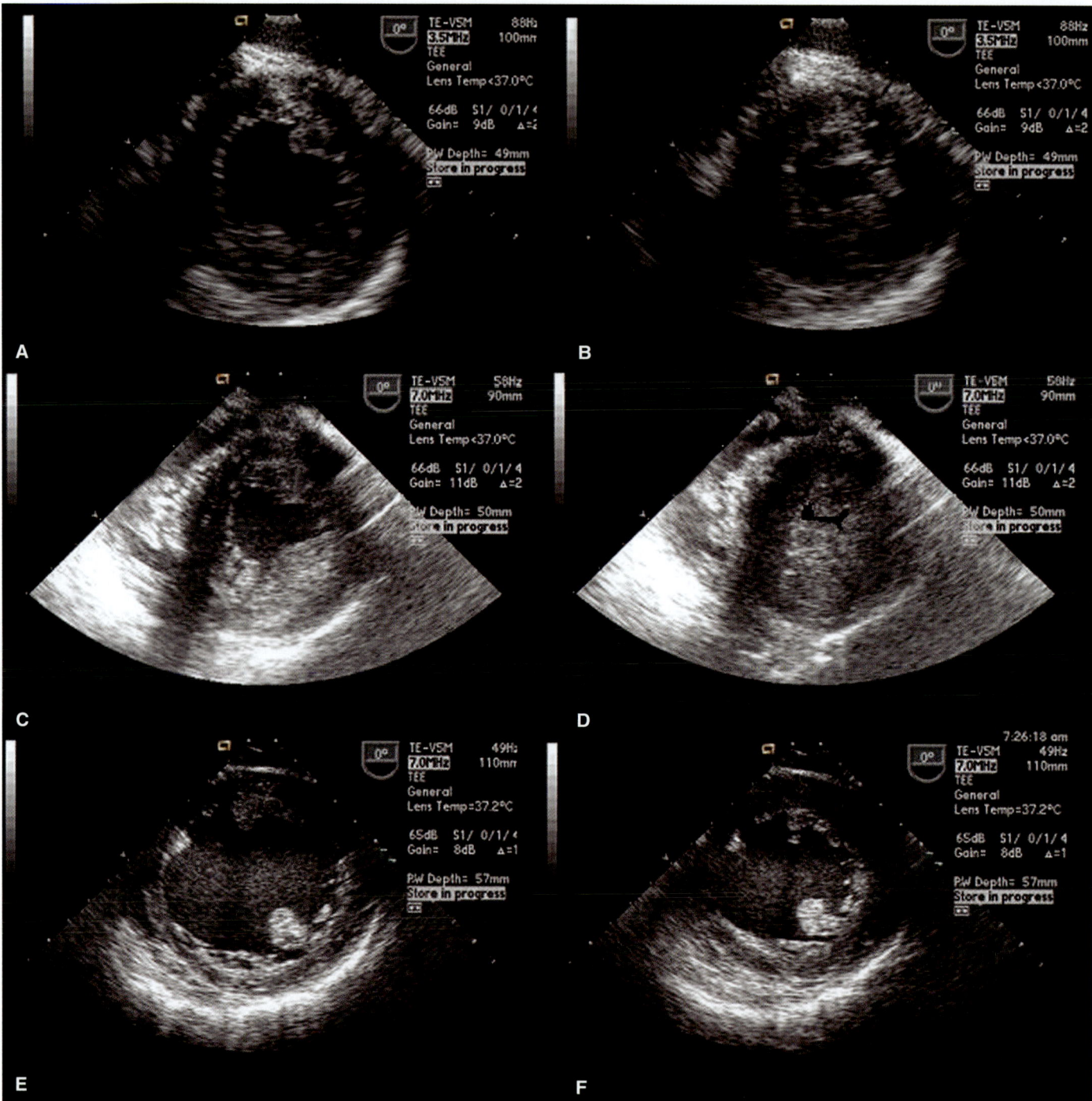

FIGURE 40-1 Transgastric view of the left ventricle (LV). Shown, from top to bottom, are three different LVs in diastole and systole. Note the relationship between segmental function or volume load and end diastolic area (EDA) and end systolic area (ESA)—black cavity inside the LV. Normal LV segments in diastole (A) and systole (B). Normal LV in diastole (C) with small EDA, and almost absent LV cavity in systole (D), typical of severe hypovolemia. Large EDA (E), and ESA (F), typical of severe LV dysfunction.

INDICATIONS

- Various organizations including the American College of Cardiology, the American Society of Anesthesiologists, the Society of Cardiovascular Anesthesiologists, and the American Society of Echocardiography have published indications for the intraoperative use of transesophageal echocardiography. Those indications that are supported by the strongest evidence are known as category I indications.[1,2]
- Category I indications:
  - Heart valve repair
  - Most congenital heart surgery that requires cardiopulmonary bypass
  - Surgical intervention for endocarditis, particularly with extensive disease or inadequate preoperative evaluation of disease severity
  - Repair of ascending aortic dissection with possible aortic valve involvement
  - Evaluation of life-threatening hemodynamic disturbances in which ventricular function is unknown
  - Pericardial window procedures
  - Hypertrophic obstructive cardiomyopathy repair
  - Placement of intracardiac devices
- Other indications such as removal of cardiac tumors, cardiac aneurysm repair, or pulmonary embolectomy are supported by relatively weaker evidence and are considered category II and III indications.
- At our institution, we have an additional indication that we refer to as the "WTH" indication. It's when you don't know "what the heck" is going on, or your patient doesn't appear to be responding to anything you give. That's about the time we make a dash for our magical TEE probe and take an early look rather than wait for the patient to become unstable or code!

CONTRAINDICATIONS

- Relative contraindications to probe insertion include patients with a history of the following:[1,3]
  - Previous upper gastrointestinal (GI) surgery (recent surgery is an absolute contraindication)
  - Significant hiatal hernia
  - Odynophagia
  - Dysphagia
  - Previous neck or mediastinal radiation
  - Recent upper GI bleed
  - Thoracic aortic aneurysm
  - Unstable cervical spine
- Certain conditions and diseases of the esophagus, such as strictures, varices, diverticula, tumors, esophagitis, or Mallory-Weiss tears, also make probe insertion a relative contraindication.
- Many of these relative contraindications can be assessed with a good old fashioned preoperative history and physical examination. Always remember to review the medical record and talk to the patient, if possible, prior to shoving a probe into the patient's esophagus.
- It's probably a good idea to avoid TEE in patients with dysphagia, previous neck or mediastinal radiation, or esophageal stricture until they have been seen by a gastroenterologist. If a TEE examination is a must, then consider using a pediatric probe. But remember, always by "scared" of the risk of esophageal perforation.

COMPLICATIONS

- Inserting TEE probes into an esophagus may be risky business. The following are all potential complications of probe insertion:[4,5]
  - Dental injury or oral trauma
  - Endotracheal tube displacement
  - Upper GI hemorrhage
  - Pharyngeal, esophageal, and gastric perforation (be on the lookout for this in patients with a history of neck or mediastinal radiation, dysphagia, and esophageal strictures)
  - Swallowing dysfunction (much more common than we think!)
  - Bronchial/aortic compression in infants

THE PROBE

- Transesophageal echoes are performed on both pediatric and adult patients. The standard adult TEE probe tip (the largest portion) measures approximately 14 × 11 mm in size and 100 to 110 cm in length. Pediatric scopes usually measure 11 × 8 mm in diameter and 70 to 75 cm in length (Figure 40-2).
- TEE probes consist of an endoscope-like device that houses a transducer at its tip. The transducer is responsible for emitting and receiving ultrasound waves.
- Both adult and pediatric probes can be quite pricey. On average the cost of a new TEE probe can range from $24,000 to $45,000 depending of the type of the probe. Needless to say, *handle with care!* You're holding the equivalent of a good car in your hands.
- Proper care of the probe can eliminate cross-contamination among patients and help save tens of thousands of dollars in repair cost annually.

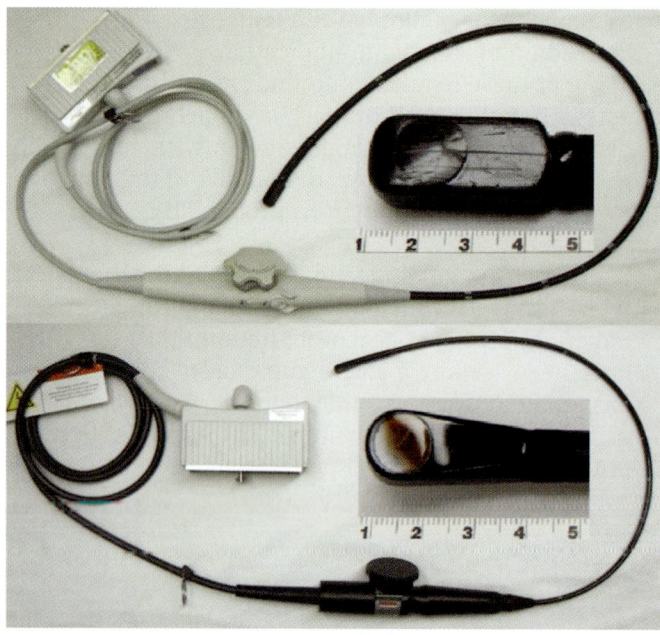

FIGURE 40-2 Top: Adult TEE probe. Note magnified detail of TEE probe tip. The round area at the tip contains all ultrasound elements aligned in a plane perpendicular to the long axis of the probe (image at 0 degrees). Once the multiplane button is pressed, these elements rotate, allowing an image to be generated anywhere between 0 and 180 degrees. Bottom: Pediatric TEE probe. Note magnified detail of TEE probe tip. All probes have a module that connects to the ultrasound machine, the handle with all probe controls, and finally the probe itself, ending with the ultrasound (US) elements at the tip.

- Certain general maintenance measures should be universal:
  - Regular visual inspections of the probe after each use
  - Probe disinfection after each use according to the manufacturers recommendations; go to http://www.gehealthcare.com/usen/service/docs/TEEProbeCareChart_FNLB.PDF

EQUIPMENT

Proper Probe Insertion

The basic echocardiography unit consists of a TEE probe, monitor, recording unit (VCR or digital recorder, and images are stored in the hospital echocardiography laboratory or similar), computer unit and probe connecting ports, and a control panel where image and signal processing occurs (Figure 40-3).
- TEE probe insertion must be done in a gentle fashion. To begin with, empty the contents of the

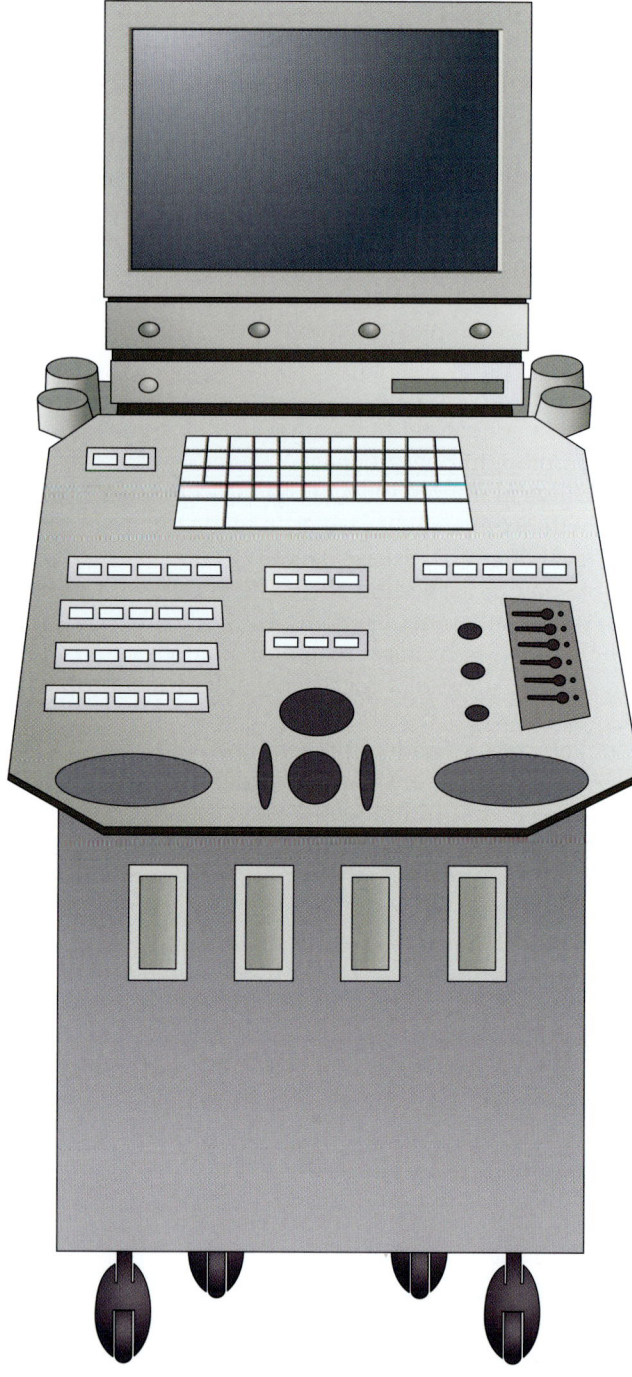

FIGURE 40-3 Ultrasound machine. Monitor at top, recording unit below, to follow keyboard. Under the keyboard are ultrasound docking ports. There are many types and sizes of machines with different capabilities and computing power.

stomach with an orogastric tube. Remember, sound waves travel well through fluids but poorly through air, and sometimes during mask ventilation a fair amount of air is insufflated into the stomach.

- In a patient who has not received any muscle relaxant, probe insertion may initiate gagging and cause the patient to bite down on the probe. To prevent this, you can get patients deeper under general anesthesia prior to probe insertion, or administer muscle relaxants.
- A good way to prevent probe damage is by the routine use of bite guards. We like to place the bite guard onto the probe prior to insertion. Placing the bite guard into the mouth of an asleep patient prior to probe insertion may make maneuvering and inserting the probe more difficult.
- Generously lubricate (hydrosoluble lubricant) the TEE probe tip, and insert the transducer in the midline of the oropharynx. To help facilitate easy passage you should lift the mandible anteriorly with your other hand. Do not lift the jaw by placing pressure on the lower teeth; you might regret it when some teeth come flying out! (Figure 40-4)
- Make sure the probe knobs are NOT in the locked position and then *gently* advance the probe, the keyword here being "*gently.*" Very little force is actually required to advance a properly positioned TEE probe.
- If you're experiencing any difficulty or resistance, *do not force the probe forward*, remove it and start all over. It might just be a matter of repositioning the patient, applying more lubrication, or providing a little more mandibular displacement.
- Throughout this process it's imperative that you also maintain a close watch on the patient. Remember, most of these patients are receiving general anesthesia at this point and will display some degree of hemodynamic instability.

Probe Manipulation

- So now that you managed to get the probe in, how the heck do you control this thing? The tip of the probe is somewhat like the head of a slithering snake in that it has the ability to turn and bend in multiple planes.
- On the handle of the adult TEE probe you'll find two knobs (one large and one small), two buttons used to lock each of the knobs in place, and a button

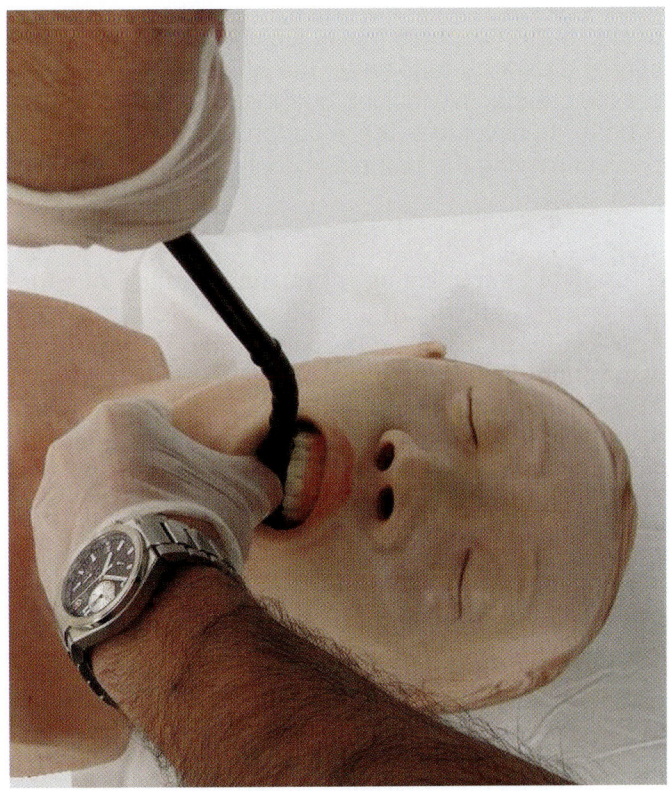

FIGURE 40-4 Left: Lateral view of TEE probe insertion in an anesthetized dummy. We place bite block over the probe and keep it close to the probe handle. Once the probe is inserted, we place the bite block between the teeth. In an awake or sedated patient the bite block must be placed before probe insertion. Right: Operator's view. Note the hand performing an upward displacement of the jaw by pulling the jaw up and NOT the teeth!

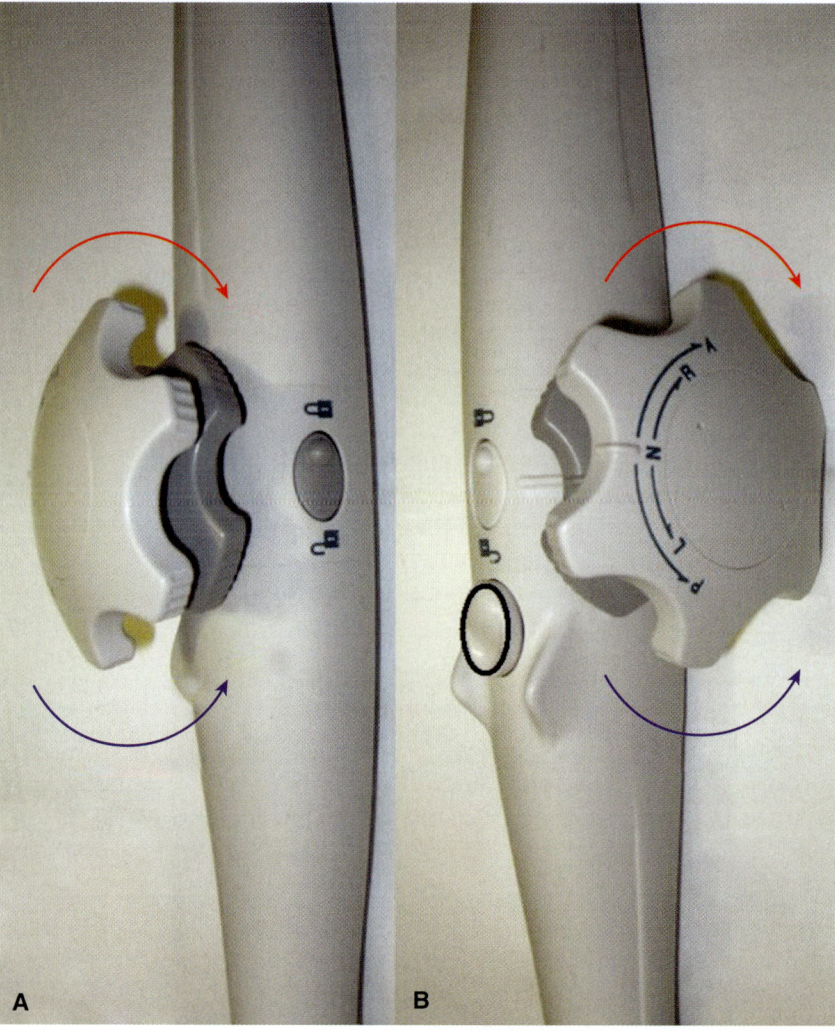

FIGURE 40-5 TEE probe handle and controls. Top of the images is the machine end, and bottom is the probe end of the TEE handle. Left (A) and right (B) side view of the probe handle. Large pale gray wheel controls the anterior flexion (anteflex/*red arrow*) and posterior flexion motion (retroflex/*blue arrow*) of the probe tip. The dark gray wheel controls the left and right lateral flexion of the probe tip. By pushing the probe forward or pulling it back the TEE tip will advance or withdraw. The whole handle can be turned to the left of right, and the TEE tip will follow. The black circled button controls the multiplane. The light and dark buttons under the wheels are their respective locking buttons. It is better to never lock these buttons to prevent moving the probe accidentally with them locked.

used for "multiplaning" or rotating the ultrasound elements at the tip of the TEE probe (Figure 40-5).
- Never insert a TEE probe that is in the locked position; this runs the risk of some serious esophageal scraping!
- Prior to messing around with these buttons and knobs, you can obtain various images by simply advancing and withdrawing the probe (Figure 40-6).
- You can also rotate the probe to the left by turning the handle counterclockwise (to the left) and to the right by turning clockwise (to the right).
- The large knob allows you to flex the tip of the probe anteriorly and posteriorly (anteflex and retroflex), whereas the smaller knob bends the tip of the probe to the right and left.
- The button used for multiplaning essentially allows us to rotate the ultrasound beam (0 to 180 degrees) and view various "cuts" of the tissue we are examining.
- For example, there is an apple sitting on a tabletop and we wish to examine its interior. Using a

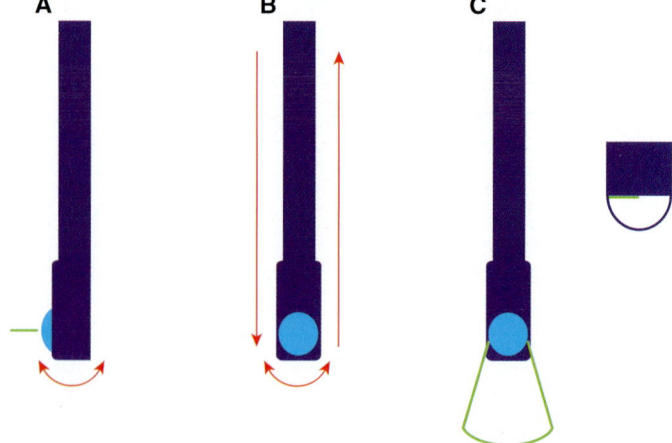

FIGURE 40-6 TEE probe tip in lateral (A) and anterior (B,C) view. (A) Red arrow indicates anteflex, and retroflex motion (large/light gray handle wheel control). (B) Probe advanced, and withdrawn from the esophagus, also the flex to the right and flex to the left motions (small/dark gray handle wheel control). (C) Zero-degree ultrasound plane shown in green.

knife we can cut the apple in half from left to right through a horizontal plane (referred to as 0 degrees). We could also cut the apple from top to bottom through a longitudinal plane (90 degrees). If we choose to, we could make a variety of "cuts" between 0 and 180 degrees and obtain multiple views of the interior of the apple. The multiplaning feature does the same thing; it allows you to alter the plane in which sound waves are emitted, just like your hand controls the angle at which you cut into the apple. You can obtain these various angled cuts by pressing on the button, which in turn rotates the transducer elements. The exact degree change is displayed on the monitor. Turning the transducer 180 degrees provides a reverse image of that obtained at 0 degrees.
- In summary,
  - TEE probes can be advanced/withdrawn
  - TEE probes can be turned to the left/right
  - The tip can be bent anteriorly/posteriorly and/or bent right/left
  - Transducer elements can be multiplaned (0 to 180 degrees)

ULTRASOUND PHYSICS

- Like most clinicians, you probably assumed that once you got into medical school you would never have to bother with any of those mind-boggling physic concepts and equations. Well, guess what? You were wrong! It's time now, boys and girls, to revisit some of those old classroom physics lessons. This time around, however, shouldn't be as bad, because we'll just stick to the basics.
- Sound waves are essentially mechanical pressure waves that can be characterized by their wavelength (λ), frequency (f), and velocity (v).
- Human beings are capable of hearing sound waves with frequencies between 20 and 20,000 Hz. *Ultra*sound waves are those sound waves whose frequencies lie above this range. Ultrasound waves produced by TEE transducers typically have frequencies between 3.5 and 7 million Hz (MHz).
- The relationship among wavelength, frequency, and velocity can be seen in the following basic equation: $\lambda = v/f$.
- Sound waves tend to travel faster through denser material. Sound wave velocity through human soft tissue is approximately 1,540 m/s.
- Altering the frequency of the transmitted ultrasound waves can have a significant effect on image acquisition. Increasing the frequency of ultrasound waves allows for greater image resolution. However, an increase in frequency also decreases the penetrance of the waves. One must therefore balance the need for greater resolution with the expense of decreased depth of penetration.
- Piezoelectric elements are the source of all ultrasonic wave production within a transducer. They can be seen as energy converters capable of converting electrical signals into mechanical vibrations and hence sound waves. The opposite is also true: they are capable of receiving ultrasonic waves and converting them into electrical energy.
- Once an ultrasonic wave is emitted, it interacts with tissues in four ways: reflection, refraction, scattering, and attenuation.
- Ultrasound machines process the timing, intensity, and phase of reflected waves in order to form an image.
- Besides providing topographic information, most modern TEE machines are also capable of providing information regarding velocity and direction of blood flow via Doppler echocardiography.
- The *Doppler effect* describes the increase in frequency of sound waves as an object moves toward a receiver, and the corresponding decrease in frequency as the object moves away from the receiver. We all experience this effect in real life on a daily basis, whether we're waiting on the platform for the good old New Jersey Transit trains or while we're flagging down a cab in the city and hear the honking cars pass by. In the case of Doppler echocardiography, the "trains" and "honking cars" are actually red blood cells scattering the ultrasound waves we shoot at them, and in turn altering the frequencies of the reflected waves. This Doppler *shift* is dependent on the velocity of blood flow.
- Ideally speaking, we would like to be parallel to blood flow when measuring its velocity. This is not always possible, but if we maintain an angle of less than 20 degrees to the direction of blood flow measurements will be accurate enough.
- All flow is the result of pressure gradients, and since we now have the ability to measure velocity via the Doppler equation, we can then use the simplified Bernoulli equation to determine the pressure gradient (mm Hg) generated: Pressure = 4 (Velocity)^2.
- The ability to measure pressure gradients comes in handy when assessing the degree of valvular stenosis. Larger pressure gradients are associated with greater degrees of stenosis under most circumstances.
- Various modes of echocardiography are available; however, the two-dimensional (2D) mode is currently the most frequently used (Figures 40-7 and 40-8).
- A 2D image is produced by moving an ultrasound beam through a given plane rapidly and displaying the processed information simultaneously in order to create an image.

- Most TEE transducers are capable of capturing 30 to 60 images per second (frame rate = 30 to 60 Hz; seen in the right upper corner of Figure 40-8). The higher the frame rate the less motion artifact you will see.
- Two other commonly used modes in echocardiography are pulsed-wave Doppler (PWD) and continuous-wave Doppler (CWD). Both modes are used to measure velocity and direction of blood flow (Figure 40-9).
- PWD allows you to make these measurements in specific locations that you desire, whereas CWD obtains these measurements along a "line of sight" of an ultrasound beam.
- Both modes have their advantages and disadvantages. However, in general terms, CWD is capable of measuring higher velocities (>2 m/s) than is PWD.
- If you've ever glanced at a monitor screen to see an ultrasound image with some blue, red, or maybe even green color displayed on it, then you've seen what is known as color-flow Doppler.
- Color-flow Doppler is probably one of the coolest modes around. It displays both flow and 2D imaging together simultaneously. The colors are indicative of the direction of flow in relation to the transducer. Flow toward the transducer is red, and flow away from the transducer is blue (these settings can be changed).
- Color-flow Doppler is a form of PWD and therefore cannot measure higher velocities accurately. In fact with very high velocities, some funky stuff starts to happen with the colors. Reds change to blues, and blues to reds, a phenomenon known as aliasing. Pretty psychedelic stuff, huh! (Figure 40-10)

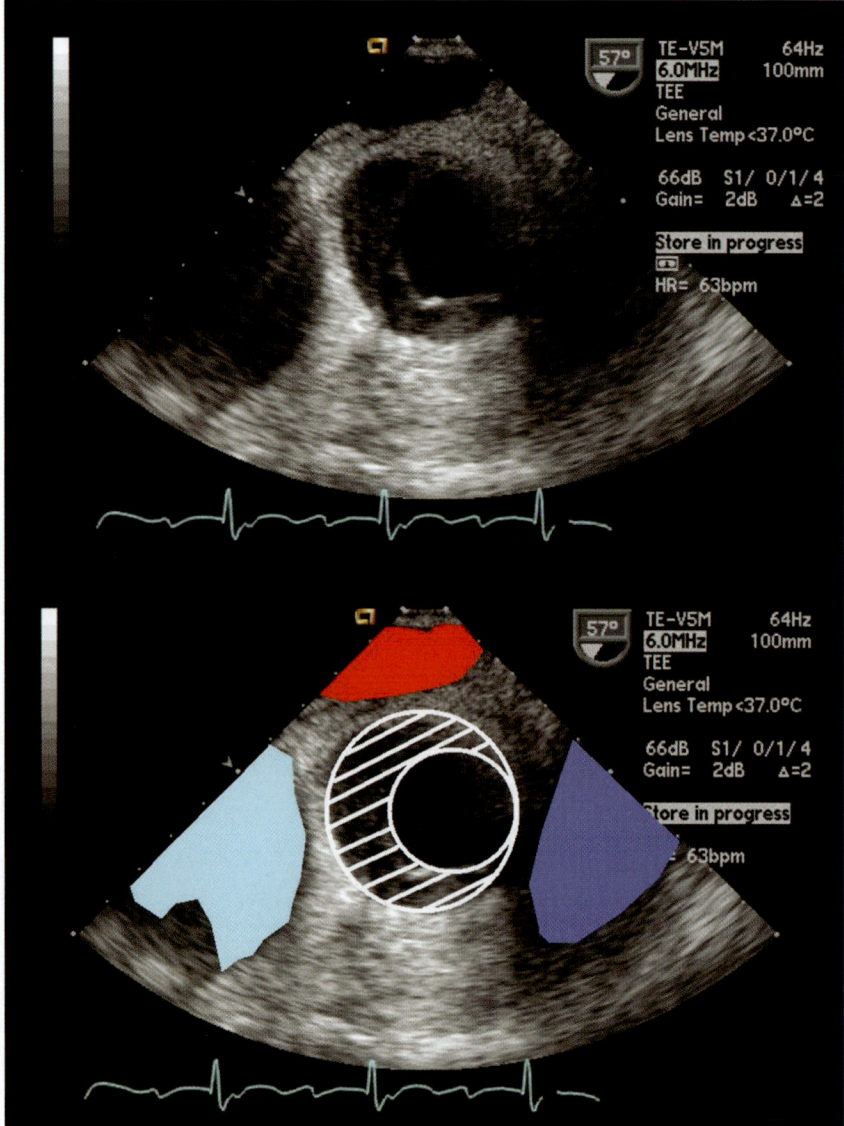

FIGURE 40-7 Two-dimensional short axis view of the ascending aorta with aortic wall dissection. Cartoon: large white circle is the aortic wall; small white circle is the true aortic lumen; white shaded area is the dissection lumen; left atrium is in red; right atrium is in light blue; and a portion of the main pulmonary artery is seen in dark blue.

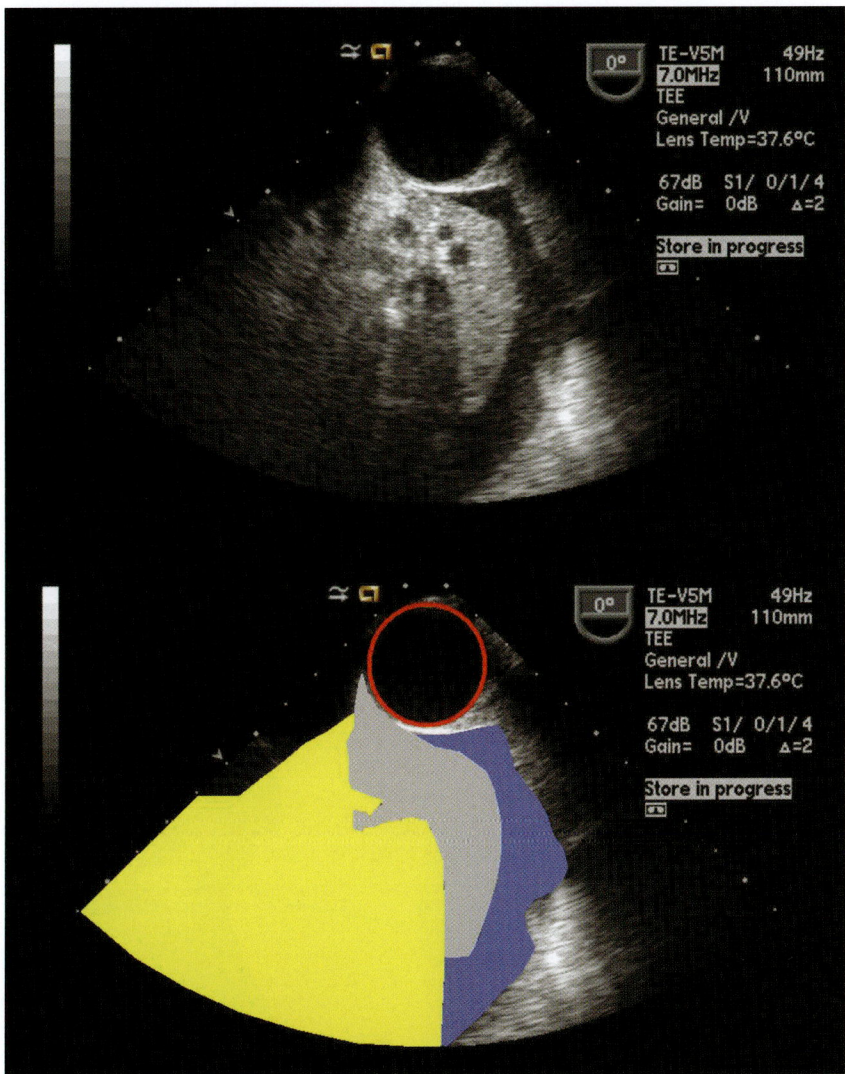

FIGURE 40-8 Two-dimensional short axis view of the thoracic aorta (*red circle*), and the corresponding cartoon at the bottom. Note a left pleural effusion (*blue*), partial left lung atelectasis (*light gray*), and normally aerated left lung (*yellow*).

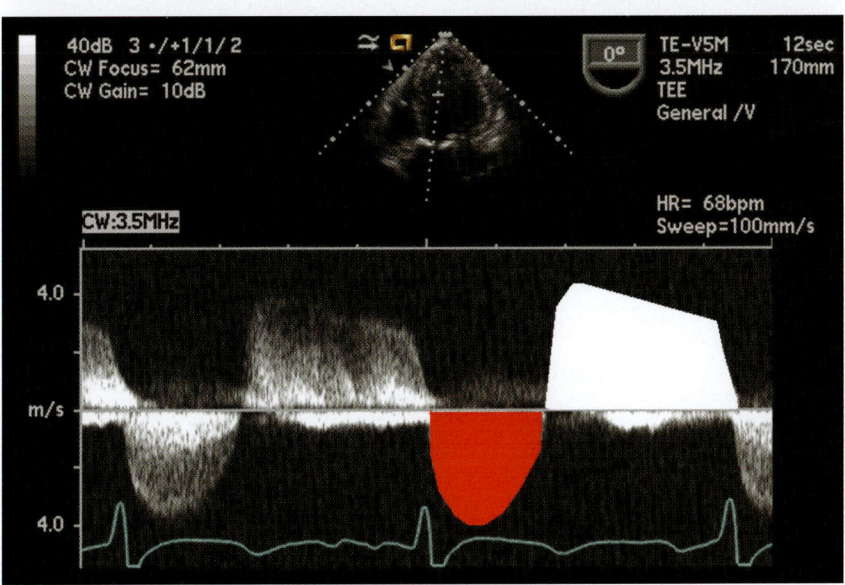

FIGURE 40-9 Continuous-wave Doppler (CWD) scan through the aortic valve. The TEE probe tip was placed deep in the stomach and the tip anteflexed until a deep transgastric view of the LV was obtained after the CWD button was pressed in the echo machine console. In this scan the velocity scale was set at 4 m/s (left side of the image) and the image sweep at 100 mm/s to be able to see more detail. At zero meters per second we have our baseline; elements inscribing below represent red cells moving away from the transducer. If the red cells are toward the transducer, we will see the tracing above the baseline. The image shows a patient with severe aortic stenosis (*red colored area*) with 4 m/s flow in systole (see ECG) across the aortic valve and mild aortic insufficiency (*white*) as well.

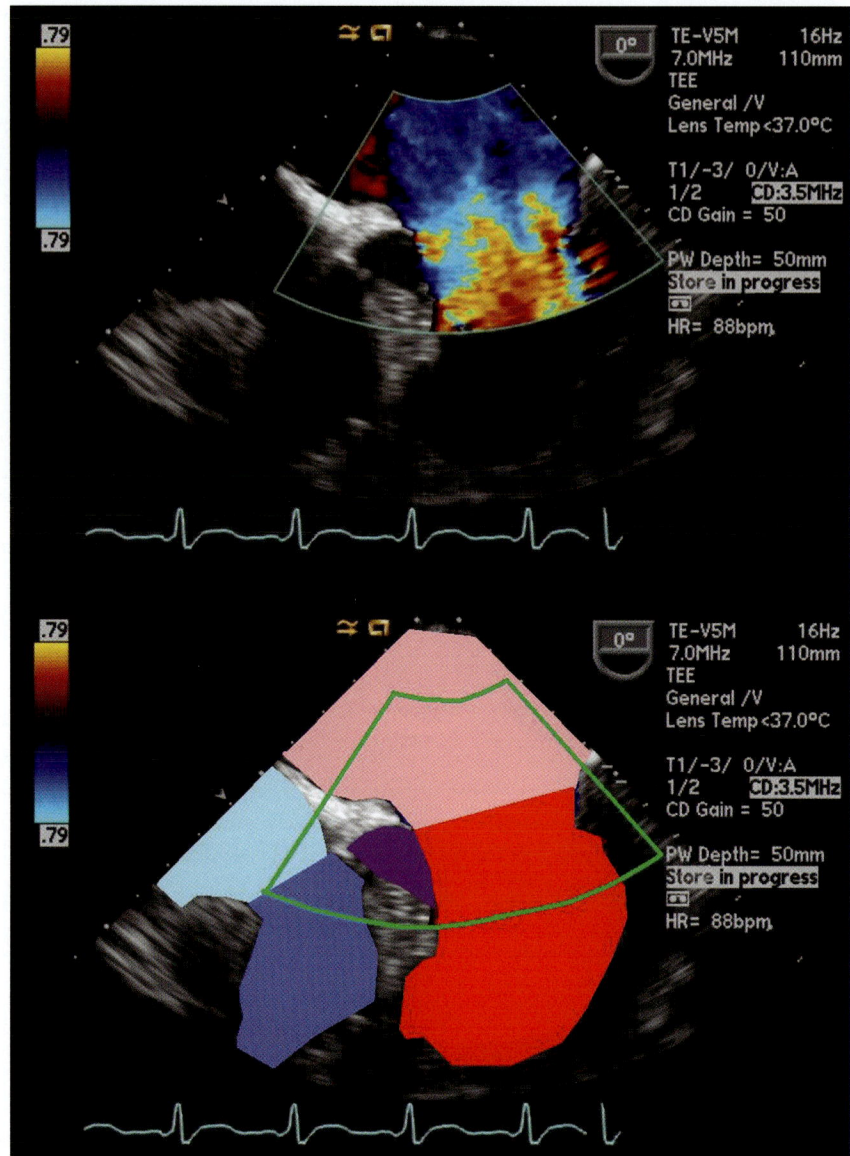

FIGURE 40-10 Midesophageal four-chamber view. CFD showing normal mitral inflow pattern. Cartoon LA in pink; LV in red; CFD sector in green; RA in light blue; RV in dark blue.

ASE/SCA 20 STANDARD VIEWS

In 1999, the American Society of Echocardiography (ASE) and the Society of Cardiovascular Anesthesiologist (SCA) published their guidelines for performing a comprehensive intraoperative TEE exam.[6] The guidelines include 20 standard images that comprise a comprehensive examination; go to http://www.asefiles.org/multiplanetee.pdf.

The only thing that is somewhat outdated on those guidelines is the way the left ventricle segments are currently named;[7] go to http://circ.ahajournals.org/cgi/reprint/105/4/539 (Figure 40-11).

With 20 different views to obtain, you might be asking yourself, "Where do I start?" There really is no "correct" place to start. Many clinicians prefer to begin their imaging with the structure that is to be operated on or of main concern (e.g., aortic valve, left ventricle). It's best to confirm that the patient actually has a problem before the surgeons open his/her chest! Others like to begin by getting a glance at the left ventricle and observing its function—or lack of, in many cases. Let's focus on the imaging of some important structures and the relevance of doing so.

Left Ventricle

- In an ideal world, everyone we put to sleep would have a left ventricle that's nice and strong and capable of tolerating all the anesthetics agents we expose it to. Not the case! Unfortunately, in the real world, we're presented with all sorts of sluggish hearts that require our expertise for protection. TEE can be thought of as our "top-of-the-line" monitoring system for the heart. Our main goal

when imaging the left ventricle is to assess both global and segmental systolic function. In terms of segmental systolic function and ischemia monitoring, we can use a standardized model that divides the left ventricle into 17 segments (Figure 40-12).
- We can also get an idea of coronary artery territory and visually inspect each of these segments for *both* movement and thickening (Figures 40-13 and 40-14).
- Any segmental wall motion abnormalities can be graded using the following qualitative grading scale:
  - 1 = normal motion (>30% thickening)
  - 2 = mildly hypokinetic (10–30% thickening)
  - 3 = severely hypokinetic (<10% thickening)
  - 4 = akinetic (does not thicken)
  - 5 = dyskinetic (paradoxical movement during systole)
- You will notice that many clinicians have developed a trained eye when it comes to evaluating global systolic left ventricle (LV) function. Essentially, they visually assess different cross sections of the LV in order to come up with a relatively accurate estimate of ejection fraction. More quantitative ways of evaluating global systolic function also do exist. A transgastric midventricular short axis view of the LV can be used to measure what is referred to as the *fractional area change* (FAC) and *fractional shortening* (FS). FAC utilizes LV area and FS utilizes LV diameter. Both equations basically make inferences on LV function by comparing the change in size of the LV from diastole to systole.

We can also calculate the *ejection fraction* by measuring the LV in a three-dimensional way; pretty complicated stuff![8] (Figure 40-15)

Aortic Valve

- The aortic valve is a semilunar valve composed of three cusps (noncoronary, right coronary, left coronary) (Figure 40-16).
- Like the other valves of the heart, one of the main functions of the aortic valve is to ensure unidirectional blood flow. We therefore want to assess the valve for the presence of any regurgitation and its overall leaflet motion.
- Color Flow Doppler (CFD), once again, aids us in the assessment of the presence/severity of any regurgitant jets. Both the overall size of these jets as well as the degree to which they extend into the LV can be seen with CFD.
- The presence and severity of stenotic aortic valves can also be evaluated with our magical TEE probe. Slide down to the midesophageal position to obtain a short axis view of the aortic valve. From this view, the valve should look like the classic Mercedes Benz sign. Use some of those fancy buttons on the TEE machine to freeze the image during systole. You can then trace the maximum orifice of the valve and allow your machine to calculate its area (Figure 40-17).
- Aortic valve areas less than 1 cm^2 are considered "severe" stenosis, whereas those less than 0.7 cm^2 are considered "critical" stenosis.
- Another way to assess stenotic aortic valves is by sliding your probe down to the transgastric position and obtaining a long axis view of the valve. Using CWD, you can measure the velocity of blood flow through the stenotic portion of the valve. Once you've obtained this value, plug it into the simplified Bernoulli equation, Pressure gradient = 4 (Velocity)^2, to get your pressure gradient. Severe aortic stenosis is characterized by peak gradients greater than 64 mm Hg.
- Keep in mind that severe stenosis can still be present without markedly elevated peak pressure gradients and velocities. This occurs most commonly in the face of poor LV function. Sluggish LVs are incapable of producing significant pressure gradients!

Mitral Valve

- The mitral valve is composed of two leaflets, an anterior and posterior. These leaflets are joined at two points—the commissures (anterolateral and posteromedial).
- Mitral regurgitation is best assessed with color flow Doppler by looking for regurgitant jets flowing into the left atrium during systole. The severity of regurgitation can be graded as 1+ (mild) to 4+ (severe) (Figure 40-18).
- The evaluation of mitral stenosis is similar to that of aortic stenosis. CWD can be used to measure the velocity of blood flow through the mitral valve during diastole. Plug that value into the simplified Bernoulli equation like before and you got yourself a transvalvular pressure gradient.
- Another way to accomplish this is by actually measuring the area of the stenotic orifice, or planimetry, but this can be very tricky. Play with the machine so that you freeze the image (this time in diastole) and trace the orifice. A mitral valve area <1 cm^2 is severe.

Tricuspid and Pulmonic Valve

- These valves can be best assessed in the four-chamber and right ventricle (RV) inflow-outflow views.
- While we are in the area, it's also not a bad idea to take a quick look at the interatrial septum. Often you will find a patent foramen ovale (25% of the general population) or undiagnosed atrial septal defect (Figure 40-19).
- The easiest way to check is to scan the whole inter-atrial septum with CFD.
- Pericardial effusions are usually easy to recognize because fluid around the heart looks black if unclotted and gray (like liver) if clotted—a bit trickier to see! (Figure 40-20).

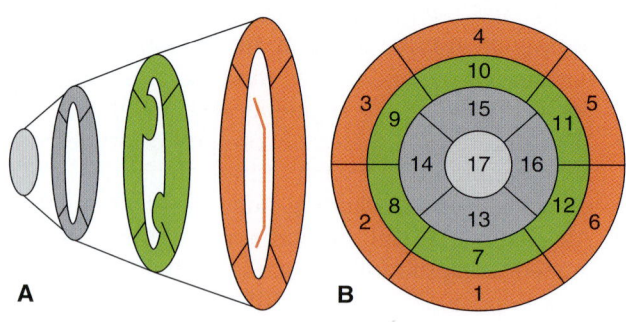

FIGURE 40-11 LV 17 segment model. (A) The LV is divided into three equal regions, the base (*red,* where the mitral valve is), the middle (*green,* where the papillary muscles are), and the distal portion (*blue*). The distal region includes the apical cap (*gray*). (B) LV 17 segments: 1 = basal anterior; 2 = basal anteroseptal; 3 = basal inferoseptal; 4 = basal inferior; 5 = basal inferolateral; 6 = basal anterolateral; 7 = mid-anterior; 8 = mid-anteroseptal; 9 = mid-inferoseptal; 10 = mid-inferior; 11 = mid-inferolateral; 12 = mid-anterolateral; 13 = apical anterior; 14 = apical septal; 15 = apical inferior; 16 = apical lateral; 17 = apical cap.

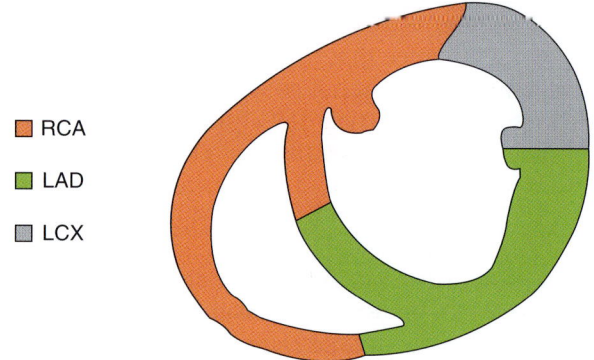

FIGURE 40-12 The LV transgastric middle short axis view allows assessment of the main coronary circulation to the heart as all main coronaries have territorial representation in this view. LAD (*green*) = left anterior descending coronary; LCX (*blue*) = left circumflex; RCA (*red*) = right coronary artery.

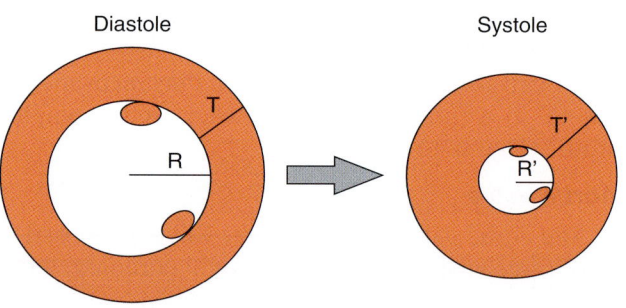

FIGURE 40-13 Normal regional wall motion must include radial shortening (R→R') *and* wall thickening (T→T'), as shown in this cartoon of the LV transgastric middle short axis view.

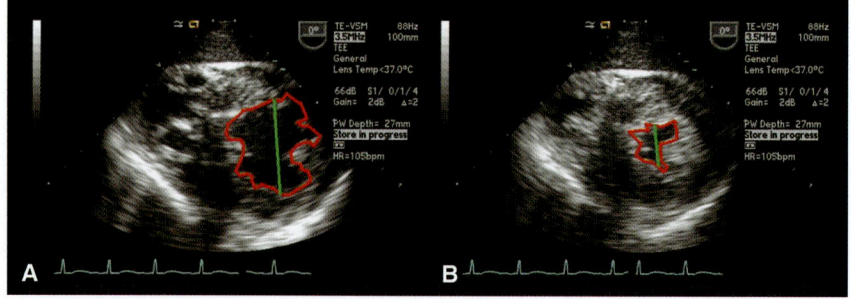

FIGURE 40-14 LV transgastric middle short axis view with diastolic (A) and systolic (B) fractional area change (FAC) concept shown in red and fractional shortening (FS) shown in green.

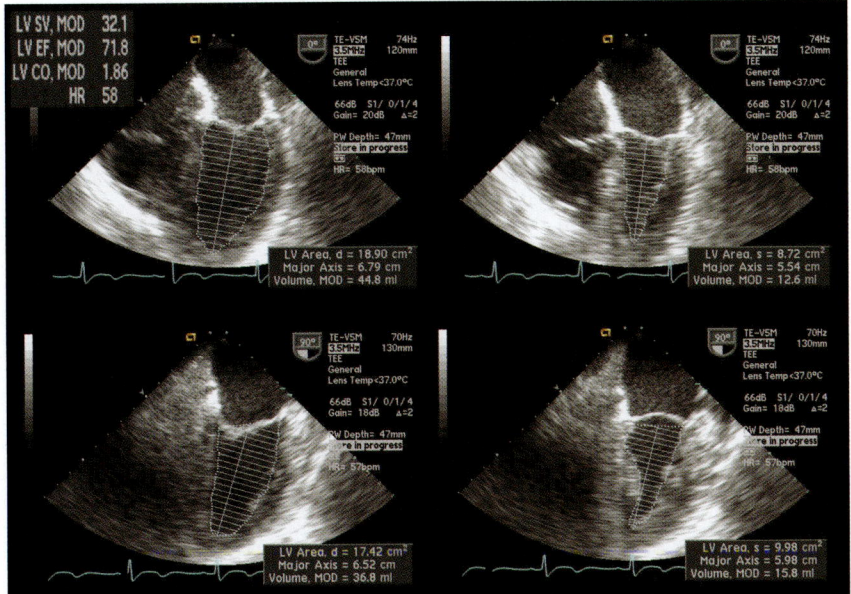

FIGURE 40-15 Calculation of the ejection fraction (EF) by measuring the LV cavity in diastole and systole in the four-chamber and two-chamber mid-esophageal views. We trace the endocardial borders, input the data in the echo machine, and like magic we have the EF! The machine also calculates the stroke volume and multiplies it by the heart rate and we got the cardiac output!

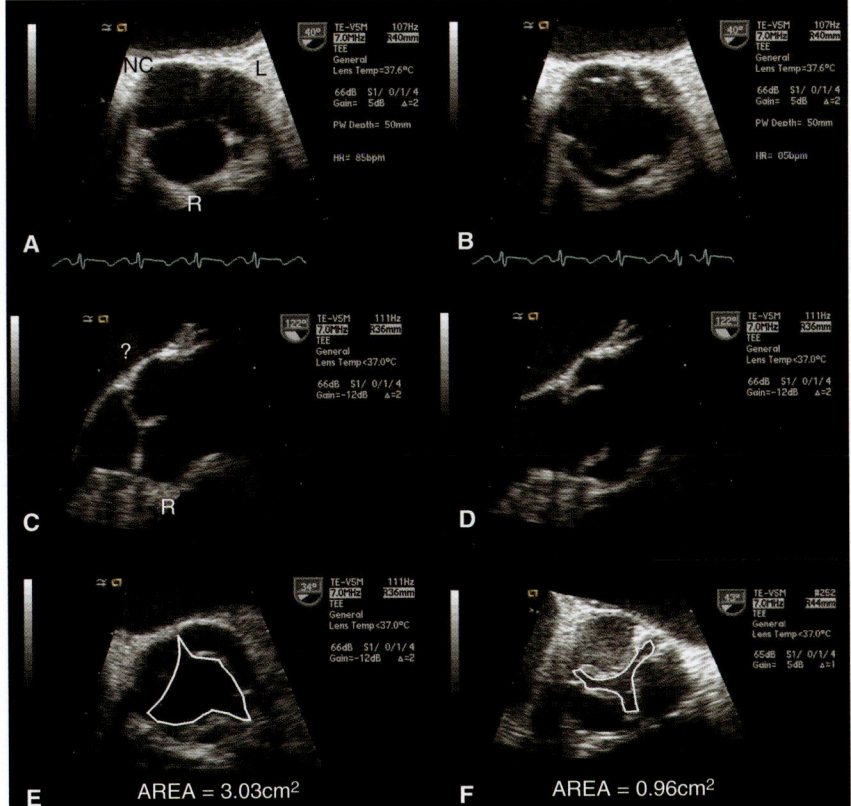

FIGURE 40-16 Zoom views of the aortic valve (AV). Mid-esophageal AV short axis (A,B,E,F) and long axis view (C,D). (A) Normal AV in diastole. L = left coronary cusp; R= right coronary cusp; NC = noncoronary cusp. (B) Normal AV in systole. (C) Normal AV in diastole. In this view it is difficult to know which coronary cusp is on top ("?"), the "NC" or the "L". (D) Normal AV in systole (very mild restriction in leaflet opening). (E) Mild restriction in AV opening. (F) Severe aortic stenosis.

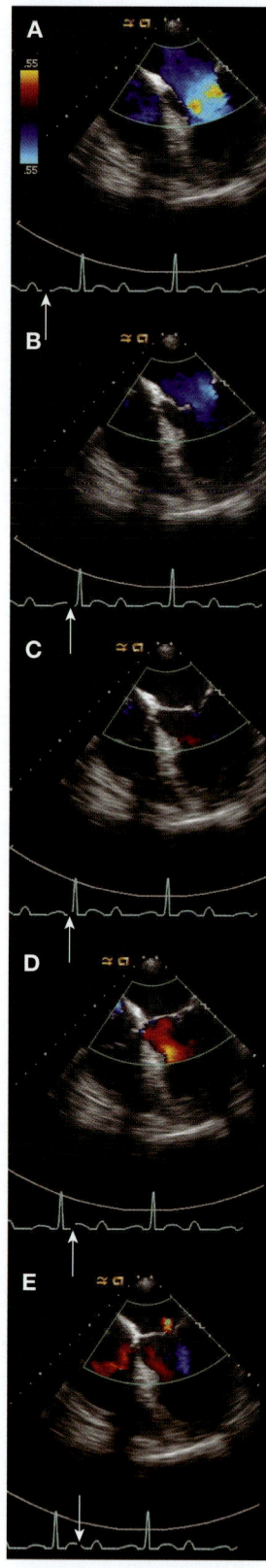
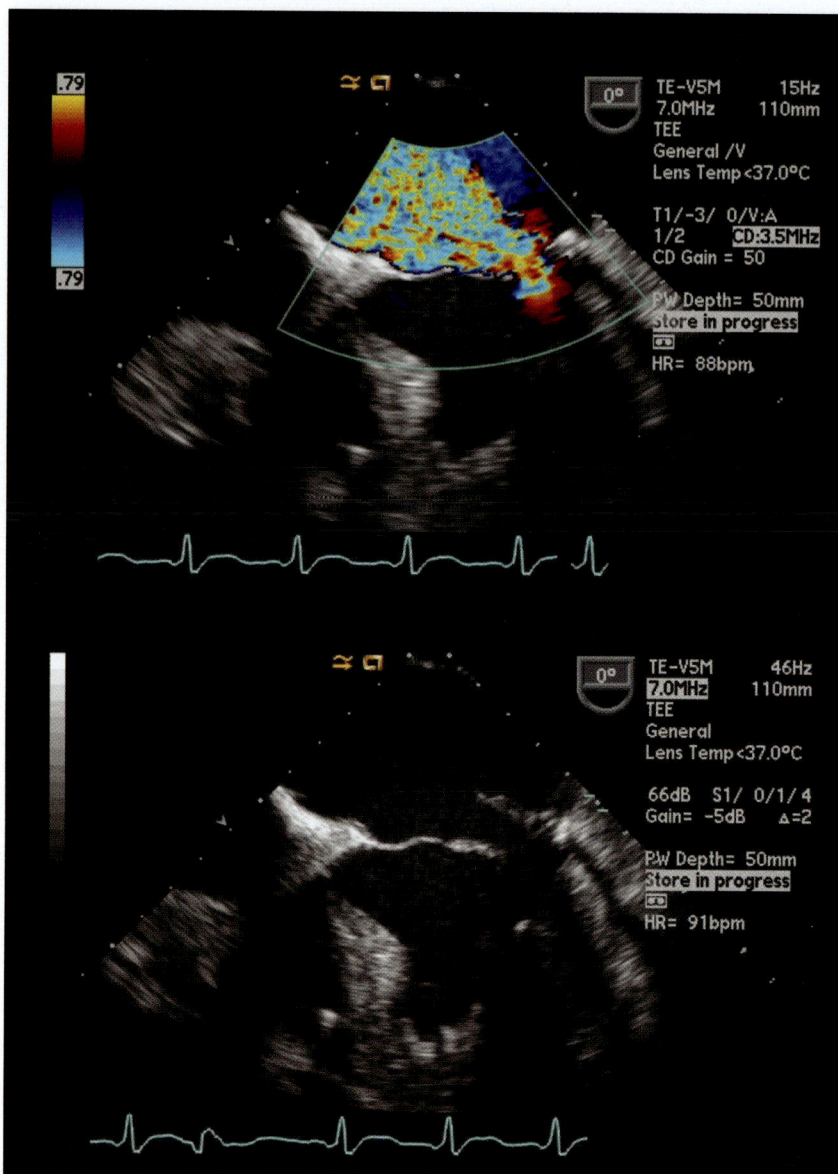

FIGURE 40-18 Mid-esophageal four-chamber view in systole. Top: CFD across the mitral valve notes severe mitral regurgitation (MR) jet directed toward the interatrial septum. Bottom: Note the lake of coaptation of the mitral valve leaflets due to rupture chords in the posterior mitral valve (MV) leaflet.

FIGURE 40-17 Mid-esophageal four-chamber view showing a normal cardiac cycle sequence (follow ECG and *white arrow*) and mitral inflow by CFD. (A) Early diastole, passive LV filling (*blue*). (B) Atrial contraction and second wave of ventricular filling (*blue*). (C) End diastole. (D) Ventricular systole and ejection. Note red in LV outflow tract (LVOT) area. (E) Late systole. Note trace of mitral regurgitation.

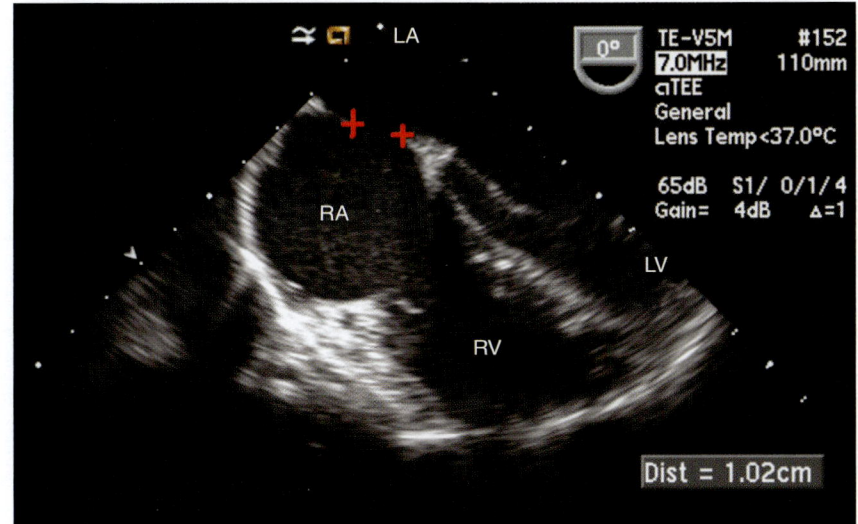

FIGURE 40-19 Mid-esophageal four-chamber view. Secundum atrial septum defect measuring 1.02 cm in this plane.

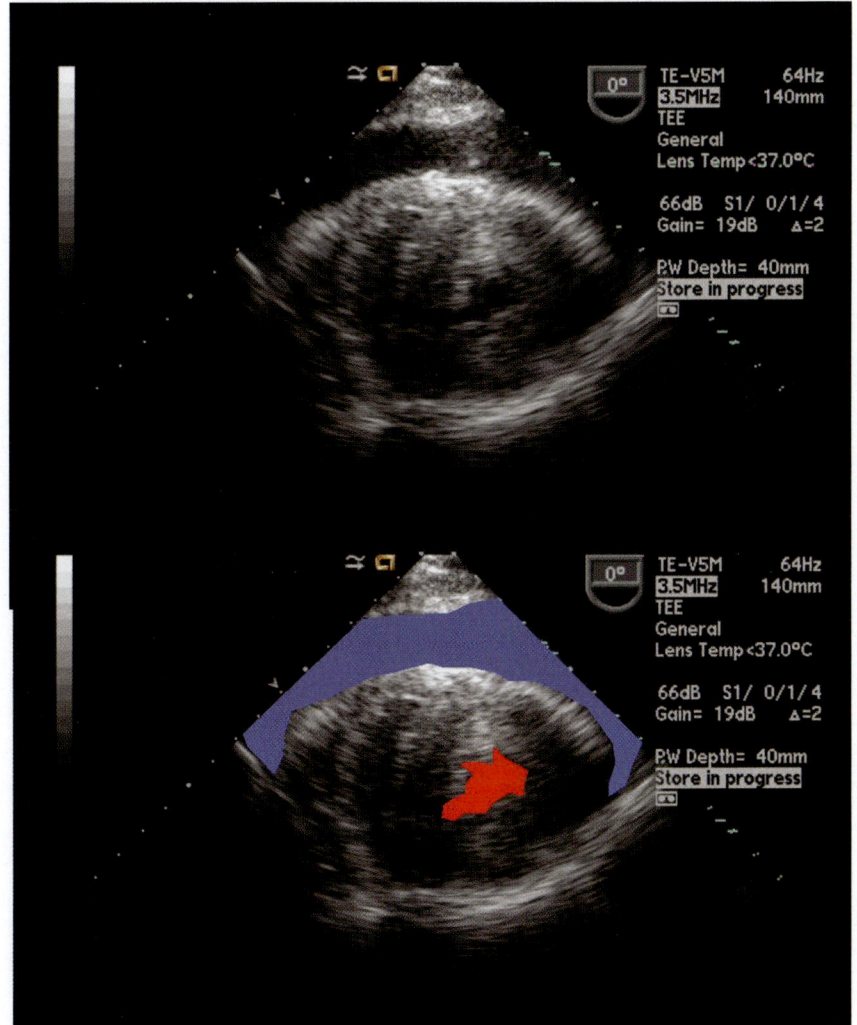

FIGURE 40-20 Transgastric middle short axis view of the RV and LV during systole with a large (>1 cm thick) pericardial effusion. Bottom image: Effusion shown in blue and LV cavity in red.

EPIAORTIC (EAU) AND EPICARDIAL (EUS) ULTRASOUND

- As amazing as TEE is, it still has its limitations. One of these limitations is its inability to image the distal ascending aorta and parts of the aortic arch. This is where epiaortic and epicardiac ultrasounds come into play (Figure 40-21).
- During these examinations we usually manage the ultrasound machine while the surgeon manages the surface probe (Figure 40-22).
- Atherosclerotic disease of the aorta is pretty common in patients presenting for open heart surgery. Manipulation of these plaques is a significant source of atherosclerotic emboli, which have been shown to be a major cause of perioperative stroke and morbidity/mortality in patients undergoing cardiac surgery. Our epiaortic ultrasounds allow us to tread carefully in this war zone by identifying a safe location to cannulate and clamp the aorta.
- The ASE/SCA has published recommendations for a comprehensive epiaortic exam that includes five views of the ascending aorta and aortic arch.[9]
- Once you've completed the comprehensive examination, you'll be able to assess the severity of aortic atherosclerotic disease.
- Remember: not all plaques are equal. Various studies have shown that certain plaque characteristics are more associated with neurologic injury than others. These characteristics include:
  - Plaque height and/or thickness >3 mm
  - Presence of mobile components
  - Ascending aortic location

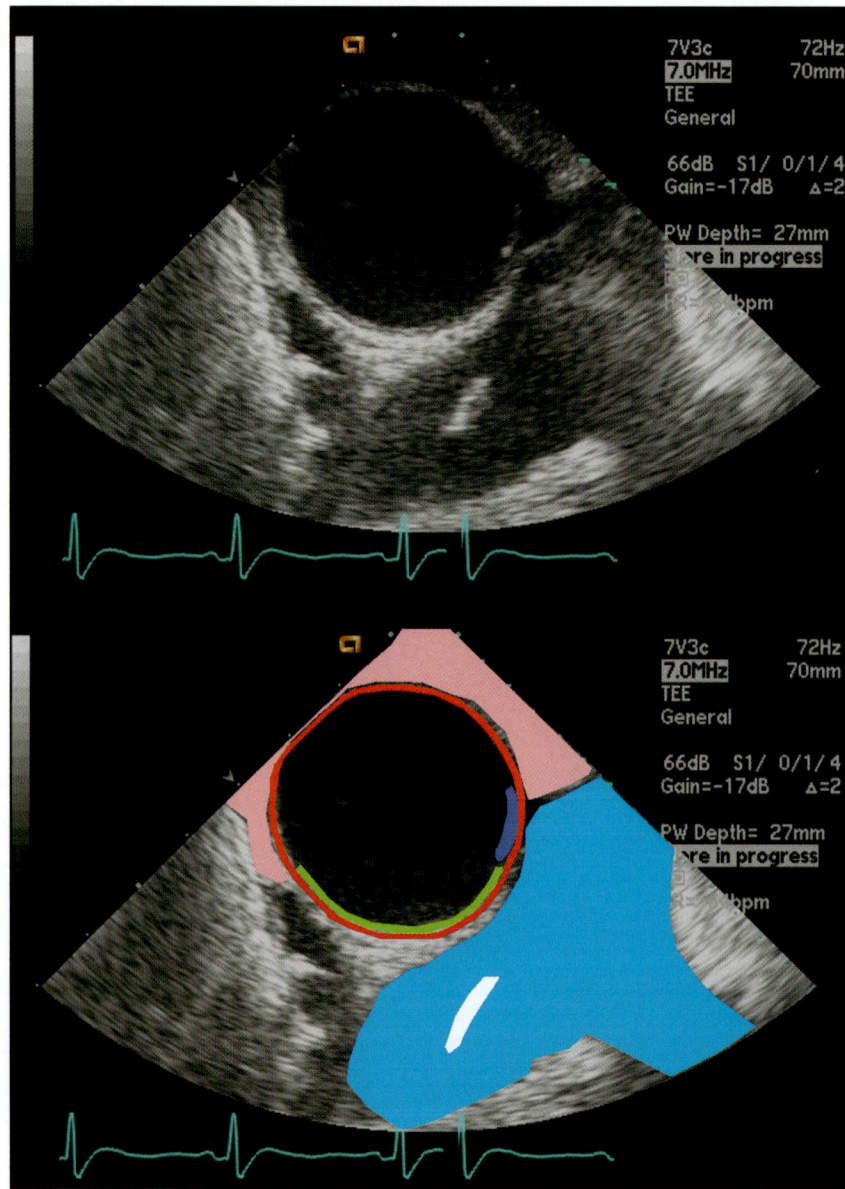

FIGURE 40-21 Epiaortic ultrasound examination showing some intimal thickening in the posterior wall (*green* in the cartoon), and a short segment in the right lateral wall of a 1-mm-thick plaque (*dark blue*). Ascending aorta in short axis in red; main pulmonary artery and initial portions of left and right pulmonary artery (PA) in light blue; the segment of the PA catheter can be seen as well in white. Saline was poured into the chest cavity to give some distance between the transducer and the aortic anterior wall (*pink*); otherwise imaging the anterior wall is very difficult.

Chapter 40 TEE LOOK! IT'S A BIRD...IT'S A PLANE...NO, IT'S TEE MAN!

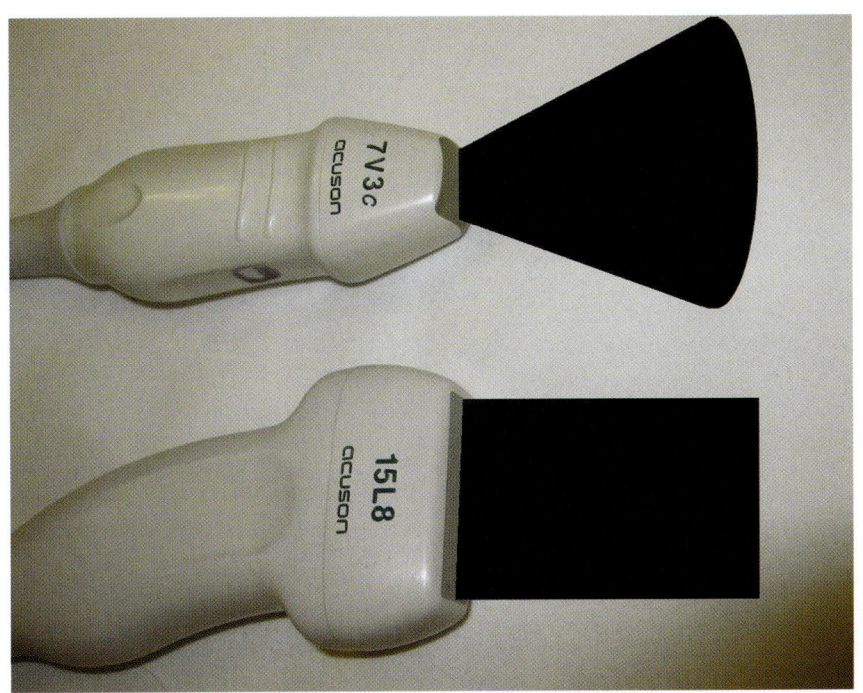

FIGURE 40-22 There are many surface ultrasound probes. For epiaortic ultrasound (EAU) a high frequency is preferable. Shown are a 3- to 7-mHz phased array probe (top) and an 8- to 15-mHz linear array probe (bottom) and the corresponding ultrasound plane shape they can generate. You have to move the actual transducer to scan the area you are interested in, as there are no handle controls, in contrast with the TEE probe.

TRANSTHORACIC ULTRASOUND

- Whatever you've learned thus far for TEE can also be applied to transthoracic echocardiography (TTE). The images, however, are tougher to acquire since you are imaging through the chest wall. Lots of useful images can be obtained via this relatively noninvasive technique.
- If you ever get the chance to mess around with one of these machines, you'll discover that there are five major transthoracic windows to the heart. They are the parasternal long and short axis windows, the apical window, the subxiphoid/subcostal window, and the suprasternal window (Figures 40-23 and 40-24).
- By progressing further down into the abdomen, you'll be given a peak at the liver, spleen, and abdominal aorta (Figure 40-25).
- Once you become oriented to the different windows, you'll begin to understand just how useful this new skill of yours really is. The relative noninvasive nature of this examination will allow you to shine like a star in all sorts of settings including the ICU and ER.
- Just remember, though, that it takes time and interest to be good at this. Be patient, and make friends with the experts in your service and the echo lab. Pretty soon, you'll be the one teaching others!

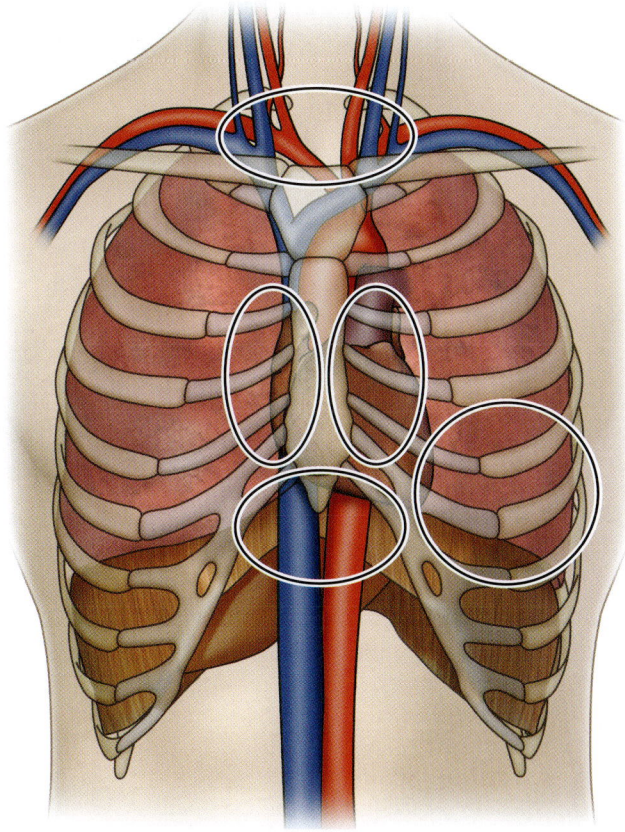

FIGURE 40-23 Main transthoracic echocardiography windows. Almost always you will be able to get a couple of them. Lower frequency probes are better because the heart is a bit further away.

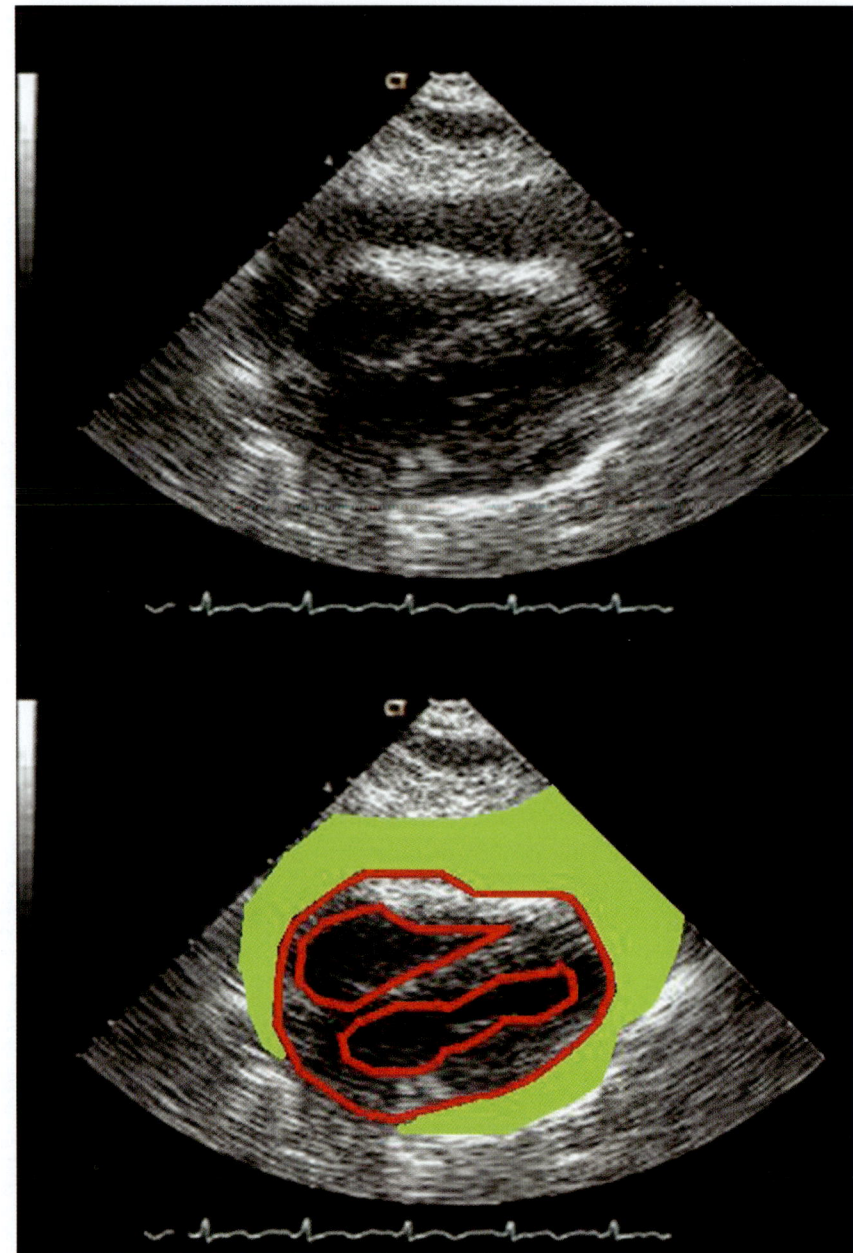

FIGURE 40-24 Transthoracic echo through the subxiphoid window in an obese patient demonstrating a large pericardial effusion (*green*). The heart is shown in red.

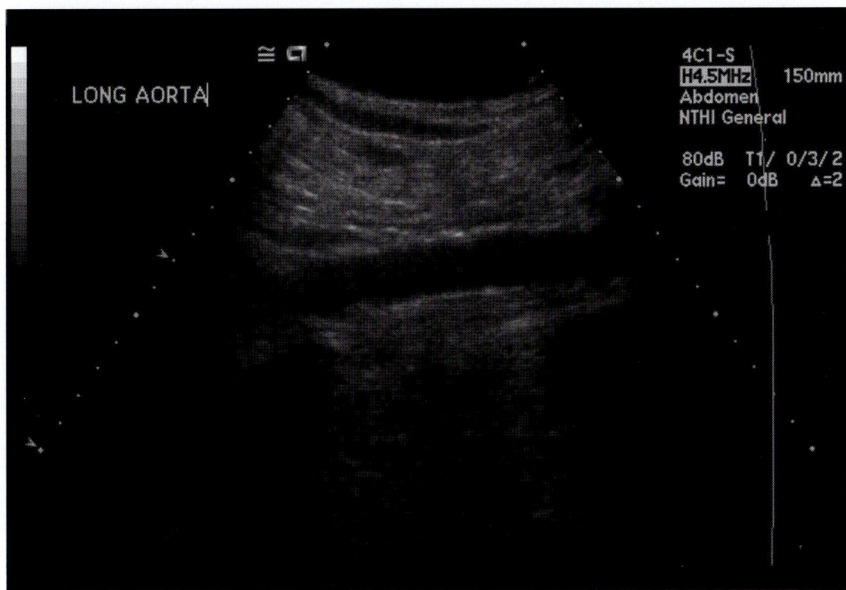

FIGURE 40-25 Transabdominal ultrasound showing the abdominal aorta in long axis.

CONCLUSION

- We should think of ourselves as ultrasonographers, with TEE being only a part of what we can image. Refresh your basic anatomy and remember that every patient is different.
- You really don't need to memorize TEE angles to obtain certain images because very few patients actually read the anatomy book! Just follow the anatomical connections and the images obtained will make sense.
- Remember to visit the University of Toronto TEE webpage at http://pie.med.utoronto.ca/TEE/TEE_content/TEE_standardViews_intro.html.
- Once you start to do echo studies, record your baseline examination so you have something to compare; also if your department is going to bill for the service, you must record and store the study.
- Connect the electrocardiogram to the echo machine and you will be able to time events and also look at the ST segment, rhythm, bundle branch blocks, pacer rhythm, etc.
- Don't do your examination in a hurry. Evaluate the heart regionally and globally before making any diagnosis or you will make mistakes.
- Try to correlate your echo and the clinical picture and remember that myocardial infarction, myocardial stunning, myocarditis, motion artifacts, and bundle branch blocks can cause regional wall motion abnormality (RWMA), but a sudden, severe decrease or cessation of segmental contraction is almost always due to myocardial ischemia.
- Eyeball the RV and LV systolic function, and try to "calibrate your eye" by seeing echoes with the cardiologist at the echo laboratory at your institution, or in the OR with your local experts, the cardiac guys!
- See educational videos (tons on YouTube).
- Ask lots of questions, read about the topic, and test yourself with the experts.
- Talk to your cardiac surgeon to correlate TEE with actual anatomy!
- As you shall see, TEE can give you a lot of information and be lots of fun!

REFERENCES

1. Practice guidelines for perioperative transesophageal echocardiography. An updated report by the American Society of Anesthesiologists and the Society of Cardiovascular Anesthesiologists Task Force on Transesophageal Echocardiography. *Anesthesiology* 2010;112:1.
   Guidelines outlining both indications and contraindications to the use of TEE.
2. ACC/AHA/ASE 2003 guideline update for the clinical application of echocardiography: summary article. *J Am Soc Echocardiogr* 2003;16:1091–1110.
   Provides evidence based recommendations for the use of echocardiography for various pathological states.
3. Kallmeyer IJ, Collard CD, Fox JA, et al. The safety of intraoperative transesophageal echocardiography: a case series of 7200 cardiac surgical patients. *Anesth Analg* 2001; 92:1126–1130.
   Case series reporting the incidence of intra-operative TEE complications.

4. MacGregor DA, Zvara DA, Treadway RM, et al. Late presentation of esophageal injury after transesophageal echocardiography. *Anesth Analg* 2004;99:41–44.
   Describes two case reports of delayed presentation of esophageal injury following TEE.

5. Maslow A, Bert A, Schwartz C, et al. Transesophageal echocardiography in the noncardiac surgical patient. *Int Anesthesiol Clin* 2002;40:73–132.

6. Shanewise JS, Cheung AT, Aronson S, et al. ASE/SCA guidelines for performing a comprehensive intraoperative multiplane transesophageal echocardiography examination: recommendations of the American Society of Echocardiography Council for Intraoperative Echocardiography and the Society of Cardiovascular Anesthesiologists Task Force for Certification in Perioperative Transesophageal Echocardiography. *Anesth Analg* 1999;89:870–884.
   Ultimate guideline for performing a complete TEE examination, with pictures and all!

7. Cerqueira MD, Weissman NJ, Dilsizian V, et al. AHA scientific statement. Standardized myocardial segmentation and nomenclature for tomographic imaging of the heart: a statement for healthcare professionals from the Cardiac Imaging Committee of the Council on Clinical Cardiology of the American Heart Association. *Circulation* 2002;105:539–542.
   Provides a blueprint for identifying myocardial segments. Essentially allows all of us to be on the "same page" when referring to the myocardium.

8. Odell D, Cahalan M. Assessment of left ventricular global and segmental systolic function with transesophageal echocardiography. *Anesthesiol Clin* 2006;24:755–762.
   Tips on how to evaluate the global and segmental ventricular function.

9. Glas KE, Swaminathan M, Reeves ST, et al. Guidelines for the performance of a comprehensive intraoperative epiaortic ultrasonographic examination: recommendations of the American Society of Echocardiography and the Society of Cardiovascular Anesthesiologists; Endorsed by the Society of Thoracic Surgeons. *Anesth Analg* 2008;106:1376–1384.
   Ultimate guideline for performing a complete epiaortic ultrasound! Also contains great pictures.

SUGGESTED READING

GE Healthcare. TEE probe care. http://www.gehealthcare.com/usen/service/docs/TEEProbeCareChart_FNLB.PDF
Recommendations for proper TEE probe care.

Sonora Medical Systems. Care of the transesophageal probe. http://www.4sonora.com/news/press/TEE_Probe_Care_Rev_3a1c.pdf.
Recommendations for proper TEE probe care.

Toronto General Hospital. Virtual transesophageal echocardiography. http://pie.med.utoronto.ca/TEE/TEE_content/TEE_standardViews_intro.html.
Great interactive Web site to learn about TEE.

CHAPTER 41
THE SWAN SONG

JOCHEN STEPPAN
MARY BETH BRADY
NANHI MITTER

> Hear the music, the thunder of the wings,
> Love the wild swan.
>
> Robinson Jeffers,
> *Love the Wild Swan*, (1930s)

INTRODUCTION

The pulmonary artery catheter, or Swan-Ganz catheter, is named in honor of its inventors Jeremy Swan and William Ganz. We wonder how they came up with that one!

Legend has it that Swan had the idea of attaching a balloon at the tip of a catheter to float it through the bloodstream, after observing sailboats offshore at Santa Monica. He realized that boats with a spinnaker in front of the main mast had a great speed advantage over the ones with classic sails. This triggered the idea for the original design of a catheter with a balloon to float through the blood (pretty impressive imagination on his part). The design was later refined by Ganz who added a thermistor probe for measurement of cardiac output—not sure what he was watching while coming up with this idea.

The Swan-Ganz catheter expands the monitoring capability of the anesthesiologist manyfold. In addition to administering medications and fluids, it provides readings of the central venous pressure, the pulmonary artery pressure, the pulmonary artery occlusion pressure (PAOP), otherwise known as wedge pressure, or the pulmonary capillary wedge pressure (PCWP). Furthermore, you can measure cardiac output and mixed venous oxygen saturation, either intermittently or continuously depending on which version of the catheter is used. But what to make of all those numbers? And, in the area of evidence-based medicine, does it improve patient care and safety? In the world of evidence-based medicine, the jury is still out. The debate about whether patients with pulmonary artery (PA) catheters fare better than their cohorts without has waged for years and still wages today. That said, there are two kinds of people in the world: those who love the PA catheter and those who hate the PA catheter with equal passion. But no matter which side you choose, you will need to know the contraindications, complications, how to place it, when to place it, how to troubleshoot, and most importantly, how to interpret all the numbers. Keep in mind, it isn't just the numbers but how you interpret these numbers that really makes the difference.

INDICATIONS

Unfortunately, the official guidelines from the American Society of Anesthesiologists (ASA) are somewhat vague. As per the ASA practice guidelines from 2003, PA catheters should be considered for patients who present with significant organ dysfunction or major comorbidities that entail an increased risk of hemodynamic disturbances or instability. The decision to place a PA catheter should be based on the hemodynamic risk of the individual case rather than surgical setting-related recommendations.

Sounds like a lot of double speak, I know. It is a lot of double speak. To simplify things, a PA catheter should be considered in order to monitor:
- Cardiac function
- Filling pressures
- Volume status
- The effects of ionotropic support

But in the words of one of my mentors, "There is only one reason to put in a PA catheter, and that is to determine the cause of hypotension." You see, if we can manipulate cardiac function, filling pressures, volume status, etc., we should be able to raise the patient's blood pressure. And really that's the best and easiest way to look at it because do we really care about monitoring filling pressures and volume status? Bottom line: if the patient is hypotensive and you are unable to figure out why, a PA catheter can be very helpful. (The pro-TEE fraction argues that transesophageal echocardiography [TEE] is the best way to determine the cause of hypotension.)

CONTRAINDICATIONS

Well, all is relative, but ignorance is definitely not bliss. The number-one contraindication in terms of PA catheters is not having a clue as to what you are doing or how to interpret the information. If this means you, definitely keep reading. Usually patients who have plenty of relative contraindications are the ones who are getting a PA catheter, so always think "risk/benefit" and before you float this catheter keep in mind the following:

- If you do not know how to interpret the Swan numbers or how to place a Swan, it is not a good idea to float a Swan.
- Patients with pulmonary hypertension are at increased risk of PA rupture.
- Floating the Swan through the right heart can cause a right bundle branch block, which leads to a complete heart block if superimposed on a preexisting left bundle branch block (unless of course a pacing device is in place).
- In pediatric cases you may need an extra-small Swan, and kids tend to have holes in their hearts that result in Swans migrating into unintended chambers.
- Clots in the right atrium or ventricle are at risk of dislodging and causing pulmonary emboli—never a good thing.
- Surgery on the right side of the heart causes interference in the surgical field.
- Heparinization can cause uncontrolled bleeding in the case of the dreaded pulmonary artery rupture.
- Postpneumonectomy patients are at risk of perforation of the arterial stump on the side of the pneumonectomy.

COMPLICATIONS, OR WHEN THE SWAN BECOMES THE UGLY DUCKLING

Floating a Swan always bears the potential for severe complications, so keep them in mind and your head in the game. Do not get fooled by "just a routine" Swan. The best treatment is prevention and knowledge.

- PA rupture is certainly the most devastating complication. It classically presents with the inability to get a wedge tracing, damped wave forms, blood in the endotracheal tube in the intubated patient or hemoptysis in the awake patient, hypotension, tachycardia, or the never subtle cardiovascular collapse. If this sounds like a nightmare, believe us it is. But if you find yourself in the middle of this nightmare, take a deep breath and do the opposite of what instinct tells you to do. Most providers want to deflate the balloon, but no, just like in a horror movie, don't do it. If you suspect rupture of the PA, keep the balloon inflated in an attempt to tamponade the bleeding. Turn the patient onto the side of the bleeding lung to avoid spillage into the intact lung and/or consider lung isolation with a double lumen tube (just be careful because of the now-bloodied airway!). Also, you might consider informing a colleague in thoracic surgery—yes, thoracic surgery. You see, these complications go one of two ways: the first is that of watchful waiting in hopes that the balloon tamponades the bleeding and all is well. The second, again a bit of a nightmare, requires surgical repair, and yes, this is not trivial surgery.
  - Since we are chatting about this horrible complication, it is probably worth mentioning the patients who are at higher risk of rupture. Unfortunately, these patients are the ones who are getting a PA catheter. They are the elderly, those with pulmonary hypertension, and those anticoagulated, and for whatever reason females tend to rupture more often than males.
- Arrhythmias reveal everything from premature contractions, right bundle branch block (RBBB), ventricular tachycardia (Vtach) to ventricular fibrillation (Vfib) (yes, welcome back to the nightmares). When confronted with this you have two options: either withdraw the catheter or swiftly pass through the right ventricle (RV) into the PA.
- Knotting of the PA catheter during the floating process (rare but it can happen). The good news is it is usually worth a publication.
- And, of course, the usual culprits of central venous cannulation: bleeding, infection, pneumothorax, and carotid puncture.

EQUIPMENT AND PERSONNEL

- Secure airway: When asked to place a Swan, ask, "Does this patient need to be intubated first?"—same idea as mentioned in the chapter about central venous pressure (CVP).

- Two practitioners: You will need another set of hands and eyes; floating a Swan is a task for at least two people. You need two sets of eyes, two pairs of hands, and two heads. Hopefully with all that, at least one person will monitor the patient. (Not joking here; PA catheters can be very distracting, so make sure someone is paying attention to the patient, not just to all the PA catheter hullabaloo).
- Communication: Clear communication and understanding among team members is a must, especially regarding the balloon inflation and deflation. (Ever hear about closed loop communication? You definitely need it here.) We know you know this, but always, yes always, advance with the balloon inflated, withdraw with the balloon deflated. NEVER the other way around, or yes, you will find yourself in that nightmare!
- Introducer: Prior to insertion you will need to place an introducer, preferably in the right internal jugular (IJ) vein (shortest and straightest route), but it can be done from pretty much all major central line insertion sites (Figure 41-1).
- A Swan-Ganz catheter—sounds simple, doesn't it? Not so. There is a big market out there with lots of different models, from the regular Swan to the more fancy ones with continuous mixed venous oxygen saturation, continuous cardiac output, or pacing capability. Just pick one! Or your institution will do so for you (Figure 41-2).
- A sleeve, so the catheter can be adjusted afterward while being inside this sterile field.
- At least two transducers to follow CVP and PA pressure tracings.
- Full barrier protection, including sterile field, gowns, gloves, and a cap. Actually for a Swan you want to be *extra* sterile; just think about where it is going—right into the heart. So better be sterile given the potential for catastrophic infectious complications if you place those nasty bugs directly into the heart or onto a heart valve.
- Extra stuff: Don't forget all those little things like suture material, flush syringes, and a small syringe for the balloon.
- Really extra stuff: In case you are having a tough time you can consider a C-arm or TEE for guidance, but they are usually not needed.

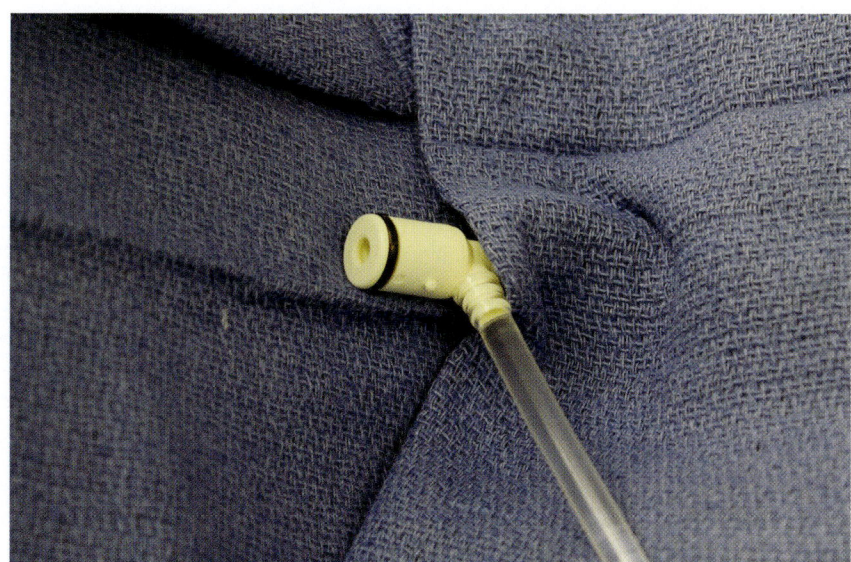

FIGURE 41-1 Introducer sheath in right jugular vein, covered by sterile towels.

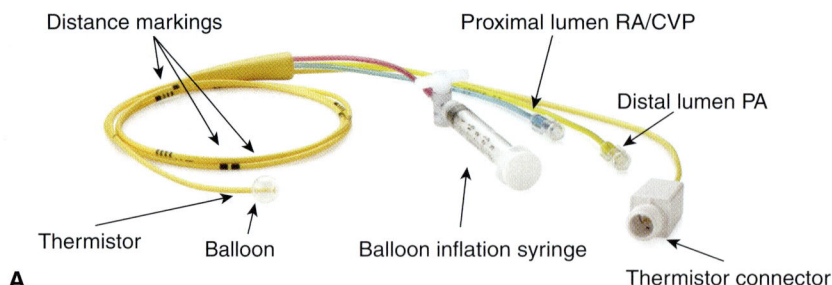
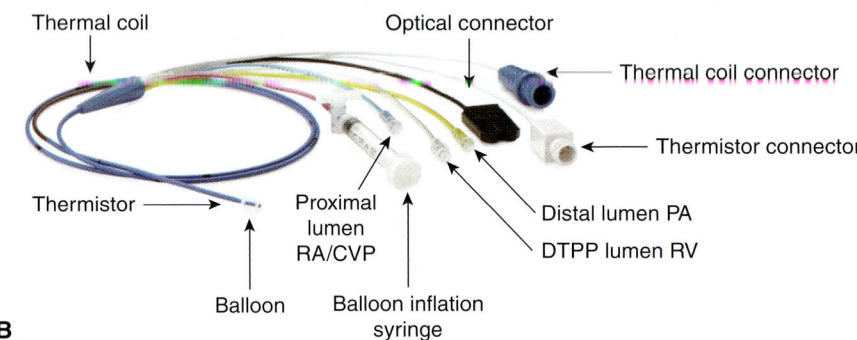

FIGURE 41-2 Examples of pulmonary artery catheters. (A) Multiflex pulmonary artery catheter: the standard version. (B) OptiQ advanced sensor catheter: the fancy version. (Reprinted with permission of ICU Medical, Inc.)

INSERTING A SWAN

A few thoughts before we get started. Floating a Swan for every patient with severe cardiac disease is becoming more and more uncommon. On the other hand, pretty much every patient with significant cardiac disease gets a TEE probe placed intraoperatively. Nevertheless, the TEE is far from replacing a Swan as it is just not practical. This is especially true in the ICU, when you cannot keep a TEE in all the time. So even if you might not need it in the OR, consider your ICU colleagues (but keep it to yourself; "use in the ICU" is never the right answer on the orals!).

Once in place, a Swan provides you a lot of different pieces of information, and it is easy to get distracted by them or to be lost in interpretation. Never forget that the most important task is to keep the patient safe! Always make sure that the patient is stable and remember your ABCs. Keep in mind that the numbers have to be in the right context; your job is not simply documenting them but also interpreting them in the hemodynamic setting for each individual patient.

ANATOMY

A river runs through it, so it always starts with a good history. Know the circulation and the river on which you wish your Swan to float.

Look for contraindications in your particular patient and other scenarios that might pose problems for a smooth float, such as:
- Patients with a history of heart surgery as a child (modified anatomy)
- Superior vena cava syndrome (aka the road block)
- Other congestion in the lumen, such as pacer wires and port lines
- Septal defects, which can reroute your catheter into the left heart
- Right heart surgery, which might require repositioning during the surgery
- Tricuspid vegetations or clots; you don't want to dislodge them directly into the lung.

TECHNIQUE

Time to get some hands dirty but not the patient, so gown and glove up!

The introducer is already in place, and the venous position is confirmed. First you want to get your patient out of the Trendelenburg position and into a level position or slightly rotated to one side to facilitate floating.

Take the PA catheter out of the sterile packaging without contaminating it, and thread it through the sheath and lock it at 80 cm (one bold and three thin marks). Pay attention to the correct orientation of the sheath with the locking mechanism toward the patient (Figure 41-3).

You can either flush all lines yourself and cap them with a stopcock so it doesn't drain and air reenters the lumen (see Figure 41-4), or you can hand the end of the Swan to a team member to flush it for you and connect it to the transducers. Remember, this part of the catheter is now unsterile, so make sure not to touch anything beyond the sheath at the 80-cm mark (Figure 41-4).

Also check the balloon to make is sure it is intact (Figure 41-5).

One of the more common mistakes of not getting a proper tracing is due to incorrect transducer connections. Make sure the transducers are properly hooked up and are zeroed. The CVP port is attached to the CVP transducer, and the PA port is attached to the PA catheter. Sounds easy, but everyone makes this mistake at least once. To confirm this, you can zero them independently and visually confirm that the transducer and the tracer on the screen correspond, you can gently wiggle the tip of the catheter and check that the correct reading changes, or you can zero both at the level of the patient's chest and elevate the PA port straight in the air (30 cm) while keeping your CV port at the level of the chest (your PA tracing should now read 20 mmHg and your CVP still 0; if the numbers are switched, so are your transducers; if the numbers are way off, re-zero, flush, or switch transducers). You can also occlude the tip of the PA port, and on the monitor you should be seeing a diagonal straight line with increasing pressure on the monitor.

Lay the catheter out so that the curve of the Swan mimics the route through the heart. For example, if you start with the right internal jugular (IJ), the Swan should form a counterclockwise curve and pointing upward toward the 11 o'clock position (Figure 41-6).

Take another good look at the patient and the monitors to make sure everything is stable before you start; a disconnected endotracheal tube (ETT) cannot wait and makes floating a Swan obsolete (sounds trivial, but it happens).

Insert the Swan through the diaphragm of the sheath, and if no resistance is encountered, slowly advance to 20 cm. The tip should be in the superior vena cava (SVC) above the right atrium (RA) and you will see a central venous pressure tracing (Figure 41-7A).

Now inflate the balloon with the provided syringe, using 1.5 cc of air. Again use closed-loop communication, say "inflate balloon," and listen for verbal confirmation "balloon inflated"; the same is true for deflation. Yes, this is very important because failure to communicate can have serious consequences when you introduce foreign bodies into a beating heart. Also, withdrawing a Swan with the balloon inflated can lead to catastrophic consequences—use your imagination; remember the nightmare?

Advance the catheter in small increments, watching the pressure tracing. Also listen to the pulse oximetry and advance in synchrony with every heartbeat. This guarantees that the heart valves are open while you pass them and you really "float" the catheter with the blood flow.

In a simplified world, changes should happen every 10 cm. So at 30 cm expect to see the RV tracing and say "RV"; sometimes I say "LV" at this point just to see if people are paying attention. Again, communication is key (Figure 41-7B).

Now that you are in the RV, the chance for ectopy and heart block increases, so be on the lookout. If you encounter them in the RV outflow tract, consider increasing your speed to pass this danger zone.

Advance further until you see a jump in diastolic pressure and reach the PA at roughly 40 cm (Figure 41-7C). At this point you have two choices: you can either advance it a few centimeters into the PA, let the balloon down, and leave it there (using the PA diastolic as a surrogate for the wedge pressure), or you can advance further until you get a wedge tracing (Figure 41-7D) and let the balloon down afterward (higher risk of complications, especially PA rupture). There are two schools of thought behind this, and it really depends on what information you need for the case (we'll address this later).

Slide the sheath all the way over the catheter and connect it to the introducer. Make sure that after all that excitement you do not inadvertently push the catheter in or pull it out during this process; the sheath tends to stick to the catheter and the connector at the end can be stubborn. Lock the sheath to the catheter (Figure 41-8).

One more thing: make sure you deflate the balloon! Congratulation you just floated a Swan; nicely done!

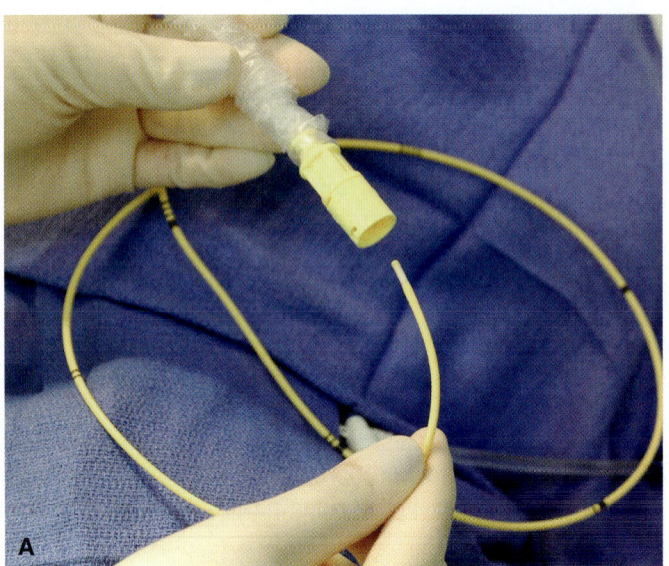
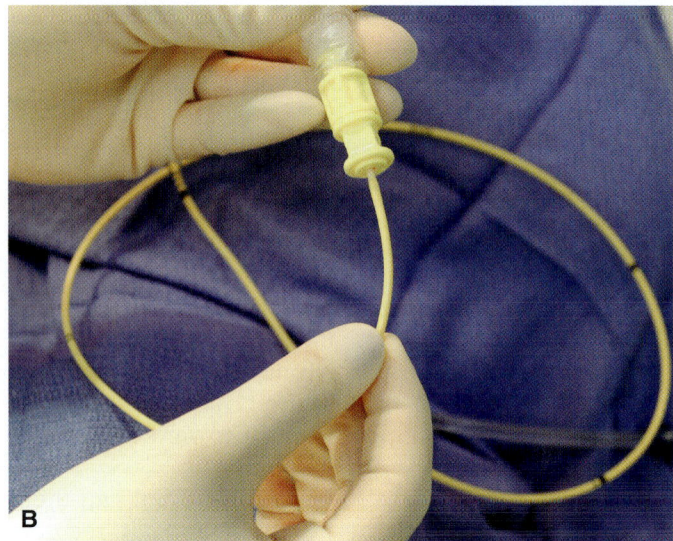
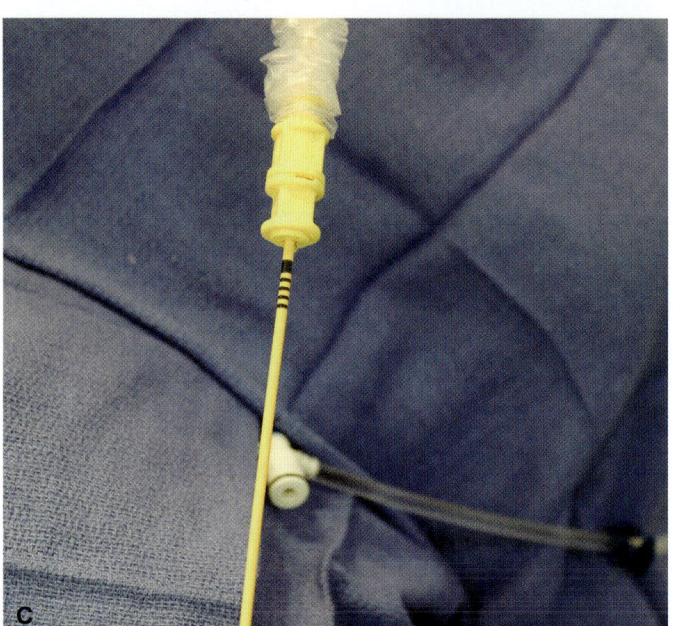

FIGURE 41-3 Threading the sheath onto the pulmonary artery catheter. (A) Oops, that's the wrong end! (B) Yep, that looks better! (C) Correct position of the sheath locked in place at 80 cm.

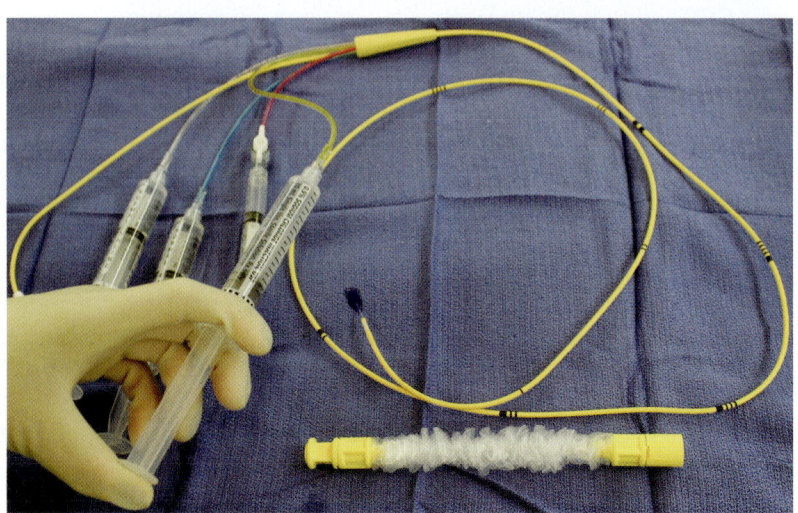

FIGURE 41-4 Sterile flushing of the different lumen with normal saline. Note the sheath lying below the catheter.

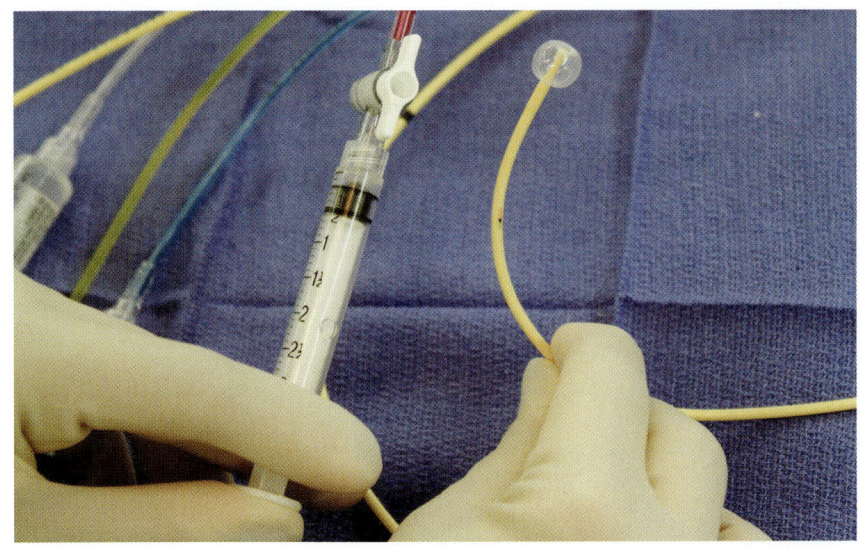

FIGURE 41-5 The balloon is checked and ready to go. Don't forget to deflate before insertion; otherwise you will have a tough time pushing it through the introducer sheath.

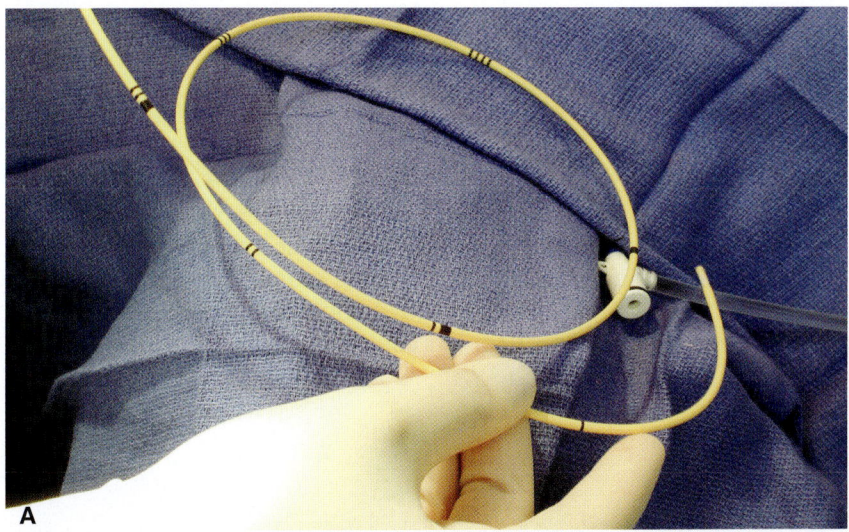

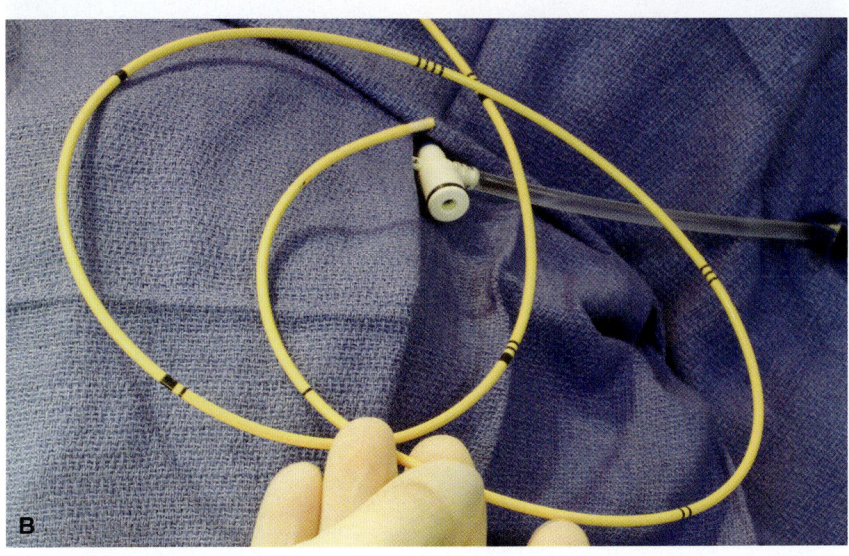

FIGURE 41-6 To make floating easy, try to mimic the route the catheter has to travel inside the veins. (A) Correct positioning: the catheter forms a counterclockwise curve, with the tip pointing upward toward the 11 o'clock position. (B) The "pretzel": you will have a tough time floating the catheter into the lungs when you start out with the tip facing away from its destination.

A Right atrial/central venous pressure (RA/CVP)

2 to 6 mmHg
Mean 4 mmHg
a = atrial systole
c = backward bulging from tricuspid valve closure
v = atrial filling, ventricular systole

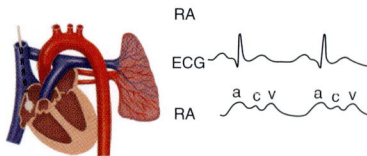

C Pulmonary artery

Systolic pressure (PASP)
15–25 mmHg
Diastolic pressure (PADP)
8–15 mmHg
Mean pressure (MPA)
10–20 mmHg

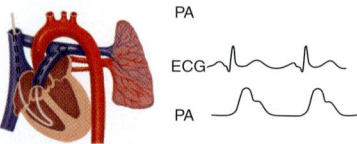

B Right ventricular

Systolic pressure (RVSP)
15–25 mmHg
Diastolic pressure (RVDP)
0–8 mmHg

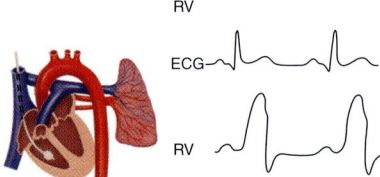

D Pulmonary artery occlusion pressure (PAOP)

Mean 6–12 mmHg
a = atrial systole
v = atrial filling, ventricle systole

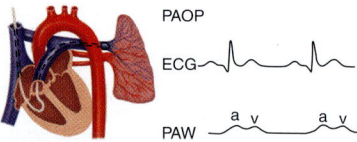

FIGURE 41-7 Illustrations of the different pressure tracings you will encounter, with the corresponding catheter positions. (A) Pulmonary artery catheter inside the right atrium with depiction of a central venous pressure tracing. (B) The pulmonary artery catheter is now past the tricuspid valve, inside the right ventricle. Note the higher systolic pressure inside the ventricle (15 to 25 mmHg). (C) A sudden jump in the diastolic pressure indicates that the pulmonary artery catheter has traveled inside the pulmonary artery. (D) A typical wedge pressure tracing (or pulmonary artery occlusion pressure tracing), which serves as a surrogate for left ventricular preload. (Reprinted with permission of ICU Medical, Inc.)

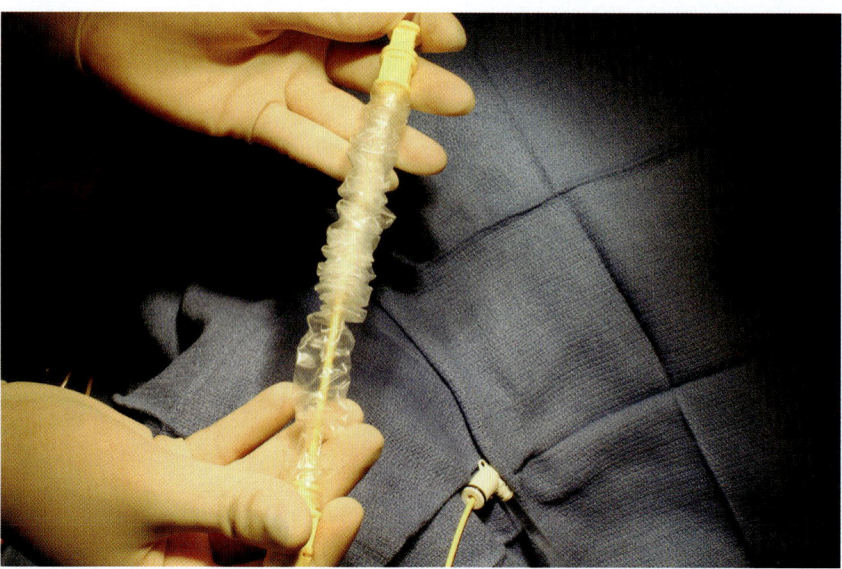

FIGURE 41-8 Slide the sheath over the catheter and lock it in place. Be careful not to advance the catheter when you do so and make sure the balloon is deflated!

TROUBLESHOOTING: WHEN THE SWAN WON'T GO OR THE WAVES LOOK FUNNY

- Remember, common things are common, so when you do not get a waveform check your transducers first and make sure they are attached correctly and zeroed.
- If those are working properly and you are not able to float the Swan in the RV, take down the balloon, pull the catheter out, and make sure the balloon still inflates.
- Realign the Swan so the curvature follows the direction you are intending it to go (or if this does not work, just point it in the complete opposite direction; don't ask why, just do it).
- Recheck the patient's position, making sure that he or she is slightly head up, with the right side down.
- Consider using a new catheter or inject cold saline. Sometimes after you have tried for a long time the catheter gets warm and very soft, making it harder to float directly. The cold saline will stiffen the soft catheter.
- Other things to consider if the Swan won't float into the RV are to let the patient take a deep breath, if the patient is awake ("sucking the Swan toward the PA"), or if the patient is on the vent, consider detaching for a short moment; just make sure you put the patient back on again!
- You can also give a fluid bolus to fill the heart and vasculature.
- Remember to advance in synchronicity with the heartbeat.
- If the C-arm or TEE is available, you can consider using it for guidance.
- Be mindful not to advance the catheter too far, when you are searching for a wedge tracing. Especially in the patient with mitral regurgitation (MR), large V waves can mimic the PA tracing, making it hard to identify correctly and leading to over-threading of the PA catheter with the potential to cause PA rupture. In this case you should consider overlying the arterial and PA waveform to confirm that they peak in unison, while in patients with MR and large V waves, the wedge waveform will show a shift to the right compared with the arterial tracing. Therefore, some practitioners recommend not floating the Swan past 55 cm for a normal-size adult.
- Lastly, if it took you so long that the surgeons have already opened the chest, you can ask them for assistance to guide to Swan with their fingers in the field.

EXPERT ADVICE

- Beware the Swan that comes to you from the ICU or other faraway places. In fact, always mistrust the Swan that comes from somebody else. It has nothing to do with implying that you are the only one in the world who can handle a PA catheter properly (which might be true), but it is always better to be safe than sorry. Always check the depth of the Swan; if it advertently migrated to 70 cm and you try to inflate the balloon in a tiny pulmonary vessel, you will have a lot of explaining to do (remember the nightmare?). Kinks, tangled lines, loss of caps or (partially) pulled catheters are all very common, especially after transport. Also, last but not least, always know the status of the balloon: up or down!
- Not every Swan needs to be wedged. Most times the PA diastolic pressure corresponds sufficiently with the wedge pressure, which in turn corresponds to the left atrial (LA) pressure, which corresponds to the LV end-diastolic pressure, which is a surrogate for LV end-diastolic volume, and this correlates to wall stretch, also known as preload. So no need to chase a wedge pressure and risk PA rupture in an already sick patient, right?
- Not every patient needs a Swan, for example, a patient with extensive cardiac history who is scheduled for a herniotomy. Sure, a PA catheter could help manage cardiac complications, but is this worth the risk in a low-risk surgery? Points to consider: there should be no big fluid shifts, the patient should be extubated after the completion of surgery (if general anesthesia is used), there should be no ICU stay afterward, the patient has otherwise no major comorbidities, and the surgeon is experienced and fast (hopefully). It is probably not a good idea to expose the patient to a risk of PA rupture. Let's make it even worse and the patient is a Jehovah's Witness and you can't transfuse. This is a sticky situation.
- Even if you don't need a Swan, others might. This is not an uncommon scenario in the cardiac OR. Let's take, for example, a patient arriving for heart surgery, with a history of end-stage renal disease but relatively good ventricular function for bypass. Sure, you can manage this patient in the OR with a TEE and without a Swan, but what about your colleagues who have to manage the patient in the ICU afterward? Evaluating fluid status without urine output can be very challenging. Probably a good idea is to place the Swan in the OR under maximal sterile conditions and in a controlled setting, before the patient's status becomes more unstable after a big surgery.

- Infusion into the sheath: One of the most underappreciated dangers that we subject our patients to is transporting them from the OR to the ICU. This is especially true with all the lines, tubes, poles, infusions, and more. It is not uncommon that lines get tangled, dislodged, or pulled. In the case of a Swan you don't even need to pull it out all the way to render it useless. Consider this: you just transferred your patient to the ICU, when not even a minute into signout you see the blood pressure dropping. After troubleshooting the transducers and making sure that everything is connected, you begin treating the patient with pressors and fluids, but the patient does not respond. What went wrong? The patient has been fairly stable in the OR, so what is different now? Finally, somebody realizes that the Swan with the epinephrine infusion was pulled out a few centimeters, just far enough so that the proximal port is now infusing into the sheath instead of the patient; this is bad news.

WHAT DO YOU DO WITH THE DIGITS?

First of all, never jeopardize the patient's safety just to get a number!

In order to interpret the numbers, you need to know what the "normal" values are:

Parameter	Normal Values	Units
Right atrial pressure	2–6	mmHg
Right ventricular pressure	15–25/0–8	mmHg
Pulmonary artery pressure	15–25/8–15	mmHg
Wedge pressure	6–12	mmHg
Left ventricular end diastolic	4–12	mmHg
Cardiac output	4.5–7.5	l/min
Cardiac index	2.8–4.2	l/min/m^2
Stroke volume	50–110	ml/beat
Systemic vascular resistance	900–1400	dynes·s·cm^{-5}
Pulmonary vascular resistance	150–250	dynes·s·cm^{-5}

Always know two things about your patient with a PA catheter:
1. The normal PA pressures
2. The PA pressure compared to the systemic pressure

Bear in mind that the "normal" numbers above might not be the normal numbers for your particular patient. Also, always interpret PA pressures in relation to the systemic blood pressure. PA pressures can reach half the systemic values (or higher) fairly rapidly, especially in hypotensive patients.

Now let's talk about specific basic terms for interpretation of the Swan numbers, starting with the concept of transmural pressure. Basically this means that the transmural pressure of the heart (also known as filling pressure, the one you like to know) is the result of the pressure inside the heart (the one you measure) minus the extracardiac pressure (not measured easily). Normally the extracardiac pressure (in diastole) approximates zero, and therefore the transmural pressure (filling pressure) can be approximated by measuring the intracardiac pressure alone. For example, a wedge pressure of 15 mmHg if taken out of context sounds like a reasonable surrogate for adequate volume status, but if your patient is in cardiac tamponade and the pressure around the heart is 13 mmHg, your real wedge suddenly becomes 2 mmHg, which is not quite enough preload for the heart to support the circulation; no wonder the patient is in shock. It can be tricky to use a pressure as a surrogate for a volume; therefore, one must be familiar with the concept of transmural pressure gradient in order to determine the true filling pressure inside the heart.

Next on the list is the Starling curve, or more precisely the Frank-Starling curve (Frank is yet another one who, like Ganz, doesn't get mentioned frequently). The Starling curve gives you information about the compliance of the heart. Compliance is the relationship between change in volume and corresponding changes in pressure. If the compliance of the heart is very high, intracardiac pressures will not increase by much, even if the volume increases significantly—like a thin balloon. On the other hand, in a less compliant heart, changes in volume will lead to large increases in intracardiac pressures—like a thick rubber tire. A classic example would be the patient with aortic stenosis who has a very thick (rubber tire–like) ventricle, and has decreased compliance. In this patient, low-volume states correspond to high-pressure numbers. Again, measuring a wedge pressure of 15 mmHg in this patient could mean that he/she is severely dry and needs fluid resuscitation.

Let's take, for example, a random patient and use the Swan to figure out why the patient is hypotensive. Now that we have a Swan in place we can measure a cardiac output and the calculated systemic vascular resistance (SVR) to see if the problem is due to decreased peripheral resistance (like septic shock). In this example, the

SVR seems adequate but cardiac output is low. We know the heart rate, so we can calculate stroke volume, which is determined by contractility, preload, and afterload. One way to differentiate them is to give a fluid challenge to increase the wedge pressure by maybe 10% and measure the cardiac output again. If the CO increases significantly, chances are your patient is dry and the wedge pressure is too low for your patient. If the cardiac output is unchanged, chances are that you are dealing with a problem of contractility and an inotrope should be considered next. If, on the other hand, the CO falls significantly, chances are the heart is overfilled and you actually have to lower the preload.

The bottom line is that interpretation of all the numbers a PA catheter gives you can only be done in the context of your specific patient. There is no such thing as absolute numbers for everyone, especially since the patients who get a PA catheter are the ones with abnormal physiology; otherwise, you probably would not need to place it in the first place.

SUGGESTED READING

Abreu AR, Campos MA, Krieger BP. Pulmonary artery rupture induced by a pulmonary artery catheter: a case report and review of the literature. *J Intensive Care Med* 2004;19(5):291–296.

Chittock DR, Dhingra VK, Ronco JJ, et al. Severity of illness and risk of death associated with pulmonary artery catheter use. *Crit Care Med* 2004;32(4):911–915.

Evans DC, Doraiswamy VA, Prosciak MP, et al. Complications associated with pulmonary artery catheters: a comprehensive clinical review. *Scand J Surg* 2009;98(4):199–208.

Iberti TJ, Fischer EP, Leibowitz AB, et al. A multicenter study of physicians' knowledge of the pulmonary artery catheter. Pulmonary Artery Catheter Study Group. *JAMA* 1990;264(22):2928–2932.

Keusch DJ, Winters S, Thys DM. The patient's position influences the incidence of dysrhythmias during pulmonary artery catheterization. *Anesthesiology* 1989;70(4):582–584.

Leibowitz AB, Oropello JM. The pulmonary artery catheter in anesthesia practice in 2007: an historical overview with emphasis on the past 6 years. *Semin Cardiothorac Vasc Anesth* 2007;11(3):162–176.

Moore RA, Neary MJ, Gallagher JD, et al., Determination of the pulmonary capillary wedge position in patients with giant left atrial V waves. *J Cardiothorac Anesth* 1987;1(2):108–113.

Practice guidelines for pulmonary artery catheterization: an updated report by the American Society of Anesthesiologists Task Force on Pulmonary Artery Catheterization. *Anesthesiology* 2003;99(4):988–1014.

Sandham JD, Hull RD, Brant RF, et al. A randomized, controlled trial of the use of pulmonary-artery catheters in high-risk surgical patients. *N Engl J Med* 2003;348(1):5–14.

Sandham JD. Pulmonary artery catheter use—refining the question. *Crit Care Med* 2004:32(4):1070–1071.

Shah MR, Hasselblad V, Stevenson LW, et al. Impact of the pulmonary artery catheter in critically ill patients: meta-analysis of randomized clinical trials. *JAMA* 2005;294(13):1664–1670.

Vender JS. Pulmonary artery catheter utilization: the use, misuse, or abuse. *J Cardiothorac Vasc Anesth* 2006;20(3):295–299.

CHAPTER 42

ANESTHESIA FOR THE CARDIAC CATHETERIZATION LAB

WILLIAM GRUBB
DANNY CHAUNG

Nearly all men can stand adversity, but if you want to test a man's character, give him power.

Abraham Lincoln

INTRODUCTION

Most common catheterization lab procedures require that the patient remain comfortable and immobile during the procedure. It is like trying to have your children sit still at a movie theater. These procedures can include:
- The placement and testing of an automatic implantable cardioverter-defibrillator (AICD)
- The "mapping" of the conduction system for detection of aberrant pathway(s)
- Radiofrequency ablation catheters for treatment of conduction system abnormalities
- Sedation for anxious patients during catheterization/angioplasty
- The hybrid lab combining percutaneous procedures with cardiothoracic surgical procedures

Most procedures are primarily accomplished under light sedation with midazolam and minimal narcotic. It is important to exclude certain cases from sedation, such as:
- Morbidly obese patients (body mass index [BMI] > 30)
- Patients who have had recent meals (full stomach)
- Mallampati class IV airway (any indication of difficult airway)
- Patients with symptomatic congestive heart failure
- Procedures in areas where there is lack of support or monitoring equipment, especially areas without formal recovery areas postprocedure (e.g., postanesthesia care unit [PACU])
- Procedures performed without a clinician trained/experienced with conscious sedation
  - Therefore, all supervising persons need advanced cardiac life support (ACLS) certification.
  - All physicians need conscious sedation training and experience in order to render patients unconscious in an operative suite.

Intravenous medications used for sedation in the cath lab can include:
- Titrated boluses of diphenhydramine, midazolam, fentanyl, or meperidine
- Propofol infusions
- Dexmedetomidine infusions
- Combinations of small boluses of etomidate and propofol infusions

As most readers of this book will be familiar with the use of bolus injections for sedation procedures and the use of propofol infusions, our emphasis is on the use of the newer sedation medication, Precedex (dexmedetomidine). Precedex is an α_2-adrenoreceptor agonist with sedative properties that is used because it does not cause respiratory depression. It can cause bradycardia and hypotension. It is not given to patients with advanced heart block, and it needs to be dose adjusted for patients with renal failure, diabetes, or hepatic failure. A report of the experience of the cardiology service by Williams et al.[1] at the Atlanta VA Medical Center describes the use of infusions of 0.4 to 0.6 μg/kg/h. Any hypotension in patients was treated with infusions of phenylephrine.

AICD PLACEMENT AND TESTING (SHORT CATH LAB)

Many cardiologists rely on the use of anesthesia services for brief periods of time during AICD placement and testing. This complex interaction between the cardiac and anesthesia team necessitates a preprocedure interview/evaluation of the patient by the anesthesia team covering the lab. After placement of monitors, initial sedation can be administered by the cardiology team during the percutaneous placement of central venous access and lead placement. As described above, our hospital requires a "sedation" training course for these physicians.

During catheter placement, cardiologists usually administer fentanyl and midazolam. Our catheterization labs are equipped with all necessary airway access equipment and anesthesia machines to facilitate incorporation of the anesthesia team into the area in case of an airway issue prior to testing of the device (Figure 42-1).

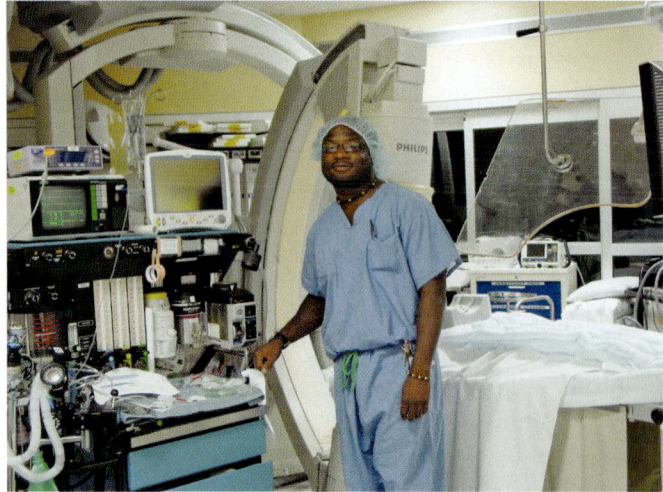

FIGURE 42-1 Anesthesia monitors viewed from the foot of the patient. The patient's head will be in the C-arm of the fluoroscopy unit behind the anesthesia technician.

THE ANESTHESIA TEAM MAY BE BECKONED

During the Actual Cutdown or Generator Pocket Placement

The request for deeper sedation is infrequent but may require additional injections of a benzodiazepine coupled with possible airway support. In our service, an anesthesia/respiratory tech is on site and trained to help with airway management requiring the insertion of oral or nasal airways. The placement of the percutaneous lead is often done using venous cutdown access usually via a left internal jugular (IJ) cutdown. This can occasionally precipitate an arrhythmia, possibly resulting in an urgent anesthesia intervention.

During Subsequent Tests of the Generator

If a patient has medical problems or respiratory issues that exceed the needs of a minimal airway support system, the "short cath lab infantry" is called in for additional airway management during the formation of the generator pocket and subsequent testing of the AICD generator. Occasionally, the patient with congestive heart failure (CHF) cannot tolerate lying flat for the placement of the device, and the anesthesia team is requested to administer general anesthesia. The team needs to remain available for other problems including the development of hypotension secondary to induced or recalcitrant arrhythmias.

When "anesthesia" arrives at the battle scene, the patient is observed for current oxygenation/airway support, and if necessary, a deeper state of sedation is accomplished through the use of small amounts of etomidate, or if tolerated, the addition of propofol infusions.

If the procedure has progressed flawlessly with minimal sedation administered by the cardiology team, the anesthesia team may be requested only for the testing of the AICD. If the patient is sleeping upon arrival, it is important to try to assess the need for additional sedation by communicating with the patient to determine the current state of awareness. The testing of the device will produce intense muscle spasms and require complete amnesia for patient comfort. It is always crucial to review what has already been given by the primary team and know when this was injected. Testing the AICD requires the induction of ventricular tachycardia.

Do not forget to have the staff remove any jewelry from the patient to protect the skin from burns during cardioversion.

The patient should have R2 pads placed during the setup procedure. It is important to know where they are placed and to test this equipment prior to the procedure.

During AICD testing, the cardiologist induces ventricular tachycardia and allows the device to detect the arrhythmia, and subsequently shock the heart with a preset electrical discharge. The strength of the electrical discharge for internal cardioversion is usually around 25 J. The length of time the AICD device witnesses the arrhythmia prior to successful cardioversion is an important measurement of the competency of the device. This time period is recorded in milliseconds. Longer time intervals between detection and discharge are not acceptable. The system may not be successful because the impedance of the leads is not correct or the leads have not closely approximated viable cardiac tissue. If this happens, the patient will need external cardioversion with R2 pads.

These are the variables associated with the testing of the device and usually determine the amount of time the patient needs to be unconscious (amnestic). With a rebreathing mask established, and in the presence of preexisting sedation, a single dose of 0.5 to 0.8 mg/kg of propofol (lean body weight) is usually adequate to provide comfort to the patient during the cardioversion.

With each induction of ventricular tachycardia and subsequent cardioversion, up to 10% of the cardiac output is lost. If the patient has a cardiomyopathy or has had a recent myocardial infarction (MI), it is important to expect clinical symptoms of failure that may require diuretics or inotropic support. It is also important to note that in a patient with low cardiac output, circulation time is decreased and the time for a drug to work is prolonged; therefore, one must be patient with onset of effect and titrate carefully prior to rebolusing the patient. The respiratory depression from sedation coupled with the loss of pulmonary blood flow from the myocardial depressant effects of our anesthetics determines whether the next step in management may occasionally necessitate intubation. We are the ultimate fail-safe for these patients and need to act wisely and communicate clearly with our medical colleagues in such clinical scenarios!

ABLATIONS (THE "LONG CATH" LAB)

The previously described relationship between the cardiology team and the anesthesia team must be redefined for the care of the patient presenting for radiofrequency (RF) ablation. These cases are performed by a separate team in our institution. As they are elective procedures, they are assigned to a "long cath" lab team.

The RF ablation procedure is tedious to perform and painful for the patient, requiring prolonged immobility and sedation. There is increased use of fluoroscopy to guide multiple catheters, and often an increased need for deep sedation for the insertion of multiple femoral sheaths. Many complex mappings and subsequent ablations require the use of intraatrial echo requiring an additional uncomfortable catheter that can be extremely hot.

Ablation produces heat and often requires the use of an esophageal temperature probe mandating general anesthesia with an endotracheal tube (ETT). The temperature probe serves as a safety mechanism to prevent the occurrence of an esophageal ulcer. Most ablation patients require a depth of sedation/analgesia that requires airway support and possibly paralysis. Remember, if you had this RF ablator in your chest you'd be moving around like a kid in a movie theater, too.

An exception is the patient who presents for "retouching" of previously ablated areas, or has a small well-defined ectopic area. For these patients an laryngeal mask airway (LMA) or ETT may not be necessary, and the procedure can be accomplished with minimal sedation. Our service often uses a propofol continuous infusion to establish patient comfort and relies on an oral or nasal airway with an oxygen rebreathing system to enhance FiO_2. The end-tidal CO_2 can be monitored from a distance (with the anesthesia staff behind a lead protected shield), thus eliminating radiating exposure to the anesthesia provider. Figure 42-2 demonstrates the

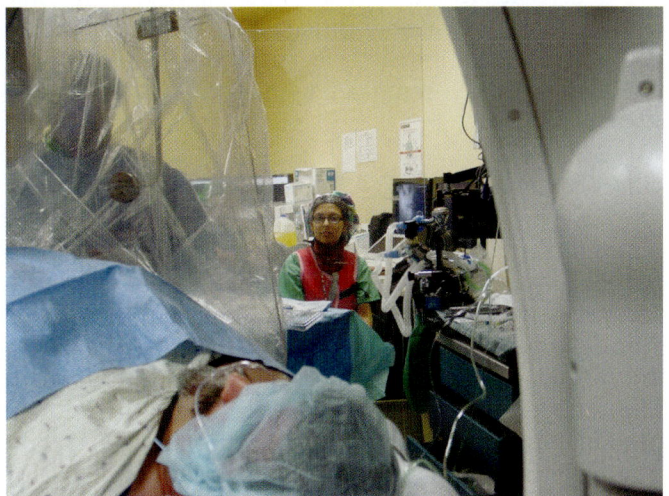

FIGURE 42-2 Anesthesia staff behind clear "lead" screen behind the cardiologist.

ideal locations and geographic relationships between the C-arm, cardiologist, patient, and anesthesia provider.

Some of the ablations are much longer, particularly those involving the entire roof of the left atrium. In these cases, the extent of the RF lesions requires a prolonged commitment from the team.

Water-cooled RF catheters require constant irrigation at the tip of the RF probe. These catheters use a basal infusion rate of 2 mL/h. The amount of irrigation infused during lesioning is dependent on the operating temperature of the probe, which is determined by the energy output utilized during the lesioning. The irrigation rate is directly (electronically) linked to the probe output. If the output is >30 W, 30 ml/min irrigation is received by the patient, causing significant extra volume. In patients with a history of CHF and dilated cardiomyopathy, the use of diuretics at the end of the procedure is often necessary.

Often the RF burns are performed for hours, and the patient may need diuretics to mobilize fluids during the post-RF lesioning period. Because these patients are potentially fluid overloaded and have poor cardiac function after being cardioverted, it may be advisable to observe the intubated patient post-lesioning or perhaps obtain an arterial blood gas (ABG) measurement prior to extubation at the end of the case.

The ablation of the left atrium is technically difficult and requires prolonged patient immobility. This is so demanding that many centers have used high-frequency jet ventilation (HFJV) during the ablation. A study by Goode et al.[2] at the University of Pittsburgh noted that at their institution, when left atrial (LA) ablations were performed with general anesthesia (GA) ETT with the use of the HFJV, there was less motion of the posterior LA with fewer tendencies for RF catheter dislodgment. Interestingly, the HFJV group had a more efficient procedure requiring less cath lab time when compared to matched controls.

STEREOTACTIC CATHETERIZATION LAB

A new form of the ablation cath system utilizes a magnetic field to guide the tip of the RF ablation catheter through the diseased cardiac tissue. The position of the catheter is then confirmed with fluoroscopy. Movement within the magnetic field affects the position of the catheters. These systems use software to drive powerful magnets positioned near the patient. It was developed to guide a catheter using a remote console with the assistance of magnetic fields to pull the catheter to precise locations and hold it there. Software maps the diseased heart and the magnets allow for the safe positioning of the catheter near the precise location of the conduction system malfunction. The position of the patient and the necessity for the field to remain motionless requires the use

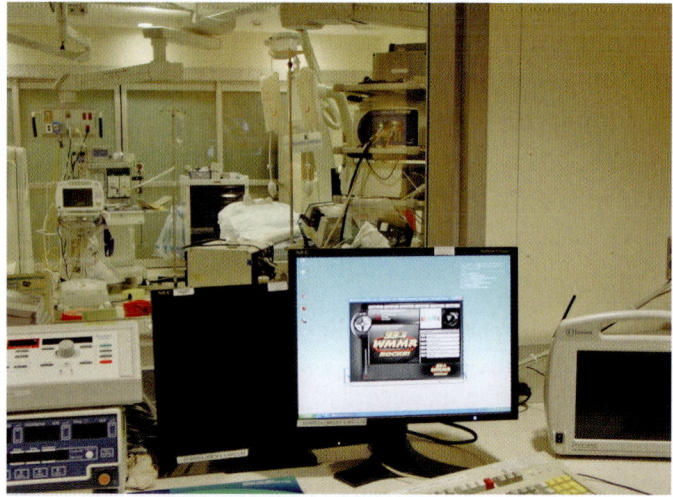

FIGURE 42-3 View from the control room: the remote monitor in right lower screen; the patient's head will be facing the control room (center).

of general anesthesia and neuromuscular blockade. There is a certain time requirement for new operators to become proficient. The learning curve often plateaus after several hundred ablations. Recently constructed labs are equipped with remote monitors in the lead-lined control rooms, so that the patient can be observed from a distance without exposing the anesthesia team to radiation. Trust us, this book has humor, but we have no jokes to make about radiation exposure. Remote monitoring of an intubated patient is possible. Figure 42-3 shows the view of the remote monitors from the radiation-protected control rooms of the stereotactic lab.

HYBRID CATHETERIZATION LAB

The hybrid cath lab functions as a complete operating room. This allows the patient to receive the catheterization, coupled with the potential for open chest surgical repair if the unthinkable happens or if the procedure cannot be corrected via percutaneous catheter techniques.

There should be ample room in the lab for complete teams of anesthesia, radiology, and vascular/thoracic surgery.

RADIATION SAFETY IN THE CATHETERIZATION LAB

The basic premise of the anesthesia provider in the cath lab is to create the safest possible environment for the patient and also for all OR personnel.

The first consideration is that any female patient of reproductive age is documented to be pregnancy test negative for this admission. The responsibility here is twofold, in that not only is avoidance of many anesthetic agents an important issue, but also the risk of radiation exposure needs to be fully considered.

Most cath labs are constructed to have the anesthesia equipment at the head of the patient. This is because of the professional history of the anesthesia care provider's desire to control the airway and stay away from anything below the clavicle. A quick look at the design of the fluoroscopic (C-arm) machine usually shows us that the "skirts" on the image intensifier are designed to protect the radiologist/cardiologist from scatter of the x-ray beam. There are often no skirts on the cephalad portion of the intensifier. For this reason, scattered x-rays are actually sent toward the patients head and toward the anesthesia provider if he or she remains at the "head" of the table (Figure 42-4).

As suggested above, the anesthetic technique requires minimal airway maintenance, and the anesthesia team remains distant from the patient to limit the total time of radiation exposure. An ideal cath lab anesthetic is one that can be managed from a distance but does not preclude the simplest of airway techniques. Ideally, the anesthesia provider can sit in the "antechamber" (DJ booth), the lead-lined monitoring room, with the technicians who are running the x-ray equipment. The use of a portable x-ray shield with a full floor screen is seen in (Figure 42-5). This can be used if you feel you have separation anxiety from the patient.

If the anesthesia provider is called upon to participate directly in the area of the image intensifier, there is the need to constantly wear a full posterior wrapped lead-lined x-ray garment and lead glasses. X-rays can penetrate through your skin and your eyes. Even with conventional eye glasses, x-rays can penetrate into your corneas and cause damage.

This allows the provider to turn freely in the areas around the C-arm to get to the necessary anesthesia equipment to support the patient. Because full wrap lead is worn, the provider can go in and out of the control room. The provider cannot rely on or expect the cardiologist to delay the progress of the case to allow time for the anesthesia personnel to adjust the anesthetic in any way. In fact, you must remember that the responsibility for your own safety is yours! Again, this need for the anesthesia personnel to come out of the antechamber and into the x-ray field makes it unacceptable to have a pregnant female conducting the anesthesia. Also, since the provider will have already spent many extra minutes in the immediate area of the C-arm, it is actually mandatory that a thyroid collar cover the anterior neck, and that there be no abilities for the x-ray to penetrate an incomplete chest wall lead protection system.

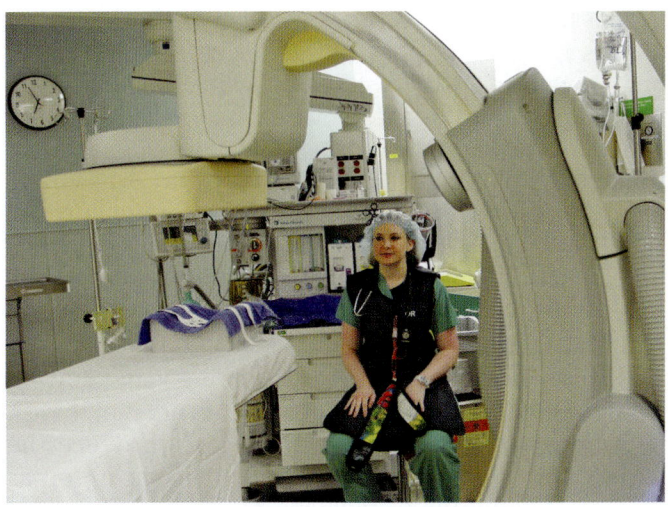

FIGURE 42-4 An improper place to conduct anesthesia in the cath lab; the radiation can travel toward the legs, and the neck and eyes are not protected.

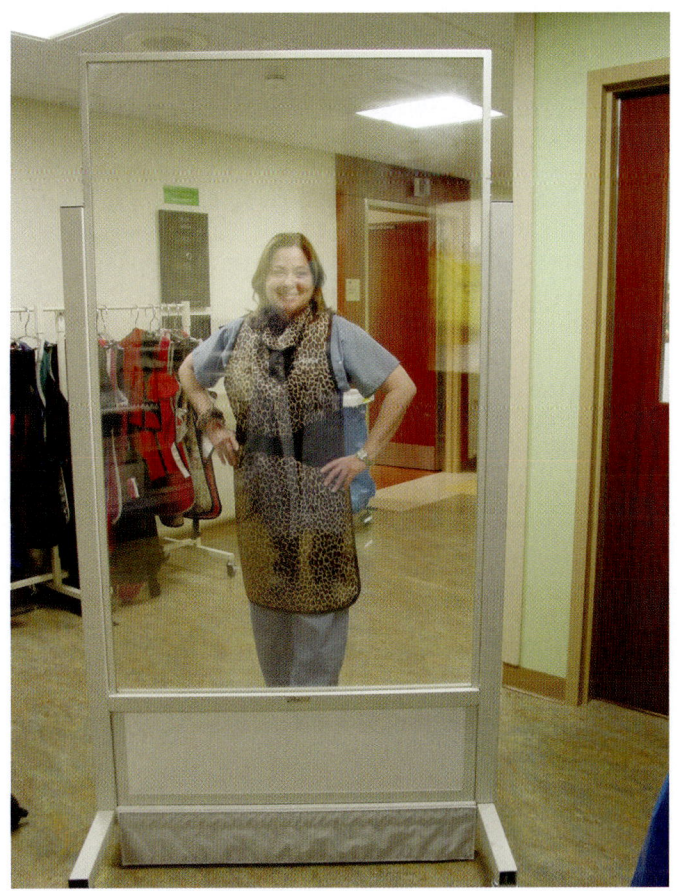

FIGURE 42-5 Staff behind an excellent "lead" screen, with full-wrap lead shielding when stepping out to work closer to the C-arm. Note the skirt on the floor protecting the feet and lower legs.

The Food and Drug Administration (FDA) Web site[3] defines radiation injuries as specific to the area of the body involved. It is well documented that workers wearing lead in a 6-foot radius of the image intensifier are still at risk of eye exposure, which leads to cataract formation. Public health policy defines x-ray exposure in rads absorbed at the skin. Here is a list of the effect of toxic x-ray exposure:
- 300 rads: minor skin changes
- 600 rads: erythema and swelling
- 1500 to 2000 rads: moist desquamation

Reports of patient skin damage in the cath lab were most frequently associated with RF cath ablation cases. It is important to note that these cases produce the largest amount of radiation. Legislation is in process that will require the display and recording of the total amount of radiation exposure a patient receives during each procedure and during each hospitalization (i.e., duration, rate, and cumulative). Newer legislation will require the provider to know the radiation dose rates for specific fluoroscopic systems and for each mode of operation during the clinical protocol. These dose rates will be derived from measurements performed. These policies may be specific for each institution.

The cath lab personnel should be aware of the following general guidelines for ensuring safety in the presence of a C-arm fluoroscopic device:
- Shielding and lead aprons: most shields are rated in equivalencies to a thin lead layer. Safe shields are rated 0.5-mm equivalency or above and most glass shields exceed this amount.
- The smaller side of the C-arm is the camera (x-ray tube). This is the side of the device where there is the most scatter of the radiation. Since the image intensifier is usually placed above the patient, the greatest amount of scatter and danger to the health care personnel is under the table or on the smaller side of the C-arm. There are often lead aprons on the image intensifier side of the equipment, further reducing the amount of radiation emitted from the field toward OR personnel.
- The beam can be "collimated" (reduced in size) to decrease the amount of scatter away from the region of radiographic interest generated.
- Pregnant women do not belong in the C-arm suite, and breast tissue of women is at risk and should be well shielded. Women also remain more sensitive to the effect of radiation on the thyroid.
- TIDS: time, intensity, distance, and shielding determine the effects of radiation.

CONCLUSION

The cath lab is a dynamic setting where the anesthesia provider is a necessary component to provide the patient comfort and safety while recognizing the risk of prolonged radiation exposure.

REFERENCES

1. Williams L, Bloom H, Atlanta VA Hospital. Moderate sedation pioneers for atrial fibrillation ablations, Atlanta VA Medical Center, Atlanta, GA. *EP Lab Digest* 2010;10(1):23.
   Discusses the use of Precedex sedation in patients presenting for atrial fibrillation ablation procedures.

2. Goode JS, et al. High-frequency jet ventilation: utility in posterior left atrial catheter ablation. Department of Anesthesiology, Atrial Arrhythmia Center University of Pittsburgh, Pittsburgh, Pennsylvania. *Heart Rhythm* 2006; 3(1):13–19.
   Discusses the role of high-frequency jet ventilator ventilation to minimize the movement of mapping and ablation catheters in the cardiac patient.

3. Food and Drug Administration Web site. http://www.fda.gov/Radiation-EmittingProducts/default.htm
   This federal report details proposed radiation safety regulations for the health care industry.

CHAPTER 43

PORT ACCESS SURGERY: ALL FEAR MINIMUS MAXIMUS—MINIMALLY INVASIVE PORT ACCESS HEART SURGERY

JONATHAN KRAIDIN
MARK ANDERSON
STEVEN H. GINSBERG

Sleep after toil, port after stormy seas
Ease after war, death after life does gently please.
    Edmund Spenser, *The Faerie Queene* (1590)

WHAT MAKES THESE CASES DIFFERENT?

Nearly 100 years after the first successful cardiac operation was performed, port-access valve surgery offers the potential for reduced postoperative pain, recovery time, and cost, while providing a favorable cosmetic result compared to a conventional sternotomy approach. Anesthesia for port access surgery is complex, so this chapter just covers the basics.

INDICATIONS

- Mitral valve surgery
- Aortic valve surgery
- Tricuspid valve surgery
- Atrial septic defect (ASD) repairs
- Atrial mass excision
- Ventricular mass excision

Contraindications

- Many of the serious complications are vascular in nature.
- Preoperative imaging with a CT angiogram of the chest with iliofemoral runoff is particularly useful to avoid any misadventures.

COMPLICATIONS[1]

- Atrioventricular (AV) block
- Bleeding from port sites
- Bleeding from lung adhesions
- Right phrenic nerve palsy
- Atelectasis
- Perforation of aortic wall
- Coronary sinus injury

BENEFITS

- Improved cosmesis
- Reduced operative complications
- Reduced pain
- Decreased blood transfusions[2]
- Lower infection rate when performed through a thoractomy
- Faster recovery
- Reduced hospital costs

SETUP

- Setup needs to be done in the room with strict sterile technique. It takes a little more time, so plan accordingly. Organization is key!
- You have a choice of using a steerable or nonsteerable coronary sinus catheter with an 11-French (F) introducer. This is used for the retrograde cardioplegia.
- The pulmonary vent uses a 9F introducer. This is used to vent blood from the left ventricle through the pulmonary circulation.
- Flush all ports with saline.
- Prepare the ultrasound and a sterile probe cover for scanning the internal jugular vein.
- Cover everything up until the patient arrives (Figure 43-1).

You will need to monitor the systemic blood pressure, coronary sinus pressure, and pulmonary pressures.

If you are using the EndoClamp, you will need two systemic blood pressures (right and left radial pressures) and a line for measuring the pressure at the tip of the endoclamp. This is a total of five pressures (Figure 43-2).

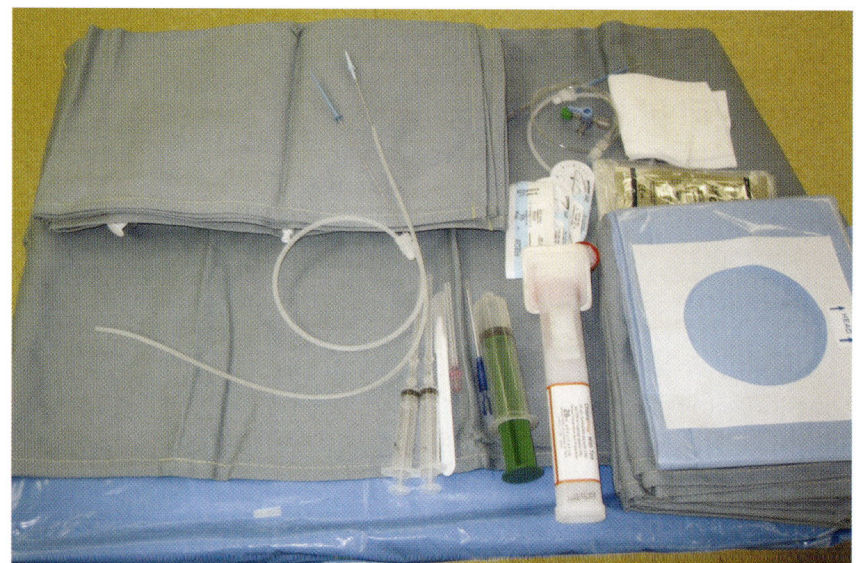

FIGURE 43-1 Table setup.

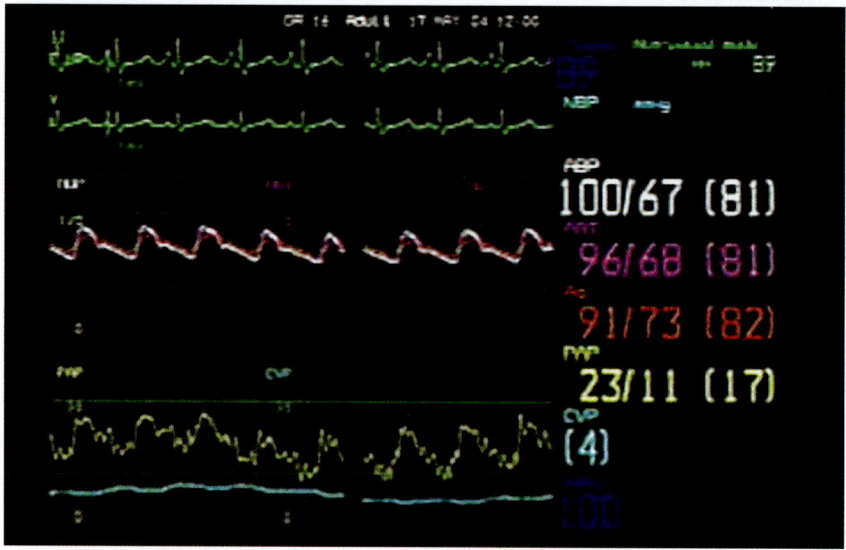

FIGURE 43-2 Monitor with five pressures.

LINES NEEDED FOR PORT ACCESS SURGERY

- Coronary sinus catheter
- Pulmonary vent catheter
- Femoral venous line
- Ascending aorta or femoral arterial cannula
- EndoClamp

PRELIMINARY LINES, INDUCTION, LUNG ISOLATION, AND ECHO

- Start with an arterial line and a good IV.
- Everything after the right internal jugular (RIJ) approach is exponentially more difficult. If one is not able to get access at the neck, the chance of getting the coronary sinus catheter in the right spot is slim.
- If the surgeon is using an endoclamp (it clamps the aorta from within the vessel), you will need a right and left radial arterial line. The right arterial line is the most important for monitoring occlusion of the innominate artery. If you cannot get a right-side pressure line, you will not be able to safely use the endoclamp.
- Don't forget to put on the defibrillator pads. They need to be out of the surgical site, and the current path needs to go through the heart.
- Right lung isolation makes the surgical approach easier; it is not absolutely necessary. A bronchial blocker usually suffices. If the patient is shorter than 5'3", a double-lumen tube might be a better choice, as it can be difficult to reliably isolate the right side with a blocker.
- During the line placement the anesthesiologist will be sterile, so additional personnel are required to monitor and care for the patient.
- A preliminary echo is done to verify the pathology. The surgeon should be present. If there has to be a modification to the surgery, a port-access procedure may not work. You do not want to spend the time placing all of these lines only to find out the valve is normal!
- Assess the coronary sinus anatomy while performing the echo and think about your approach.

INSERTING THE BIG ACCESS LINES

- The insertion of the neck lines and the deployment of the coronary sinus catheter can take some time. This is especially true if you are just learning how to do this. Tell the surgeon to do something for the next hour.
- The RIJ approach is the best for the placement of the coronary sinus catheter. This is the one that everyone fears. You do not want to mess up the RIJ, so you want to get in and get out as fast as possible. The use of the vessel ultrasound device allows you to easily hit the vessel and verify that the wire is intravenous (Figures 43-3 to 43-6).

The pulmonary vent is nothing more than a fancy pulmonary catheter that has been modified to suck blood out through it with a vacuum-assisted pump controlled by the perfusionist (Figure 43-7).

After you have inserted the introducers, give the patient 5000 U of heparin. This prevents clots from forming within the introducers; more importantly, it prevents clots from forming in the coronary sinus and vent catheter.

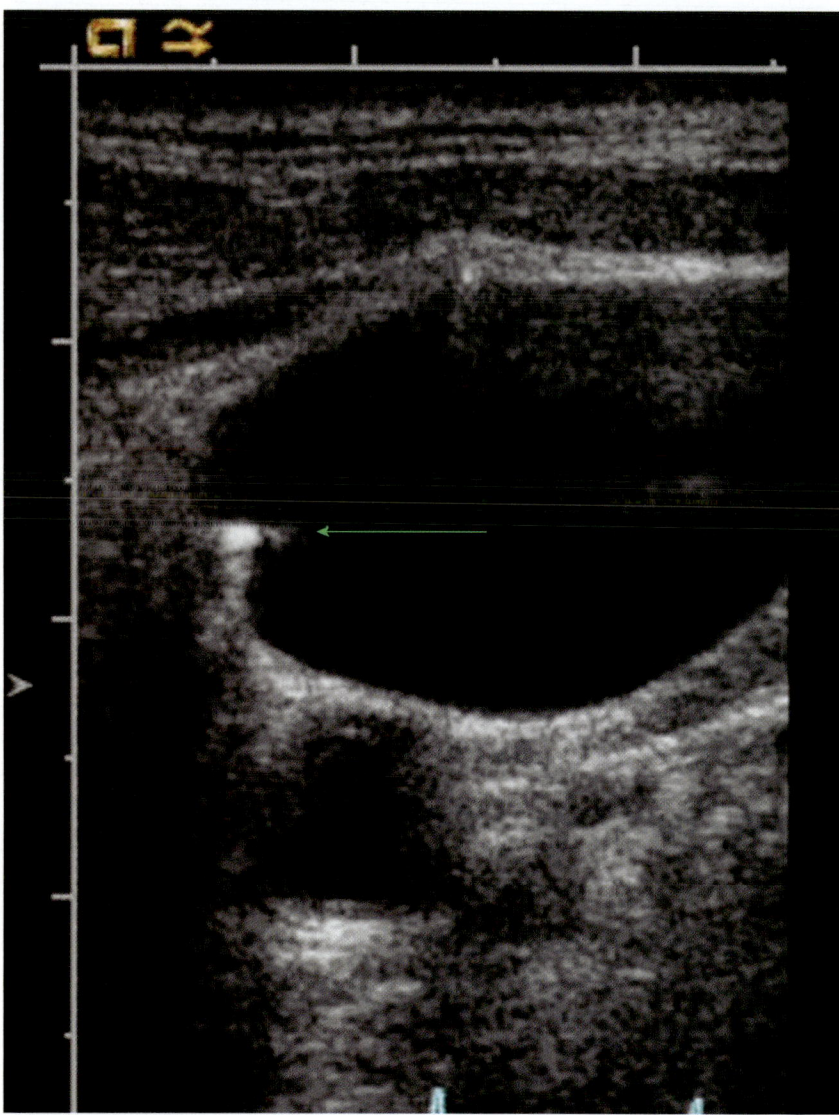

FIGURE 43-3 Wire seen within the internal jugular vein.

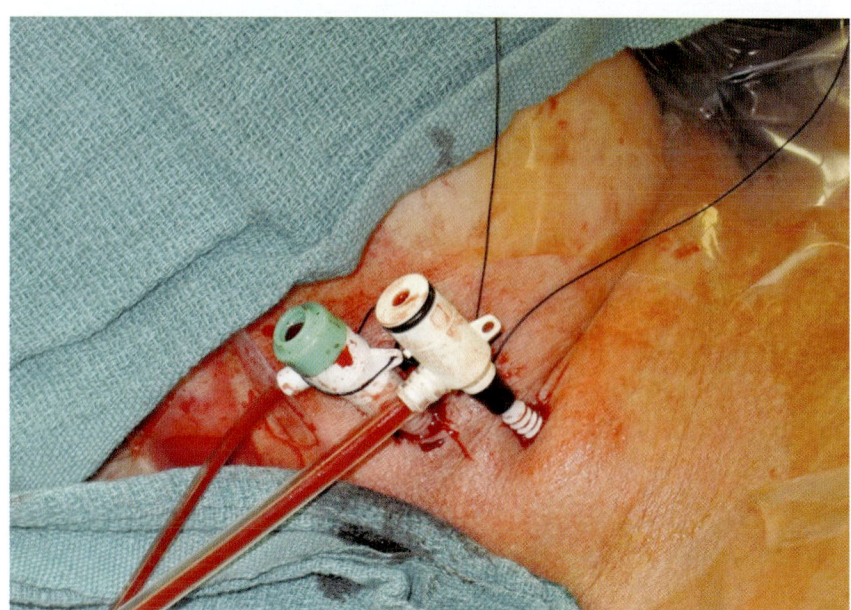

FIGURE 43-4 Green is the 11F coronary sinus introducer. The other is a 9F introducer for the pulmonary vent. Note the purse string around the 11F introducer.

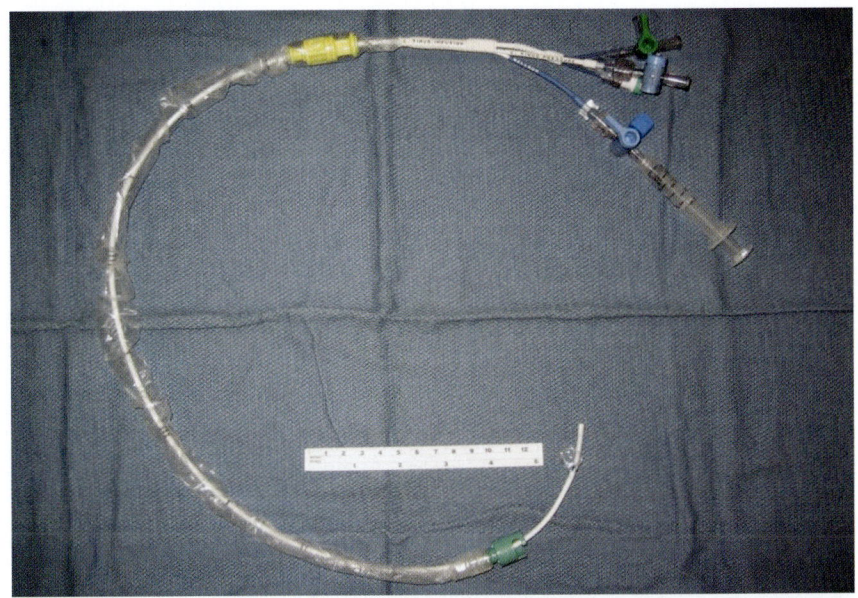

FIGURE 43-5 Coronary sinus catheter.

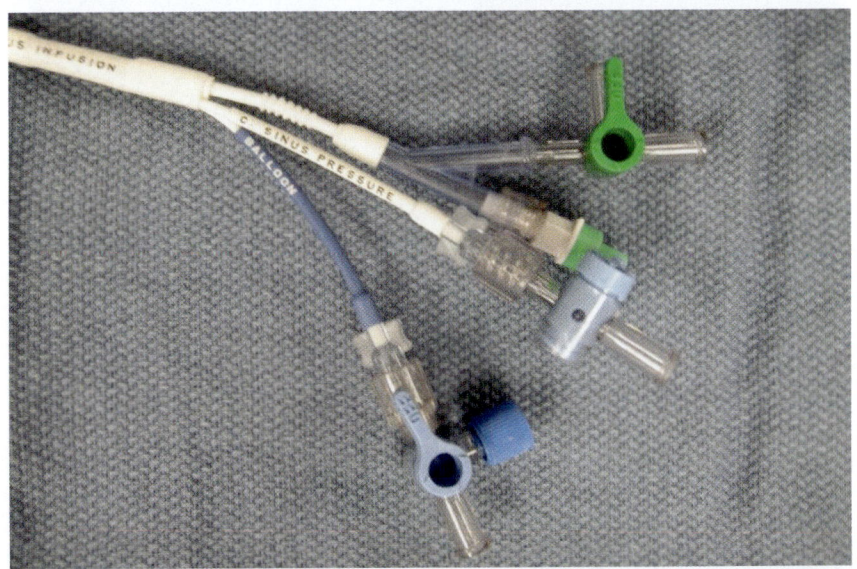

FIGURE 43-6 Coronary sinus catheter ports from top down: cardioplegia line, sinus pressure, and balloon.

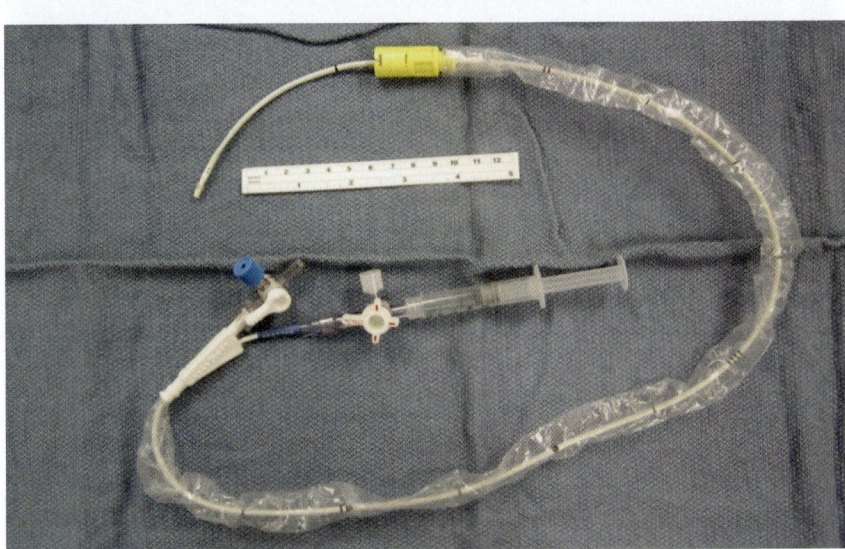

FIGURE 43-7 Pulmonary vent.

INSERTING THE CORONARY SINUS: DRUM ROLL

- A transesophageal echo (TEE) is absolutely necessary to place the coronary sinus (CS) catheter. Almost all of the time, fluoroscopy is unnecessary.[3]
- The short axis view is the easiest image to obtain, but the least helpful. Get good at seeing the CS in a modified bicaval view between 110 and 125 degrees (Figure 43-8).

If you can get a double-barrel view of the inferior vena cava and the coronary sinus, you should have a good shot at getting the catheter in place in no time at all (Figures 43-9 and 43-10).[4-6]

- Getting the coronary sinus catheter in place requires slow deliberate movements in concert with the TEE. When a ¼ to ½ cc of saline results in a ventricularized waveform, you have successfully positioned the catheter in the coronary sinus.

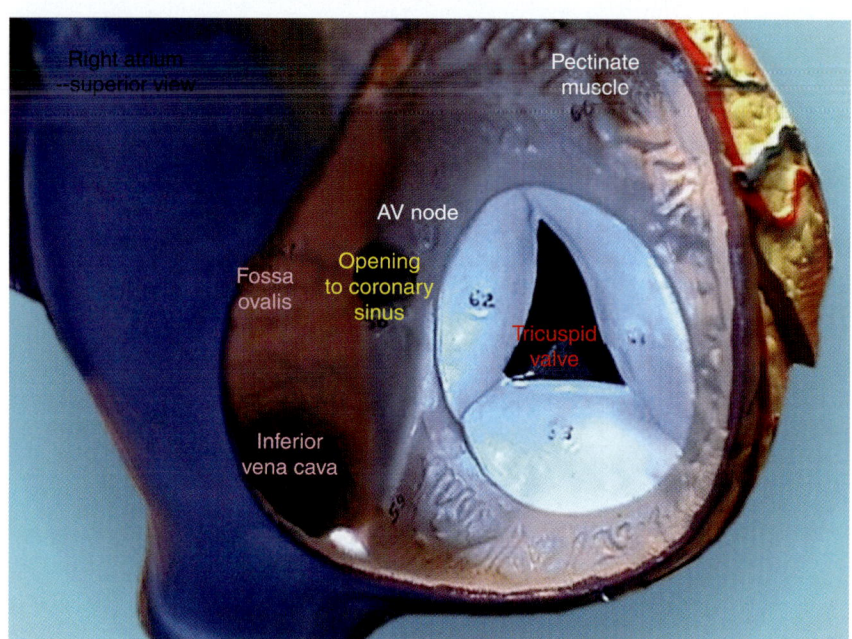

FIGURE 43-8 Relationship of coronary sinus to the tricuspid valve and inferior vena cava (IVC).

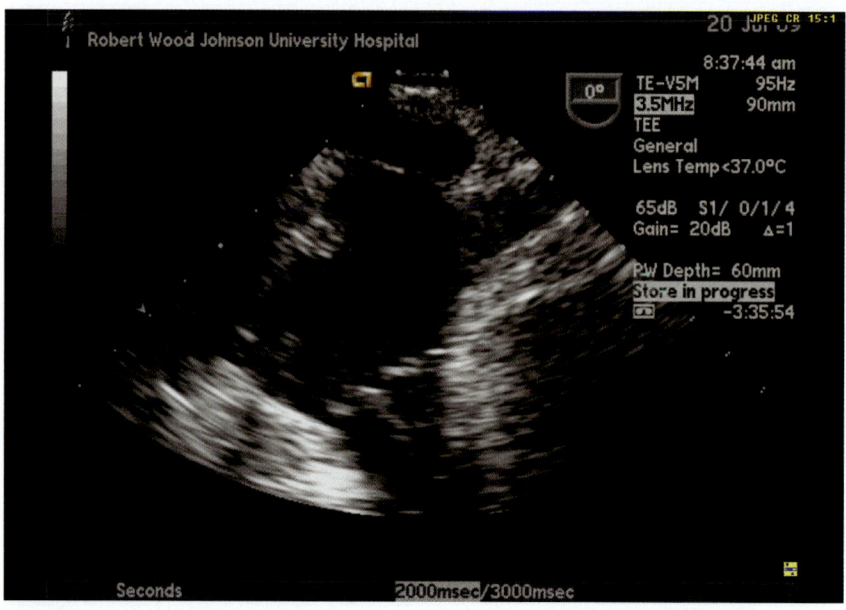

FIGURE 43-9 View of coronary sinus with a deep four-chamber view.

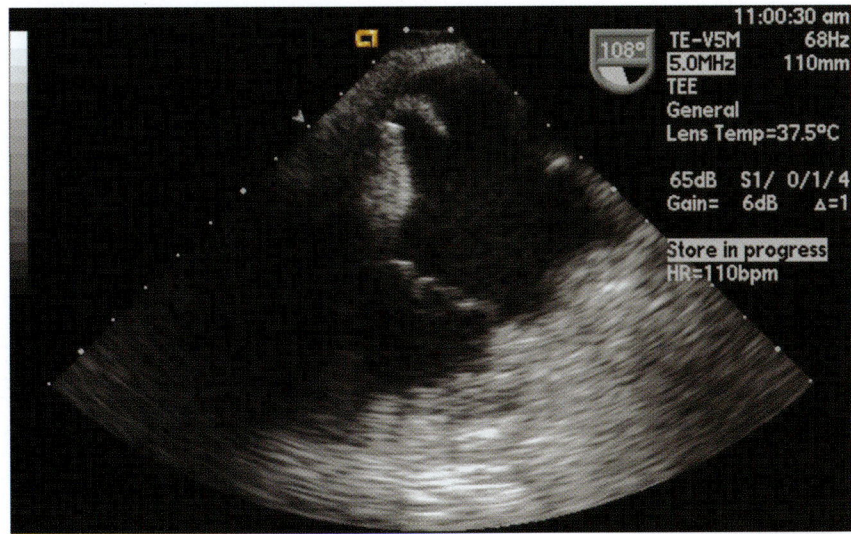

FIGURE 43-10 Double barrel formed by coronary sinus and IVC.

FLOATING THE PULMONARY VENT CATHETER

- The pulmonary vent is a glorified pulmonary catheter that actively drains blood from the left side of the heart through the pulmonary circulation.

- When you get a pulmonary tracing, use the TEE to verify that the catheter is just past the main pulmonary artery (Figures 43-11 to 43-14).

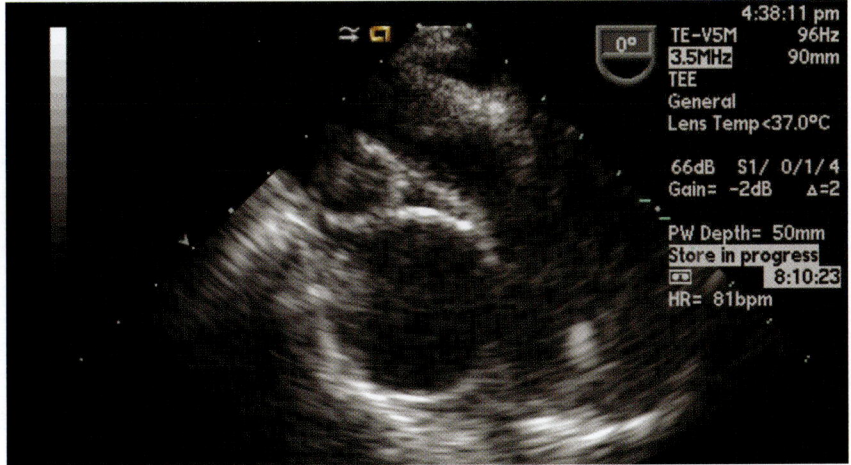

FIGURE 43-11 Pulmonary vent tip seen in the right pulmonary artery, just past the main pulmonary artery.

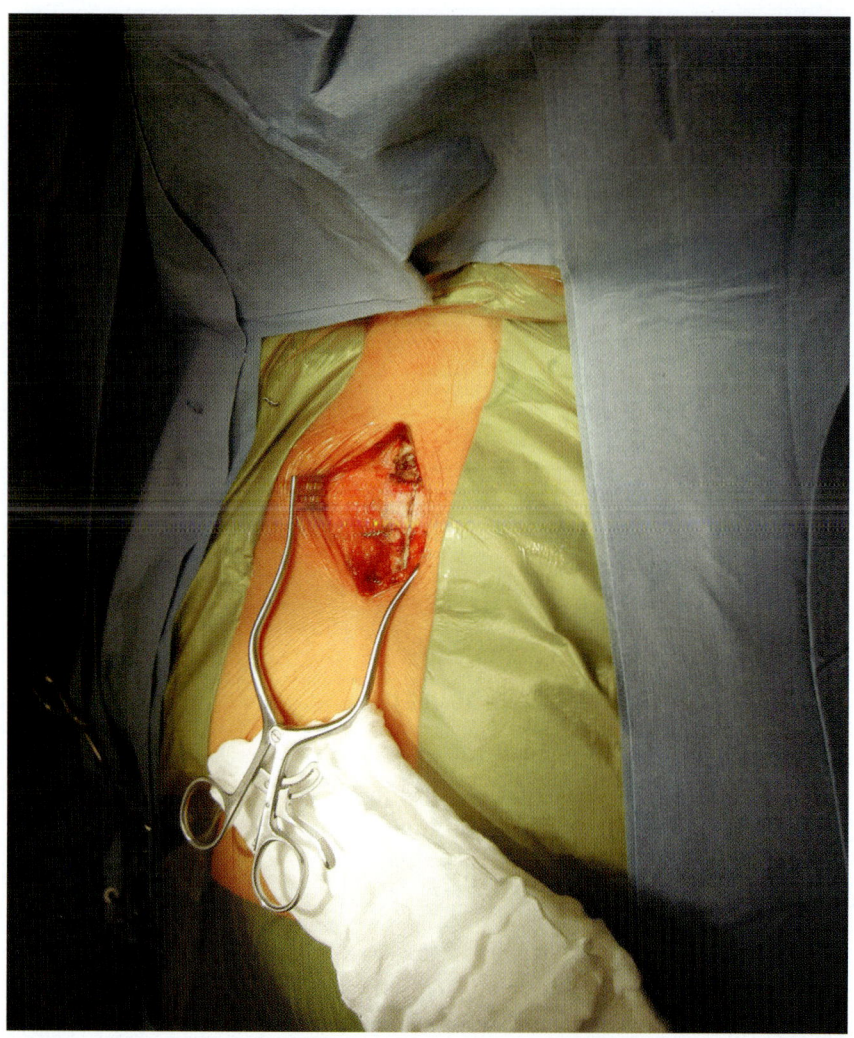

FIGURE 43-12 Mini-sternotomy on a redo; now that's a small incision.

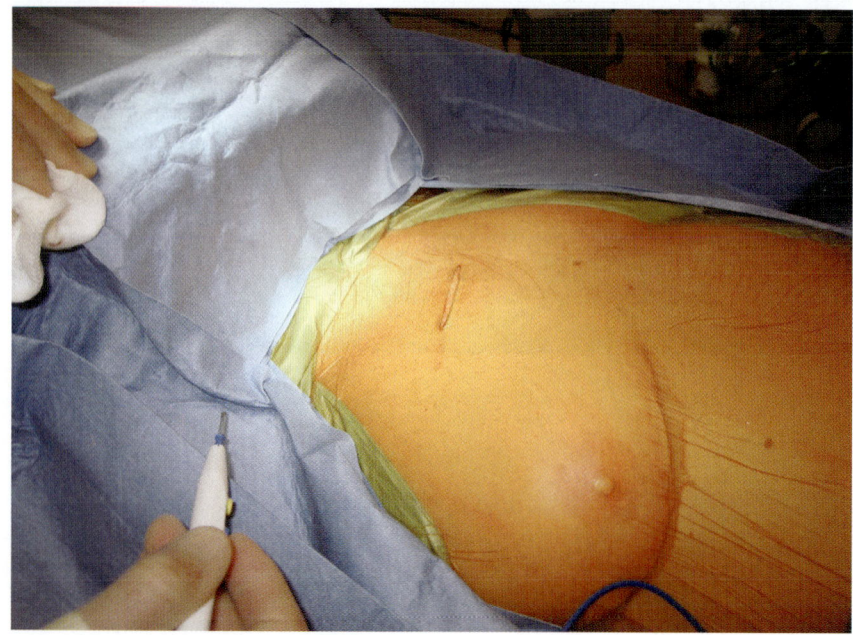

FIGURE 43-13 Mini-aortic valve through a thoracotomy approach; now that's a really small incision.

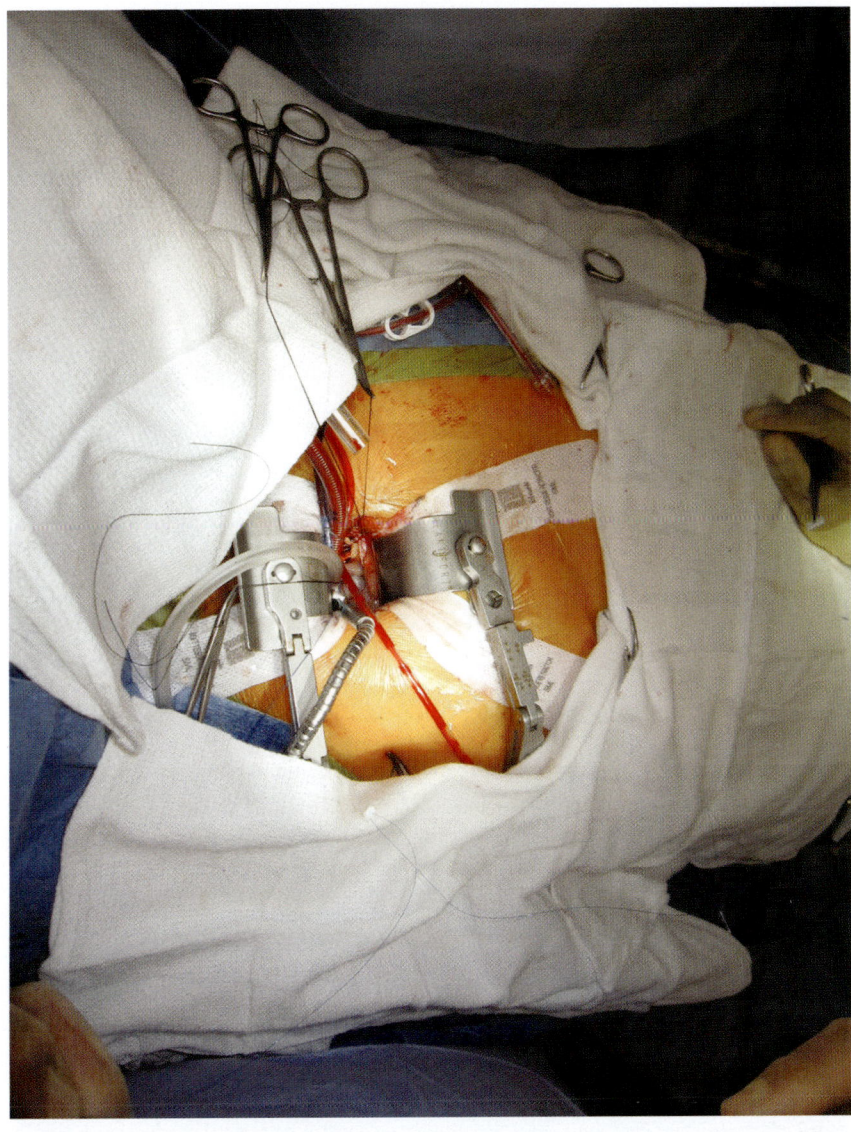

FIGURE 43-14 Mini-aortic valve using a thoracic approach with instruments in place: a tight fit.

SURGICAL LINES: VENOUS AND ARTERIAL ACCESS

- The surgeon dissects out the right femoral vein.
- If femoral venous access is not possible, consider a transthoracic approach.
- A wire is inserted into the femoral vein and threaded up into the right atrium. One uses the TEE to confirm the position.
- Make sure the wire does not go through a patent foramen ovale.
- The venous cannula is inserted through the femoral vessel and threaded into the right atrium. The tip will rest at the superior vena cava (SVC)-atrial junction (Figures 43-15 and 43-16).
- Arterial access is via either the femoral artery or aorta.
- If femoral arterial access is not possible, consider a transthoracic approach utilizing the ascending aorta or the axillary artery.
- Use the TEE at the midesophageal level to confirm that the wire is in the aorta if the surgeon is obtaining femoral access. This line is used to perfuse the body (Figure 43-17).
- If the EndoClamp is going to be used, the wire and catheter are inserted through the femoral artery. The position just above the aortic valve is confirmed with TEE (Figure 43-18).

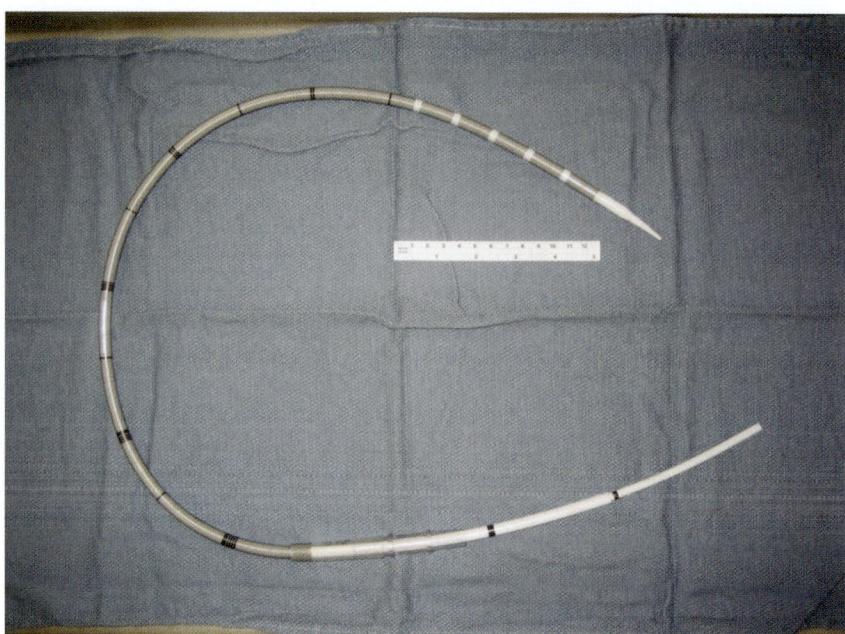

FIGURE 43-15 Edwards Quickdraw™ multi-orifice venous cannula.

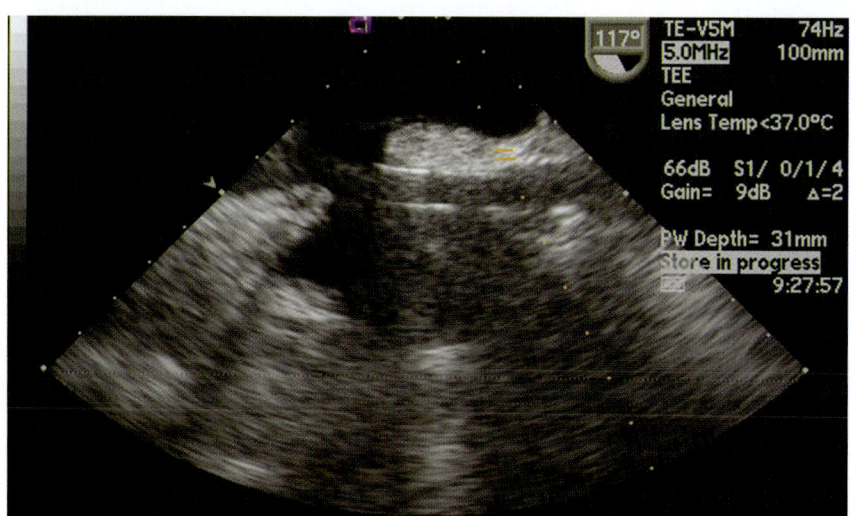

FIGURE 43-16 Tip seen on TEE at atrial-SVC junction.

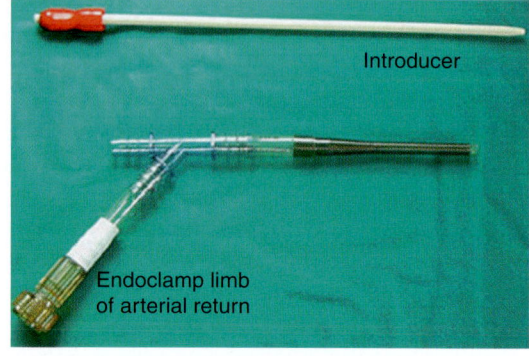

FIGURE 43-17 Arterial line.

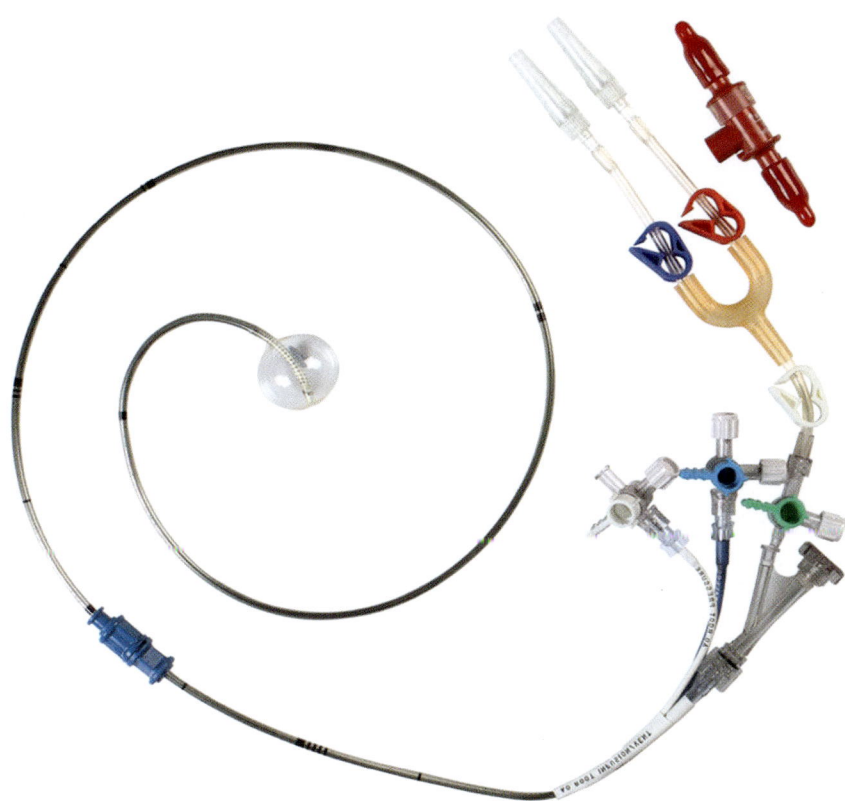

FIGURE 43-18 EndoClamp.

ENDOCLAMP

- The endoclamp allows one to stop the aortic blood flow by occluding the lumen with an endovascular balloon. It is used for mitral valve surgery.
- It is inserted through the femoral artery over a wire.
- It is positioned just distal to the aortic valve at the sinotubular junction by visualizing it on TEE while monitoring the right, left, and root pressures. The balloon will be filled after the initiation of cardiopulmonary bypass (CPB).

INITIATION OF CPB

- Like other pump cases, the perfusionist cools and empties the heart.
- Antegrade cardioplegia is given into the aortic root by the surgeon. The surgeon uses an external cross-clamp.
- Retrograde cardioplegia is given through the coronary sinus catheter.
- Blood is vented out of the left atrium and ventricle with the pulmonary vent catheter.
- If the surgeon is using the EndoClamp, antegrade cardioplegia is given through this line and no external cross-clamp is used.

SURGERY

- Watch for left ventricle (LV) distention when antegrade cardioplegia is given, since the surgeon cannot see the left ventricle.
- If the EndoClamp is used, make sure it does not migrate and block the innominate artery.
- The surgery itself is basically the same, except that it is now done through a very small hole instead of a large sternotomy.

REFERENCES

1. Mohr FW, Falk V, Diegeler A, et al. Minimally invasive port-access mitral valve surgery. *J Thorac Cardiovasc Surg.* 1998;115:567–571.
   This is a comprehensive article for those who want to know more about port-access surgery. It also includes a broader list of complications associated with the surgery.
2. Grossi EA, Galloway AC, Ribakove GH, et al. Impact of minimally invasive valve surgery: a case controlled study. *Ann Thorac Surg.* 2001;71:807–810.
   This gives a broader list of the benefits associated with the surgery.
3. Applebaum RM, Cutler WM, Bhardwaj N, et al. Utility of transesophageal echocardiography during port-access minimally invasive cardiac surgery. *Am J Cardiol.* 1998; 82(2):183–188.
   How to acquire the views necessary for port access surgery.

4. Miller GS. *Coronary Sinus Catheter Placement.* Irvine California: Edwards Life Sciences; 2009.
   A great book on coronary sinus catheter placement.
5. Coddens J, Deloof T, Thendrickx J, et al. Transesophageal echocardiography for port-access surgery. *J Cardiothorac Vasc Anesth.* 1999;113:614.
   Numerous TEE views for port access surgery.
6. Clements F, Wright SJ, Bruijn N. Coronary sinus catheterization made easy for port-access minimally invasive cardiac surgery. *J Cardiothorac Vasc Anesth.* 1998;12:96.
   Details on guiding the coronary sinus catheter for port access surgery.

PART VII

BRAINIACS

CHAPTER 44
ICP MONITORING

MARK R. ETTINGER
ADAM SCHIAVI

INTRODUCTION

Intracranial pressure (ICP) monitoring is not something that anesthesiologists are tasked with doing very often. Most patients who come to the operating room after closed head injury are undergoing a procedure in which their cranial cavity will be opened, thus obviating the need for ICP monitoring. And patients who do have an ICP monitor in place are often considered too unstable for the OR. However, there are instances in which patients are brought to the OR for procedures after closed head injury or subarachnoid hemorrhage during which it is important to monitor and treat any elevations in ICP. It is a task we must take very seriously, as the primary determinant of outcome in patients with closed head injury is control of ICP and maintenance of adequate cerebral perfusion pressure. And although this task is usually in the hands of the intensivist or neurosurgeon, in the operating room, you, as the anesthesiologist, are at the controls. So let's take a test flight into the ICP sky, so your next flight in the OR will be a smooth one.

INTRACRANIAL PRESSURE

Intracranial Contents and the Monro-Kellie Doctrine

- As the intracranial vault is essentially a closed box, its volume is fixed and constant. The Monro-Kellie doctrine, proposed in the early 19th century, describes the following relationship:
  - v.intracranial (constant) = v.brain + v.CSF + v.blood + v.mass lesion
- All of these compartments are fluids and, therefore, noncompressible. A rise in the volume of any one compartment will lead to a rise in ICP unless there is a corresponding decrease in the volume of one of the remaining compartments.
- In the normal brain, small changes in the volume of blood, brain, cerebrospinal fluid (CSF), or a mass lesion will lead to small changes in ICP. This occurs until a critical volume is reached, at which point very small changes in volume lead to a large increase in pressure (Figure 44-1).[1]

CSF AND ICP

- CSF surrounds the brain and spinal cord and is thought to function as a shock absorber in the central nervous system (CNS). It may also serve an immunologic function analogous to the lymphatic system. It circulates in the subarachnoid space, between the pial and arachnoid membranes of the meninges.
- CSF is normally clear and colorless with a pH of 7.33 to 35 and specific gravity of 1.007.
- Total CSF volume in an adult is approximately 150 mL.
- CSF production is about 450 mL/day, which means that CSF is turned over approximately three times every day.
- Normal ICP in an adult is 7 to 15 cm H_2O.[2]

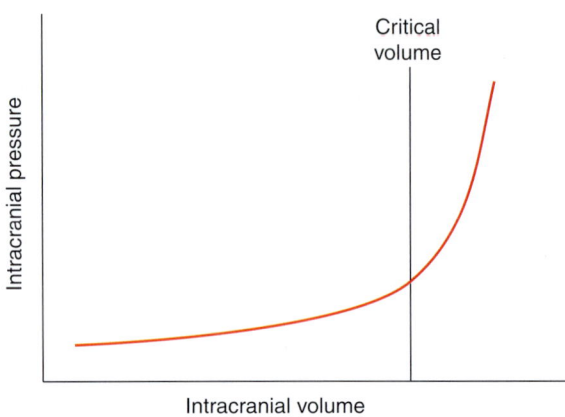

FIGURE 44-1 Intracranial pressure-volume curve.

CEREBRAL PERFUSION PRESSURE AND CEREBRAL AUTOREGULATION

- Secondary brain injury (i.e., injury that occurs after the initial trauma) is due in part to cerebral ischemia. This ischemia is usually due to decreased cerebral blood flow as a result of a decreased perfusion pressure. The critical parameter for brain function postinjury is actually not ICP but rather adequate cerebral blood flow (CBF) to meet metabolic demands.[2]
- CBF depends on cerebral perfusion pressure (CPP), which is related to ICP by the following relationship:
  - CPP = MAP − ICP (MAP = mean arterial pressure)
- The normal adult's CPP is >50 mmHg. *Cerebral autoregulation* is a mechanism by which large changes in systemic blood pressure produce only small changes in CBF. This allows the normal brain to maintain the necessary blood flow over a wide range of arterial pressures. In the normal brain, CPP has to drop below approximately 40 mmHg before CBF is impaired.[3]
- The primary goal of ICP control is to maintain adequate CPP.

INTRACRANIAL HYPERTENSION (IC-HTN)

- IC-HTN is defined as the persistent elevation of intracranial pressure above 20 mmHg for greater than 5 minutes in a patient who is not being stimulated.[4]
- IC-HTN may be due to any of the following conditions:[1]
  - Cerebral edema
  - Hyperemia: the normal response to head injury; thought to be due to vasomotor paralysis and loss of cerebral autoregulation
  - Traumatically induced masses:
    - Epidural hematoma
    - Subdural hematoma
    - Intraparenchymal hemorrhage
    - Depressed skull fracture
  - Hydrocephalus due to obstruction of CSF outflow or absorption
  - Hypoventilation
  - Systemic hypertension
  - Venous sinus thrombosis
  - Increased muscle tone and Valsalva maneuvers as a result of agitation or posturing
  - Status epilepticus
- Most centers have established criteria for treating ICP >20 mmHg[5]

CONSEQUENCES OF INCREASED ICP

Signs and Symptoms[1,2,6]

- The most common symptom of increased ICP is headache.
  - Generalized in nature, worse at night and when patient is recumbent
- Vomiting
  - Interestingly, the vomiting associated with increased ICP is usually not associated with nausea
- Blurred vision or diplopia
- Motor or sensory deficits
- Symptoms vary depending on chronicity of the increase in ICP
  - Chronic, progressive increases usually result in mild symptomatology, and frequently patients have no symptoms at all.
  - Acute rises in ICP often manifest as delirium or patients become obtunded, and there are often signs of brainstem compression.
- Physical exam findings[1,6]
  - Papilledema
  - Lumbar puncture (LP): opening pressure is elevated. Measured by hooking a manometer to the LP needle and documenting the pressure reading at the fluid column's highest point.
    - It is absolutely essential that one perform a fundoscopic exam prior to performing a lumbar puncture in a patient with suspected intracranial hypertension. If there is papilledema, a CT scan must first be obtained to verify that there are no signs of a noncommunicating hydrocephalus. Performing an LP in patients with noncommunicating hydrocephalus may lead to rapid herniation and death.[1,6]
  - Cranial nerve deficits: CN III, VI, and VII
  - Cushing's triad
    - Hypertension, bradycardia, and respiratory irregularity

- Observed in the advanced stages of intracranial hypertension and usually signals impending herniation

Herniation Syndromes[6]

- Brain is supported by dural folds that prevent undue movement within the cranial cavity.
  - Falx cerebri: sickle-shaped dural fold that separates the two cerebral hemispheres
  - Tentorium cerebelli: tent-shaped dural fold that separates the occipital lobes from the posterior fossa structures
- There are four major types of herniation (Figure 44-2)
  - Cingulate herniation
    - Mass lesions in the supratentorial space cause a pressure gradient driving ipsilateral brain tissue (cingulate gyrus) to herniate under the falx cerebri
    - Usually displacement of the lateral ventricles as well
    - No clinical signs and symptoms specific to this syndrome
  - Uncal herniation
    - Most severe and most common herniation syndrome
    - Usually seen with lesions of the middle cranial fossa
      - ▲ Epidural hematoma
      - ▲ Subdural hematoma
      - ▲ Temporal lobe contusions and neoplasms
    - Mass in the middle fossa causes the uncus, the most inferomedial structure of the temporal lobe, to herniate between the brainstem and tentorial edge into the posterior fossa.
    - Medial displacement of the brainstem may cause compression of the brainstem against the tentorial edge. This produces a notch known as *Kernohan's notch*.
    - Clinical syndrome
      - ▲ Progressively impaired consciousness
      - ▲ Dilated ipsilateral pupil
      - ▲ Contralateral hemiplegia
  - Central transtentorial herniation
    - Occurs with mass lesions far from the tentorium (unlike uncal herniation, which occurs from mass lesions proximate to the tentorium)
    - Downward displacement of the diencephalon and midbrain through the tentorial opening
    - Clinical syndrome
      - ▲ Bilateral pinpoint pupils
      - ▲ Cheyne-Stokes respirations
      - ▲ Obtunded
      - ▲ Loss of vertical gaze
  - Tonsillar herniation
    - Generally results from acute expansion of posterior fossa lesions
    - May result from an ill-advised lumbar puncture in patients with a supratentorial mass and noncommunicating hydrocephalus
    - Tonsil of the cerebellum herniates through the foramen magnum, compressing the medulla
    - Clinical syndrome
      - ▲ Cardiorespiratory impairment
      - ▲ Hypertension
      - ▲ Cheyne-Stokes respirations
      - ▲ Impaired consciousness
      - ▲ Decerebrate or decorticate posture possible

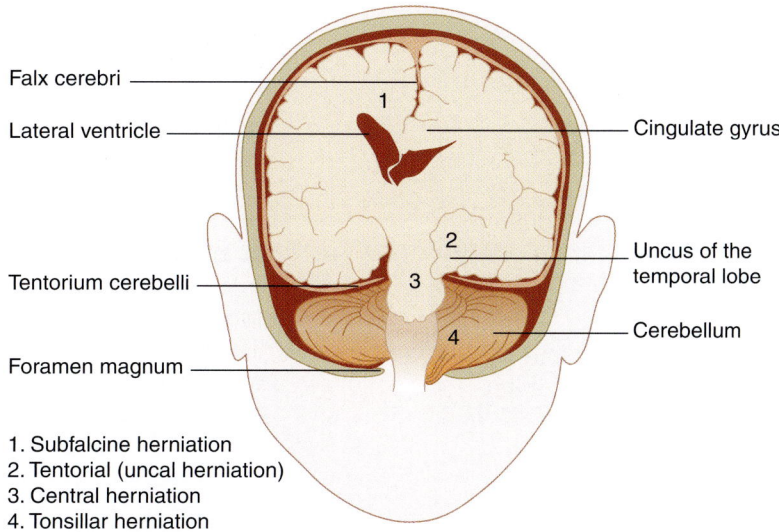

1. Subfalcine herniation
2. Tentorial (uncal herniation)
3. Central herniation
4. Tonsillar herniation

FIGURE 44-2 Herniation syndromes. (Drawn by Kelly Brenan Rothschild.)

INTRACRANIAL PRESSURE MONITORING

Indications for ICP Monitoring

- Increased ICP is the most significant factor determining morbidity and mortality in patients with neurosurgical disorders.[5,7]
- There are no clinical indicators in the early phases of rising ICP to help forestall a further rise. The clinical indicators usually occur in the end stages and are therefore of little use to help prevent the consequences of increased pressure.
- The two most common clinical conditions in which ICP monitoring is indicated are closed head injury and subarachnoid hemorrhage.[1]
- In closed head injury, ICP monitoring is of particular relevance because outcomes have been shown to directly correlate with cerebral perfusion pressure, of which ICP is a key component (Table 44-1).[2]
- Neurologic criteria for ICP monitoring: severe head injury (Glasgow Coma Scale (GCS) score <9 after CPR) and either:[1,5]
  - A: An abnormal admitting head CT, or
  - B: A normal CT, but with two or more risk factors

TABLE 44-1 Indications for ICP Monitoring

Indications for ICP Monitoring	Risk of Raised ICP
Severe head injury (GCS 3-8)	
• Abnormal CT scan	50-60%
• Normal CT, age >40 or mean arterial BP <90	50-60%
• Normal CT scan, no risk factors	15%
Moderate head injury (GCS 9-12)	
• If anesthetized/sedated • Abnormal CT scan	Approx 10-20% will deteriorate to severe head injury
Mild head injury (GCS 13-15)	
• Few indications for ICP monitoring	Only around 3% will deteriorate

- Risk factors include age >40, SBP <90, and decerebrate or decorticate posturing on motor exam.
- In patients with a GCS <9, even patients with a normal CT and no risk factors will still have a 15% incidence of elevated ICP, so many centers will monitor ICP in all patients with a GCS <9.[4]
- Contraindications to ICP monitoring include an "awake" patient (neurologic exam can be used for monitoring) and coagulopathy.

Types of ICP Monitors (Table 44-2)[1,8]

- Intraventricular catheter (Figures 44-3 to 44-5)
  - An open-ended conduit is placed directly into the lateral ventricle.
  - "Gold standard" for ICP monitoring
  - Allows for continuous ICP monitoring and periodic drainage of CSF to treat IC-HTN. Also allows for CSF sampling to assess for signs of meningitis or ventriculitis
  - Medications can be administered through a ventricular catheter, such as thrombolytic agents in the case of intraventricular hemorrhages or antibiotics in the case of ventriculitis.
  - Disadvantages include an increased risk of infection, difficult to place at times, and risks of hemorrhage and damage to brain tissue during placement.
  - Transducer must be readjusted each time the patient's head is moved
  - Placement[1]
    - An area of scalp typically 11 to 12 cm posterior to the glabella and 2 to 3 cm lateral of midline is prepped. The right side is usally chosen because it is less likely to be the dominant side in the patient and usually easier for a right-handed operator.
    - An incision is made in the scalp that penetrates through to the cranium.
    - A handheld drill is used to pentrate the cranial cavity down to the level of the dura.
    - A small incision is made into the dura, and the catheter is passed approximately 6 to 7 cm at an angle ideal for depositing the catheter into the lateral ventricle near the foramen of Monro.
    - The scalp is then sewed around the catheter and the catheter is hooked to a pressure transducer and manometer.

TABLE 44-2 Types of ICP Monitors

Device	Advantages	Pitfalls
Intraventricular catheter	Gold standard of accuracy Allows drainage and sampling Allows ICP control Inexpensive	Most invasive Can be difficult to place Catheter can be occluded by tissue Needs repositioning with head position change Potential for infection
Subarachnoid bolt/screw	Quickly and easily placed Does not invade brain tissue Allows sampling of CSF Lower infection rate	Blocked by swelling brain Catheter can be occluded by tissue Must be balanced and recalibrated frequently
Subdural/epidural catheter/sensor	Least invasive Easily and quickly placed	No CSF sampling or drainage
Fiberoptic probe	Can be placed in the subdural, subarachnoid, intraventricular, or intraparenchymal spaces Easily transported Minimal artifact and drift Low risk of infection No need to adjust for patient position	Cannot be recalibrated after placed High cost Easier to break/damage

- The catheter is hooked to a three-way stopcock that will allow for two essential functions of the intraventricular catheter:
  - When the stopcock is open to the transducer, it will read and display the intracranial pressure transduced at the catheter tip.
  - When the stopcock is open to the manometer, it will allow continuous drainage of CSF at a pressure determined by the level of the manometer.
- Subarachnoid bolt
  - Hollow screw that goes into the skull abutting the dura. The dura is penetrated, allowing CSF to fill the bolt and equalize with the pressure in the subarachnoid space.
  - Lower risk of infection than an IVC, prone to errors that include ICP underestimation, misplacement of the screw, and occlusion by debris
- Intraparenchymal wire
  - Wire that contains a microtransducer at the tip of a flexible wire
  - Placement is very easy. An incision is made into the scalp and then a 4-mm hollow screw is inserted into the skull. The wire is then passed through the screw into the brain parenchyma.
  - Device does not allow for CSF sampling or drainage
  - More accurate than a subarachnoid bolt
  - One additional advantage over an IVC is that it does not need to be recalibrated after placement, regardless of patient positioning
  - While their measurements are typically accurate, after a few days values begin to drift and eventually become grossly inaccurate.
- Complications of ICP monitors include infection, hemorrhage, and malfunction (Table 44-3).

TABLE 44-3 Complications of ICP Monitors

Monitor Type	Bacterial Colonization	Hemorrhage	Malfunction or Obstruction
IVC	10–17%	1.1%	6.3%
Subarachnoid bolt	5%	0	16%
Intraparenchymal	14%	2.8%	9–40%

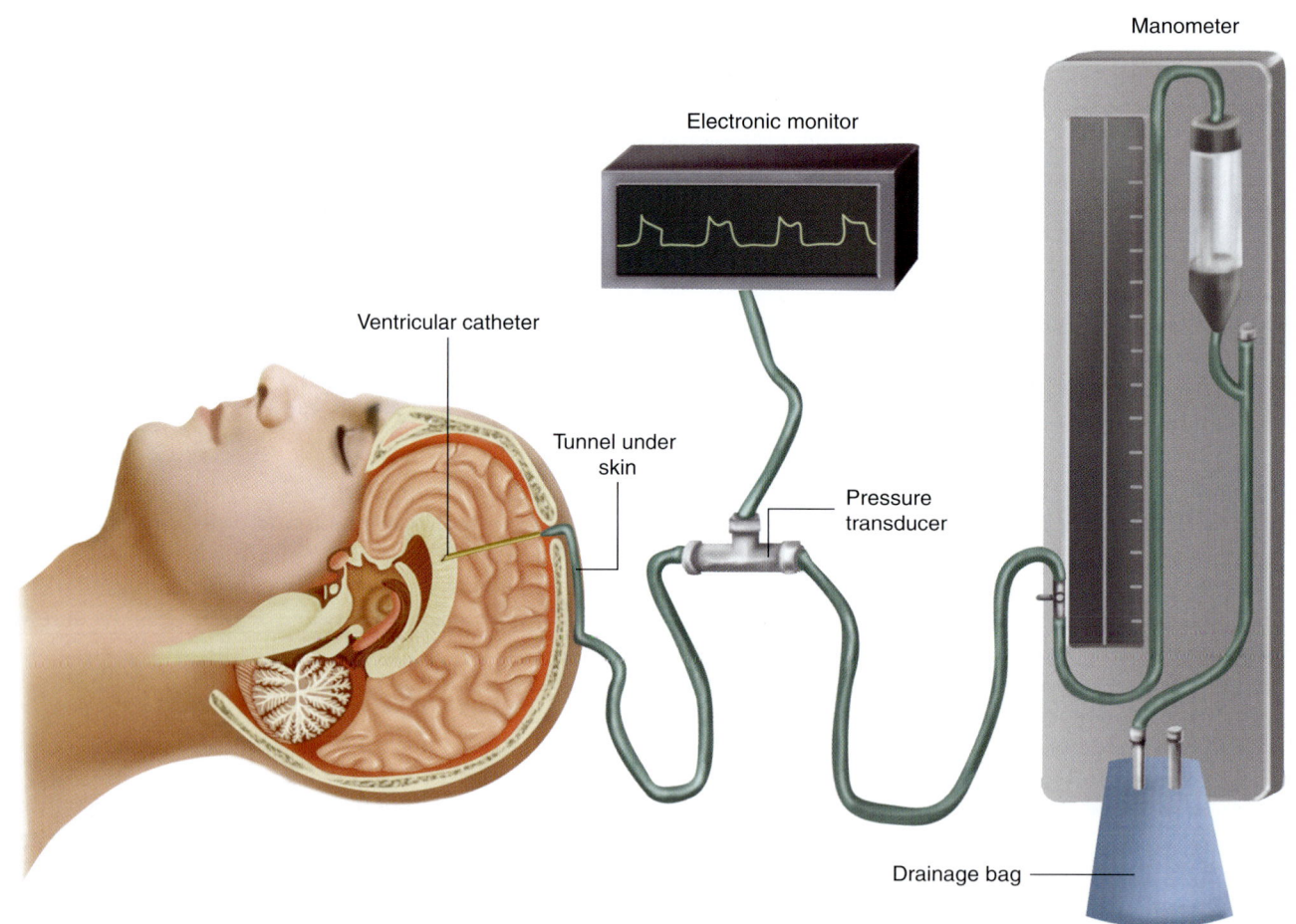

FIGURE 44-3 Key elements of an intraventricular catheter setup. (Drawn by Kelly Brenan Rothschild.)

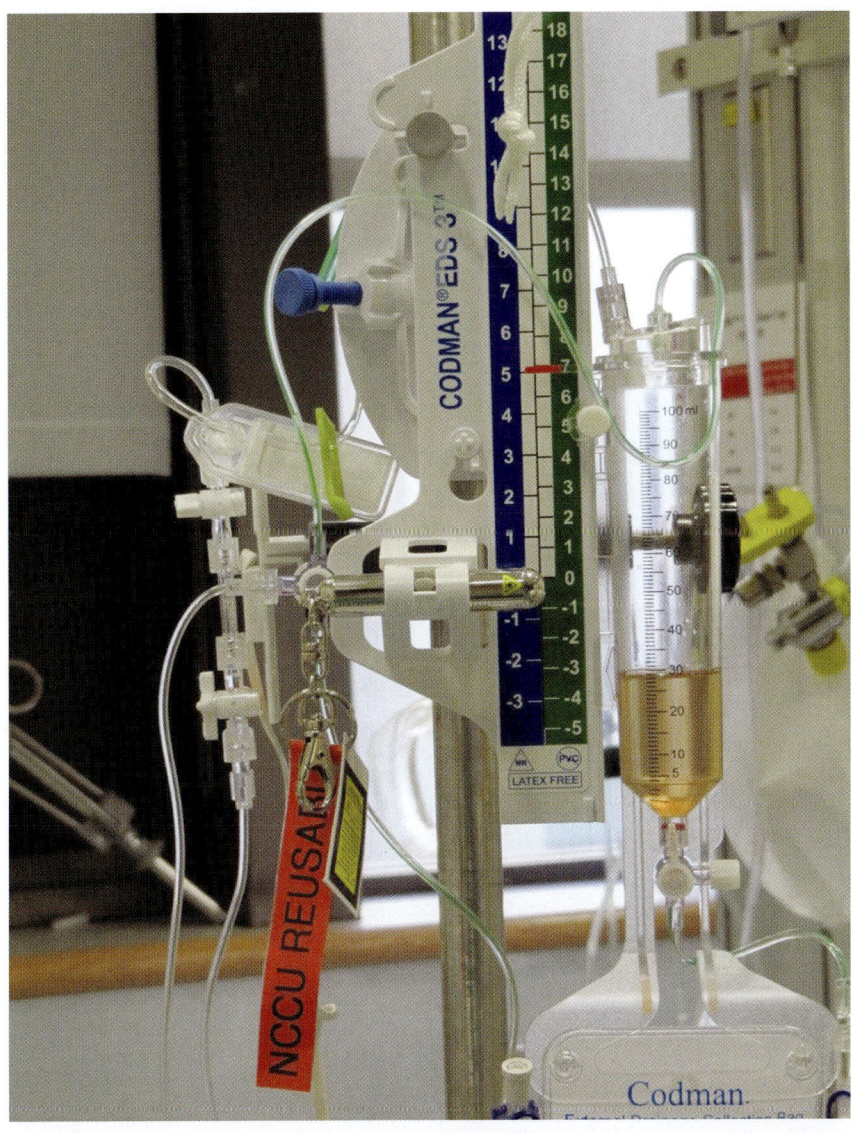

FIGURE 44-4 Codman™ external drainage device.

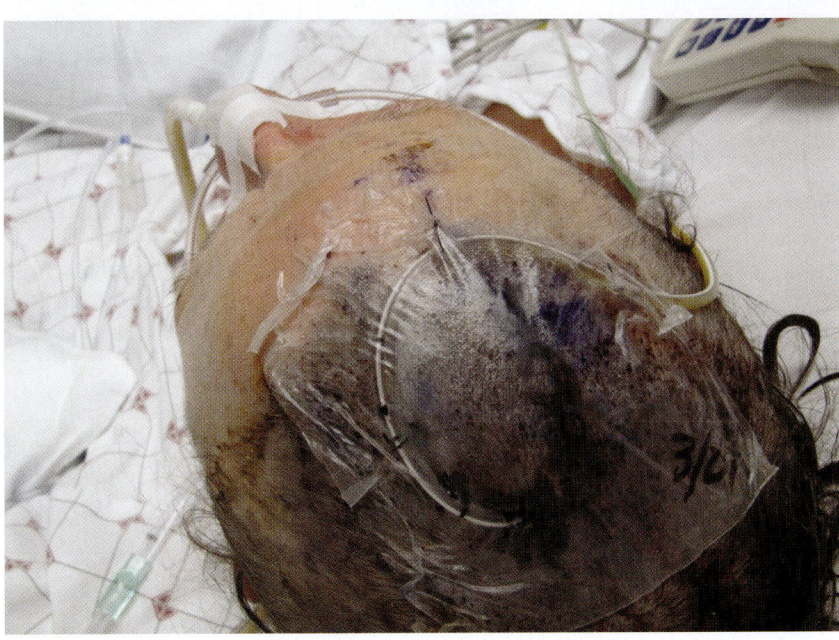

FIGURE 44-5 Patient with a left frontal ventricular catheter.

The Normal ICP Waveform (Figures 44-6 and 44-7)

- The normal ICP waveform, the waveform that occurs with normal blood pressure and the absence of intracranial hypertension, is rarely seen, since ICP is usually only monitored when it is elevated.[9]
- The normal ICP waveform includes two main peaks:[1]
  - A large 1- to 2-mmHg peak corresponding to the *arterial systolic pressure* wave, with a dicrotic notch
  - Followed by a smaller peak corresponding to the central venous "A" wave from contraction of the right atrium

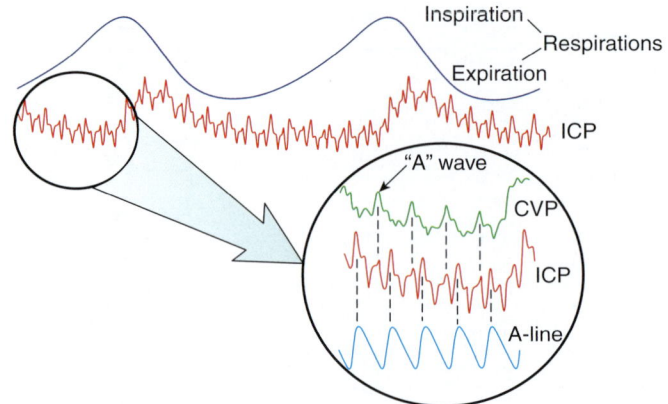

FIGURE 44-6 ICP waveform showing its characteristic two peaks corresponding with arterial pressure and the CVP "A" wave.

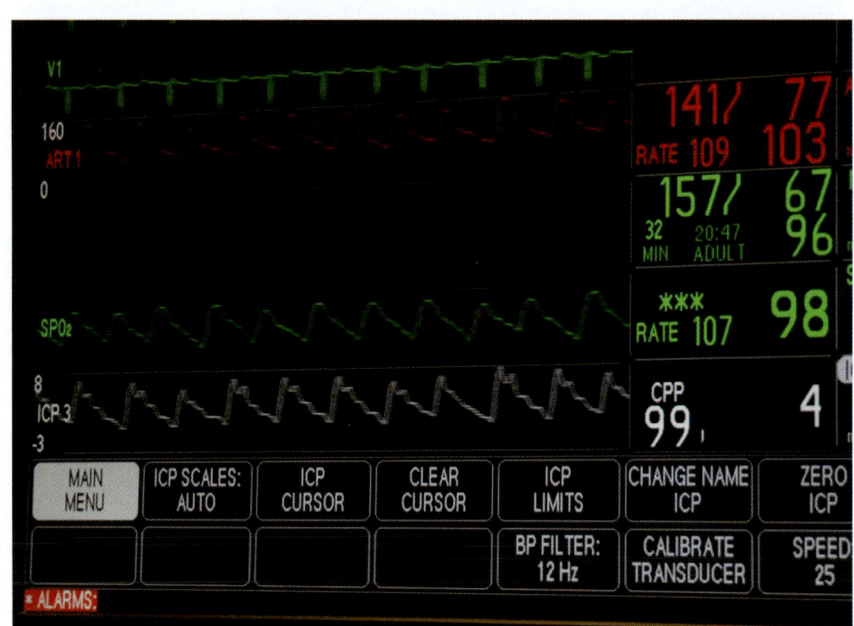

FIGURE 44-7 ICP waveform in a patient with an intraventricular catheter after subarachnoid hemorrhage. CPP is calculated by subtracting ICP from MAP.

Common IVC (Intraventricular Catheter) Pitfalls[1,8]

The following are common pitfalls that occur with external ventricular drainage devices. Some of them also apply to ICP monitoring in general:

- Air filter on drip chamber gets wet
  - Fluid cannot drain freely into drip chamber (the pressure is no longer regulated by the height of the manometer)
  - Solution: change air filter on drip chamber
- Improper connections
  - A pressurized irrigation bag with or without heparinized saline should *never* be connected to an ICP monitor.
- Changing position of head of bed
  - You must adjust the level of the drip chamber. This is often accomplished by having a laser pointer attached to the stopcock and adjusting the chamber until the laser is level with the external auditory meatus.
- Improper pressure reading
  - It is important to remember that when the IVC is open to drain, the pressure reading will not be accurate. The pressure cannot exceed the height of the drip chamber. To get an accurate reading, you must close the stopcock to drainage and ensure that it is open to the transducer.

- Drip chamber falls to floor
  - This will cause CSF to be drained to a negative pressure vacuum. This can lead to severe overdrainage, which may result in seizures and subdural hematoma formation.
  - The chamber should be secured to a pole or the bed rail and its position checked regularly.

Troubleshooting IVCs[1]

- IVC no longer works
  - Manifestation
    - Dampening or loss of waveform
    - No fluid drains into drip chamber
  - Possible causes
    - Occlusion of catheter proximal to transducer
    - IVC pulled out of ventricle
  - Test
    - Temporarily lower drip nozzle and watch for two or three drops of CSF
  - Solution
    - Verify all clamps are open
    - Flush no more than 1.5 mL of nonbacteriostatic saline (preservative-free) with very gentle pressure into ventricular catheter
    - This should be done under sterile conditions and usually by someone experienced at the technique (neurosurgeon or neurosurgical resident).
  - If it is known that the ventricles are collapsed, then the IVC may still be OK and it may take additional time for drainage to occur.
- IVC waveform dampened
  - Manifestation
    - Loss of normal distinct peaks on waveform and change from previously observed waveform
- Possible causes
  - Occlusion of catheter proximal to transducer
  - IVC pulled out of ventricle: no fluid will drain
  - Air in system
    - Allow CSF to drain until air is expelled.
    - Do not inject fluid into system to flush air into brain.
  - Postcraniectomy
    - Due to fact that monitor is no longer in a closed space, this finding is normal.

TREATMENT OF INTRACRANIAL HYPERTENSION

- The treatment of intracranial hypertension is a very complex topic about which entire books have been written. A full discussion of treatment is beyond the scope of this chapter. What is important to know as a consultant in anesthesiology is how we can control ICP in the operating room.
- The goal of therapy is to keep ICP <20 mmHg and CPP >70 mmHg.

Routine Measures for ICP Control (Table 44-4)[1,4]

- **Respiratory**
  - Avoid hypoxia and keep PaO_2 >60 mmHg and SaO_2 >90%.
  - Keep $PaCO_2$ at low end of normal (35 mmHg). While hyperventilation is good for lowering severe acute rises in ICP, it should be avoided if possible, as a low $PaCO_2$ may compromise cerebral blood flow.
- **Cardiovascular**
  - Avoid hypotension.
  - Goal is *euvolemia*. Running patients "dry" is an outdated principle and will only make the control of hypotension difficult and compromise CPP.
  - Control hypertension (keep systolic BP <160).
- **Positioning**
  - Elevate head of bed to 30 to 45 degrees.
  - Keep patient's head straight to avoid kinking of neck veins.
  - If patient has a tracheostomy, ensure that the tape is not too tight around the neck.
- **Fluid therapy**
  - Maintenance of euvolemia is important for hemodynamic stability.
  - Central venous pressure (CVP) 8 to 12 mmHg or pulmonary capillary wedge pressure 10 to 15 mmHg
  - Fluid of choice is normal saline. Avoid hypotonic solutions such as lactated Ringer's. Avoid colloids, as their use has shown a decrease in survival after closed head injury.
  - For the treatment of hypotension, pressors are preferred over fluid boluses.
  - Osmotic agents
    - *Hypertonic saline* (3% NaCl at 0.1 to 1.0 mL/kg/h) is a good choice of fluid for treating persistent elevations in ICP. There are no specific goals for its titration, but sodium levels should be kept below 160 to 165. Similar efficacy with mannitol.
    - *Mannitol* (0.5 to 2.0 g/kg) is given in the acute setting to lower ICP. Its effect is almost immediate and lasts up to 6 hours.
    - In the operating room, the neurosurgeon will usually direct the anesthesiologist in terms of the desired therapy.
    - Osmotic therapy must be tapered after 24 hours of continuous use. The cerebral homeostatic mechanism resets to a higher osmolarity and continued use may lead to rebound intracranial hypertension.

TABLE 44-4 Summary of Measures to Control IC-HTN

Step	Rationale
General measures (should be utilized routinely)	
Elevate head of bed to 30–45 degrees	Reduces ICP by enhancing venous outflow, but also reduces mean carotid pressure (no net change in CBF)
Keep neck straight, avoid tight trach tape	Constriction of jugular venous outflow increases ICP
Avoid hypotension (SBP <90)	• Normalize intravascular volume • Use pressors if needed
Control hypertension	• Nitroprusside if not tachycardic • Beta-blocker if tachycardic • Avoid overtreatment
Avoid hypoxia (pO_2 <60 mmHg)	Hypoxia may cause further ischemic brain injury
Ventilate to normocarbia (pCO_2 = 35–40 mmHg)	Avoid prophylactic hyperventilation
Sedation	Narcotics, propofol, benzodiazepines to prevent agitation
Specific measures for IC-HTN (use these steps in successive order if there is persistently increased ICP)	
Heavy sedation (propofol, narcotics, etc.) and/or paralysis (vecuronium)	Reduces sympathetic tone and movement, both of which raise ICP
Drain 3–5 mL CSF if IVC is present	Reduces intracranial volume
• Mannitol 0.5–1 g/kg • Hypertonic saline "bullet" 23.4% 10–20 mL • Hypertonic saline infusion (3%) at 0.1-mL/kg/h	Some patients refractory to mannitol will respond to hypertonic saline
Hyperventilate to PCO_2 30–35 mmHg	Reduced pCO_2 → reduced CBF → reduced ICP

- Endocrine
  - *Glucose control* is essential to management of the acutely injured brain. Hyperglycemia has been correlated with poor outcomes after head trauma.
  - Insulin therapy to keep blood glucose levels between 80 and 140 mg/dL.
  - The routine use of glucocorticoids is not recommended for the treatment of patients with head injury or elevated ICP. However, if ICP elevations are due to mass effect from a tumor, then high-dose steroids play an important role in their control.

Measures for Documented Intracranial Hypertension[1,7,10]

- Heavy sedation and paralysis
  - Agitation, movement, coughing, and fighting the ventilator are all measures that will raise ICP.
  - Keep the patient heavily sedated with the use of sedatives (propofol is preferred) and narcotics.
  - If the patient continues to have elevated ICP after these measures, then you should administer muscle relaxant to paralyze the patient.
- CSF drainage
  - Can only be done when an IVC is in place
  - Open the IVC to drainage and set the manometer to <10 cm above the auditory meatus.
- Osmotic therapy
  - Mannitol: 0.5 to 1 mg/kg bolus over <20 minutes. May give every 6 hours and may alternate with furosemide 10 to 20 mg.
  - Keep patient euvolemic to slightly hypervolemic.
  - If patient is refractory to mannitol, use hypertonic saline: 3% NaCl at 0.1 to 1 mL/kg/h.
  - Hold osmotic therapy if serum osmolarity >320 mOsm/L.

- Hyperventilation
  - Do not use hyperventilation prophylactically.
  - Avoid aggressive hyperventilation (pCO_2 <25 mmHg).
  - Use only for short periods of time.

REFERENCES

1. Greenberg M. *Handbook of Neurosurgery.* 7th ed. Germany: Thieme Stuttgart; 2006.
2. Lang EW, Chestnut RM. Intracranial pressure and cerebral perfusion pressure in severe head injury. *New Horizons.* 1995;3:400-409.
3. Latorre JG, Greer DM. Management of acute intracranial hypertension: a review. *The Neurologist.* 2009;15(4):193-207.
4. Miller JD, Dearden NM, Piper IR, Chan KH. Control of intracranial pressure in patients with severe head injury. *J Neurotrauma.* 1992;1:317-326.
5. Guidelines for the management of severe traumatic brain injury. 3rd ed. Accessed at www.braintrauma.org/pdf/protected/Guidelines_Management_2007.
6. Regenchary SS, Ellenbogen RG. *Principles of Neurosurgery.* 2nd ed. Philadelphia: Mosby; 2005.
7. Smith M. Monitoring intracranial pressure in traumatic brain injury. *Anesth Analg.* 2008;106(1):240-248.
8. Zhong J, Dujovny M, Park HK. Advances in ICP monitoring techniques. *Neurol Res.* 2003;25:339-350.
9. Narayan RK, Kishore PR, Becker DP, et al. Intracranial pressure: to monitor or not to monitor? A review of our experience with acute head injury. *J Neurosurg.* 1982;56:650-659.
10. Wolfe TJ, Torbey MT. Management of intracranial pressure. *Curr Neurol Neurosci Rep.* 2009;9(6):477-485.

CHAPTER 45

CEREBRAL OXIMETRY— BRAIN POWER

REBECCA REEVES
EUGENIE HEITMILLER

Self-respect is to the soul as oxygen *is to the body. Deprive a person of* oxygen, *and you kill his body; deprive him of self-respect and you kill his spirit.*
— *Thomas S. Szasz*

INTRODUCTION

Another monitoring device! Why do we care about brain oxygen saturation? Brain monitoring during surgery is an extremely complicated and much debated issue. Just about everyone agrees that cerebral injury during surgery is a major source of morbidity and mortality. The fact is that the brain loves oxygen, and unfortunately does not tolerate ischemia or hypoxia very well, making it extremely susceptible to injury.

- Some studies show that serious neurologic injuries occur in up to 6.2% of patients after myocardial revascularization.
- Other studies show an incidence of postoperative cognitive decline between 40% and 60% in patients undergoing cardiac surgery.
- Hypoperfusion during cross-clamping in carotid endarterectomy surgery is a major cause of stroke.

These situations lead to functional decline, an increase in the length of hospital stays, and overall poor outcomes after surgeries that theoretically should increase functional status. Thus brain monitoring during surgery is a very hot topic, and several monitoring techniques are currently available:

- Cerebral functional state: electroencephalography and evoked potentials
- Cerebral hemodynamics: carotid artery stump pressure and transcranial Doppler
- Cerebral metabolism: jugular bulb monitoring and near-infrared spectroscopy

We're going to focus on *near-infrared spectroscopy* (NIRS), also known as cerebral oximetry or brain oximetry.

Here's how it works: "the color of life":

- Cerebral oximetry is a new application of an older technology that uses near-infrared spectroscopy to measure frontal cortical brain saturation.
- It works like a standard pulse oximeter; do you need a review? The measurement is based on absorption differences of oxygenated and deoxygenated hemoglobin. Basically, oxygenated hemoglobin absorbs more infrared light (850 to 1000 nm) and less red light (600 to 750 nm). The fraction of oxyhemoglobin can be determined and real-time changes in regional oxygen saturation can be measured.
- Like pulse oximetry, an absolute number, on a scale of 1 to 100, is reflected on the monitor, 100% being completely oxygenated hemoglobin.
- Unlike pulse oximetry, NIRS doesn't require pulsatility. It measures the saturation of an entire tissue bed (brain tissue plus arterial and venous blood). This is *mostly* venous blood (70–75%), since most of the hemoglobin is on the venous side of the tissue. The device also has a fancy-pants mechanism for compensating for wavelength-dependent scattering losses and interference from things such as fluid, tissue, and melanin. It's complicated.

- "Normal" values differ from patient to patient, but values similar to normal mixed venous saturation are frequently seen. Readings in the 60s to 70s are common. Notice in Figure 45-1 that the monitor readings of an overworked, post-call resident are splendid!
- Values are updated every few seconds.
- It is more important to get a baseline value and follow trends rather than focusing on a specific number! NIRS is more reliable for monitoring trends than are absolute values.

INDICATIONS

Two thirds to four fifths of cerebral blood flow is venous. Again, NIRS measures mainly local venous oxygen saturation. In a setting of ischemia, values decrease as the brain extracts more oxygen before function fails or permanent damage occurs. Thus, this monitor may be most helpful during operations that are associated with a decrease blood flow to the brain.

Currently, NIRS has been best studied and used regularly in the following cases:
- Cardiac surgery, to help guide flows and hemoglobin requirements during cardiopulmonary bypass, and for postoperative monitoring
- Carotid endarterectomy, because perioperative stroke is a significant risk, occurring in 5% to 8% of patients
- Intensive care unit patients, because central nervous system injuries caused by cerebral ischemia are difficult to detect in comatose or sedated patients
- Head trauma patients, for obvious reasons
- Kidney/liver to estimate absolute tissue oxygenation of these organs.

CONTRAINDICATIONS

Not very many to mention:
- Allergy to adhesives might be an issue.
- And (obviously) if placement of sensors would contaminate a sterile field—but you already knew that!

EQUIPMENT

- The monitor, about the size of a transport monitor (Figure 45-2)
    - Manufacturers and models:
        - Invos (Somanetics Corp., Troy, Michigan)
        - Fore-Sight (CAS Medical Systems, Branford, Connecticut)
        - Nonin (Nonin Medical, Plymouth, Minnesota)
        - Niro (Hamamatsu Photonics, Hamamatsu City, Japan)
- A patient, with a brain, preferably
- Disposable sensors (come in a variety of sizes to suit your patient; most are weight based for adult/child/infant/neonatal)
- Sensor cables, reusable

TECHNIQUE

- Step 1: The manufacturers recommend wiping off the patient's forehead thoroughly with alcohol pad to remove oil/debris/etc.
- Step 2: Place sensors across skin on forehead, avoiding hairline/eyebrows (unless you are offering a free eyebrow wax). Place one sensor left of midline, and the other goes directly right of midline (Figure 45-3).
- Step 3: Firmly press down sensors to ensure good contact. Easy enough!
- Step 4: Attach sensors to sensor cable, and ensure that the right-sided cable is hooked up to the right-sided sensor—obviously!

INTERPRETING THE NUMBERS

- Given the variability of baseline values between patients, a baseline should be obtained before induction of general anesthesia.
- Remember, the rationale for maintaining a high-normal mean arterial pressure (MAP) to augment cerebral blood flow and hence NIRS numbers is based on an assumption that ischemic areas of the brain have lost normal autoregulation.
- Cerebral ischemia is then determined if there is a change in baseline NIRS values of 20%. However, if baseline is less than 50%, a reduction of 15% from baseline is generally the threshold.
- Some believe that keeping all patients' MAP targets of 50 to 60 mm Hg during cardiopulmonary bypass does not prevent cerebral ischemia. Rather, individualizing MAP to target the patient's autoregulatory range may prevent cerebral ischemia during cardiopulmonary bypass.

Example: Prior to induction of general anesthesia, your patient's baseline cerebral oximetry values were 68% on the right and 66% on the left. If during cardiopulmonary bypass the value decreased to below 55%, the perfusionist should consider increasing flows or the anesthesiologist should consider transfusing red blood cells. If you were monitoring during carotid endarterectomy and saw similar dips, consider reaching for the anesthesiologist's-bail-me-out medication of choice—phenylephrine!

ACCURACY

As we said before, NIRS measures mean tissue oxygen saturation in all three cerebral compartments containing blood (arterial, venous, and capillary) and must penetrate the scalp, skull, and dura (areas that also contain some amount of blood) to get to the brain. The monitor's fancy-pants method for subtracting the noncerebral tissue works pretty well, but it isn't perfect. There can be considerable variation between patients. Thus, NIRS works better as a trend monitor. Figure 45-4 depicts the site of action of NIRS technology.

- Studies show that NIRS values correlate with transcranial Doppler measurements of cerebral blood flow.[1]
- NIRS, transcranial Doppler, and stump pressure all provide similar accuracy for detection of cerebral ischemia during carotid endarterectomy.[2]
- NIRS has also been shown to correlate with arterial and jugular bulb oxygen saturations, and thus is a useful tool for monitoring trends in cerebral tissue oxygenation.[3]
- NIRS has been shown to provide real-time continuous measurement of cerebral blood flow autoregulation.[4]

ADVANTAGES

- Simple to use
- Setup takes little time
- Noninvasive
- Does not require pulsatility, so it can be used during cardiopulmonary bypass, extracorporeal membrane oxygenation (ECMO), shock, or low flow states
- Good indicator of global decreased cerebral blood flow
  - Low perfusion pressure
  - Hypocapnia
  - Pump oxygenator-related low flow
  - Malpositioned cannulae for cardiopulmonary bypass or ECMO
  - Carotid artery disease
  - Cerebrovascular hypoxia
- Minimal training needed—a monkey could do it! But a monkey can't interpret it!

DISADVANTAGES

- Cannot detect changes in areas remote from the measurement site
- Focuses on frontotemporal region
- No "normal" measurements (absolute number) or known expected changes
- Acceptable lower limit unknown
- Anesthetic drugs that influence cerebral metabolic rate may cloud the picture

SOME OTHER STUDIES

- There have been reports of recognition of cerebral air embolisms during monitoring with NIRS.[5]
- Monitoring cerebral regional oxygen saturation (rSO_2) in coronary artery bypass patients avoids profound cerebral desaturation and is associated with significantly fewer incidences of major organ dysfunction, resulting in a hospital cost savings (shorter hospital stays, shorter intensive care unit stays, lower incidence of strokes, and less need for prolonged ventilation).[6]
- Preoperative NIRS levels reflect the severity of cardiopulmonary dysfunction and may add to preoperative risk stratification in cardiac surgery patients.[7]
- Perioperative periods of diminished cerebral oxygen delivery, as indicated by rSO_2, are associated with a 1-year Psychomotor Development Index and brain magnetic resonance imaging abnormalities among infants undergoing reparative heart surgery.[8]

THE GOOD NEWS

NIRS has many potential uses in a variety of clinical scenarios. We can expect that, in the future, more technologically advanced systems will be introduced in the market that have greater accuracy, and more studies will produce data to guide its use.

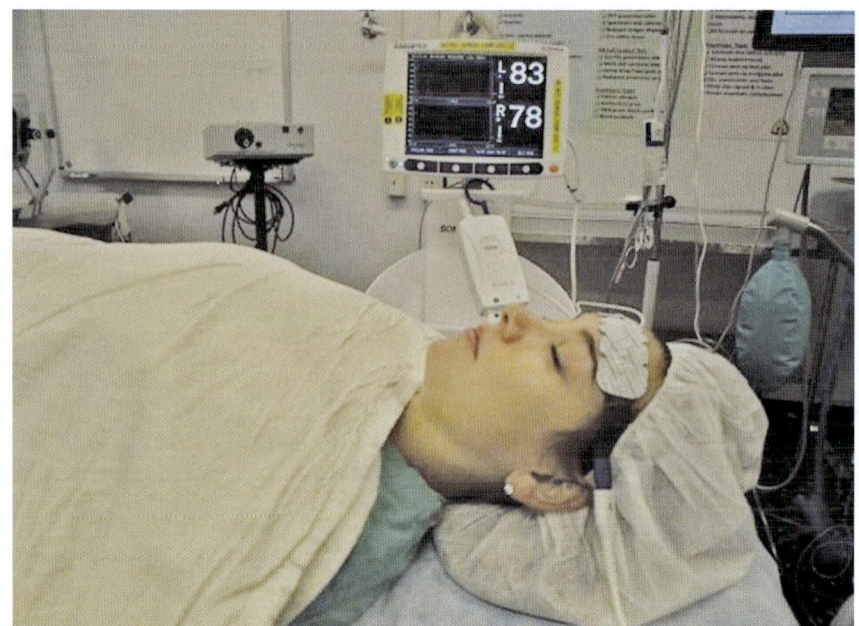

FIGURE 45-1 Near-infrared spectroscopy monitoring of a sleeping post-call resident.

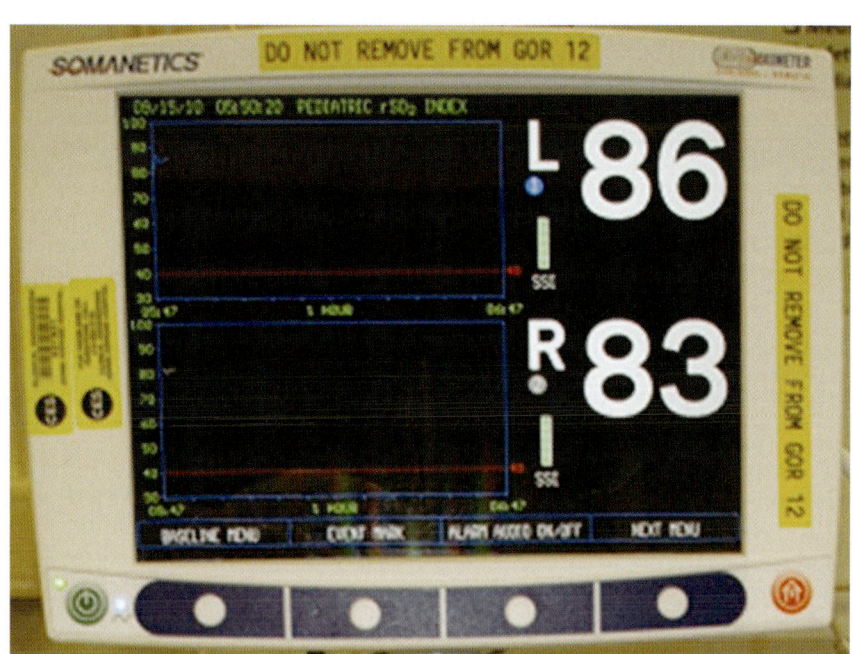

FIGURE 45-2 Near-infrared monitor display.

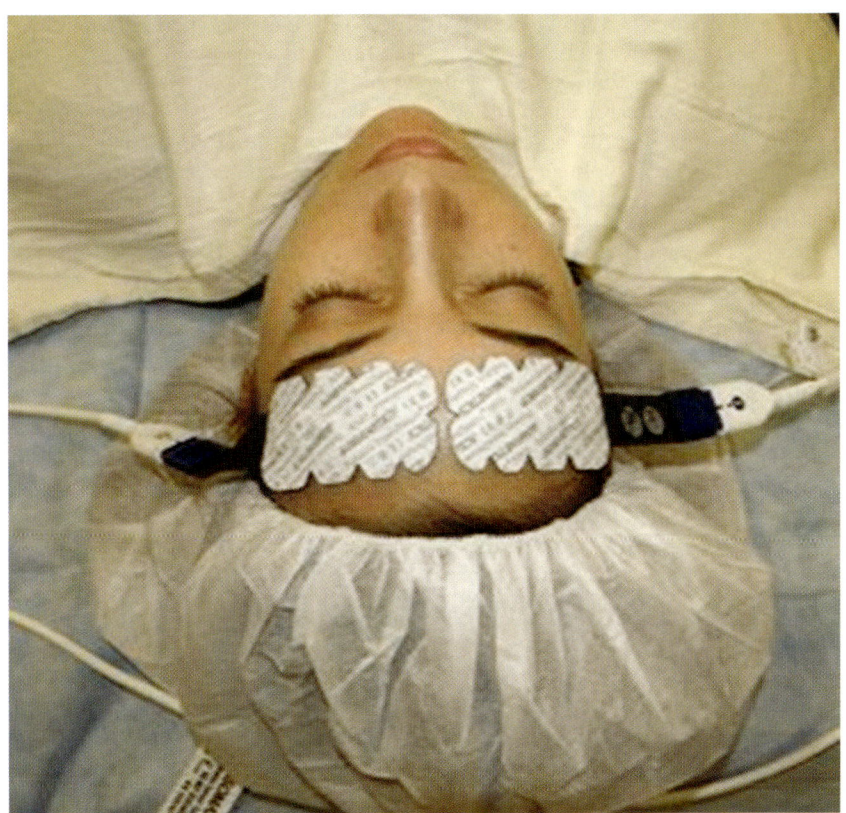

FIGURE 45-3 Near-infrared monitor sensor pad placement.

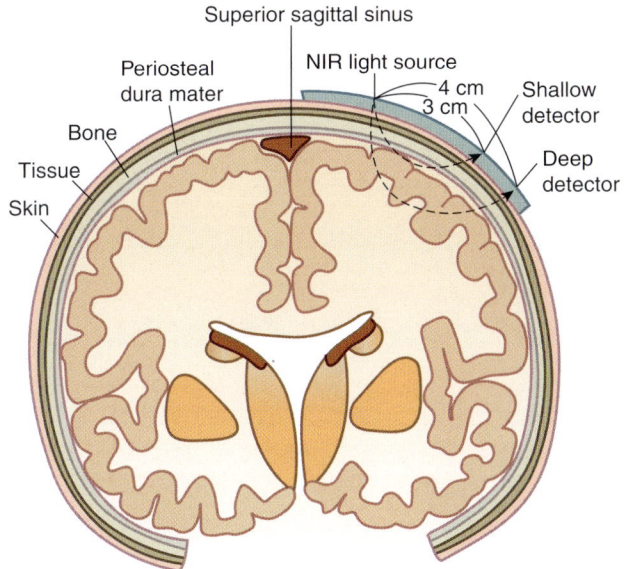

FIGURE 45-4 Near-infrared technology: site of action.

REFERENCES

1. Kirkpatrick PJ, Lam J, Al-Rawi P, Smielewski P, Czosnyka M. Defining thresholds for critical ischemia by using near-infrared spectroscopy in the adult brain. *J Neurosurg* 1998;89:389–394.
2. Moritz S, Kasprzak P, Arlt M, Taeger K, Metz C. Accuracy of cerebral monitoring in detecting cerebral ischemia during carotid endarterectomy. *Anesthesiology* 2007;107:563–569.
3. Kim M, Ward D, Cartwright C, Kolano J, Chlebowski S, Henson L. Estimation of jugular venous O_2 saturation from cerebral oximetry or arterial O_2 saturation during isocapnic hypoxia. *J Clin Monit Comput* 2000;16:191–199.
4. Brady K, Joshi B, Zwwifel C, et al. Real-time continuous monitoring of cerebral blood flow autoregulation using near-infrared spectroscopy in patients undergoing cardiopulmonary bypass. *Stroke* 2010;41:1951–1956.
5. Fischer GW, Stone ME. Cerebral air embolism recognized by cerebral oximetry. *Semin Cardiothorac Vasc Anesth* 2009;13:56–59.
6. Murkin JM, Adams SJ, Novick RJ, et al. Monitoring brain oxygen saturation during coronary bypass surgery: a randomized, prospective study. *Anesth Analg* 2007;104:51–58.
7. Herringlake M, Garbers C, Kabler J, et al. Preoperative cerebral oxygen saturation and clinical outcomes in cardiac surgery. *Anesthesiology* 2011;114:58–69.
8. Kussman BD, Wypij D, Laussen PC, et al. Relationship of intraoperative cerebral oxygen saturation to neurodevelopmental outcome and brain magnetic resonance imaging at 1 year of age in infants undergoing biventricular repair. *Circulation* 2010;1222:245–254.

SUGGESTED READING

Guarracino F. Cerebral monitoring during cardiovascular surgery. *Curr Opin Anaesthesiol* 2008;21:50–54.

Highton D, Elwell C, Smith M. Noninvasive cerebral oximetry: is there a light at the end of the tunnel? *Curr Opin Anaesth* 2010;23:576–581.

Kakihana Y, Matsunaga A, Yasuda I, Imabayashi T. Brain oximetry in the operating room: current status and future directions with particular regard to cytochrome oxidase. *J Biomed Optics* 2008;13:033001-1-14.

CHAPTER 46
MRI—DO'S AND DONUTS

ANASTASSIA GRIGORIEVA
DEBORAH SCHWENGEL

> Press close magnetic nourishing night.
> — Walt Whitman, *Song of Myself* (1891)

INTRODUCTION

Magnetic resonance imaging (MRI) has become a widely used diagnostic modality due to its unique features:
- Images in any plane (transverse, sagittal, coronal, oblique)
- Excellent soft tissue contrast without the need of intravenous contrast media
- Minimal patient preparation
- No ionizing radiation, noninvasive, and biologically inert

PRINCIPLES OF MRI

- Atoms with an odd number of protons or neutrons, most notably hydrogen, have the potential to act as magnetic dipoles.
- When subjected to a powerful static magnetic field, they align themselves with the magnetic field.
- When a pulse of radiofrequency (RF) energy is applied to the magnetic field, these atoms change their positions.
- As the pulse of RF energy is discontinued, the protons return to their original alignment (i.e., they "relax") and, as they do, they release energy.
- The release of energy over time (the relaxation time, i.e., T1 or T2) is specific for given tissues and is used to generate the MRI signal that is used to construct a computer image with excellent definition.
  - T1 is the time taken to return to the resting magnetic vector.
  - T2 is the time taken to return to the resting axial spin.
- The magnetic field is measured in tesla (T) units (1 T = 10,000 gauss). While the earth's magnetic field is approximately 0.5 gauss, MRI scanners used for clinical purposes generate a field of 0.15 to 2.0 T, and up to 8 T used in research.

DANGERS OF MRI

While the magnetic field itself is not known to produce any direct harm to humans, there are several effects of the magnetic field and RF forces that can cause injury or even death in people located in or in close proximity to the magnet or damage monitoring equipment (Table 46-1).

Burns can occur if looping or redundancy of wires occurs because it sets up a secondary electromagnetic field.

Another potential danger of MRI is quench! And, no, we don't mean getting really thirsty and longing for a cold beverage by the end of a long, busy day in MRI. MRI scanners are super-cooled with inert gases such as helium. If these cryogens escape either intentionally or unintentionally, a quench has occurred. It is usually done purposely to decommission a scanner or in an

TABLE 46-1 Characteristics of MRI

MR Force	Effect on Medical Devices	Adverse Effect
Static magnetic field—ALWAYS on	Rotational force on object	Tearing of tissues. Object attempts to align with magnetic field
Spatial magnetic gradient—ALWAYS on	Translational force	Missile effect. Acceleration of object into bore of magnet
Gradient magnetic field Pulsed during imaging	Induced currents	Device malfunction or failure
Radiofrequency field Pulsed during imaging	RF currents cause heating	Patient burns Thermal and electrical
Radiofrequency field Pulsed during imaging	Electromagnetic interference	Device malfunction Induced noise (monitors)

emergency to remove a projectile from a scanner but can rarely occur spontaneously. Features of a quench:

- Cryogens exposed to room temperature increase in pressure and rapidly become a gas.
- Ideally the exposed cryogens should egress out of the MRI scanning room via a valve to the outside environment. This is demonstrated in a You Tube video: **http://www.youtube.com/watch?v = naMuS0IR_jE&feature = related**
- A quench occurs over 5 to 15 seconds; therefore, the magnetic field does not drop immediately.
- If a quench should occur but the cryogens do not exit via the designed pressure valve, the most immediate risk to occupants of the room is asphyxiation and frost bite.
- Later, the room may become a fire hazard as flammable liquid oxygen accumulates due to the rapid drop in room temperature.
- If an unanticipated quench should occur, retrieve and stabilize the patient, and then evacuate the MRI site immediately.
- For the anticipated quench, be certain it is indicated, push the quench button, and evacuate the room immediately. *Do not touch the quench button* for any reason other than an emergency requiring MRI shutdown (Figure 46-1).
- Memorize this equation: Quench = Cold inert gas + Low oxygen = Frostbite injury + Hypoxia.
- Quench is potentially deadly and it is also very costly. It takes 96 hours to repower an MRI machine, which translates into hundreds of thousands of dollars of lost scanning time.

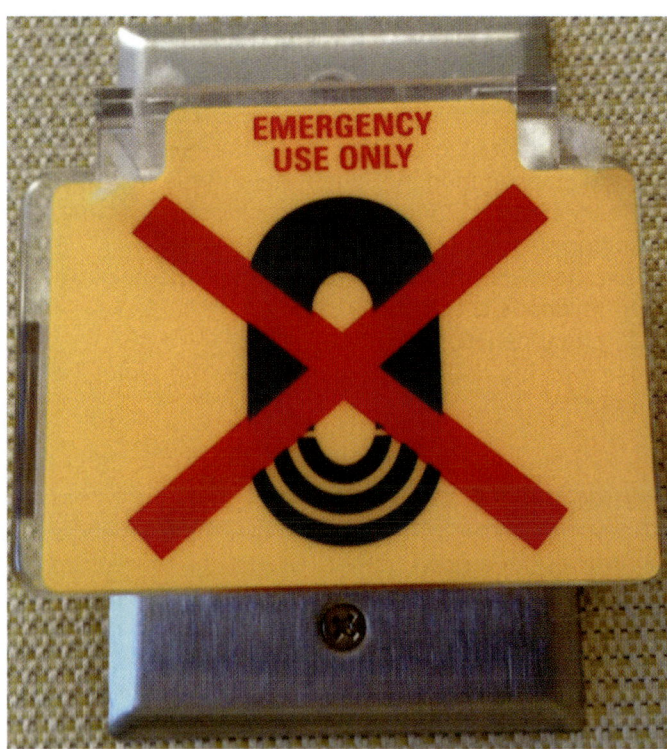

FIGURE 46-1 Quench button. Not all buttons look like this, so find out what your quench button looks like.

ANESTHESIA IN MRI

So all of this stuff is important for radiologists and MRI techs, not anesthesiologists, right? Wrong! As MRI becomes more and more popular, anesthesiologists are becoming more and more involved in providing anesthesia in the "faraway place." While many adults and small infants can tolerate lying still in a small-diameter (50 to 65 cm) hollow tube for some period of time (from 20 to 60 minutes) with or without sedation, many patients cannot. The need for general anesthesia or heavy sedation is often needed for the following patients:
- Children up to the age of 5 or even older
- Adults with claustrophobia
- Patients with significant pain
- Patients with significant comorbidities

What do you need to know when you get a "Congratulations! You are going to MRI tomorrow!" page the night before?

First, are you certified to provide anesthesia in MRI? A formal training program should be put in place for all MRI personnel to provide a safe environment for patients and practitioners. No one should be allowed to become "MRI personnel" before completing the training. At our institution, you get a capital letter "M" on your ID badge after you become certified in MRI safety. No M, no access to MRI. If your institution doesn't have such a certification program, it should! Think "systems-based practice" if you are of the 6 Accreditation Council for Graduate Medical Education (ACGME) core competencies bent.

When you arrive at the MRI area, remember to remove all things that can be damaged or sucked in by the MRI scanner, e.g., metal watch, pager, cell phone, stethoscope, ID badge, credit cards (who knew that losing lunch money was one of the MRI dangers?!) before you enter MRI zone III.

Zone III? What is that? The MRI suite is divided into four zones:
- Zone I: public zone with free access
- Zone II: interface between the public zone and the MRI suite, where all movement by non-MRI personnel is supervised by MRI personnel
- Zone III: the area within which the introduction of ferromagnetic objects may form a hazard
- Zone IV: the scanner room itself

Second, as was alluded before, MRI is one of the "faraway places," which means that you need to plan ahead. Make sure you are fully prepared to provide anesthesia with all necessary medications and resuscitation equipment if it becomes necessary.

OK, now back to you. By now you have removed all of your own ferromagnetic objects. Here are a few others to think about that have been known to sneak into the scanner room and become weapons of destruction:
- Oxygen canisters (Figure 46-2)
- Laryngoscope blades
- "Bean bags" (some may contain ferrous shot)
- Chairs
- Clipboards
- Infusion pumps
- Scissors
- Metal gurneys
- Hospital beds
- Code teams

Code teams? Huh? Oh, good, you are paying attention. Remember, that unlike you, other code team members may not be familiar with all the dangers of MRI. For some, it might be the first time in this strange place in the basement and they are loaded with all sorts of metal objects. In the event of a code during a scan, be sure that the patient is removed from the MRI suite as soon as possible and relocated to a suitable resuscitation area. Know where your resuscitation equipment is located before you start giving an anesthetic. We also keep difficult airway equipment in the MRI and other remote anesthetizing locations (Figure 46-3).

If a code occurs, put a guard at the scanning room door so that none of the code team providers accidently enters the scanning room. Remember: *The magnet is always on.* You can't help the coding patient if you are being impaled by somebody's metal pen or reflex hammer!

Next thing you need to do is to make sure that your patient is not a "man or woman of steel" and you, too: no artificial limbs, pacemakers, aneurysm clips, etc. Unless proven otherwise, pacemakers are not MRI compatible. While it's the MRI technician's job to inquire about any potential MRI no-no's present in the patient's body, it doesn't hurt to confirm with the patient that he or she doesn't have the following:
- Pacemaker made with ferrous materials
- Intracranial aneurysm clip
- Bullets or shrapnel
- Bronchial or tracheal stents
- Metal objects in the eye
- Epidural catheters

Any of these objects exposed to the magnetic field can shift, burn, or malfunction, turning a harmless test into a life-threatening emergency. If you aren't sure if an implanted device is MRI compatible, don't take the patient in the room. Refer to the manufacturer's specs to determine compatibility or go to www.mrisafety.com for the information you need. While some devices are compatible in a 1.5-T environment, they might not be proven safe in a 3-T MRI. Know which tesla strength your MRI scanner is.

Let's assume the patient has been cleared for MRI. Now it's your turn to anesthetize the patient and place him/her in the scanner. Pearls to consider:
- The induction of general anesthesia and intubation, if needed, ideally takes place in an induction room adjacent to the MRI scanner. This room can also double as a resuscitation room (Figure 46-4).
- After the patient is anesthetized and monitors are in place, he/she is then transported to the scanner on a MRI-compatible stretcher.
- Due to the limited access to patient's airway while the patient is in the scanner, a laryngeal mask airway (LMA) or endotracheal tube can be used, but an oxygen mask or a nasal cannula can be safe options too. When deciding which method of airway management to use, you should always consider your patient's underlying pathology. For example, a patient with an intracranial mass is at risk of increased intracranial pressure (ICP). This patient may decompensate with sedation and hypoventilation. Therefore, such a patient would benefit from intubation and controlled ventilation in order to avoid hypercarbia.
- Ventilation during MRI can be spontaneous or controlled, using an MRI-compatible anesthesia machine and ventilator. Long circle systems used for MRI are 20 feet long. The consequence is delayed equilibration of respiratory gases, particularly at low fresh gas flow rates. A certain amount of tidal volume will be lost in the longer circuit, making spirometric measurement at the anesthesia machine less accurate. CO_2 sampling tubings are likewise longer than in operating rooms. The result is delayed CO_2 sampling; therefore, it will take slightly longer to recognize changes in ventilation in the MRI environment.
- If your patient has an indwelling ICP monitor, it is important to determine whether this ICP monitor is MRI compatible prior to placing the patient in the scanner room. You should also consider that the ICP monitor may interfere with the quality of the MRI image, if the head is being scanned; the diagnostic value of the study may be compromised by this piece of equipment. See Chapter 44 for details on ICP monitoring.
- The choice of anesthetic—sedation versus general anesthesia—is based on several factors:
  - Patient's medical condition
  - Duration of scan
  - Special scan requirements such as positioning, the need for breath holding, or interventional procedures
  - Postanesthesia care unit (PACU) capabilities
- Either intravenous or inhalational general anesthesia can be safely used to deliver anesthesia in MRI. Consider the following points when deciding which medications you will choose:
  - Total intravenous anesthesia (TIVA) requires MRI-compatible infusion pumps or a noncompatible pump located outside the scanning room with tubing threaded through a conduit in the wall (Figure 46-5).
  - General anesthesia may be associated with shorter PACU stay compared with nurse-administered sedation, but sedation is often delivered with less costly medications.
  - PACU costs can have a significant impact on the overall cost of administering an MRI; it is therefore prudent to consider the cost of recovery time when deciding on the anesthetic technique.
  - Never compromise patient safety, comfort, or satisfaction. Maintain easy access to the patient's IV during the scan.
  - Be sure there is enough fluid in the IV bag before leaving the patient in the scanning room.
  - Like the patient needing TIVA, patients who require pumps for vasoactive infusions during the scan cannot be scanned unless extension tubing is passed through the conduit in the wall or the infusion is transferred to an MRI-compatible pump system.
    - Extension tubing should be properly primed prior to attaching it to the patient in order to avoid air embolism.
- Make sure that all of the standard American Society of Anesthesiologists (ASA) monitors (electrocardiogram [ECG] pads, pulse oximetry, blood pressure cuff) are made of MRI safe materials (no ferrous components). Looped cables or frayed insulation can cause thermal injury, so make sure all wires go longitudinally down the long axis of the patient.
- Prior to placing the patient in the scanner, make sure that all of the tubing is long enough to travel with the MRI bed.
- Make sure that the monitoring equipment outside of the scanner room is picking up all of the vital signs data (SpO_2, $ETCO_2$, BP, HR, ECG) correctly before starting the scan. The scan will cause artifact on the ECG tracing. Newer MRI-compatible monitors provide filtering modes that minimize the amount of artifact that you will see on the tracing. If you are having trouble getting an accurate HR because of artifact, use the SpO_2 as your source of HR monitoring. If you cannot tell if your patient is having a dysrhythmia, ask the MRI technologist to

stop the scan to determine if the ECG trace shows artifact or true rhythm disturbance.
- After the scan is complete and the patient emerges from anesthesia, he/she is transferred to the recovery area until standard recovery room discharge criteria are met.

Providing anesthesia in MRI can be an exciting and rewarding experience as long as it's approached with proper planning and preparation and you follow this mnenomic at all times: MRI—*M*etal *R*esults (in) *I*njury. MRI anesthesia is a pain, so if you are comfortable doing it, you become a value-added anesthesiologist. If you want to make yourself marketable (and the job market is getting tight), be the "go-to" person for MRI.

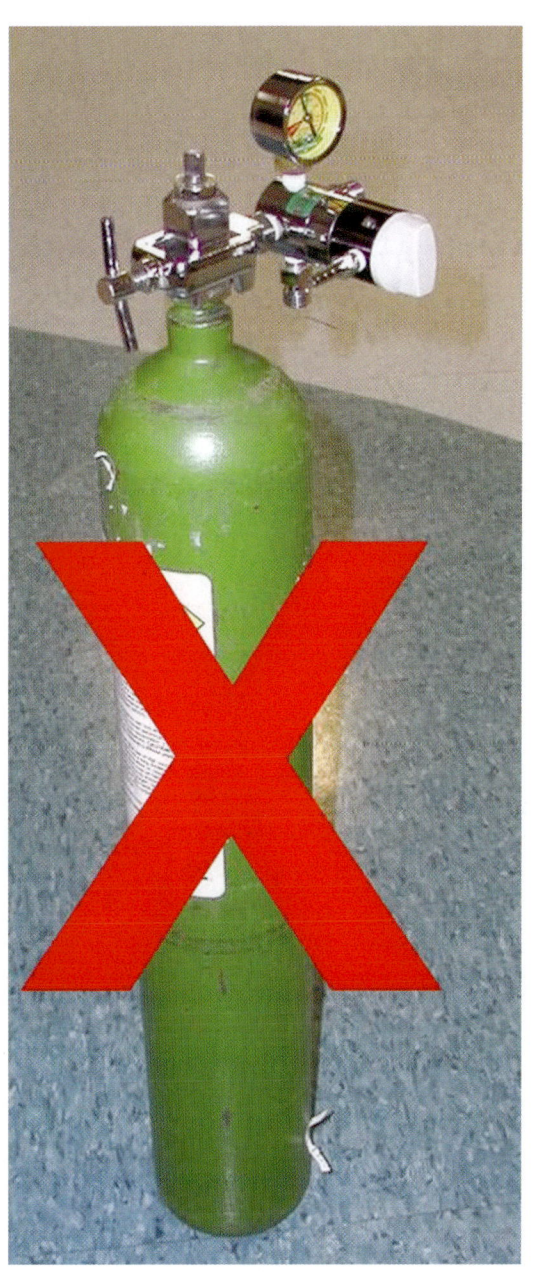

FIGURE 46-2 An iron oxygen tank, like the one shown here, must never be taken into a scanning room. It will become a missile and possibly kill someone.

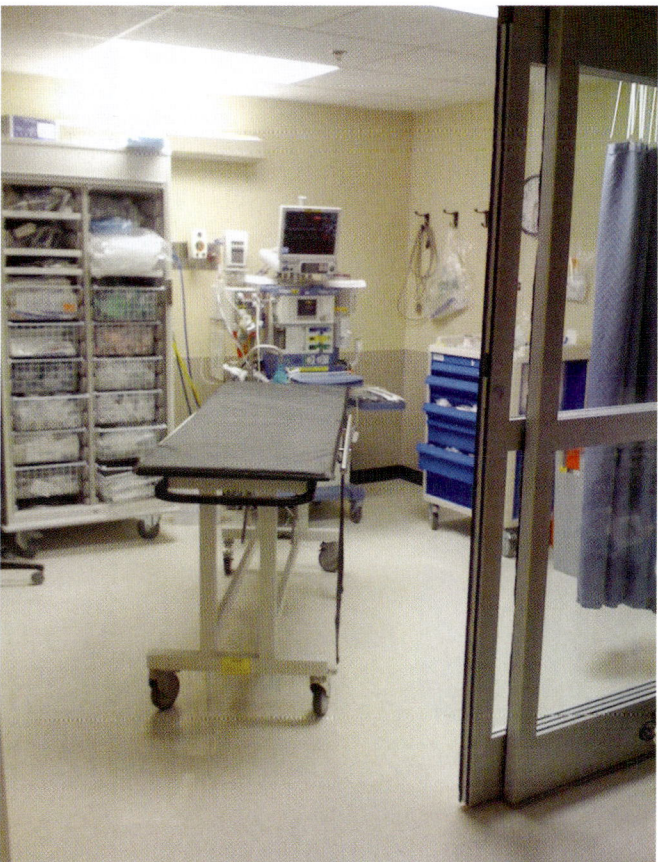

FIGURE 46-3 A designated induction room can also serve as a resuscitation area.

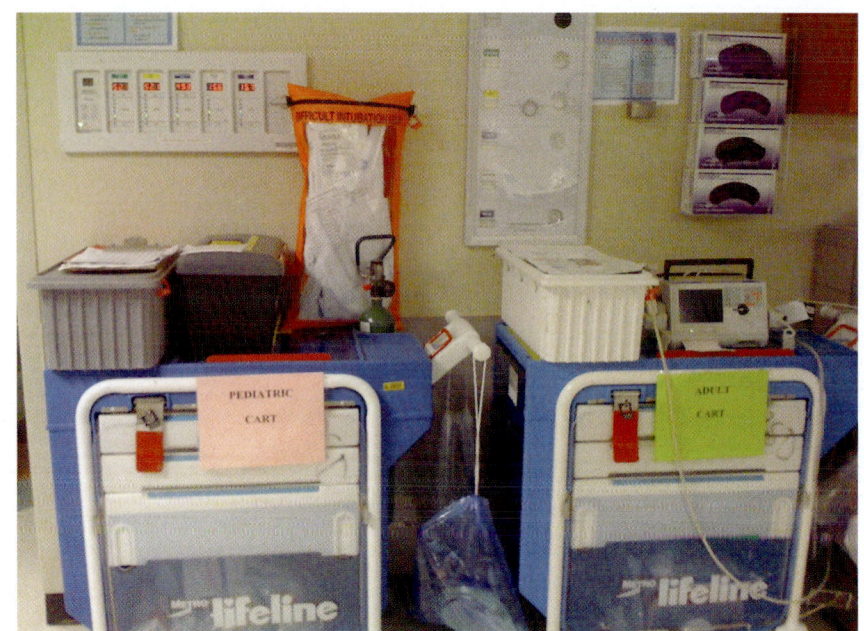

FIGURE 46-4 Standard resuscitation equipment with a difficult airway bag in the MRI suite.

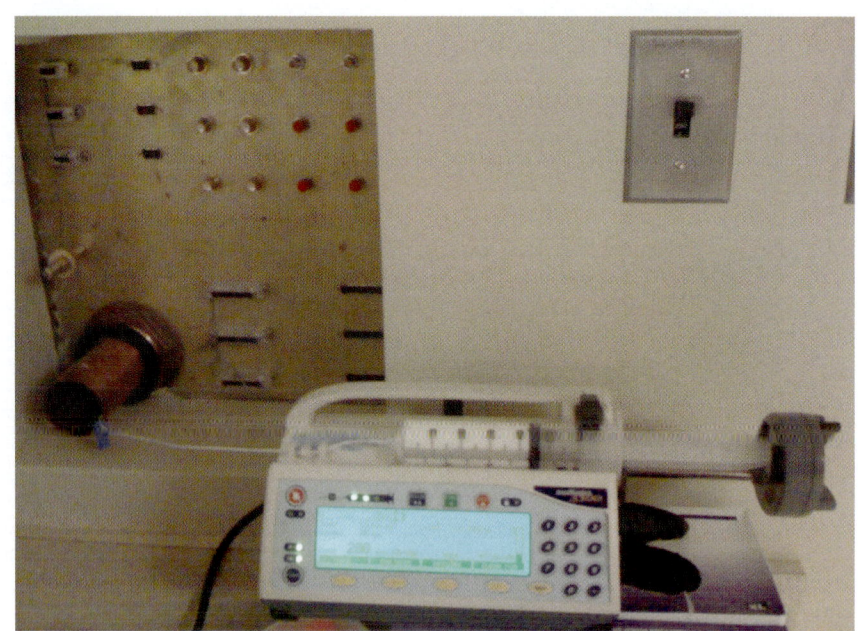

FIGURE 46-5 An infusion pump delivering propofol via extension tubing fed through a copper conduit in the wall to the scanning room.

SUGGESTED READING

Barash PG, Cullen BF, Stoelting RK, Cahalan MK, Stock MC. *Clinical anesthesia*, 6th ed. Philadelphia: Lippincott Williams & Wilkins, 2009, Chapter 34.

Serafini G, Zadra N. Anaesthesia for MRI in the paediatric patient. *Curr Opin Anaesthesiol* 2008;21(4):499–503.

Shorrab AA, Demian AD, Atallah MM. Multidrug intravenous anesthesia for children undergoing MRI: a comparison with general anesthesia. *Paediatr Anaesth* 2007;17(12): 1187–1193.

PART VIII

ROOMSMANSHIP

CHAPTER 47
GETTING STARTED

NICHOLAS B. NEDEFF
JUSTIN THAMPI
TRAVIS LEE

The secret of getting ahead is getting started. The secret of getting started is breaking your complex overwhelming tasks into small manageable tasks, and then starting on the first one.

Mark Twain

INTRODUCTION

Close your eyes for a minute and imagine that your job depends on your ability to get procedures done quickly and safely. Now open your eyes and get moving, because it does. Efficiency is the key to keep the operating rooms moving along smoothly. No matter how much a surgeon likes you, he will like you that much more if you can move quickly. There is one thing surgeons want: they want to go fast!

In accomplishing this:
- DO NOT go so fast that you become unsafe.
- DO NOT skip critical steps.
- DO NOT ignore professional behavior and treat the patient or OR staff poorly.
- DO get rid of unnecessary steps and wasted movements.

INDICATIONS

Reaching the light at the end of the tunnel: the sooner the procedure gets started, the sooner it finishes, and the sooner you get home.

CONTRAINDICATIONS

You want everyone at work not to like you. You like working late. You do not like being gainfully employed.

PHILOSOPHY OF EFFICIENCY

Trim the fat. The key is to make everything you do count. Everything should be done with speed and purpose. The goal is economy of movement.

Efficiency starts in the preoperative phase before the patient even makes it into the OR; teamwork, organization, and communication are essential.

Preoperative evaluation must include a thorough medical history and review of the chart. This includes reviewing imaging studies and laboratory tests. This evaluation must be done in a timely fashion, so that any concerns that come up can be addressed early so that the case can proceed as scheduled. Few things get a surgeon angrier than delaying or canceling an elective procedure the day of surgery when the patient is already there for issues that could have been resolved earlier. Oh, also, the patient who has been NPO since midnight and who woke up at or before the crack of dawn is probably not going to be happy either.

Get the insurance companies involved early to get preapproval for the procedure. Having to worry about funding the day of surgery only causes delays and adds unnecessary stress to everyone including the patient. Discussing finances with the patient right before you are about to wheel back to the OR isn't the fastest way to building rapport.

TEAMWORK

The team consists of the anesthesiologist, surgeon, pre- and postoperative staff, OR nurses, environmental services, and, in some cases, nurse anesthetists or anesthesia assistants. Every member of the team has an important role in keeping the OR running efficiently. And every member of the team deserves to be treated in a respectful manner.

It is important to remember that every member of the team is crucial. This includes the people in environmental services who make sure the OR gets turned over quickly. Without them the in-between time will add up and slow the flow in and out of the OR to a crawl.

GET YOUR ACT TOGETHER

The secret to success is *preparation*. Get all your supplies ahead of time. Running around looking for supplies when the patient is in the room doesn't instill confidence.

Surround yourself with good people. A well-trained anesthesia technician is a great resource. Technicians can be trained to keep track of inventory in the stockroom and OR. They can also help maintain the parade of emergency carts that we have, from difficult airway cart to the malignant hyperthermia (MH) cart. They can also help with the OR setup, from connecting the circuit to preparing invasive monitors.

Remember, a well-trained anesthesia technician is a luxury, not a necessity, and should be treated as such. Relying too heavily on your anesthesia technician will eventually show you why you shouldn't. It is important that you know just as much as the technician does about where things are and how to set them up.

Make sure you have extras with you, whether it's an IV or an A-line. We will eventually miss on the first try. Missing on the first try is less than ideal, but don't make it worse by not being ready for it. Remember, even Babe Ruth struck out.

Clean up as you go along. Leaving an area like a hurricane just passed through is bad form, and, more importantly, dangerous. Many of our messes involve sharps, and you don't want to be responsible for you or someone else getting stuck. Clean up with caution so you don't fall victim to the "dirty sharp under the drape" syndrome. Few things ruin your day faster than going to grab a dirty drape or wad of gauze and sticking yourself with a freshly used sharp.

Look before you leap. Before starting to premedicate your patient with midazolam, double-check with the rest of the team that all the paperwork is in order. Remember, teamwork and communication are important. Sedating a patient only to find out that the consent needs to be redone will lead to delays and the evil eye.

Once the patient and the chart have been checked and we have IV access that is actually in a vein, we are clear for takeoff. It's time to premedicate and head to the OR. From this point on we should be running like a well-oiled machine (See Figure 47-1). Make sure your machine is ready to go.

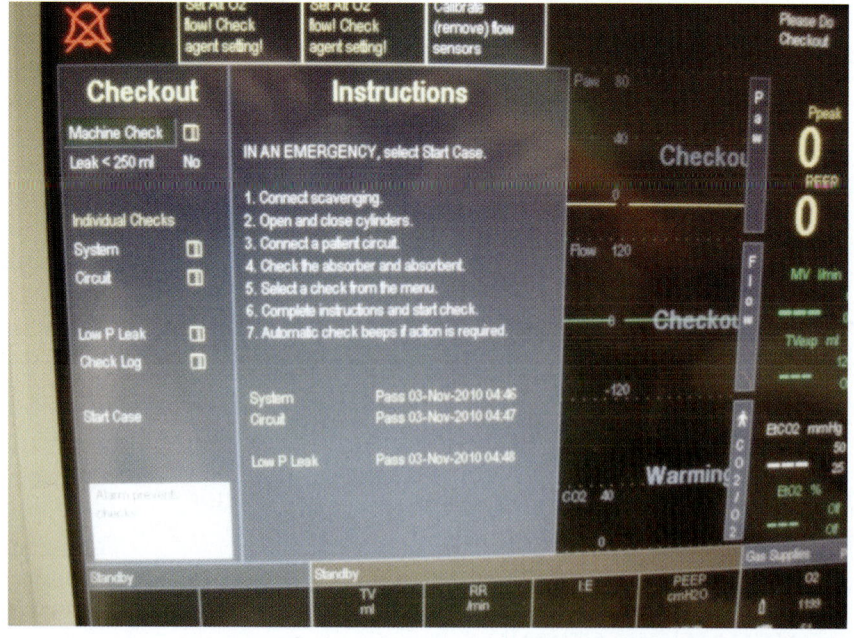

FIGURE 47-1 MACHINE: It all starts with the machine check. Yes, it takes time. No, you can't skip it. While today's machines are so reliable and seldom have problems, finding a problem is best done before a patient is anesthetized.

TECHNIQUE

You play like you practice. Prior to bringing the patient into the room, go over the case and take note of what you will need and how you plan on moving around the OR. By doing this you can see where you can combine steps and put them in a logical sequence that streamlines your movement. This will shave off several minutes from the procedure, and when you add it up at the end of a day you've saved yourself a good chunk of time.

Try to minimize the number of trips you have to take walking around the patient. It conserves time and energy. Plus if you walk around the patient five or six times when it should have been once or twice, the rest of the OR staff will think you are lost, crazy, or both.

Prior to the patient's arriving in the OR, have the monitors laid out on the bed on the side of the patient you are going to place them on (See Figure 47-2). When the patient is transferred to the OR table make sure the gown is untied so the patient does not sit up and lie down only to have to sit back up again. Start on the patient's right side and placing the appropriate electrocardiogram leads and any other monitors and then strap down the arm. Move over to the left and repeat. Now come on down to the head of the bed and start to preoxygenate for 3 to 5 minutes.

Notice how long it takes to preoxygenate. Seems like we're wasting time just standing there. Is there something we could do different? Maybe we can just skip this part? No. That is not an option. Being efficient means performing all the necessary tasks quickly, not skipping critical steps to save time. That is called being unsafe and lazy, and no one appreciates it.

Luckily, there is a high-tech solution: most ORs are equipped with a black face strap that you can use to secure the oxygen mask on the patient. By doing this you can start to preoxygenate the patient while you are putting on the monitors, which conveniently enough takes 3 to 5 minutes.

Now that you return to the head of the bed having successfully placed all monitors, your patient is preoxygenated and ready for induction. To make induction an easy one-hand operation, place stopcocks on your IV line within easy reach. This way you can load your drugs in the order you plan on giving them and just turn, push, turn, repeat.

When it comes to induction, do not take anything for granted. Always have a backup plan and a backup-backup plan. This way, when things go wrong and we are in the midst of crisis, we are prepared. Here teamwork and communication are critical; it is important to take charge of the situation and give clear instructions to the personnel you have in the room, as well as call for help.

The key is always to evaluate and analyze what you're doing so you can find ways of doing it more efficiently.

Remember, always have extras. This way if you miss on the A-line, you just grab the handy spare that you brought with you, instead of doing the walk of shame over to the supply area to get another one or asking someone to bring you another one as you hold pressure.

Clean up after yourself. Treat sharps with respect. Don't leave them lying around. As someone who has been stuck by a sharp, trust me, it is not fun.

A good anesthesiologist is not just someone who can administer a safe anesthetic. You have to look good doing it too. So act like a professional and treat the patient and the rest of the OR team with courtesy and respect. If you do this, people will want to work with you.

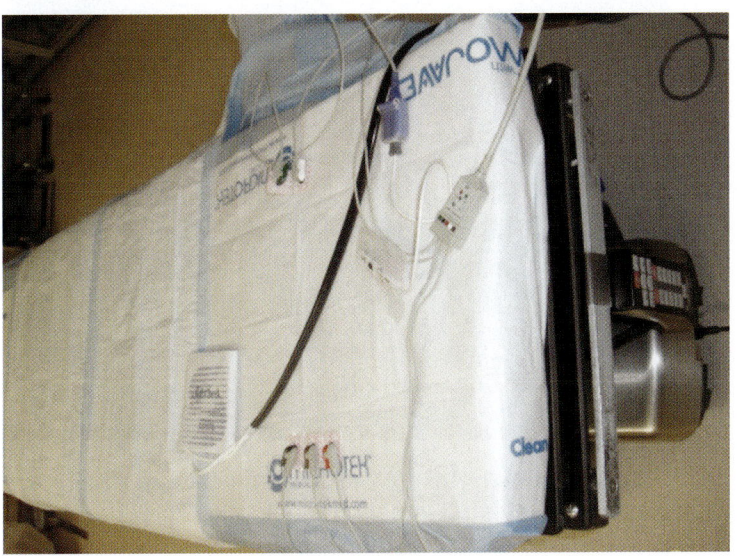

Figure 47-2 MONITORS: Monitors laid out and ready for quick application.

GLITCHES

Do not confuse cutting corners with efficiency. "Shortcut" is not a synonym for "streamline." If you mix these two up, you may find yourself try to intubate a patient who has not been preoxygenated, with a laryngoscope without a light, whose arms are dangling off the arm boards. The only thing this will do is efficiently remove you from a job.

Don't be disrespectful to the other members of the OR team. You rely on them to help get the procedures going. Treating them poorly is not right and will not get things moving. Pushing the rest of the OR team to move faster for no reason will only diminish your credibility and move you up their least favorite people list.

Treat the OR staff with respect and work with them to get procedures started in a timely manner. This way you will earn their respect, and when there is a crisis and you need to push people to move faster for a reason, they will be more likely to understand and give you their best effort.

Sometimes slow is as fast as you can go. If you have a really bad case slow down, take a minute to establish what needs to be done, prioritize, and then get after it. If you don't take that little extra time in the beginning, you will likely overlook something big and spend much more time down the road.

An efficient, organized, and motivated anesthesiologist commands respect from the patients, surgeons, and OR staff.

BEWARE OF TOO MUCH EFFICIENCY IN CERTAIN SITUATIONS

OR schedules are not written in stone. In a busy practice schedules can change frequently. Pay attention to schedule updates.

Pay attention to the patient you are seeing. Double-check the chart, the consent, and the surgical site. Sedating the wrong patient because you didn't pay attention to a change in the schedule is no fun. Communication with the OR front desk and the rest of the OR staff is key in avoiding these mix-ups and making sure everyone is on the same page.

STUFF IN MARGINS

MMAIDS: A Mnemonic for the Pregame

- *M*achine: A proper machine check is important and should be done by you, even if someone else attached the circuit to the machine for you. You should trust, but verify.

- *M*onitor: Make sure that you have all the necessary monitors in good working order prior to starting the procedure (See Figures 47-3 and 47-4).
- *A*irway: Have your airway supplies checked and laid out in an organized fashion. This includes being ready with your backup plan. Again, just because someone left a laryngoscope on top of you anesthesia machine, don't assume it works; check for yourself.
- *I*V: Have your IVs set up the way you like them, with stopcocks and the appropriate amount of extensions (See Figure 47-5).
- *D*rugs: Have your drugs drawn and appropriately stored (See Figure 47-6).
- *S*uction: You need to make sure you have it. If the time ever comes when you don't think you need it, that's when you'll need it (See Figures 47-7 and 47-8).

These simple and quick things are critical, and starting a procedure without these things being done or checked is unwise and unsafe. Being efficient is not skipping some of these steps; being efficient is doing all of it quickly (See Figure 47-9).

OAFAT: Obligatory Anesthesia, uh, Fool Around Time

This is the time from when anesthesia starts to the time we turn the patient over to our surgical colleagues.

Surgeons usually see this as wasted time, where we try and somehow intentionally slow them down. They are usually in the room repeatedly asking, "Can I start now? Can I start now?" much like a little kid in the back of a car would ask, "Are we there yet? Are we there yet?"

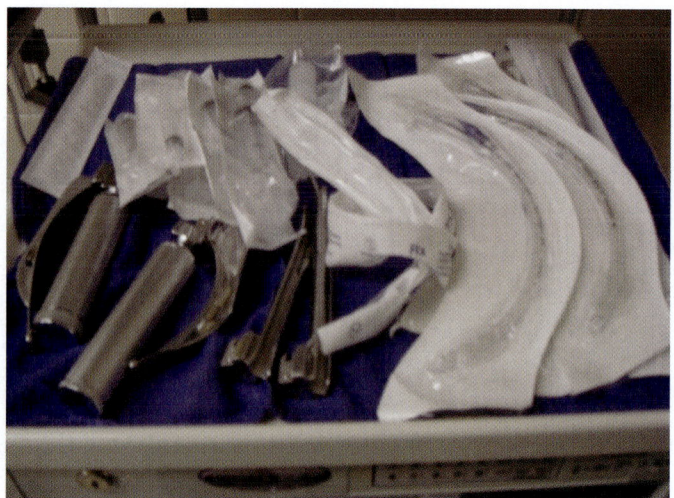

FIGURE 47-3 AIRWAY: Sometimes less is more. Having airway stuff is only the half of it. The other half is having it organized and ready to use.

Don't let the surgeons rush you when you are doing something lifesaving like securing the airway or stabilizing your patient.

At the same time, you need to move quickly and efficiently. An efficient anesthesiologist is viewed as a competent and able one. This is the kind of anesthesiologist that surgeons like to work with. Plus, it looks bad if OAFAT is longer that the surgery.

The key is to develop a starting routine that works for you and that is fast without skipping any critical steps.

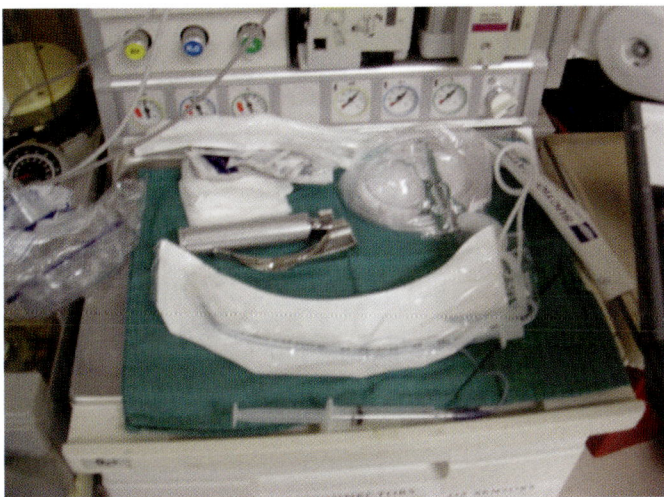

FIGURE 47-4 Airway equipment should be organized and ready to go.

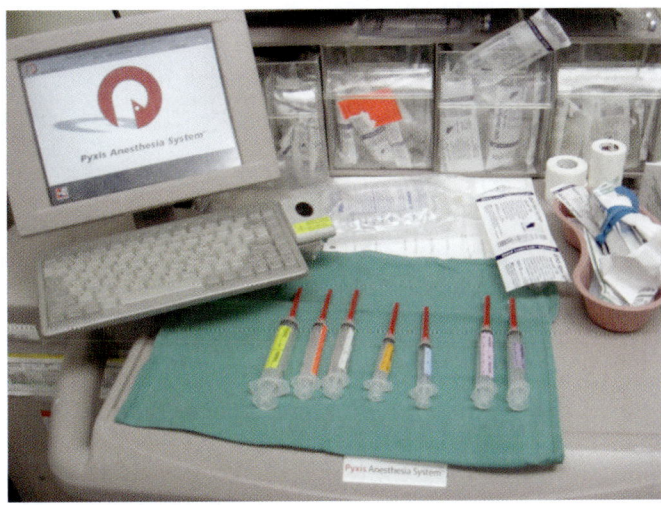

FIGURE 47-6 DRUGS: Have your drugs ready to go.

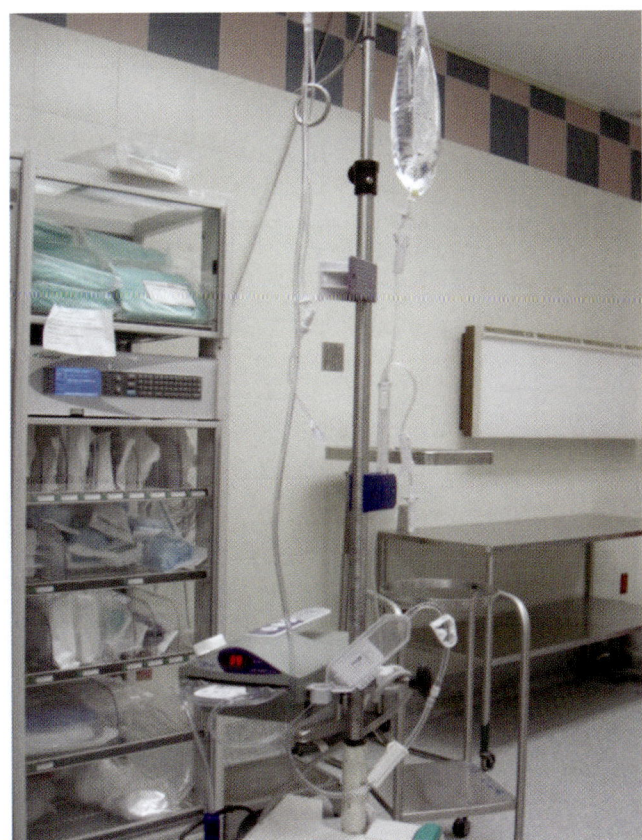

FIGURE 47-5 IV: Having your IV line setup and primed is one of the keys to being efficient.

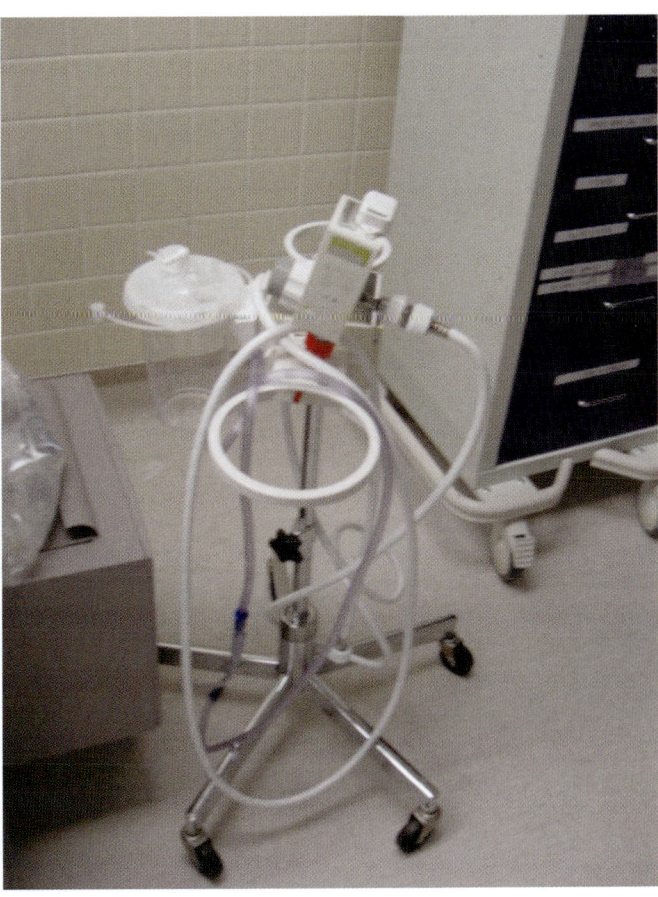

FIGURE 47-7 SUCTION: Suction ready... Not exactly!

A TYPICAL START

If you are not in efficiency mode, you will circle around the OR table several times in what to the rest of the OR staff will resemble a Chinese fire drill. Then to make up for lost time, you will likely forget to do something important such as preoxygenate your patient or double-check the suction (See Figure 47-10).

If you are in efficiency mode, you will glide across the OR from one side to the other, placing the monitors and securing the patient's arms with speed and grace. This will be followed by a smooth induction and intubation. And in doing this the patient and OR staff will sing your praises and children will want to grow up to be like you (See Figures 47-11, 47-12 and 47-13).

The important thing to remember in any and every case is that there are things you can rush and things you cannot. No matter how much of a rush there is, you always have time to stop and think before you induce.

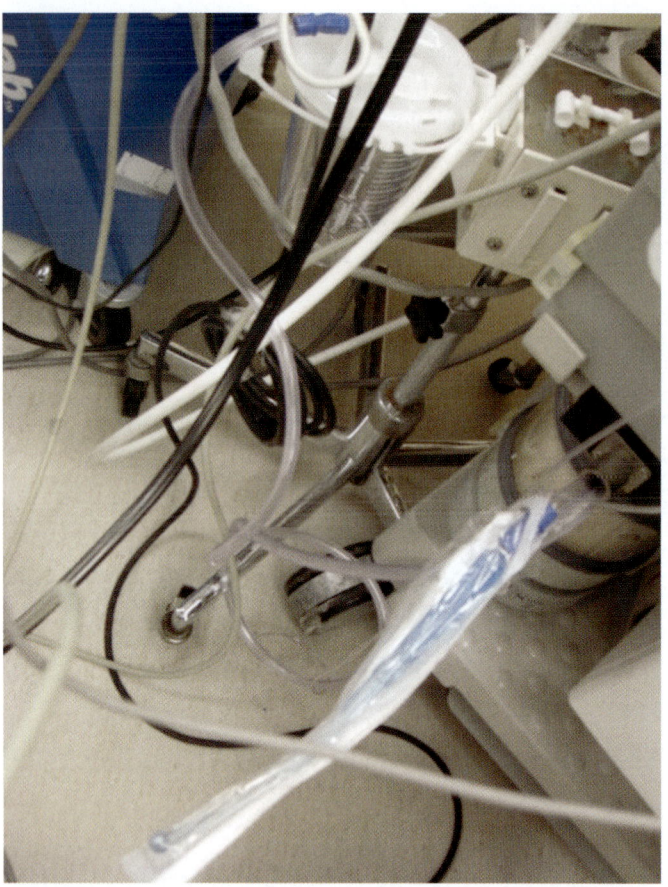

FIGURE 47-8 Suction done right.

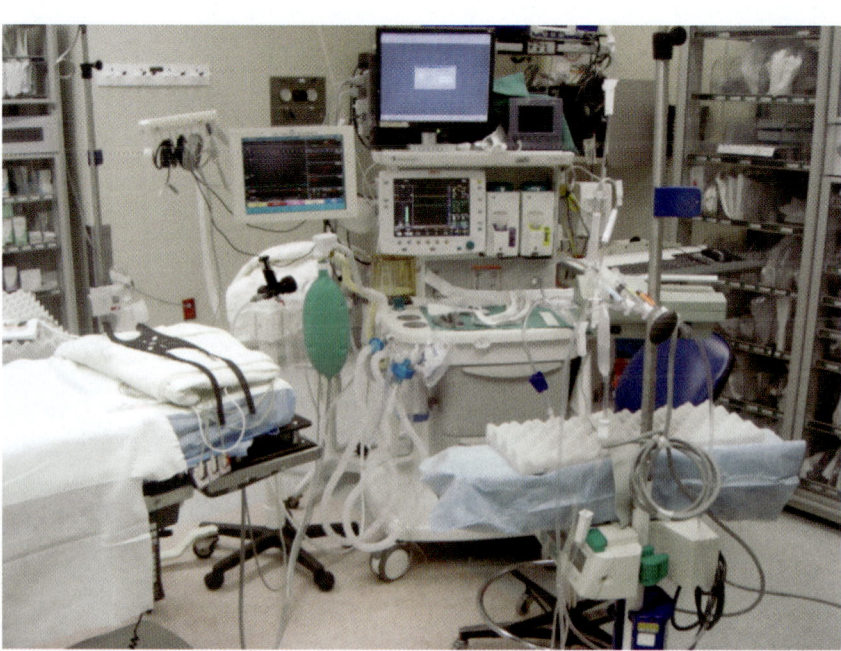

FIGURE 47-9 The OR completely ready for the next patient to come in and take a nap. Notice the right armboard already in place and the left armboard readily available for placement once the patient is moved onto the OR table.

Chapter 47 GETTING STARTED

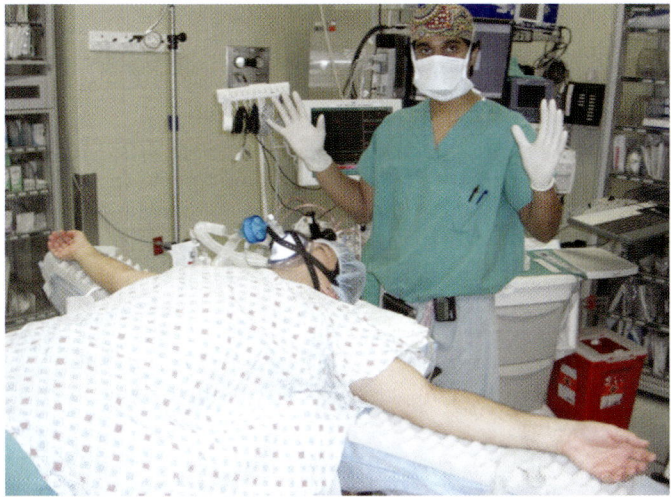

FIGURE 47-10 Look Ma, no hands! Who knew that preoxygenating could be so easy.

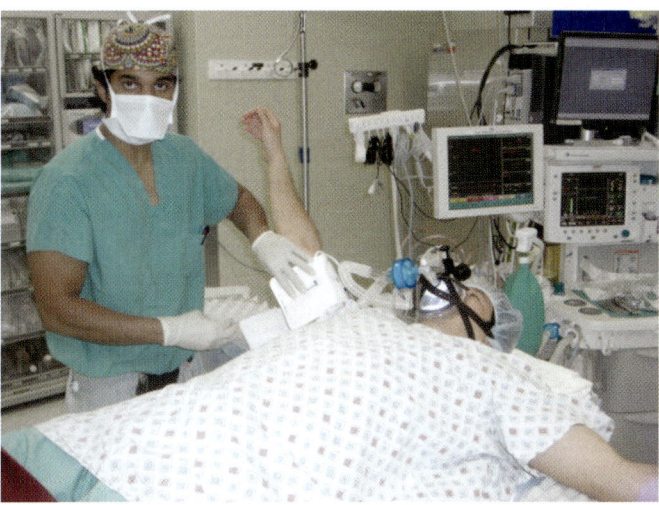

FIGURE 47-11 Next move to the patient's right and attach the appropriate monitors.

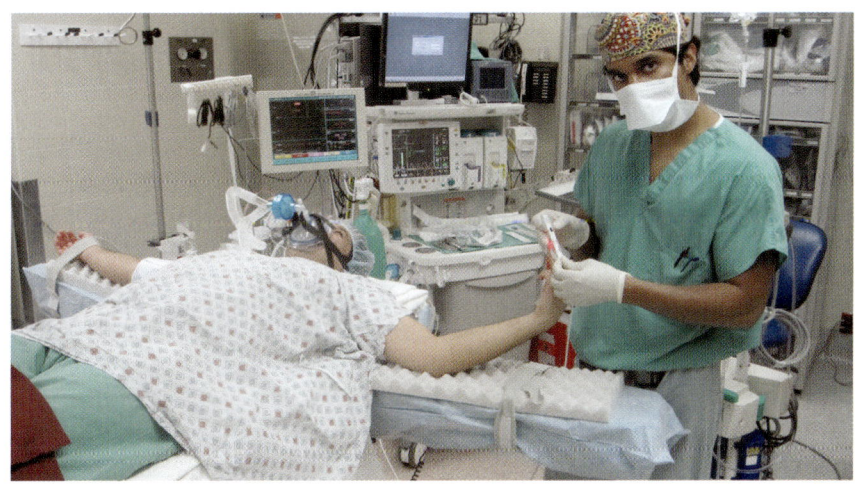

FIGURE 47-12 Then swing around to the left and finish placing the remaining appropriate monitors.

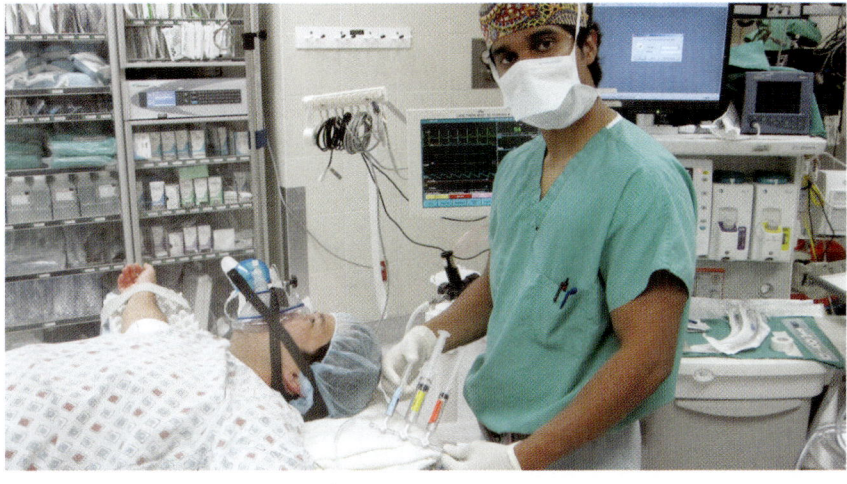

FIGURE 47-13 And now we are ready for induction. Notice that by placing stopcocks in your IV line you can easily and efficiently give your medications, with one hand. All you have to do is Twist, Push, Twist, and Repeat.

ONGOING EFFICIENCY

Efficiency doesn't stop with the induction of your patient.

Don't be greedy; share the patient. After induction, the nurses and surgeons have plenty of things they need to do to get the case going too! As long as nobody is going to get in each other's way, let them start working. For example, the nurse can start putting the Foley in while you intubate; if he or she is in your way you may need to reevaluate your technique for intubation. If you run into trouble and need help, no problem; just ask the others to stop what they are doing and give you a hand.

Remember, in order to make the OR as efficient as possible, you need teamwork and communication.

GETTING PEOPLE TO HELP YOU

To repeat, teamwork and communication are the name of the game. You can always ask some of the OR staff to help put on ECG leads or a BP cuff. The OR nurses are often just as good as, if not better than, you at placing the arm boards on the OR table and securing the arms. For example, if you are in an OR that does have a fancy high-tech facemask strap, you can ask the OR staff to hold the mask and preoxygenate while you do other things.

Keep in mind that you need to be able to function on your own and that any help you get is a luxury. If you rely too much on help, you will find yourself very inefficient when you are alone.

Make sure you know where stuff is. Spend a little time on your own to explore and familiarize yourself with the anesthesia workroom and central supply area. This way, when you do need something, you will know exactly where to go, or if you're asking someone to get you something, you'll be able to give good directions.

SUGGESTED READING

Archer T, Macario A. The drive for operating room efficiency will increase quality of patient care. *Curr Opin Anaesthesiol* 2006;9:171–176.
Great article outlining the scientific approach to redesigning the physical flow and methods of communication in the modern day operating room to improve efficiency and patient outcome.

Dexter F, Wachtel RE. Economic, educational, and policy perspectives on the preincision operating room period. *Anesth Analg* 2006;103:919–921.
Article analyzing the time between a patient entering the operating room and time of incision to determine points of inefficiency.

Masursky D, Dexter F, Garver MP, Nussmeier NA. Incentive payments to academic anesthesiologists for late afternoon work did not influence turnover times. *Anesth Analg* 2009;108:1622–1626.
A study finding that the implementation of payment to anesthesiologists for working late had no significant effect on turnover times at several times in the afternoon.

McIntosh C, Dexter F, Epstein RH. The impact of service-specific staffing, case scheduling, turnovers, and first-case starts on anesthesia group and operating room productivity: a tutorial using data from an Australian hospital. *Anesth Analg* 2006;103:1499–1516.
A tutorial examining the effect of reducing first-case delays and appropriate staff allocations to achieving greater OR efficiency.

Overdyk FJ, Harvey SC, Fishman RL, Shippey F. Successful strategies for improving operating room efficiency at academic institutions. *Anesth Analg* 1998;86:896–906.
A prospective study finding improved efficiency with proper personal accountability, streamlining of procedures, interdisciplinary team work, and accurate data collection.

CHAPTER 48
ROOMSMANSHIP

RACHEL M. KACMAR
CHRISTINE PARK

The architect should strive continually to simplify; the ensemble of the rooms should then be carefully considered that comfort and utility may go hand in hand with beauty.

Frank Lloyd Wright (1908)

Always design a thing by considering it in its next larger context—a chair in a room, a room in a house, a house in an environment, an environment in a city plan.

Eliel Saarinen, *Time* (1956)

INTRODUCTION

Right now you might be asking yourself, "What the heck is roomsmanship?" Well, basically it's all the little (and likely unnoticed) things you do in the operating room to make your job (as well as the jobs of the nurses, surgeons, etc.) a little easier. Streamlining your operating room takes practice and in some cases a little skill, but in the end it not only helps you, but also has pretty high potential to keep the patient's postsurgical life at status quo.

The categories that make up roomsmanship could (and in some cases do) fill a chapter of their own; they are that important. These are critical considerations and actions that help your procedures run smoothly and improve efficiency and flow. The topics are:
- Patient positioning
- Surveillance
- Body mechanics
- Moving a patient (to another bed, to lateral position, to/from prone position)
- Transporting a patient (from the OR to the postanesthesia care unit [PACU] or ICU)
- Line maintenance
- Troubleshooting the machine
- Setting up a rapid transfuser
- Professionalism
- Documentation

PATIENT POSITIONING (ALSO SEE CHAPTER 49)

Every procedure and every position presents its own unique danger to the patient. Even in a seemingly innocuous situation there is lots of potential for injury. Get used to checking, rechecking, and triple checking each and every time. Anesthetized patients are helpless; put yourself in their position and ask if you would be comfortable. If the answer is no, make a change.
- Don't trust anyone. If the nurses or surgeons (or surgery resident for that matter) try to "help" by tucking an arm or putting down the foot of the bed (watch the fingers!), at a minimum watch their technique. Confirm that the ulnar groove, heels, axillary rolls, and, in prone cases, the more "sensitive" areas are free of compression or sufficiently padded.
- If possible avoid any compression of pressure points. If the position or body habitus of the patient creates unavoidable contact with the bed or equipment surfaces, get familiar with the yellow foam padding or whatever equivalent is available in your OR.
- Move systematically over the patient for seemingly innocent threats. IV tubing, pulse oximetry, or blood pressure cords may be lying under the arms (again watch out for that ulnar groove). Stopcocks from IVs, central lines, and A-lines present their own hazard for injury if they stick into a patient's arm, neck, etc. for hours on end, so create a safe boundary between monitors/lines and the patient's skin.

- Return things to their rightful place. Awake patients usually assume a comfortable position on the table preinduction, so if you manipulate the neck or arms for intubation or IV/A-line/central line placement, make sure you return them to neutral (or as close to the patient-chosen position as possible). This can be very important when considering some of the elderly population with variations on arthritis, etc.
- If a patient mentions range-of-motion limitations preoperatively, have him or her assume the ideal position preinduction and attempt to maintain that position if at all possible throughout the procedure.
- Speaking of rightful places, watch out for rogue limbs. Arms (and legs) have a tendency to fall off tables or arms boards when inadequately secured. Our surgical colleagues are often unaware of the consequences when jockeying for position with an arm board, and a neglected fallen arm could potentially lead to nerve injury. Sometimes the patient's body habitus is challenging (tucking arms for a morbidly obese patient can be tricky), so use arm sleds, extra arm boards, and copious tape to secure those puppies. Getting under the drapes with a laryngoscope as a flashlight to fix things mid-procedure is a nightmare. Preventive actions go a long way.
- On the other hand, it is always better to fiddle around under the drapes and discover a problem during the procedure than to drop the drapes at the end and everyone goes "OMG, look at that!"
- Safety straps
  - The good: the leg/waist strap is a safety must, so make sure it is on, especially at the start and end of the procedure.
  - The bad: mask straps left under a patient's head for multiple hours can lead to pressure alopecia; avoid that pesky bald spot by replacing the strap with a foam donut pad. Watch out for common peroneal nerve compression by poorly positioned leg straps. It's not a good thing when a patient wakes up after a 4-hour breast reduction complaining of foot drop!
- The steep Trendelenburg position presents a myriad of issues to consider, but don't forget about the runaway patient. Periodically during the procedure make sure there is no sliding, to avoid catching the patient in your lap (Figure 48-1).
- Limit extremes. A laboring woman frequently hyperflexes her hips and knees (often at the direction of her obstetrician), which helps deliver the baby, but may lead to femoral or lateral femoral cutaneous nerve stretch and injury. Returning to neutral in between pushing episodes can save the patient from leg weakness, and you from the headache of defending your epidural as the suspected culprit.
- One trick we recently learned: when you have no choice but to put the BP cuff and IV on the same arm, run the IV tubing through the Velcro portion of the cuff. When the cuff inflates, it will compress the IV tubing and prevent backflow—amazing.

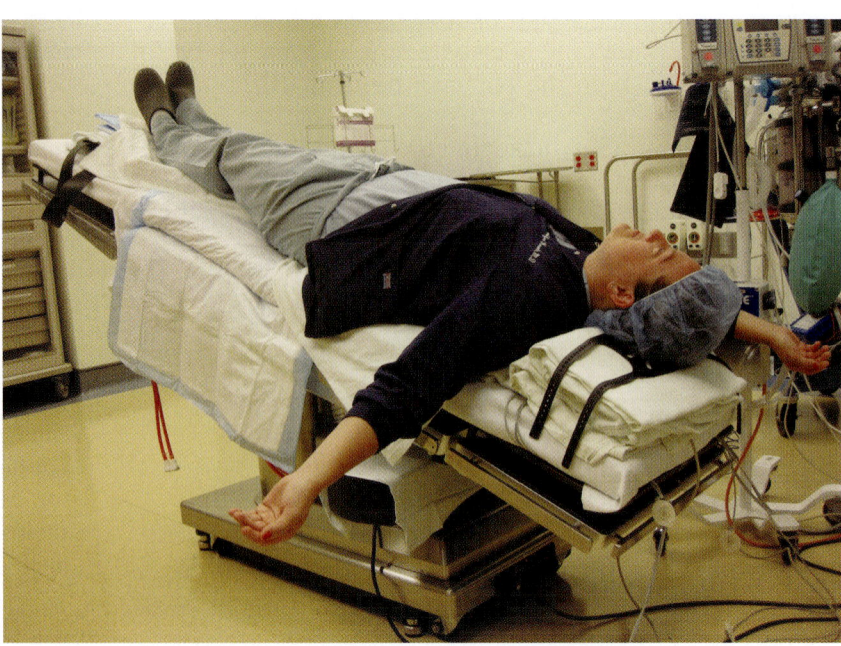

FIGURE 48-1 Steep Trendelenburg position with patient falling off bed.

SURVEILLANCE

When the first author started her residency, her attending told her that the only way she was going to kill a patient early on was by not monitoring the patient. Statements like that make an impression on CA-1s, and in a good way. Learning to monitor frequently and comprehensibly can save you from disaster. At least once a minute glance up from your OR record and train yourself to systematically go over the monitor: vitals, end-tidal carbon dioxide concentration (E_TCO_2), gas concentrations and flows, etc. Like driving, it will eventually become second nature.

- Your area behind the curtain is only one portion of the operating room environment. Surveillance must include the entire milieu: the machine, drug cart, personnel changes, the suction canisters, the lights, walls, floor, even the ceiling.
- Make sure any new additions to the OR staff—nurses, techs, neuromonitoring specialists, etc.—are aware of the plan for the case and any pertinent information about the patient's medical history.
- The monitor has sounds for a reason: to warn you when something *might* be amiss with your patient. If an alarm sounds for an SpO_2 of 74% and you see no wave form and the pulse oximeter is on the floor, consider it a better-safe-than-sorry scenario. If you can't hear over the OR soundtrack (whether it is nurses chatting, an attending surgeon yelling at the intern, or someone's iPod blaring), just turn up the alarms or pulse oximetry volume. A good rule of thumb is that you should always be able to hear your pulse ox over all other background noise in the room.
- Beware stealth IV fluid administration. If you open the fluids to flush in drugs, keep a hand on the control and then turn down the rate after sufficient time has passed. If you let go of the tubing, distractions abound, and before you realize what happened you turn around and an entire liter has emptied into the patient—and it's a renal patient. Oops.
- Take a peek at the floor every so often. Is there a large puddle of unidentifiable clear liquid? Check for leaking fluid warmer, overflow of irrigation from the surgical field, a disconnected IV that you assumed was actually delivering drugs and fluids to the patient (you know what happens when you assume…). Cover puddles with blankets or towels if there is no other cleanup option handy. No one wants a hazard for slipping, or a nidus for microshocks (don't touch anything electrical while dealing with your man-made lake).
- Speaking of fluids, also check the floor (and drapes/sheets on the bed) for blood. There can be hidden caches that are often missed when estimating blood loss (and you wondered why the patient was hypotensive). When you place an IV, make sure there is a heplock or tubing securely attached; unintentional blood-letting is frowned upon.
- One last point on fluids: look before you hang. Make sure the fluid you are administering is what you intended; 500 mL of mannitol can easily be mistaken for Hextend if you aren't careful (Figure 48-2).

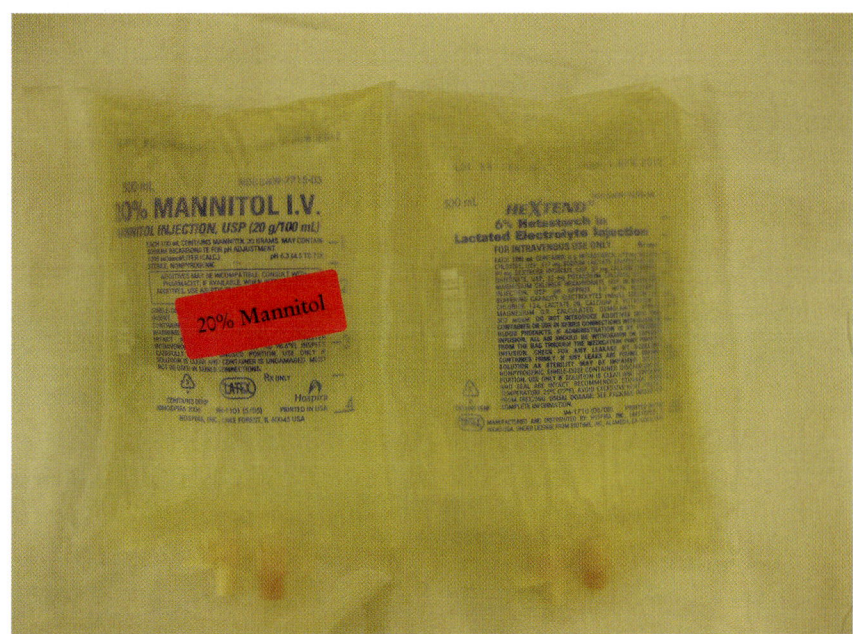

FIGURE 48-2 Hextend and mannitol bag comparison.

BODY MECHANICS

I'm not talking about the patient's body anymore; this section is for your benefit. Your lower back is going to take a beating during your career. Start taking care of it early to avoid a visit to your chronic pain colleagues later on.

- Start in preop by raising the bed to a comfortable height for pushing. There are no extra points for testing your hamstring flexibility as you maneuver down the hallway to the OR.
- When lifting patients, don't be a hero. Wait until enough help is available to safely transfer the patient from the cart to the OR bed and vice versa (and for goodness sake make sure BOTH beds are locked!). An extra 5 minutes waiting in the OR is a small price to pay for not testing the speed; your disability insurance can be processed.
- Make it a habit to investigate the chair situation as part of your morning setup. Don't settle for the cast-off stool with a broken height control; make sure to reserve one of the nice padded high-backed chairs. If you are going to be sitting for 4 hours, you need to be comfortable. Better yet, test the waters in your department about investing in massage chairs; it never hurts to ask.
- Be efficient in your movements and position. Face the chair toward the patient and monitor and look down to the chart or to use the computer. Even in a tenuous situation or emergency, efficient movements are important. No one benefits from flailing; that is how lines get pulled out and ventilators get disconnected. Move quickly and purposefully or get out of the way. And forget about the chart. Go back and catch up later.

MOVING THE PATIENT

When moving patients, you can rely on some of the basic good habits already mentioned above: plan things out, keep everything neutral, think about body mechanics.

- First take a step back. How big is the patient and how is the weight distributed? For large patients, get extra help. Extra people to lift and then position can save both your back and the patient, especially if they are anesthetized before the moving process starts. Make sure arms and legs are accounted for.
- If you can, get one of the devices made for moving patients on the cart (and under the patient) before you get into the OR. A hover-mat or similar device can be left under the patient during surgery and reused when the surgery is over.
- If the surgery requires lateral or prone position, check out the bed before moving. Are all the pads in a logical place? If the chest roll is 4 inches from the top of the bed, you are looking at a choke bar once the patient is face down; move it before flipping the patient. Make sure any bean bags are in place (and functional) before getting the patient lateral, and have your helpers hold the patient until they are inflated. If a subaxillary roll is in the cards, actually consider the size of the patient before it goes into place; one size does not fit all (Figure 48-3).
- Speaking of checking the bed, don't move the patient over until you make sure the head of the bed is actually where the head of the patient is going. Rotating 180 degrees under an anesthetized patient is just plain painful.
- The head and neck of a patient are deceptively difficult to control when flipping prone. The smoothest method we've found is to position the prone view *before* the flip. Intubate, put in the orogastric (OG) tube, temp probe, etc., and then weave those tubes through the gap in the foam of the prone view. Put the reflective base plate on with the tubes/lines coming out whichever side you eventually want them to be on. Put your right hand on top of the plate and the left hand under the head. When you flip, your right hand will be between the bed and the base and your left on top of the head. This method allows you to maintain a neutral C-spine and streamlines minor details like getting the patient hooked back up to the vent (Figure 48-4).
- Before moving, look for anything that could get yanked out of the patient if it is caught on the bed, the cart, or someone's foot, etc. This includes the endotracheal tube, IVs, A-lines, central lines, Foleys, and sequential compression devices (SCDs). Put items on the patient for transfer and disconnect where you can.
- Never move a patient with the endotracheal tube (ETT) still connected to the ventilator; a traumatic unexpected extubation is an unfortunate way to start your case or end your day.

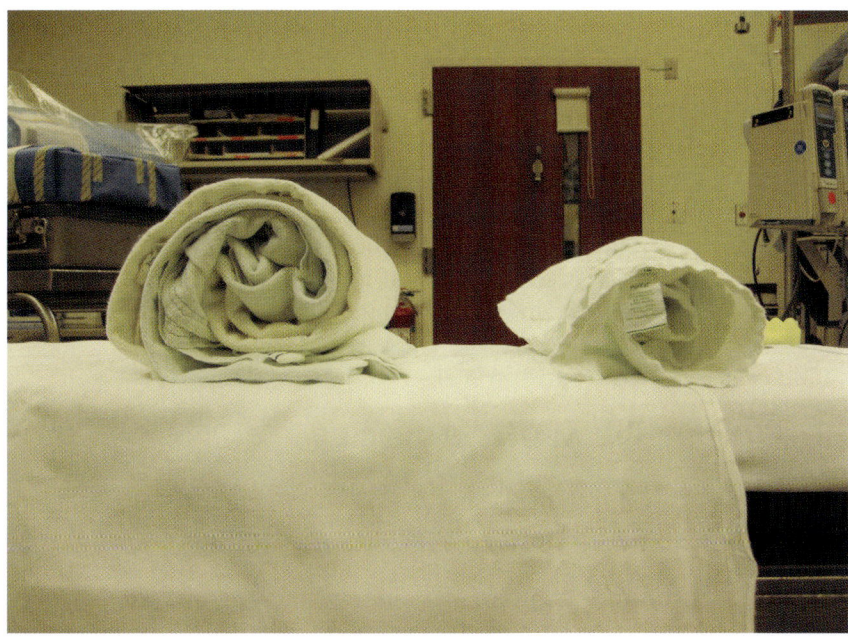

FIGURE 48-3 Comparison of chest rolls; the roll on the right is too small, but the roll on the left is a better size.

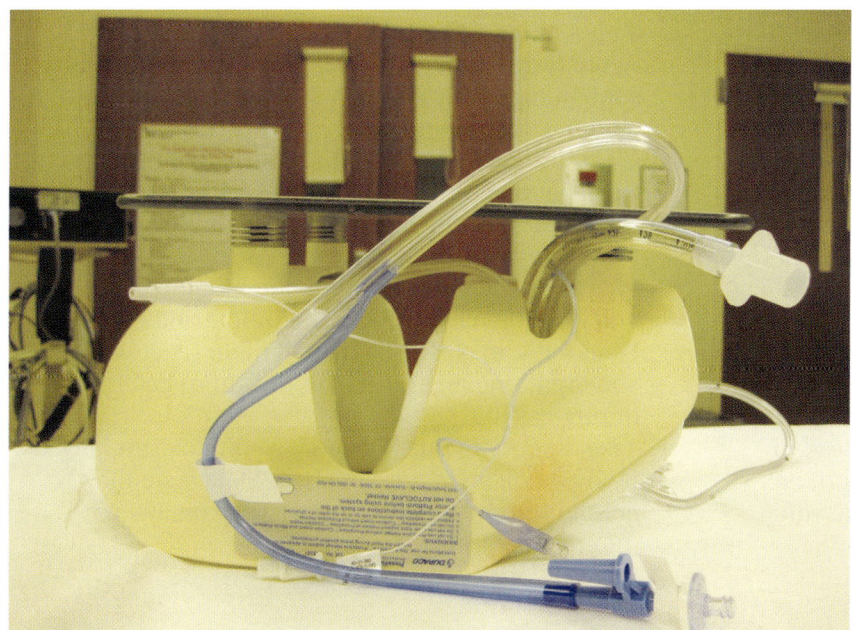

FIGURE 48-4 Mock-up of prone view with tubes positioned.

TRANSPORTING THE PATIENT

Again, this topic often gets an entire chapter because it's an important part of roomsmanship. So, briefly, here we go.

Depending on your final destination, transport can be a dangerous and stressful task. Even going down the hall to the PACU takes a few minutes and we all know how quickly patient status can change.

- Anything you would want immediately available for an emergency in the OR should be immediately available for transporting a patient to any location other than the recovery room. This includes airway equipment (new fully prepared ETT, laryngoscope and blade, oral airway, drugs for induction, muscle relaxation, hypo- and hypertension if applicable). Throw all that stuff in an extra unused suction canister (a great makeshift bucket) and keep it next to you. It's your ace in the hole when disaster strikes.
- Make sure there is a full O_2 tank on the bed if there is any possibility of administering supplemental O_2 on your journey. All those monitors you used during the procedure are still applicable during transport. Transfer the entire tram from your OR monitor to the portable monitor if possible to streamline the process. And don't forget your best monitor: you.
- If you need a ventilator after you transport, call ahead and make sure it is there waiting for you (ideally with a respiratory therapist). While you're at it, call ahead to the ICU and give the nurse vent settings; this makes you look good and saves time once you reach the ICU.
- Make friends with the anesthesia techs. If one is available to help out with transporting, life gets a lot easier. He can help set up monitors, move the patient, bag the patient, grab the elevator ahead of the bed, return things to the OR after transport, etc. And, in general, knowing the techs will make your OR time more pleasant.
- Even the cleanest, most organized setup of lines will get tangled during transport. There is no avoiding it. So, cut down on what you are taking. Disconnect extra IVs if they are heplocked. Remove temp probes and OG tubes if no longer needed.
- Don't be in too much of a rush. An unstable patient in the OR will still be unstable in the elevator, the hallway, or, God forbid, the ICU by way of the CT scanner. Wait to leave the OR until you are in control of hemodynamics (or at least at baseline for that patient).

LINE MAINTENANCE

Again, lines have a way of spontaneously tangling despite the best intentions. When you are dealing with multiple IVs, an A-line, central line(s), and, depending on the situation, an epidural, neuromonitoring leads, or a lumbar drain, all bets are off. The more organized you are, the easier your life in the OR will be.

- Label like your life depends on it. Make use of tape to label lines near stopcocks as well as near the drip chamber/flow control. Label any and all port sites that could be used for injection. Avoid the possibly catastrophic mistake of injecting something meant for an IV into an artery or the epidural space.
- Clean up slack; don't let your lines dangle on the floor. Tape lines and transducers to the bed or the Christmas tree. Loop long IV tubing and secure it with some clear tape (Figures 48-5 and 48-6).
- Plan ahead. If you know you are flipping prone and have the choice, place the A-line and extra IV in the arm closest to the OR table. That way you aren't moving lines over the entire body during the flip.
- Take a peek at your IVs every so often, especially if you are using a pressure bag. Make sure they aren't infiltrated before you try to cram 500 cc into the forearm.

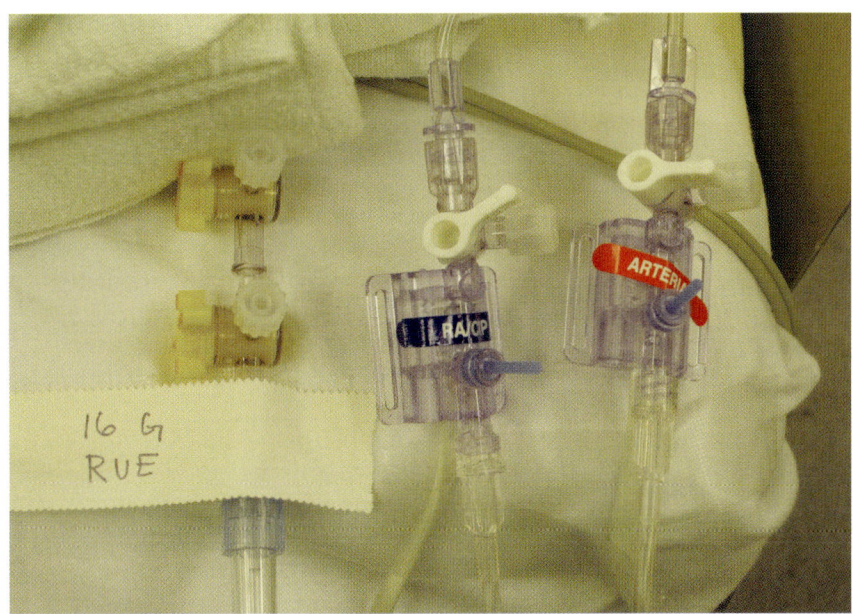

FIGURE 48-5 Labeled stopcocks.

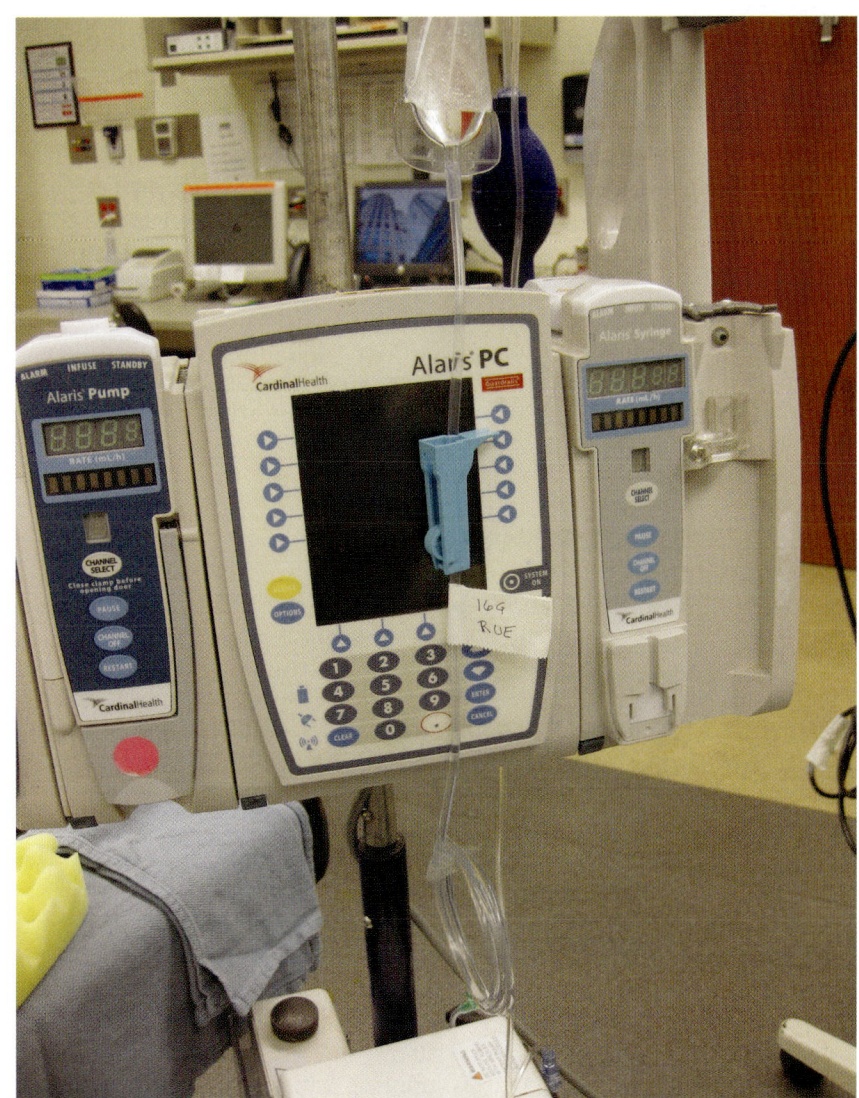

FIGURE 48-6 Line maintenance.

TROUBLESHOOTING THE MACHINE

Ninety-nine percent of the time the machine functions as designed. However, the other 1% requires quick thinking and systematic actions. Look for the horses, not the zebras; check the tube position, the cuff inflation, and the O_2 sensor, and make sure the CO_2 absorber isn't expired.

- When something malfunctions and the solution is not immediately obvious, focus on the most important thing: the patient. Hand bag if necessary, change to IV maintenance of anesthesia, and call in extra help (again, this is where having good anesthesia techs as well as reliable colleagues can make a world of difference).

SETTING UP THE RAPID TRANSFUSER

There are cases for which the rapid transfuser is part of your original game plan, but most of the time you are going to be using it (and setting it up) in a high-stress, rapidly evolving environment. Thus, it's crucial that, one, you understand how the machine works, and, two, you can quickly gather and assemble the individual components and start catching up to the waterfall of blood pouring out of your patient.

- There are different models of rapid transfers; familiarize yourself with the specific one at each hospital where you practice.
- Don't be afraid to get the rapid transfuser out early. You will have other things to occupy your time (and hands) while blood and other products are infusing: drawing blood gases, pushing epinephrine, chest compressions, etc.
- Before employing the rapid transfuser, make sure you have a functional large-bore IV or central line through which to infuse. Make sure all the stopcocks are open in the path of the rapid transfuser; a blood bath of a case doesn't have to turn into a blood bath for the entire OR.

PROFESSIONALISM

Don't take it lightly when your patient asks, "How are *you* doing this morning?" or "How did *you* sleep last night?" If you or a loved one were having the surgery, wouldn't you want a well-rested, attentive anesthesiologist in charge? Pay your patients the same courtesy. If you are expected in the OR at 7 AM, don't stay out until 2 AM at a bar. Get enough sleep, eat healthy, and exercise when you can. On the same note, if you are on home beeper call, be available, be sober, and make sure your cell phone is charged.

- When it comes to specialties, anesthesiologists by far have the easiest access to mind-altering drugs. Unfortunately, that accessibility has led to more than a few of our colleagues developing substance abuse problems. There may be better career choices for those of you with a tendency to indulge in recreational activities that give you cold sweats when faced with a urine drug test.
- Learn your fellow residents' names and the names of the surgical attendings. Avoid the typical "Hey, anesthesia" by introducing yourself at the start of each case or when you give a break or take over a procedure later in the day.
- Don't lie. Resist the temptation to shift the A-line transducer up or down as appropriate when the surgeon asks, "Is that the REAL blood pressure!!?!?!" for the tenth time in the hour. Fixing the number changes nothing about the clinical situation and benefits no one.
- If you don't have something nice to say, don't say anything at all. It's all too tempting to make a snide comment about the surgeons' skills at 2 AM when it has taken over an hour to obtain pneumoperitoneum and your attending calls into the room to find out what's taking so long. It won't make a slow surgeon get any better or faster.
- If you want to be treated with respect in the OR by our surgical colleagues, treat them likewise.
- Good communication goes both ways. If you want to be informed of what is happening in the surgical field, let the surgeons know if something is amiss on your end, and if there is anything you need them to do. Also, keep your attending up to date on any significant events, either anesthesia or surgery related.

DOCUMENTATION

All jokes about physician handwriting aside, if you can't read the record, it never happened. Invest in a good pen and start practicing your micrographia. Or if you've adopted the electronic medical record (EMR), familiarize yourself with the art of the free-text note (Figure 48-7).

- If you have nothing else ready for your first day, have a fine-point Sharpie marker in your pocket. It will be your best friend for labeling IV bags, syringes, and the premade labels for the syringes. This little secret of preparedness is amazingly useful (Figure 48-8).
- If you evaluate a patient, document it. If you check the eyes every 15 minutes during a prone procedure, make sure it is written somewhere on the record. If you evaluate a laboring patient for a fetal decel

or make a change in an epidural infusion rate, jot down a set of vitals and whatever happened while you were in the room. Make note of conversations with patients or patient families. If you draw up an emergency drug and leave it at bedside, write it down.
- Any meds or changes you make at the request of the surgeons should be recorded as such. Also note when you inform the surgeons of something.

Examples include blood-tinged urine in the Foley, decreased urinary output (UOP), lab values, and plans to administer blood products.
- Timing is critical. Be exact to the minute for drug administration, when you are called with critical lab values and when you intervene in response to a change in vitals, labs, or the clinical situation (this includes starting additional IVs, giving blood products, giving drugs, etc.).

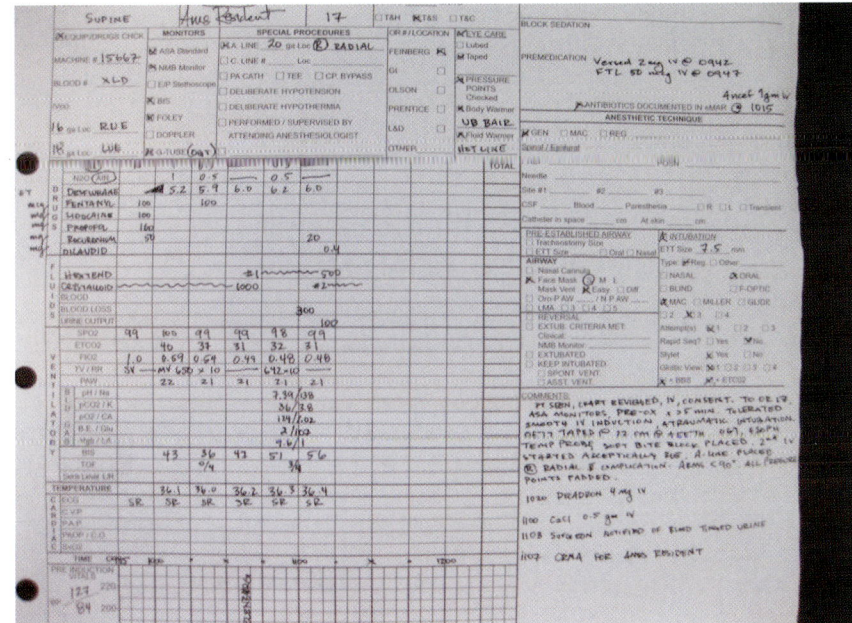

FIGURE 48-7 Neat anesthesia records.

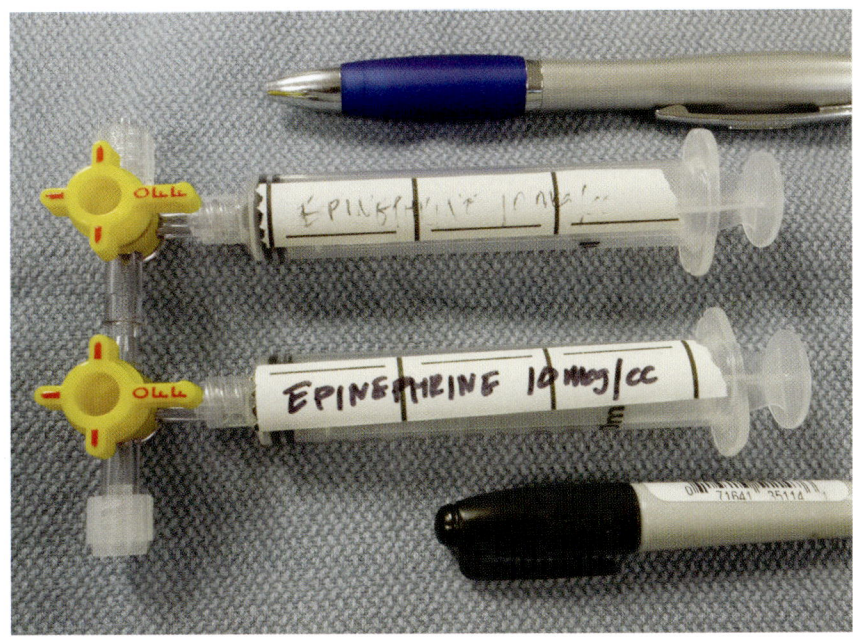

FIGURE 48-8 Pen versus Sharpie.

STORIES FROM THE OR

Drip, Drip

When the first author was a medical student, there was a previously uneventful cardiac case in which the surgeons and anesthesiologists watched helplessly as a few drips of liquid from an unnoticed ceiling pipe covered in condensation fell directly into the open chest cavity and sterile field. The procedure was completed after copious irrigation, and the patient had a relatively uneventful postoperative period involving multiple broad-spectrum antibiotics. One look up could have potentially avoided the panicky calls to risk management, patient family discussions, and concern for patient morbidity/mortality that ensued.

Boop!

When that fateful day arrives that you clamp the wrong line or leave a stopcock in the "off" position, the blood (or other products) will explode with a soft "Boop!" and the spray of blood around the room is virtually instantaneous, with everyone covered in blood and no one laughing.

The E_TCO_2 Is WHAT?

One day during a laparoscopic Roux-en-Y gastric bypass, the E_TCO_2 was slightly elevated at 37. It was brushed off as CO_2 absorption from the insufflation; the respiratory rate was increased and the value was ignored for a few minutes. A minute or two later the E_TCO_2 was in the 40s and climbing. Hand ventilating, changing the CO_2 absorbent, and further increases in respiratory rate and tidal volume (TV) provided little resistance to the ever-increasing E_TCO_2 (it peaked around 60). After entertaining the scariest scenarios (Malignant Hyperthermia [MH], thyroid storm) in the face of otherwise normal vitals, the providers finally examined the patient and found marked crepitus along the chest and neck bilaterally. A few minutes of 100% O_2 and desufflation was sufficient to bring the CO_2 back to normal range, and the case was completed uneventfully. So remember the basics (physical exam!) and the nature of the surgery when one of your monitor values just doesn't make sense.

Sabotaged!

During a liver transplant one of our fellow residents noticed that the patient's femoral A-line was no longer producing a wave form on his monitor. From the head of the bed he tried unsuccessfully to both draw back and flush the line. After several minutes of troubleshooting, he paged his attending with the update and went under the drapes to investigate. He traced the line toward its origin when he hit a roadblock: the Bookwalter retractor. A quick look down confirmed his suspicions that the surgeon clamped the arterial line to the bed and transected the tubing, leaving the remaining tubing as a conduit from the patient's femoral artery to the floor. The resident quickly stopped the bleeding and uneventfully replaced the tubing and completed the case, but a less diligent anesthesiologist may have seen an ugly case get even uglier. Never assume an equipment failure when a line or monitor suddenly and unexpectedly stops working.

Common sense is not so common.

Voltaire (1765)

SUGGESTED READING

Friztlen T. The AANA Foundation Closed Malpractice Claims Study on nerve injuries during anesthesia care. *AANA J.* 2003; 71(5):347–352.

Discussions of a group of certified registered nurse anesthetists from Minnesota about prevention of perioperative nerve injuries.

Howard SK, Gaba DM, Smith BE, et al. Simulation study of rested versus sleep-deprived anesthesiologist. *Anesthesiology.* 2003;98(6):1345–1355.

Two groups of anesthesia residents with staggered length of on-call shifts were compared in terms of psychomotor performance, mood, and subjective sleepiness. The group that started earlier had impaired performance and increased sleepiness vs. the group that started later.

Luck S. The alarming trend of substance abuse in anesthesia providers. *J Perianesth Nurs.* 2004;19(5):308–311.

This article discusses the trends of addiction in anesthesia providers, treatment options, and reentry into the clinical arena after rehabilitation.

Prielipp RC. Ulnar nerve injury and perioperative arm positioning. *Anesth Clin North Am.* 2002;20(3):351–365.

Good summary of contributing and preventative factors of this common injury.

Winfree CJ, Kline DG. Intraoperative positioning nerve injuries. *Surg Neurol.* 2005;63(1):5–18.

Description of common peripheral nerve injuries that occur despite preventative measures.

CHAPTER 49
POSITIONING 101

TEJAL MEHTA
CHRISTINE HUNTER

Thus in the highest position there is the least freedom of action.

Gaius Sallustius Crispus,
The War with Catteline (c. 40 B.C.)

INTRODUCTION

- Awake and noniatrogenically sleeping patients can adjust their position if they feel uncomfortable.
- Patients who are unconscious can't move, even in response to pain from an uncomfortable position.
- Therefore, positioning is key in preventing a pain in the neck (for you and for the patient).
- According to the American Society of Anesthesiologists (ASA) closed claims database, 15% of the cases involved nerve injury. Of these, 33% represented ulnar nerve injury, which was most frequent. Other less common sites included brachial plexus (23%) and lumbosacral nerve roots (16%).
- Even though nerve injury is a very serious complication of bad positioning, it is still possible to have a nerve injury despite the best of precautions. (No matter what a surgeon says, it's not always our fault!)

POSITIONS

Supine

- Respiratory/hemodynamic effects: These effects are fairly minimal; however, if there is a large abdominal mass present, aka pregnancy, then compression of the aorta/vena cava could result in decreased venous return to the right atrium and severe hypotension. This is best prevented by placing a "bump" behind the right flank to displace the uterus to the left and off the big vessels. Also, large abdominal girth and muscle relaxant can displace the diaphragm upward and eliminate chest wall muscle tone, causing lower lung volumes and atelectasis. Positive pressure ventilation can help negate these effects.
- Problematic IV sites: Most usual IV sites are acceptable.
- Nerves injured: Most common is the ulnar nerve, followed by the brachial plexus.
- Why? Most of the body is in neutral position including the head, trunk, and legs, but the arm position could change depending on surgical requirements, e.g., tucked, outstretched. Injury to the ulnar nerve is usually a result of direct pressure on the ulnar groove and spiral groove of the humerus. Extending the arms over 90 degrees at the shoulder could injure the brachial plexus by stretching it; even cycling a blood pressure cuff too often and too tight can cause this in a thin person.
- What can undergo necrosis if the procedure lasts a long time? The innervation sites of the ulnar nerve/brachial plexus could be affected with permanent nerve injury. Also, pressure on the heels or legs could result in ischemic injury to the affected area. This would be more pronounced in patients with peripheral vascular disease or preexisting neuropathy.
- How to prevent it? The arms should be outstretched less than 90 degrees and in supination. Elbow padding can decrease pressure on the ulnar groove, slight hip and knee flexion can reduce joint pain in these areas, and keeping the legs uncrossed and the heels padded can reduce the risk of ischemic injury. Also, keeping the head in neutral position (aligned with the spine) with an appropriately sized pillow can minimize risk of cervical spine/nerve injury as

well as focal alopecia. Eye tape is important in any position to avoid corneal abrasions. Protecting the face with a foam pillow is very useful in robotic surgery to avoid any of the robotic arms from hitting the patient's face from the other side of the drape.
- Common procedures where position is used: most laparoscopic surgeries, open abdominal surgeries, surgeries that involve the anterior portion of limbs, including knee replacements (Figures 49-1 to 49-5).

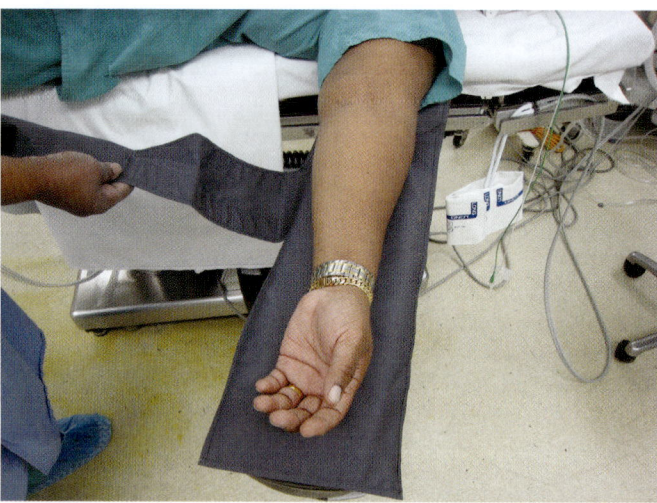

FIGURES 49-1 to 49-4 Arms should be less than 90 degrees, and proper padding at the elbows can reduce the risk of brachial plexus and ulnar nerve injuries. Look at this special strap: all in one with a Velcro strap (University of Medicine and Dentistry of New Jersey [UMDNJ], patent pending). The head should be neutral, supported by a soft pillow to prevent alopecia.

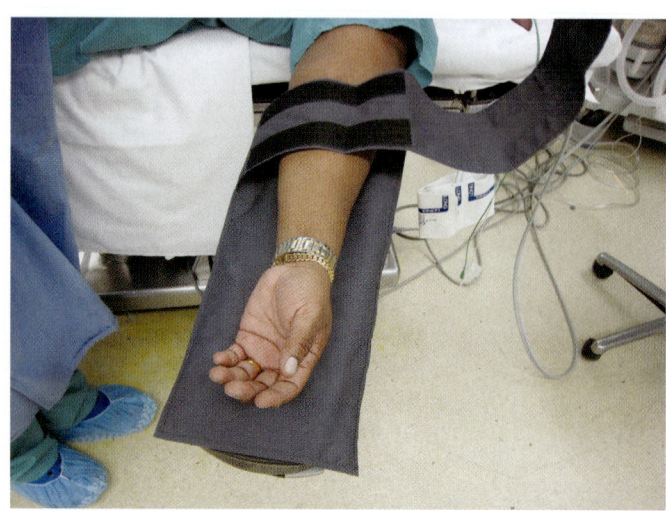

FIGURE 49-2

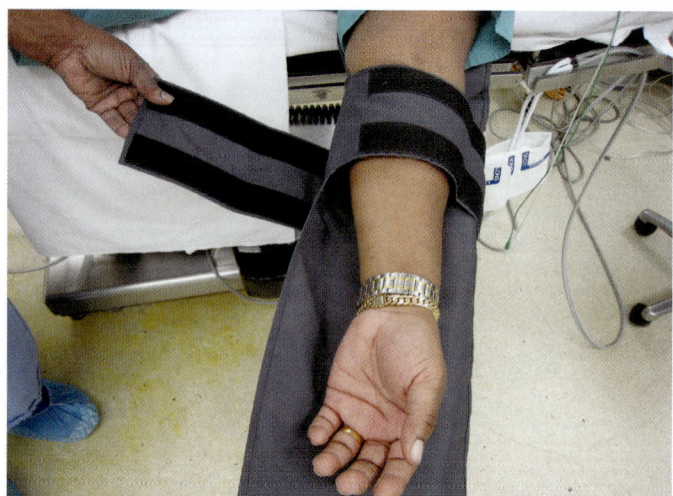

FIGURE 49-3

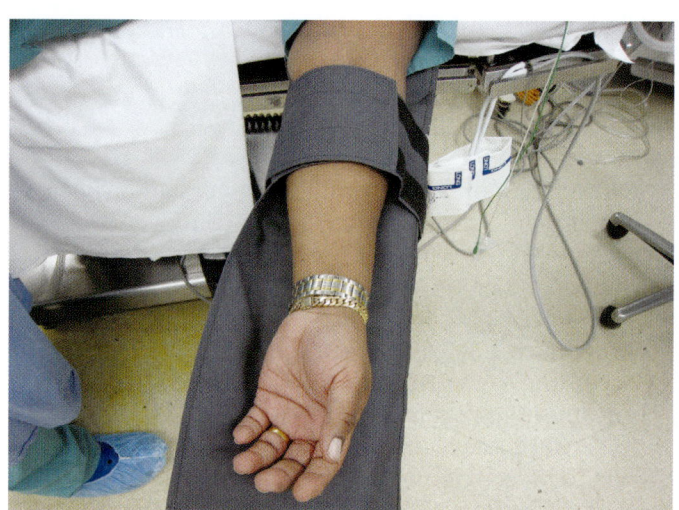

FIGURE 49-4

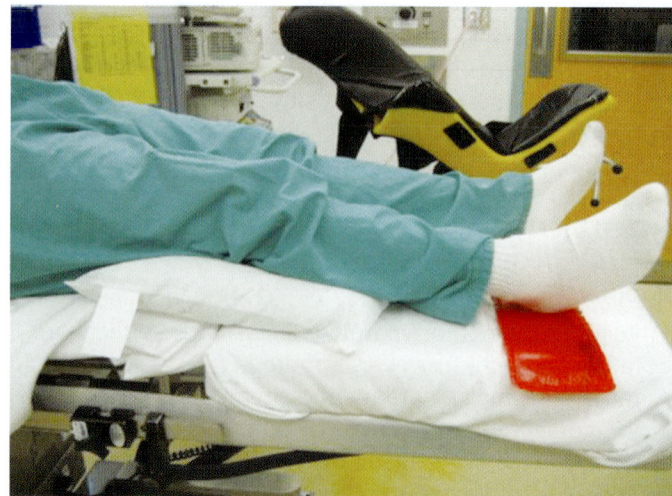

FIGURE 49-5 Side view of lithotomy position. Heels should be padded to prevent pressure ischemia, legs uncrossed, and knees slightly bent.

Prone

- Respiratory/hemodynamic effects: Similar in nature to the supine position, but with more pronounced displacement of the abdominal contents and diaphragm cephalad. Again, compression of the aorta and inferior vena cava can cause hypotension in the prone patient. Something to be extremely cautious of is that while turning a patient, the endotracheal tube (ETT) can get easily dislodged if traction is placed on the circuit. The best thing to do when turning is to disconnect the circuit just prior to the turn, and reconnect immediately upon positioning.
- Problematic IV sites: If the arms are outstretched and bent alongside the head, then IVs in the antecubitus (AC) may kink and not run. The best sites are the back of the hand or forearm. Sometimes the surgeons prefer tucking the patient's arms at the sides. Although this would allow IVs in the AC to run, one must be extra sure that the IV runs well once the patient is fully positioned. There would be no access to the IV site once the surgeon preps and drapes.
- Nerves injured: ulnar nerve, retina
- Why? Any pressure on the globe of the eye can increase intraocular pressure and occlude the central retinal artery, causing retinal ischemia and blindness. The ulnar nerve can still be compressed at the elbow.
- What can undergo necrosis if the procedure lasts a long time? The retina! If the head is in neutral position on a face pillow, pressure on the eye from the pillow itself can cause the ischemia. However, it has been shown that in prolonged surgeries, blindness can occur in association with acute blood loss, anemia, hypotension, and hypoxia, causing posterior ischemic optic neuropathy. Also, injury can occur to the ears, nose, and lips if direct pressure is applied to them. A hard oral airway placed in the mouth can occlude venous return from the tongue and cause macroglossia, obstructing the airway at the time of extubation. Facial edema is very common in the prone position, and limiting fluid administration can help minimize the airway obstruction that results. If the head is turned to one side or the other, neck pain can occur and compression of the jugular vein can impair venous return from the head, rarely causing thrombosis. Pressure injury can also happen at the inferior iliac spines, genitalia, and breasts/nipples if they are folded or have direct pressure on them.
- How to prevent it? Checking the face, at least every 15 minutes, is very important to make sure the eyes, nose, lips, and ears are free from pressure and unfolded. Elbows still need to be protected/padded to prevent ulnar injury. Breasts should be placed medially and cephalad, and care should be taken to ensure that the breasts and genitalia don't end up folded or pinched. Padding under the inferior iliac spine and rolls along the patient's sides that support the body from the shoulder to the iliac crest minimize pressure to the bony areas and help reduce venous compression by the abdomen. This also facilitates reducing the upward displacement of the diaphragm.
- Common procedures where position is used: back surgeries including laminectomies/diskectomies, any mass excisions from the back or posterior thighs, rectal/anal surgeries (positioning for this is slightly different, with the rear end up in the air and legs/head down like a jackknife, which puts more pressure at the midsection, with lessened venous return from the legs and increased pressure on the diaphragm; otherwise, it's very similar to the prone position) (Figures 49-6 and 49-7).

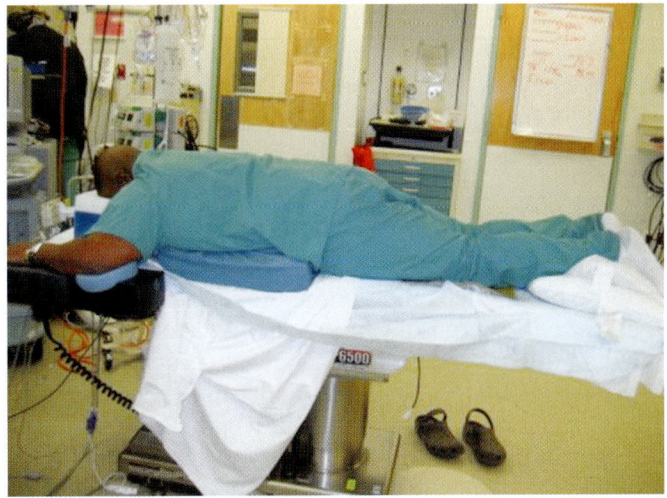

FIGURE 49-6 Prone. Bolsters should support the patient from the chest to the iliac crest, elbows padded, and knees padded and slightly flexed.

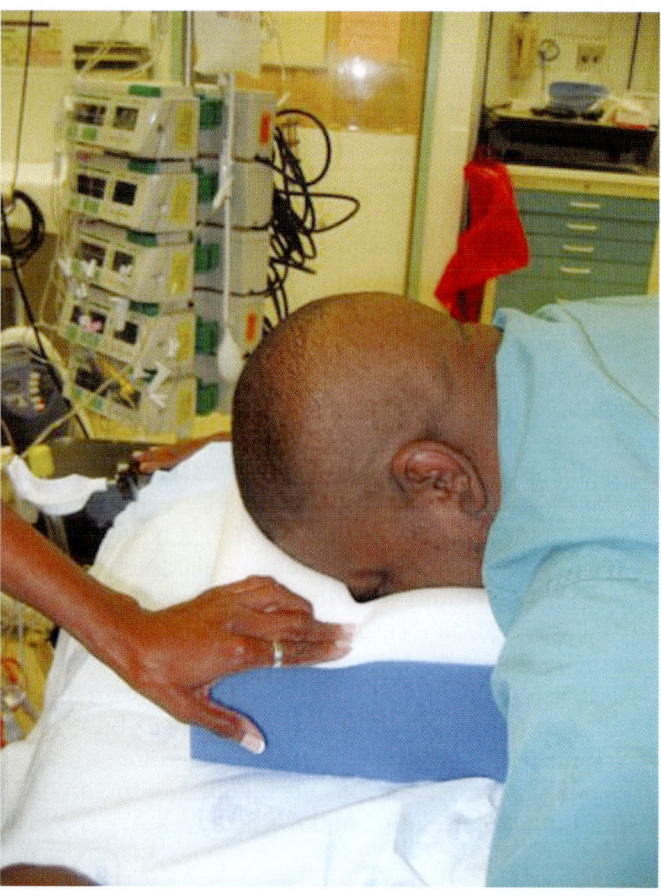

FIGURE 49-7 Head prone. Head should be neutral with eyes, nose, lips, all free from pressure.

Lateral Decubitus/Park Bench Position

- Respiratory/hemodynamic effects: These are even more pronounced than in the prone position. This is because there is a ventilation/perfusion mismatch when the dependent lung gets well perfused and poorly ventilated, while the upper lung gets well ventilated and poorly perfused. Hypotension can also occur in this position as a result of caval compression when the kidney rest is elevated.
- Problematic IV sites: femoral lines and neck lines can kink fairly easily, so it's important to make sure they are running well as soon as the patient is positioned. This is especially true in the park bench position because, although the body is lateral, the head is turned toward the ground. A neck line in the dependent side can be especially problematic. Infrequently, the upper arm may be bent and held up with a strap that can make IVs in the AC run poorly.
- Nerves injured: Mostly the brachial plexus, although the ulnar and saphenous nerves also can be affected.
- Why? The brachial plexus can be injured in a few different ways. One is if the head is turned too much to one side or the other, which can stretch the contralateral nerves. Another way is if the nondependent arm is too far outstretched with the board up in the axilla. A third way is if the chest roll is placed under the dependent axilla, which could directly compress the brachial plexus. The ulnar nerve again proves to be extra-sensitive (like my mother-in-law) if it gets compressed in the ulnar groove on the dependent arm. The saphenous nerve travels along the medial aspect of the knee and can get compressed if the two knees are kissing.
- What can undergo necrosis if the procedure lasts a long time? This depends on which part of the brachial plexus is affected. If the upper part is affected as in stretching at the neck, then potentially a "waiter's tip" deformity could result where the arm is extended, inwardly rotated, and hand flexed. Lower injuries that would occur at the axilla would affect the muscles of the hand and wrist.
- How to prevent it? The head needs to remain in a neutral position aligned with the spine. Eyes and ears should be free from pressure and unfolded. This is even more important in the park bench position as one eye may not be easily visualized. Since this position is used mainly when the head is out of reach, the head must be stabilized and the eyes/ears/nose free from pressure prior to the prep/drape. The arms are extended less than 90 degrees and placed on padded arm boards. The dependent arm should be in supination and the nondependent arm should be neutral with the axilla free. The dependent side should have a firm chest roll under it that elevates the chest and frees the axilla from pressure. Both legs should be flexed, with the dependent leg slightly behind the nondependent one and padding should be placed between the knees.
- Common procedures where position is used: hip replacements, thoracotomies (Figures 49-8, 49-9 and 49-10).

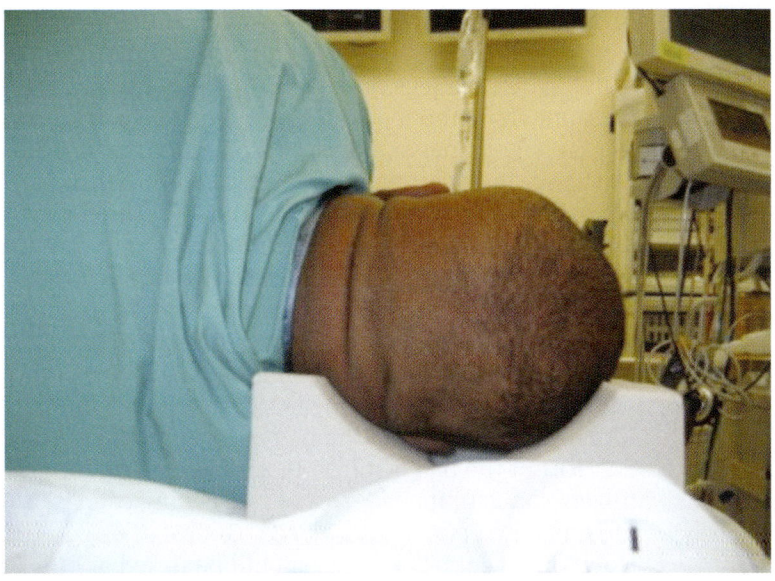

FIGURE 49-8 Head side view. Head neutral, ears unfolded, supported by a soft foam pillow.

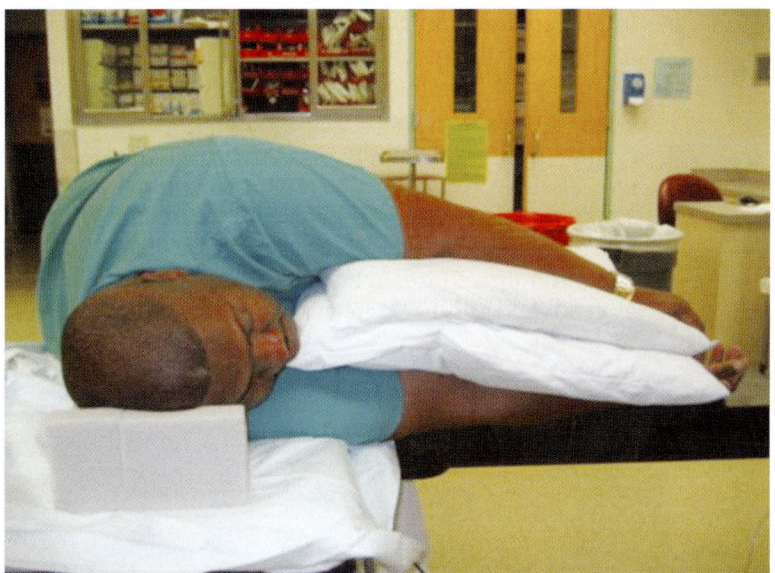

FIGURE 49-9 On side, with arms around pillow. Arms are less than 90 degrees, well padded to avoid any pressure point injuries or brachial/ulnar nerve injuries.

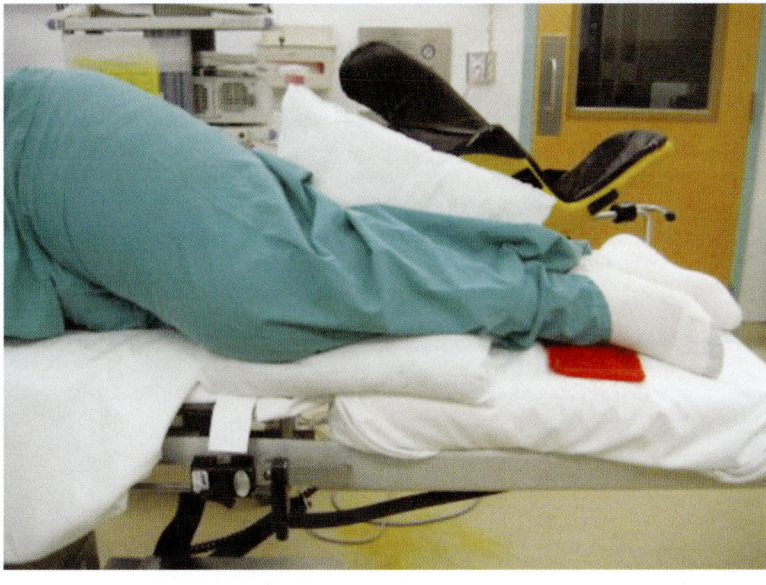

FIGURE 49-10 Legs padded on side. Knees need to be flexed with the upper leg in front of the other and a pillow placed between the knees.

Lithotomy

- Respiratory/hemodynamic effects: In this position, the patient is mostly supine with the legs up in stirrups. This enhances venous return from the legs, so hypertension could result once the legs are up. However, overzealous management of the high blood pressure during the procedure could cause hypotension at the end when the legs are brought back down and blood rushes to fill those vessels once again. Respiratory effects are similar to that in the supine position, unless the patient has a large panniculus that gets displaced upward when the legs are in position. This would push the diaphragm further cephalad, causing a decrease in lung volumes. This can even be seen during cardiac surgery when the legs are raised temporarily for the vein harvest preparation. A modification of this lithotomy position is used in Da Vinci prostatectomies where the patient is placed in the steep Trendelenburg position. According to Gallagher et al.,[1] this causes blood to rush cephalad, producing profound edema of the face, sclera, and airway. Extreme caution should be used when extubating these patients.
- Problematic IV sites: Usually the patient's arms are tucked at the sides or outstretched on arm boards, so upper extremities are fair game. Femoral central lines may kink once the legs come up.
- Nerves injured: As always, ulnar and brachial plexus are still possibilities. This time, the others mostly involve the legs including the sciatic, peroneal, and saphenous nerves.
- Why? When the legs are placed in the stirrups, pressure along the medial side of the knee can affect the saphenous nerve, pressure along the lateral side can affect the peroneal nerve, and if the hamstrings are overstretched, as with extra flexion at the hip, then the sciatic nerve can be injured.
- What can undergo necrosis if the procedure lasts a long time? Innervation sites of the above nerves could be affected, which include mostly the lower leg and foot areas. A devastating crush injury can occur if the patient's fingers have slipped in between the gap that forms when the foot of the bed is brought down. As this part of the bed is raised to a neutral position, the fingers can get pinched, sort of like getting caught in the hinge of a door as it's closed. Ouch!
- How to prevent it? The legs should be flexed at the hips and knees (no more than 90 degrees at the hips) to prevent stretching of the sciatic nerve. The rest of the legs, the medial and lateral sides of the knees/thighs, should be free from contact with the supports. Regardless, the supports should be padded in case contact occurs during the procedure. Patients who don't have padding of their own (thin body habitus), smokers, and those undergoing long surgeries are more prone to get neuropathies from this position.
- Common procedures where position is used: gynecologic and urologic surgeries (Figures 49-11 to 49-14).

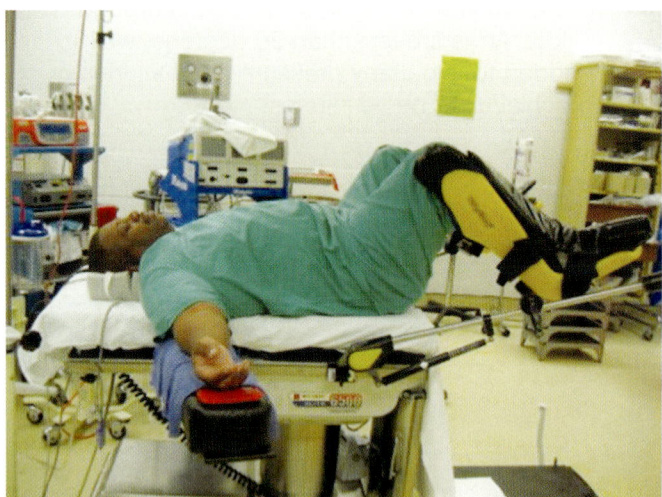

FIGURE 49-11 Side and front view of lithotomy position.

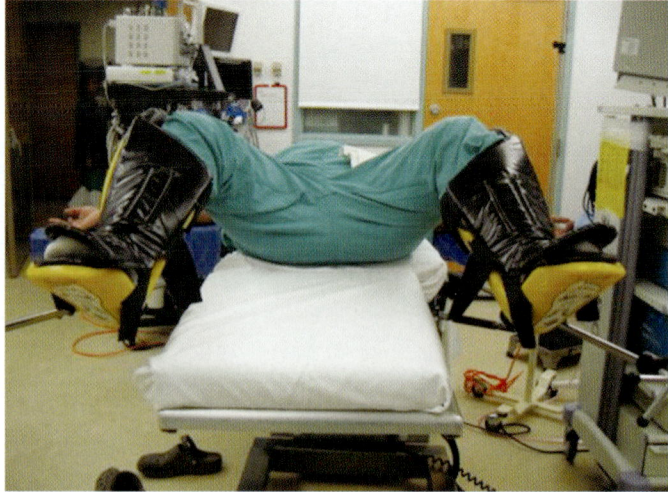

FIGURE 49-12 Hips and knees flexed less than 90 degrees to prevent sciatic stretch.

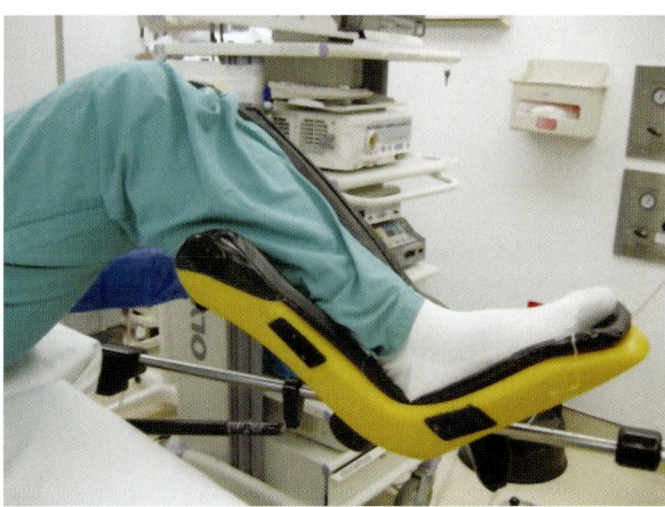

FIGURE 49-13 Lateral knee of one leg in litho. Medial and lateral knees free from pressure, heels padded, everything padded.

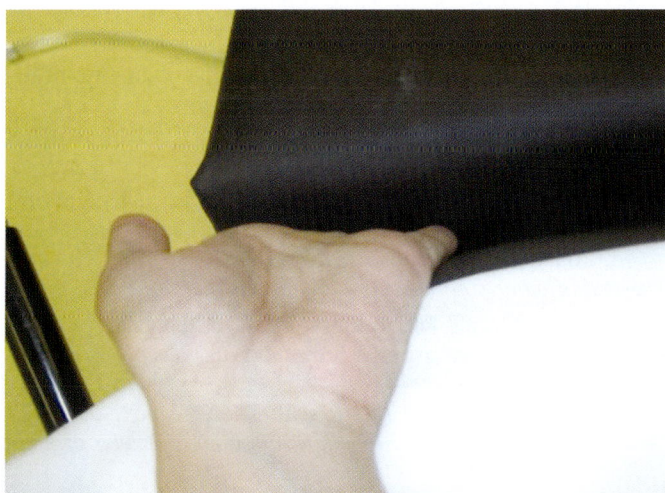

FIGURE 49-14 Can you hear the snap, crackle, and pop of the metacarpals?

Sitting/Beach Chair Position

- Respiratory/hemodynamic effects: This head-up position promotes hypotension by pooling blood away from the heart and head while at the same time minimizing blood loss and decreasing intracranial pressure. Respiratory physiology mimics that of a patient sitting or standing, with improved lung volumes secondary to abdominal contents remaining in the abdomen. While in the sitting position, the patient's back is 90 degrees to the floor, in the beach chair position the back is more like 30 to 45 degrees. You can imagine that the hemodynamics and lung physiology would be somewhere in between the sitting and supine positions, depending on the degree of the recline. Extreme head flexion can obstruct venous drainage from the tongue, pharynx, and palate, leading to airway edema and obstruction.
- Problematic IV sites: If arms are bent at the elbows, then antecubital IVs may not run.
- Nerves injured: ulnar, brachial plexus, sciatic, and brain!
- Why? Excessive stretch at the shoulders from the weight of the arms can injure the brachial plexus. This is not as much of an issue in the beach chair position since the arms are not hanging down at the sides. Supports used at the elbows for either position can put pressure on the ulnar nerve. The weight of the patient's entire torso is on the rear end, which can put pressure on the ischial spine and sciatic notch. Again, not as significant in the beach chair position since the weight of the torso is partially distributed to the back. *Warning:* Any intracardiac shunt that allows blood to go from the right side to the left side is an absolute contraindication to this position! Anytime the surgical site is above the heart, the patient is at risk for an air embolus. This is especially true in the sitting position. An air embolus can travel from the venous circulation directly across the shunt and up to the brain, causing a stroke. Severe hyper/hypotension, atherosclerotic disease, and severe cervical stenosis are all relative contraindications.
- What can undergo necrosis if the procedure lasts a long time? The innervation sites of the ulnar, brachial plexus, and sciatic nerves. The sciatic nerve supplies sensory innervation to much of the leg, as well as motor to the thigh, leg, and foot.
- How to prevent it? Padding at the elbows is very important, with care taken that it doesn't compress the ulnar nerve. Extreme flexion of the head should be avoided at all costs. The knees should be flexed and the buttocks padded to avoid sciatic stretch injuries. We would recommend placing a central catheter at the junction of the superior vena cava and the inferior vena cava to facilitate aspiration of venous air embolism should it occur. (Full detection and treatment guidelines are available elsewhere.[2])
- Common procedures where position is used: mainly for posterior fossa craniotomies (Figure 49-15).

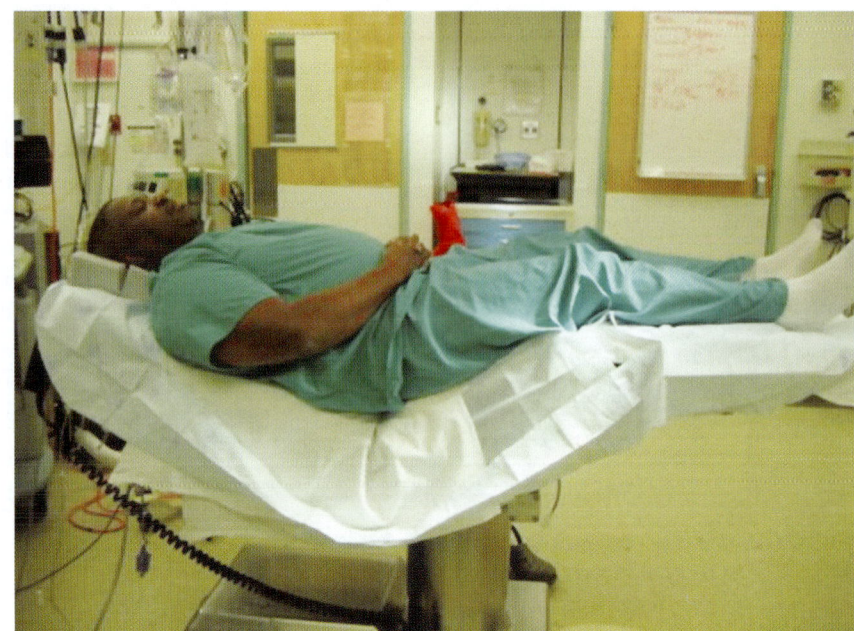

FIGURE 49-15 Ahh…the beach chair position.

CASE REPORT

A 52-year-old woman had a rhinoplasty done in the supine position that lasted approximately 3 hours. Care had been taken to pad the elbows and to make sure the arms were less than 90 degrees. The head was in neutral position on a foam pillow without any folding of the ears, the eyes were lubricated and taped by the surgeon, and the legs were uncrossed. When the patient woke up, she started complaining of pain in her heels. Upon examination, it was found that she had bilateral ulcers from improper padding. So far, no litigation process has been started, but it certainly could be. Remember to pad, pad, pad!

REFERENCES

1. Ginsberg S, Kraidin J, Chung P. The Da Vinci Code for Anesthesiologists, in Gallagher C, Lewis M, Schwengel D. *Core clinical competencies in anesthesiology*. New York: Cambridge University Press; 2010, p 203.
2. ASA Task Force on Prevention of Perioperative Peripheral Neuropathies. Practice advisory for the prevention of perioperative peripheral neuropathies. *Anesthesiology* 2000;92:1168–1182.
   The ASA writes their recommendations on how to position patients.

SUGGESTED READING

Cassorla L, Lee J-W. Patient positioning and anesthesia. Section IV: Anesthesia management. In: *Miller's anesthesia*, 7th ed. Oxford: Elsevier Science; 2010; pp 1151–1170.
Miller is the go-to book for nearly everything. This is no exception.

Gale T, Leslie K. Anesthesia for neurosurgery in the sitting position. *J Clin Neurosci* 2004;11(7):693–696.
This review article gives all the details you need to know about the sitting position.

Martin JT. The prone position: anesthesiologic considerations. In: Martin JT, ed. *Positioning in anesthesia and surgery*, 2nd ed. Philadelphia: WB Saunders; 1987.
The rest of what you need to know about the prone position.

Prielipp RC, Morell RC, Butterworth J. Ulnar nerve injury and perioperative arm positioning. *Anesthesiol Clin North America* 2002;20:589–603.
This article addresses all the do's and don'ts about the ulnar nerve. It also describes in detail the how and why of what happens.

Stambough JL, et al. Ophthalmologic complications associated with prone positioning in spine surgery. *J Am Acad Orthop Surg* 2007;15(3):156–165.
Blindness being the scariest of the neuropathies, this article describes it in detail.

Winfree CJ, Kline, DG. Intraoperative positioning nerve injuries. *Surg Neurol* 2005;63:5–18.
This article not only describes the potential mechanisms of injury to nerves, but also how to diagnose and treat the different possible nerve injuries.

CHAPTER 50
HANDOFF IN THE OR

LUKE S. THEILKEN

Because the monk is free, his state transcends all expression, predication, communication and knowledge.
Theravada Buddhists,
The Pali Canon (500 B.C.)

But we are not monks! We need to communicate.
Note: We have two chapters in a row on handoffs. This is on purpose, handoffs are *so* important.

INTRODUCTION: THE HANDOFF IN AVIATION

The condition or period in which control or surveillance of an aircraft is transferred from one control center to another is called the handoff. I recently heard a surgeon telling a patient that the "pilot" was canceling the procedure, as he frowned at me, so I figured this was appropriate.

The objective that I have for this short chapter is for you to feel comfortable with patient handoffs during shift/team change by learning a systematic approach to giving and receiving information in an organized fashion.

BACKGROUND

- Change of providers is commonplace in medicine, but the chance for error may be most extreme in an operating room or ICU setting. (Anesthesiologists/anesthetists may change several times during a prolonged procedure.) An analysis of sentinel events by the Joint Commission on National Patient Safety Goals found that poor or inadequate communication is a major source of up to 25% of all medical errors. Handoffs tend to be verbal, rushed, unstructured, and interrupted by the nature of the OR environment (Figures 50-1 and 50-2).

- Most importantly, very little structured time is dedicated to handoffs during anesthesia resident training.
- Most studies have looked at shift-to-shift handoff of multiple patients in a longer-term care setting (inpatients, ICU patients), and these handoffs tend to be somewhat cyclical. In contrast, anesthesiologists more typically perform a handoff on just one to three patients who are all undergoing current acute care. Once a handoff occurs, it's rather unlikely that the original anesthesiologist will resume care of the patient during the same operation.

MORE ABOUT HANDOFFS

- A *handoff* is defined as "the transfer of information (along with authority and responsibility) during transitions in care across the continuum; to include an opportunity to ask questions, clarify, and confirm." The primary objective of a handoff is to provide accurate information about a patient's care, treatment, current condition, and any recent or anticipated changes. The information communicated during a handoff must be accurate in order to meet patient safety goals.
- Many anesthesiologists feel that they have either given or received inappropriate handoffs during patient care in the operating room. This may include critical information such as allergies or airway issues on induction, but it may also be information related to the plan for emergence and postoperative care. Due to the number of complicated and lengthy procedures, as well as significant comorbidities in the patient population we see, it is critical to realize that patient care handoffs ensure continuity of care and to perform them in an organized and complete manner, preferably in the OR and face to face.
- Remember that handoffs are equally important for situations in which there is also a change of venue,

such as operating room to recovery room or ICU. Handoffs in these situations also frequently occur to other care providers, from physician to nurse, for example, or between physicians of different specialties.
- Risks of handoffs: We have all been given the handoff by a colleague that basically consists of something like "halfway through case, easy intubation, patient cruising," and then discovered that the patient is anemic, hypotensive, allergic to 20 medications, has an ejection fraction (EF) of 25%, etc. It is not fun to try to sort that out, and that is a dangerous situation for the patient. Of course this is an extreme example. A poor handoff could involve something as simple as an improperly positioned arm or a Bair hugger that was never turned on. Poor handoffs can result in duplication of tasks, the loss of key information, and misunderstandings of all kinds.
- Benefits of handoffs: On the flip side, good handoffs represent an opportunity to review the patient's course with a fresh perspective. By offering your incoming colleague the opportunity to ask questions (or by asking questions yourself when you take over a case), good things can happen. New information can come to light. Potential errors can be detected. Prior management decisions can be reassessed and confirmed or modified. So the patient is diabetic and had a blood sugar of 70 earlier today and has been progressively hypotensive despite an adequate hemoglobin? Oh that's right, we haven't checked a blood sugar in a while.

SOLUTION

- Currently, there are no national or American Society of Anesthesiologists (ASA)-sanctioned guidelines that relate to the patient handoff, but certainly there is important work being developed in this arena.
- When I accept a handoff, I like to go into the operating room with the person signing out to me so that I can get an overall picture of how the patient was preoperatively, as if I were the person who interviewed the patient. I ask the primary anesthesiologist the same questions I would ask the patient. I view the induction, intubation, and line placement, and I go through the anesthetic record up to the current time. I discuss any relevant postoperative plans for the patient, including emergence and disposition. This makes it easier to take over the 14-hour spine case at hour 12! (Figure 50-3)
- Try to find a few minutes of time where you will be interrupted by a minimum of distractions. If so much is going on that this is impossible, you should seriously consider whether this is an appropriate, and safe, time for a handoff to occur!
- The timing of the handoff should be reasonable. When it's late and you still have reading to do for a lecture tomorrow, it's tempting to handoff the case to a colleague, even as the last few sutures are being placed. Whether it was a 20-minute carpal tunnel release or a 3-hour colectomy, think about whether your incoming relief will have adequate time to get acclimated in order to take good care of the patient.
- We currently use a system known as I-SBAR that can be applied for handoff to residents, certified registered nurse anesthetists (CRNAs), or attendings relieving for breaks, lunch, or at the end of the day. The acronym I-SBAR stands for *I*ntroduction, *S*ituation, *B*ackground, *A*ssessment, *R*ecommendation.
- This system may be most adaptable to the perioperative period. It is important to note that hand-offs should be done consistently, in as controlled an environment as possible, and with ample time for questions as well as feedback. Studies have shown that the most consistent transfers of information have been in a combination of written and verbal form.
- When providing a handoff as the patient transitions to postoperative care, remember to include both your resident or attending colleague as well as the nurses. Ideally, this would occur with everyone present at once (Figures 50-4 and 50-5).
- In general, people seem to forget the "Recommendation" component of the I-SBAR for fear of not wanting to tread on a colleague's toes. Nevertheless, don't leave it out. Recommendations are just that, they aren't commands. If you found that the blood pressure responded more readily to crystalloids at the beginning of the case compared to the end, definitely let your colleague know that. Offer your thoughts about whether you think continuing fluids would be good versus whether and why you think you're reaching the limits. At the very least, it gives your colleague a starting point from which to develop his or her own strategy.

WHAT INFORMATION NEEDS TO GO IN A HANDOFF?

- Introduce yourself if you don't know the person to whom you are giving report.
- Patient information:
  - Name
  - Age

- Type of surgical procedure and indication
- Allergies
- Outpatient medications
- Past medical and surgical history
- Pertinent physical exam findings, including preoperative vitals and weight
- Pertinent labs, ECG findings, other tests/studies: echo, cath, stress test, etc.
- Airway exam
- Intraoperative events:
  - Premedication given
  - Antibiotics given (and need for re-dosing of said antibiotics!)
  - Type of anesthetic: general anesthesia (GA), monitored anesthesia care (MAC), regional combined with GA or MAC
  - Type of induction and agents used
  - Ease of mask ventilation: use of oral airway?
  - Intubation: blade used, grade of view, any difficulties
  - IV access, A-line, central line
  - Other monitoring: somatosensory evoked potentials, motor evoked potentials
  - Range of BP and HR; medications given and result
  - Significant events related to surgical procedure: difficulties, surgical plan, special requests from surgeon, upcoming changes/expectations
  - Estimated blood loss, urinary output
  - Blood products given or available (know the type and screen/cross status!)
  - Amount of narcotics used
  - Plan for reversal and extubation
  - Disposition of patient from OR: PACU, ASU, ICU
- Miscellaneous
  - Anesthesia attending for the case
  - Amount of drugs that were signed out and what needs to be returned to pharmacy. (It's a terrible sinking feeling to be tallying the totals at the end of a case and find a discrepancy. And the pharmacy will be not be excited about this either.)
  - Whether or not orders have been entered for PACU
  - If there are more cases to follow and if drugs have been prepared
- Introduce person taking over to the OR team

This may seem like a long list, but in reality it only takes a few minutes to stand in the operating room and discuss these key points face to face. And those few minutes can really make your life easier.

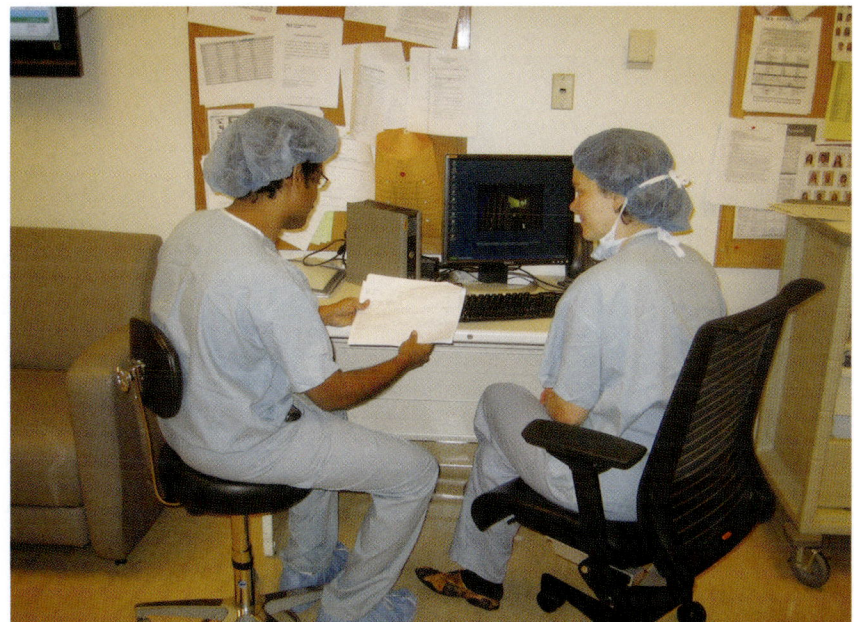

FIGURE 50-1 An example of a handoff, while using written notes and face to face. It is not in the OR and therefore leaves the team vulnerable to errors.

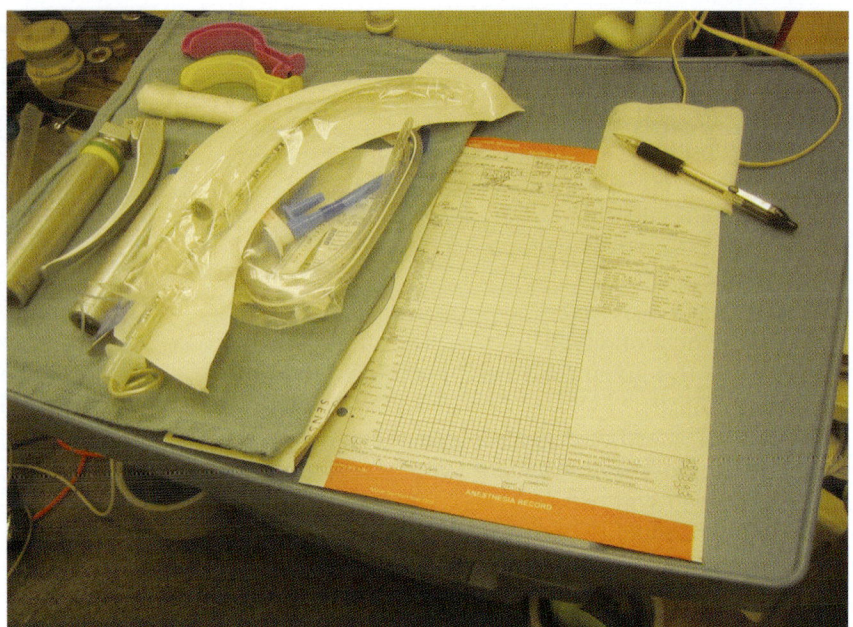

FIGURE 50-2 The patient has just been induced. While the attending has signed the chart, the record is not up to date. Always leave plenty of time for charting to be completed so there is nothing missed!

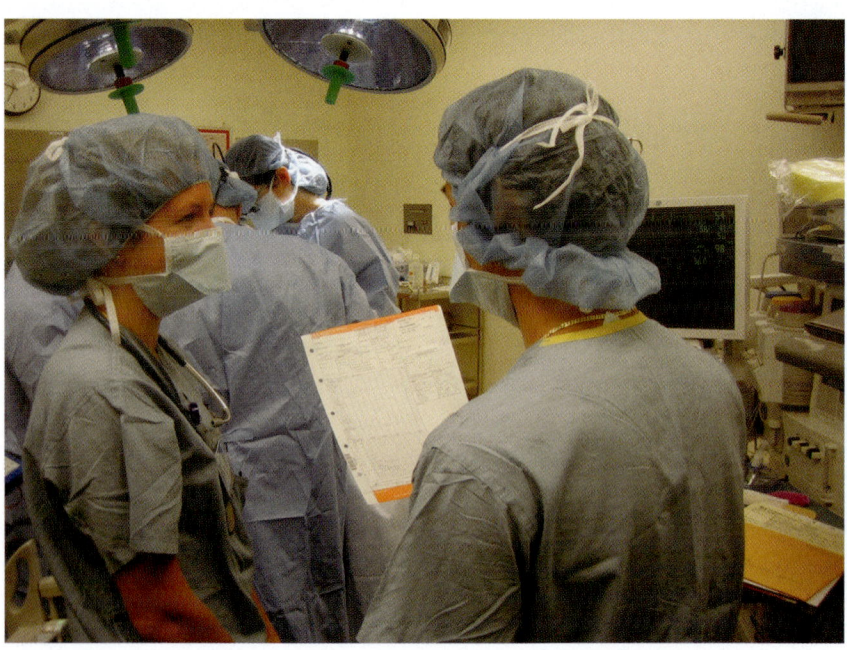

FIGURE 50-3 The handoff here is face to face and in the OR. The record is used as a cue, and the patient's chart is available to help answer any questions. The surgical team in the background is aware of the change of personnel.

Chapter 50 HANDOFF IN THE OR

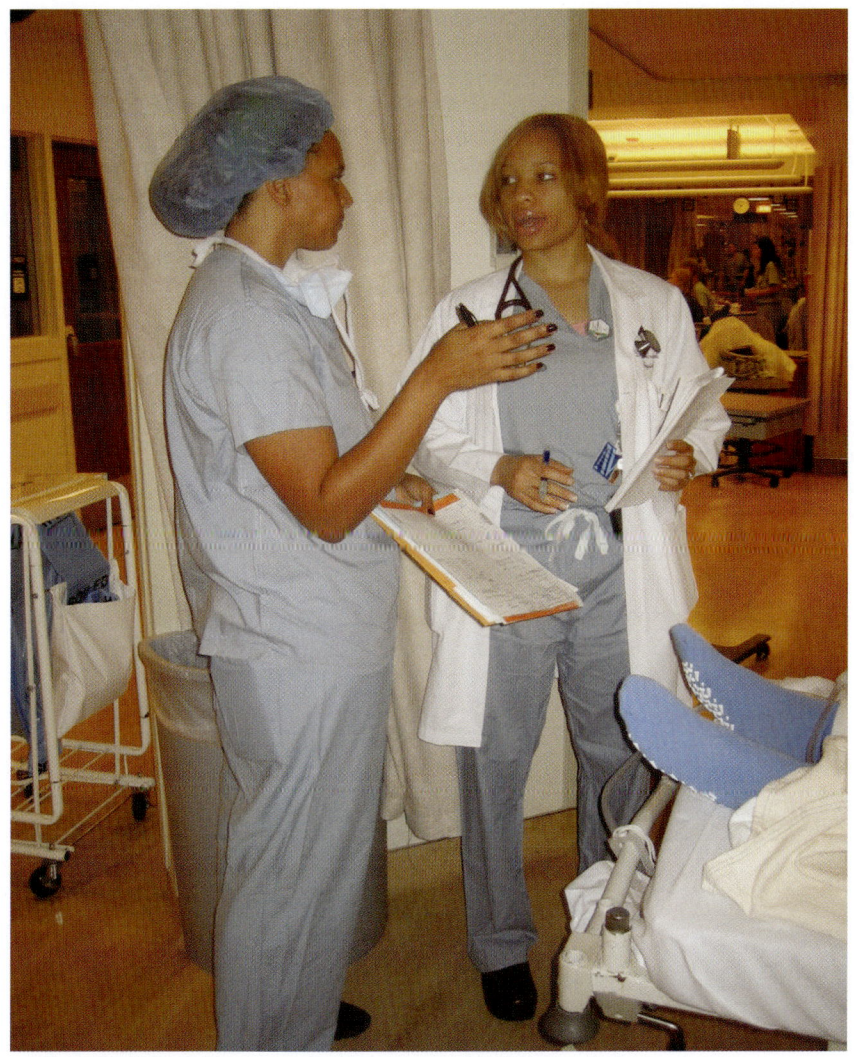

FIGURE 50-4 This picture is an example of resident handoff in the PACU at the end of the case. Again, the record is used as a cue to discuss all pertinent history as well as intraoperative events, current needs, and the to-do list, and disposition of the patient (seen here with blue socks).

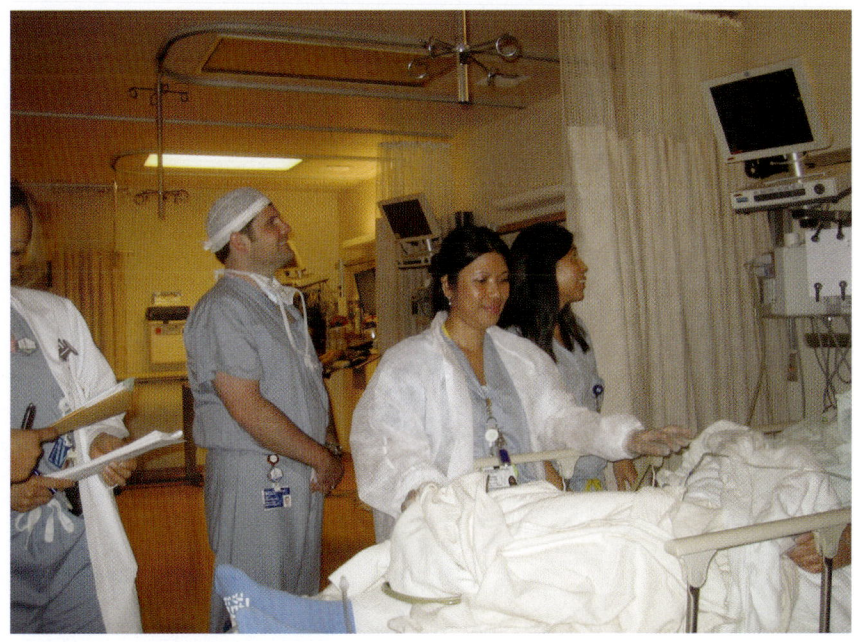

FIGURE 50-5 In the recovery room, the attending anesthesiologist, residents, PACU nurses, and the patient are seen here, all on the same page, happy with the outcome of the case.

SUGGESTED READING

Joint Commission on National Patient Safety Goals. http://www.jointcommission.org/standards_information/standards.aspx.
Standardizing handoffs remains a priority. The Joint Commission on National Patient Safety Goals contains specific guidelines for the handoff process, many drawn from other high-risk industries, and includes interactive communications, up-to-date and accurate information, limited interruptions, a process for verification, and an opportunity to review any relevant historical data.

Keyes C. Coordination of care provision: the role of the "handoff." *Int J Qual Health Care* 2000;12:519.
A short case report that details the unfortunate chain of events that had devastating consequences when information was not exchanged between providers. Everyone has heard of this type of situation. It demonstrates the need for coordination of case, as well as follow-up.

Patterson ES, Roth EM, Woods DD, Chow R, Gomes JO. Handoff strategies in settings with high consequences for failure: lessons for health care operations. *Int J Qual Health Care* 2004;16(2):125–132.
Compares handoff strategies, or what constitutes the handoff, in areas where mistakes may have devastating consequences. The authors completed an observational analysis of 21 handoff strategies in four different high-impact settings: NASA, nuclear power plant, railroad dispatch, and ambulance dispatch. Learning from what constitutes an effective handoff in these settings can be applicable to the safe care of patients in the hospital.

Patterson ES, Wears RL. Patient handoffs: standardized and reliable measurement tools remain elusive. *Jt Comm J Qual Patient Saf* 2010;36(2):52–61.
This article discusses the difficulty in standardizing what makes a handoff, and how to evaluate the handoff. It outlines seven primary functions of handoffs with specific interventions or improvements. The authors point out that the diversity in handoff measurements is due to the lack of consensus of what function the handoff serves and what information it should include.

CHAPTER 51

DON'T DROP THE BALL: A STANDARDIZED HANDOFF

JANA JANCO
MARGIT KAUFMAN
STEVEN H. GINSBERG
JONATHAN KRAIDIN

The single biggest problem in communication is the illusion that it has taken place.

George Bernard Shaw

Editors' note: We have included two chapters in a row linked to handoffs. This is such an important issue in anesthesia that it merits the emphasis.

INTRODUCTION

While many ORs are kept dark for cases, anesthesiologists don't like to be in the dark about their patients. So when time comes for your fellow anesthesiologist to relieve you so you can rush out to the gym or local watering hole, don't forget to give an appropriate sign out. The Institute of Medicine reported that 44,000 to 98,000 patients die in U.S. hospitals each year because of medical errors, with errors occurring during transitions of patient care being frequently cited as problematic.

While it's easy to say "lap. chole., will be done soon," most coworkers will need more information to treat the patient appropriately. It is not only fellow anesthesiologists who want to be "in the know," but also the postanesthesia care unit (PACU) and intensive care unit (ICU) nurses who take over from you. So go ahead, find your inner chatterbox, and spill the beans.

TALKING THE TALK INTRAOPERATIVELY

- Just start at the beginning: How old is the patient (big difference between a 90-year-old and a 9-month-old), male or female (sometimes hard to tell under all those drapes), and what procedure is your friendly surgeon performing today.
- Let's dig a little deeper: Did the patient have any previous medical problems? Let your colleague know about important medical problems such as coronary artery disease, diabetes, etc. Why did you write that they are an ASA IV?
- Abnormal labs (that K+ of 6.0 is under control, right?) and allergies all get mentioned.
- How did induction go? Can you ventilate this patient? How was the intubation? Did you call for the difficult airway equipment or could you see the patient's epiglottis from across the room? What size tube do you have in there and where is it taped? What are your ventilator settings?
- What medications were given? Are you using a lot of emergency drugs or does your record have train tracks for blood pressure and heart rate? Does the

patient need antiemetics, or when do I need to give more antibiotics?
- Add it all Up: Grab your calculator—what are your totals? Did you really give 10 L of saline? How much blood is in the bucket? Are you labeling the bags when you hang them? Is each IV numbered separately or can you trust just one numbering system? How much urine, and should it really be red? Don't forget how much fluid; for example, the cardiologist infused during an ablation.
- Do it together; check it out together. Is the endotracheal tube in the correct position? How many twitches does the patient have? Is the patient going to be paralyzed for the next week? What IV access is there? Is it working or is there a puddle of saline on the floor? Size and location are important. Is my main IV antecubital and the patient in the lateral decubitus with that arm bent? Are all the monitors OK, or is the pulse oximetry reading the O_2 saturation in the room instead of the patient's finger? Are all the pressure points padded, or does the surgical resident have his elbow in your patient's eye socket? If the patient is lucky enough to have a regional block, how high does it go (hopefully not C1)?
- Don't forget the little or big things, such as how are you keeping this patient warm? If they hit the aorta during surgery, is there blood available?
- What are the extubation plans? Are they ready to close? What will you need for transport? Did you preorder that vent you need in PACU?
- Did you remember to introduce yourself to the surgeon and circulator when taking over to avoid the usual "hey anesthesia?"
- Clean up; leave everything neat and clean before you leave the room. Remember your roomsmanship.

It's helpful if your department creates a standardized way of handing off information, but if it doesn't exist create one for yourself and stick to it. The Joint Commission on Accreditation of Healthcare Organizations (JCAHO) has come up with the rather forgettable acronym SBAR: *S*ituation, *B*ackground, *A*ssessment, *R*ecommendation.

WE MADE IT TO RECOVERY!

Everything your anesthesia colleague wants to know, the PACU staff wants to know.
- Give the basics: Age, gender, and what procedure just took place.
- Tell them why you are so great: What type of anesthesia did you do? Was it a quick monitored anesthesia care (MAC) case, or has this been a 20-hour marathon general anesthesia case?
- Heads up: Any problems with the airway? Did you show your skills as an airway expert, or was this the hardest intubation ever?
- "I can't feel my feet": Does your patient have a regional block, catheter in place, or paralyzed after we lost the motor evoked signals?
- "Houston, we have a problem": What other medical problems does this patient have? Is he on 10 L of oxygen at home? Is he diabetic and you were pushing insulin all day? Then maybe we should check a blood glucose. Is this a dialysis patient? Can we put the blood pressure cuff on the arm with the fistula?
- "I feel a little itchy": Does the patient have any allergies?
- "Wow, all your patients come out pain free." How much pain meds did you give in the OR? What other medications were given (antiemetics, antibiotics)?
- "Can I have your numbers?" What were your totals for intravenous fluids (IVFs), blood products, estimated blood loss, urine?
- Don't hold back now. Any other issues that you are dying to tell the nurse: temperature, intraop problems, the latest discussion about last night's show on TV?
- "Can I go home yet?" What pain meds or antiemetics can the patient have if he or she feels miserable? Is there anything the patient needs to do before being discharged?
- Did you give blood and do you have any labs that you have drawn and are awaiting results? Should I call?
- Did the patient ambulate preop? Is the patient going home today?

THE RECOVERY ROOM HANDOFF

Handoff Communication: Patient Care Endorsing in the PACU

- ☐ Patient age/gender
- ☐ Language barriers
- ☐ Type of operation
- ☐ Type of anesthesia: endotracheal tube (ETT), laryngeal mask airway (LMA), mask
  - ☐ Any airway concerns?
  - ☐ Still intubated? Plan?
- ☐ Check level of regional block
  - ☐ When was it was dosed?
- ☐ Past medical history
- ☐ Go over any blood products given or pending
- ☐ Any intraop lab results?
- ☐ Any labs pending?
- ☐ Any blood sugar issues?
- ☐ IVF administered:
- ☐ IV sites (gauge, location):
- ☐ Urine output:
- ☐ Estimated blood loss (EBL)
- ☐ Intraop problems or issues:
  Did the patient require O_2 preop? ☐ Yes ☐ No
  Is this a dialysis patient? ☐ Yes ☐ No
  If yes, when was the dialysis?
- ☐ Any allergies?
- ☐ Medications that the patient takes
- ☐ When you last gave which antibiotics

Operating Room

Issues related to hemodynamics:
- ☐ What narcotics did you give? _____
- ☐ Which antiemetic did you give? _____
- ☐ Report your plans for analgesia:
- ☐ If regional technique, call pain service.

If there are no other cases in your room, then go back and straighten up the room and check in with the physician in charge.

TALKING THE TALK: "WE HAVE GOT A SICK ONE FOR THE SURGICAL INTENSIVE CARE UNIT (SICU)"

Sometimes you will take the patient straight to the ICU from the OR, and these nurses are going to want just as complete of a rundown as did the PACU staff.

- Give all the basic information that you gave the PACU nurse but also much more.
- Why are there 14 bags on your pole? What drips is your patient on? Is epinephrine really up that high? What are the concentrations of the medications?
- A little extra hardware: Did this patient come back with some extra equipment such as pacemakers, balloon pumps, left ventricle assist device (LVAD) machines, or did the patient lose some things along the way (like a spleen or a kidney)?
- How are we keeping the intubated patient comfortable? And why did we not extubate?
- Did you give blood and do you have any labs that you have drawn and are awaiting results?
- "Oh, I forgot to mention: the patient speaks only Russian!"
- Did I just give a stick of paralytic and forget to tell the nurses?
- Do you want to mention that you have been giving Neo boluses during transport?

Everyone likes to be "in the know," so keep it coming; your coworkers and your patients will be much happier (and you can feel better while you are lying poolside relaxing).

THIS IS OUR CARDIAC ICU HANDOFF

CARDIAC SURGERY

Handoff Communication

Date:

OR Phone Report

Procedure
__CABG X
__Off Pump
__AVR
__MVR
__Minimally Invasive
__Aneurysm Repair
__Transplant

Surgeon: _____
Anesthesiologist: _____

Height:
Weight:
Allergies:

☐ On ☐ Off Pacer
☐ Balloon Pump
☐ LVAD
☐ RVAD
☐ BIVAD
☐ Impella

Drips:
___Amicar
___Milrinone
___Norepinephrine
___Epinephrine
___Insulin
___Nitroglycerine
___Clevidipine Butyrate (Cleviprex®)
___Vasopressin
___Amiodarone
___Dobutamine
___Fenoldopam

Sedatives:

___Dexmedetomidine (Precedex)
___Propofol
Family Contact Person:
Family Contact #:

Anesthesiologist Please Fill Out:

☐ Yes ☐ No   Fast Track?
Intubation: Easy   Difficult
____Last hematocrit
____Last Platelet Count
____Last Glucose   ____@Insulin given
____Last K^+
____# Albumin
____cc of Cell Saver
____Units of PRBC
____Units of FFP
____Units of Platelets
____Urine Output

☐ Yes ☐ No Any K^+ supplement given?
☐ Yes ☐ No Lasix given?
☐ Yes ☐ No Amiodarone load?
☐ Yes ☐ No Milrinone Load?

Past History:
☐ Pulmonary
☐ HTN
☐ DM
☐ Stroke
☐ Renal/Dialysis
☐ Rapid Recovery Planned

Time from Arrival to Extubation: ____hr____min

NOTES FROM THE FRONT

Studies have found that a pure verbal handoff, like a children's game of telephone, consistently resulted in a loss of all data, and note taking resulted in a loss of 31% of the data. But a structured printed form, such as the example above, combined with a verbal handoff resulted in minimal data loss. Sigh, more paperwork added to the mix. But get into the game because it's a JCAHO mandate!

A standardized handoff does not replace common sense. If you feel something is important, mention it.

Don't assume the receiving team is as comfortable with the patient as you were. You may be signing out the patient to someone with much less experience or perhaps even more. Always ask if there is something unclear or if something needs clarification. The person receiving the handoff may feel intimidated by you (Figure 51-1).

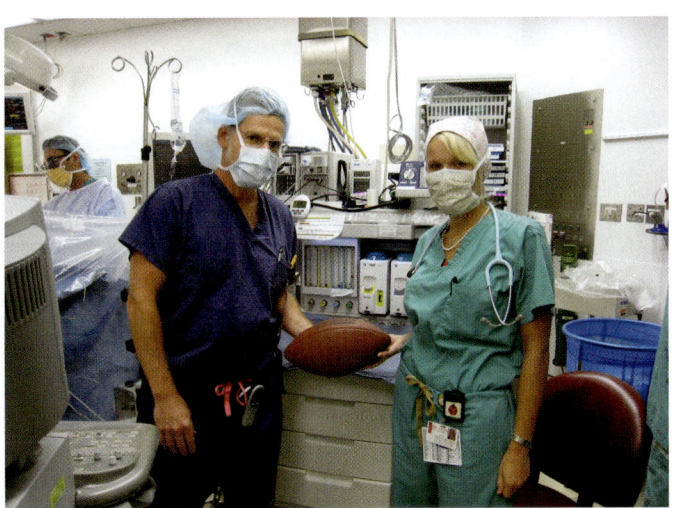

FIGURE 51-1 The handoff.

SUGGESTED READING

JCAHO. Improving handoff communications: meeting national patient safety goal 2E. *Joint Perspect Patient Safety* 2006; 6(8):9–15.

Since the release of these patient safety goals in 2006, health care organizations have been pushing for standardized handoffs between caregivers "including an opportunity (for providers) to ask and respond to questions."

Pothier D, Monteiro P, Mooktiar M, Shaw A. Pilot study to show the loss of important data in nursing handover. *Br J Nurse* 2005;14(20):1090–1093.

Three different handoff communication styles were observed and the amount of data loss was recorded. A written handoff with verbal communication amounted to minimal data loss.

Riesenberg LA, et al. Residents' and attending physicians' handoffs: a systematic review of the literature. *Acad Med* 2009;84(12):1775–1787.

A systemic review of the literature found many articles describing negative consequences of poor handoff, yet little research has been done to describe best practices. The authors called for more high-quality handoff outcomes studies focused on systems factors, human performance, and the effectiveness of structured protocols and interventions.

Smith AF, Pope C, Goodwin D, Mort M. Interprofessional handover and patient safety in anaesthesia: observational study of handovers in the recovery room. *Br J Anaesth* 2008; 101:332–337.

A British description of intraoperative handoffs between anesthetic providers. It shows how informal handoffs are routinely performed, but the use of a standardized transfer of care can possibly lead to safety gains.

Solet DJ, Norvel M, Gale RH, Frankel RM. Lost in translation: challenges and opportunities in physician to physician communication during patient handoffs. *Acad Med* 2005;80: 1094–1099.

A description of internal medicine residency patient handoffs, which concluded that precise, unambiguous, face-to-face communication is the best way to ensure effective handoffs of hospitalized patients. The authors also describe the challenge to educate residents on the skill of communication.

CHAPTER 52

ANESTHESIA INFORMATION MANAGEMENT SYSTEMS: GEEK SQUAD TO THE OR STAT!

JUSTIN LONG
RAFAEL M. RICHARDS

> Measure what is measurable, and make measurable what is not so.
>
> *Galileo*

INTRODUCTION

Anesthesiologists may spend more time on charting than almost any other activity or procedure during an anesthetic case. Do not dismiss this as idle busywork. The anesthesia record is one of the most important by-products of your performing a safe anesthetic. This document will linger on long after you have completed the case, and it has the potential to help you financially if done properly or cost you millions if not.

"You mean you forgot to document CO_2 after placing an endotracheal tube, and a few minutes later the patient had a cardiac arrest" Oops. How can you deny a goosed endotracheal tube now? Lesson from risk management 101: If it's not documented, it never happened. Complete and accurate records may save your career if any complication occurs. Good charting is essential for your livelihood, for risk management, and for patient care. Do it well!

EVOLUTION OF THE ANESTHESIA RECORD

- The first anesthesia chart was used by Harvey Cushing and E.H. Codman. They found that writing vital signs down during administration of ether led to better outcomes for patients. That is, patients died less often.
- The anesthesia record now reflects a detailed and continuous account of drugs, fluids, and blood products administered, and procedures undertaken. It also includes the observation of cardiovascular responses, estimated blood loss, body fluid output, and data from physiologic monitors during the course of the anesthesia.
- In the 1980s, the first automated record-keeping software and systems were developed. The functionality and rate of implementation of anesthesia information management systems (AIMS) have markedly risen over the past decade.
- AIMS are now complex integrated systems that have been shown to improve patient care and, in some cases, the financial performance of a department.

A recent study showed that, in the United States, AIMS have become increasingly installed in academic anesthesia departments since 2007.[1]

DEFINING AIMS

What they are:
- Anesthesia information management systems (AIMS) are electronic data collection, storage, and display systems used as a substitute for pen-and-paper anesthesia record-keeping.
- AIMS may also be called the electronic anesthesia drug record (eADR), the electronic medical record (EMR), the medication administration record (MAR), or simply by the name of the software vendor.
- AIMS can be stand-alone systems or integrated modules of a hospital-wide clinical information system.

What they do:
- AIMS facilitate the collection of anesthesia-related, perioperative patient data from patient monitors and the anesthesia machine. These data may be:
  - Vital signs: either from user entry or transferred from the monitors
  - Medications: usually from user entries, but also from the monitor in the case of inhaled agents or possibly even from an infusion pump
  - Patient information: entered by clinician
  - Events during the procedure (e.g., in room time, induction, time-out time, incision, tourniquet time, insufflation time, time finished)
  - Procedures: from user entry
  - Billing documentation (e.g., presence of an attending, type of anesthetic, actual surgical procedure done)
  - Required documentation (e.g., narcotic reconciliation, postoperative disposition)

What they do not do:
- AIMS are not going to make you a more knowledgeable, vigilant, and competent anesthesiologist.
- AIMS are not "intelligent," and do not have capacity for medical decision making. While some vendors state that their AIMS provide clinical decision support, this means that it provides access to or graphically displays an interesting subset of data to a clinician so that the clinician can analyze this data.
- Some AIMS have "smart" alarms or "intelligent" advisories. Again, this represents marketing jargon. If any AIMS did provide medical advice, the FDA would have it removed from the market immediately for practicing medicine. You still have to be a good clinician; otherwise, there would be dire consequences if the system goes down.
- AIMS are not autopilots that can administer anesthesia for you. While there are closed-loop anesthesia delivery systems that automatically maintain general anesthesia by pharmacokinetic models, these are not approved for use in the U.S.
- AIMS are not a panacea for underlying administrative, infrastructural, staffing, or other issues that hinder efficiency of anesthesia delivery.
- No studies have shown that AIMS improve anesthesia clinical efficiency, reduce anesthesia workload, or reduce turnover time between cases.

BENEFITS OF AIMS

While each of the studies cited below refers to unique implementations of AIMS in a specific institution, the benefits generally fall in two categories: financial or care related:
- Reducing anesthesia-related drug costs[2]
- Increased anesthesia billing and capture of anesthesia-related charges[3]
- Increased hospital reimbursement through improved hospital coding[4,5]
- Improvement of the data quality of the intraoperative anesthesia record[6,7]
- Support training and education of the anesthesia work force[8]
- Support of clinical decision making[9]
- Support of patient care and safety[10]
- Enhancement of clinical studies[11]
- Enhancement of clinical quality improvement programs[12]
- Support of clinical risk management[13]
- Monitoring for diversion of controlled substances[14]

Currently there are no AIMS that take advantage of all of the above benefits.

DRAWBACKS OF AIMS

The transition from a paper chart may not be easy, and it has the potential to introduce new problems:
- Need for additional information technology (IT) staff and 24-hour IT support
- Anesthesia personnel may not easily accept the electronic switch because it may alter what has been familiar for their practice as an anesthesiologist.

- AIMS mercilessly record everything, whether or not they are true reflections of how the patient is doing. On paper, the pulse-oximetry readings with poor waveforms can be omitted and the aberrant blood pressures can be retaken before being recorded to the chart.
- Hardware costs: computers, servers, and the stuff between that makes it all work
- Software licenses: the program you use for the charting and for translating your record into another electronic chart
- Changes in the way your time is billed

EQUIPMENT FOR AIMS

- Workstation: your computer, keyboard, and mouse
- Anesthesia machine and monitors (devices)
- Server: for storage of the device and clinical data
- Software: glue that translates data between devices, server, and workstation
- Network: to connect devices, server, and workstation
- Paper chart: when things really are not working out

MODUS OPERANDI OF AIMS

What is the magic that makes this data integration system work? The main thing that an AIMS does is integrate continuous machine generated data (medical devices) with human (clinician) entered data and display this on a single screen.

- Device data from the monitor or ventilator are collected by physical connection and translated to human readable form. Depending on the specific vendor, this device data translation occurs locally or on a remote server.
- Human-entered data, including observations, medications, and procedures, are manually entered by the anesthesiologist via keyboard and mouse at a workstation in the OR.
- Both the device data and human data are sent over the network to a server that integrates these data streams.
- The combined (human and machine-entered) data are sent back to the OR and displayed on the workstation for visual review, creating the electronic chart (Figure 52-1).

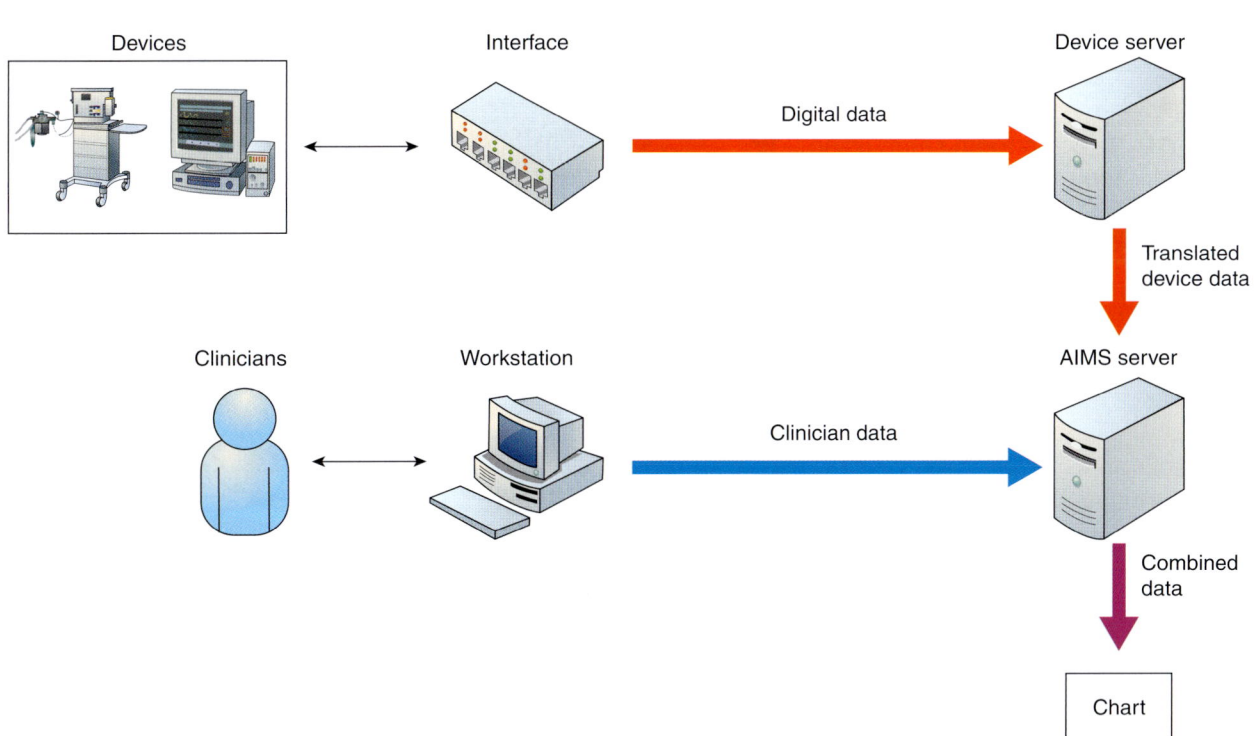

FIGURE 52-1 Modus operandi of AIMS.

HOW TO USE AIMS

There are many vendors and types of AIMS, so the advice here is limited to the use of a generic system. When you're getting your room ready in the morning, your room checklist may look something represented by the acronym SOAPMIT: Suction, Oxygen, Airway, Pharmacology (drugs), Machine, IV, Technology (computer)(Figure 52-2).

Once the patient is in the room, there is a lot to do:

- Wheel the patient in, side-rail down, and lock the bed against the OR table.
- Click on the computer to tell it that you and the patient are in the room.
- Dedicate yourself to the patient. You have to get the patient safely from one bed to another, connect your monitors, and start preoxygenation. The patient is the number one priority and must always be our focus.
- Do not turn your back on the patient and become completely preoccupied with charting (Figure 52-3).
- Induce anesthesia, do the block, or set up for monitored anesthesia care (MAC). All of this has to be held in your short-term memory for later charting. To help, do not throw away used syringes or vials until you have made sure the drug has been correctly charted.
- Once the patient is safely tucked in and the procedure has started, you may begin to enter everything you have been doing. Many things must be done from your memory; do your best!

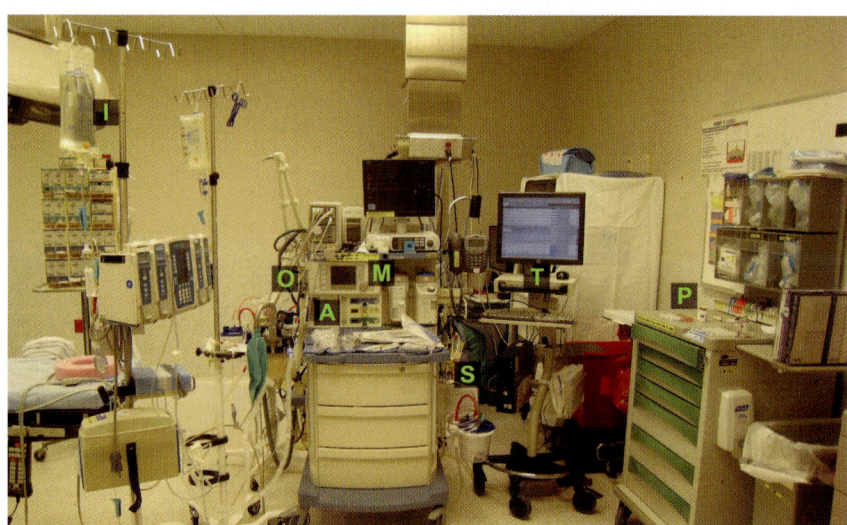

FIGURE 52-2 Basic room setup using the SOAPMIT method.

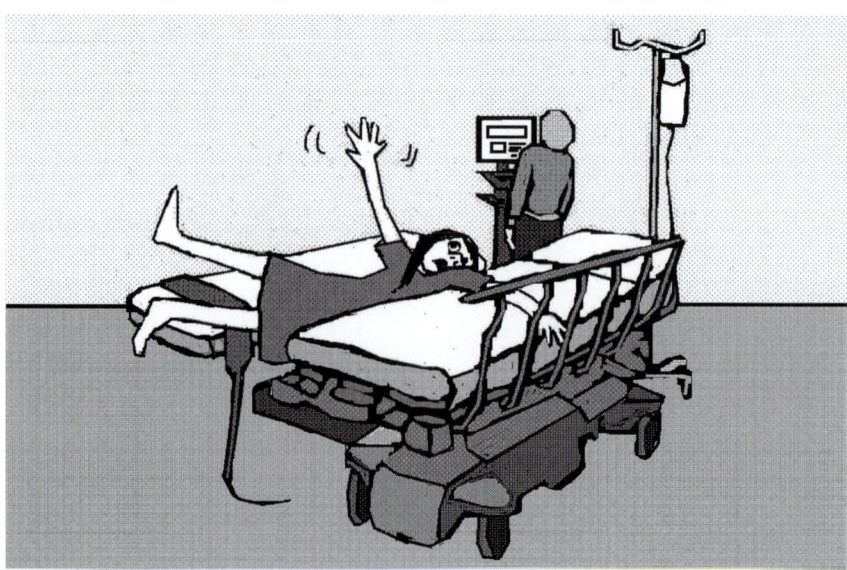

FIGURE 52-3 Crossing the gap can be a really tricky prospect for some patients.

Tips for Charting

- Do not click on things that most closely match what you did. If there is no choice that describes exactly what you did, then free text it somewhere in the chart.
- Do not get distracted with the other diversions that a computer can offer (Figure 52-4).
- Do not forget to chart the things you do for the patient that will also save you trouble with risk management later (e.g., padding, eye protection). These may not be elements of the chart that are required by the software.
- Attempt to split your induction dosing into the way it was done. For example, lidocaine, propofol, and rocuronium are not always given in the same minute, so try not to chart them this way. It is often difficult because the drugs are not always pushed by you, but try. It shows you cared.
- Even though you may start charting after incision, do not forget that your antibiotics should be timed before incision, as long as you gave them this way.
- Try to make a point of adding things to the chart that have occurred during the case. It is best when the surgeon turns to you to say, "We just opened the IVC," that there is some record of the time this occurred. The only record is likely to be yours. The computer will not prompt for every piece of information that you should ever include in a chart.
- Remember that your computer and charting software are the equipment for one of your procedures, so if it is not working, somebody should help you. The answer does not always need to revert back to paper, though that is usually a practical option.

Once the case is over:
- You are busy with emergence and extubation, and the charting again falls behind.
- Now, in one of the most likely times for complications, the tendency is to turn your back from the patient and chart that there were no complications. Just think about what you are saying versus what you're doing! Ensure all is well before you take the time to chart (Figure 52-5).

Now you click that you are leaving the OR and transporting the patient to the PACU or ICU:
- Do not take a field trip across the unit for a computer. This leaves your patient unsupervised.
- Finish charting and close the case (Figure 52-6).

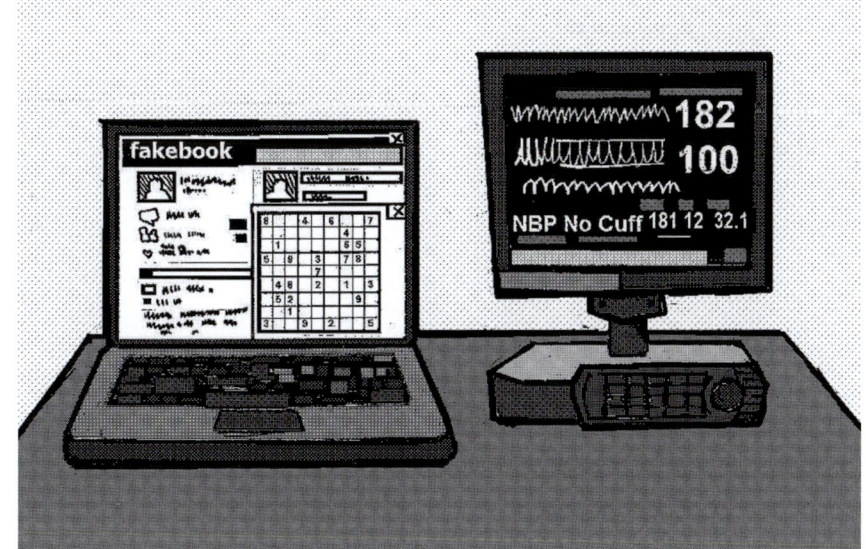

FIGURE 52-4 Just one more puzzle and you can push that amiodarone.

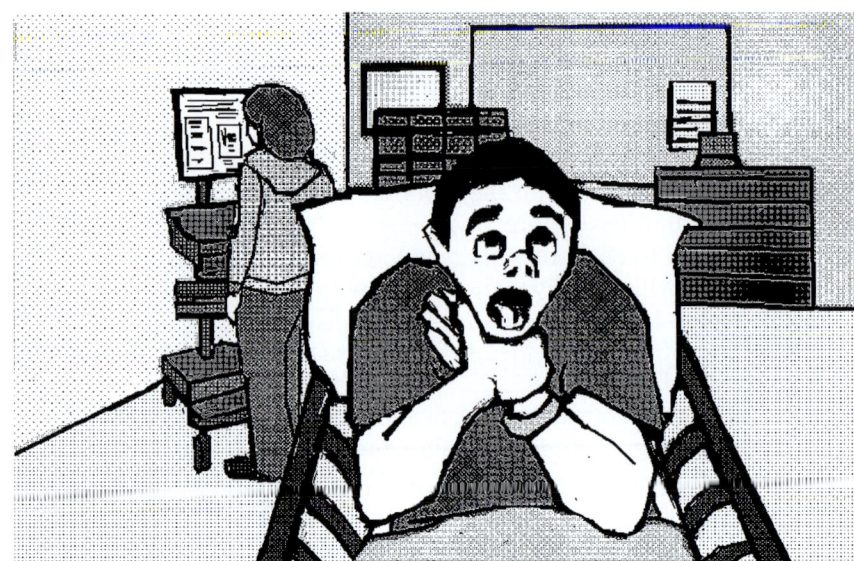

FIGURE 52-5 When the patient can't speak, they can't tell you they need help.

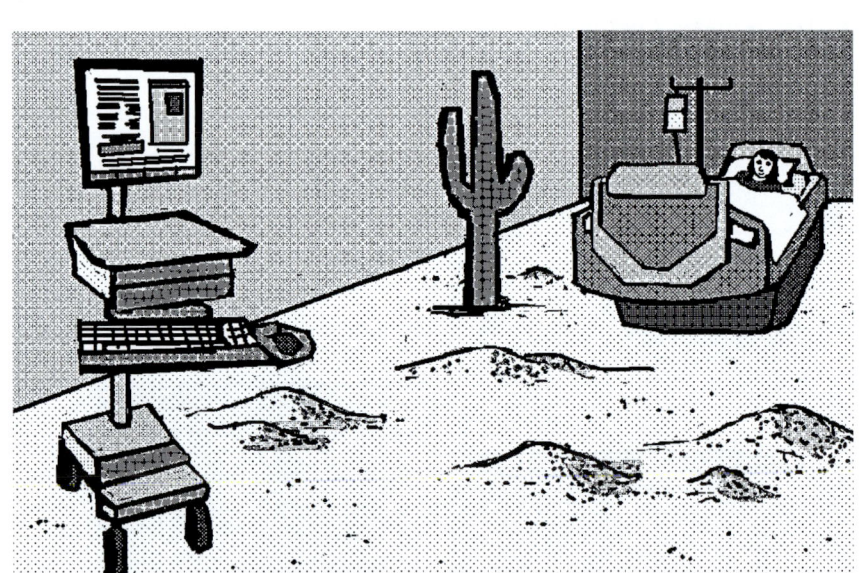

FIGURE 52-6 Sometimes the computer can be so far away that it can feel like a desert separates you from your patient.

CONCLUSION

- While not required by regulation, AIMS use is on the rise, and may very well be arriving at an OR near you.
- The benefits of an AIMS are limited only by our imagination, so we should all strive to think of new ways for the AIMS to benefit our patients.
- No matter how many ways there are to monitor patients and record these monitors, do not forget to actually watch the patient as the most important monitor.

ACKNOWLEDGMENTS

Cartoons courtesy of Mia Klimchak. Technical drawings are by one of the authors.

REFERENCES

1. Egger-Halbeis CB, Epstein R, Macario A, Pearl RG, Gunwald Z. Motivations for and barriers to anesthesia departments to adopt Anesthesia Information Management Systems (AIMS) in the US. *Anesth Analg* 2008;107(4):1323–1329.
2. Gillerman RG, Browning RA. Drug use inefficiency: a hidden source of wasted health care dollars. *Anesth Analg* 2000;91:921–924.
3. Reich DL, Kahn RA, Wax D, Palvia T, Galati M, Krol M. Development of a module for point-of-care charge capture and submission using an anesthesia information management system. *Anesthesiology* 2006;105:179–183.
4. Martin J, Ederle D, Milewski P. CompuRecord; a perioperative information management system for anesthesia. *Anasth Intensivmed Notfallmed Schmerzther* 2002;37:488–491.
5. Meyer-Jark T, Reissmann H, Schuster M, et al. Realisation of material costs in anaesthesia. Alternatives to the reimbursement via diagnosis-related groups. *Anaesthetist* 2007;56(4):364–365.
6. Cook RI, McDonald JS, Nunziata E. Differences between handwritten and automatic blood pressure records. *Anesthesiology* 1989;71:385–390.
7. Devitt JH, Rapanos T, Kurrek M, Cohen M, Shaw M. The anesthetic record: accuracy and completeness. *Can J Anesth* 1999;46:122–128.
8. Edsall DW. Computerization of anesthesia information management: users' perspective. *J Clin Monit Comput* 1991;7:351–358.
9. Merry AF, Webster CS, Mathew DJ. A new, safety-oriented, integrated drug administration and automated anesthesia record system. *Anesth Analg* 2001;93:385–390.
10. O'Reilly M, Talsma A, VanRiper S, Kheterpal S, Burney R. An anesthesia information system designed to provide physician-specific feedback improves timely administration of prophylactic antibiotics. *Anesth Analg* 2006;103:908–912.
11. Hollenberg JP, Pirraglia PA, Williams-Russo P, et al. Computerized data collection in the operating room during coronary artery bypass surgery: a comparison to the hand-written anesthesia record. *J Cardiothorac Vasc Anesth* 1997;11:545–551.
12. Röhrig R, Junger A, Hartmann B, et al. The incidence and prediction of automatically detected intraoperative cardiovascular events in noncardiac surgery. *Anesth Analg* 2004;98:569–577.
13. Feldman JM. Do anesthesia information systems increase malpractice exposure? Results of a survey. *Anesth Analg* 2004;99:840–843.
14. Epstein RH, Gratch DM, Grunwald Z. Development of a scheduled drug diversion surveillance system based on an analysis of atypical drug transactions. *Anesth Analg* 2007;105:1053–1060.

SUGGESTED READING

Hirschtick R. Copy-and-paste. *JAMA* 2006;295(20):2335–2336.

CHAPTER 53

DECODING SURGEON SPEAK

SARAH OLSON RECK
CHRISTINE PARK

It takes two to tango is a common idiomatic expression which suggests something in which more than one person or other entity are paired in an inextricably related and active manner, occasionally with negative connotations. The phrase recognizes that there are certain activities which cannot be achieved singly—like arguing, fighting, making love, dancing the tango.

The tango is a dance which requires two partners moving in relation to each other, sometimes in tandem, sometimes in opposition. The meaning of this expression has been extended to include any situation in which the two partners are by definition understood to be essential—as in a marriage with only one partner ceases to be a marriage.

Wikipedia

INTRODUCTION

The relationship between surgeons and anesthesiologists is codependent; they cannot do their jobs without each other. We coexist in operating rooms around the world, with the common goal of obtaining the best outcome for the patient. Part of this relationship involves understanding why members of the other specialty do certain things. A good example of this is the surgeon who tells you that his/her nonemergency add-on has been NPO since midnight. Surgeons understand that for the case to go, this is a necessity. In order to maintain this relationship, part of our job as anesthesiologists is to understand why the surgeon is asking you to do certain things during a procedure or what is going on during the case when he/she makes certain statements.

The job of an anesthesiologist is to be vigilant at all times. This applies not only to the patient's vital signs, but also to the events happening on the other side of the drape. When a trochanter is accidently placed into the inferior vena cava at the start of a laparoscopic procedure (this does happen), the surgeons may be so busy trying to stop the bleeding that they forget to tell you what happened. While not ideal, if you are paying attention to the surgical procedure, you will likely detect this yourself and not wonder why you are suddenly pushing sticks of phenylephrine.

This chapter describes things commonly heard in the operating room that have a bearing on your management of the patient and why the surgeon is saying them. The bottom line is that communication is the key to working together (Figure 53-1).

Surgeon: What is the blood pressure?

Anesthesiologist: The MAP is 73.

Surgeon: I want the systolic blood pressure less than 100.

- Surgeons seem to frequently ask about the blood pressure and request that it be higher than what it actually is, but in certain cases, namely ENT and orthopedic cases, the technique of hypotensive anesthesia may be employed in order to help minimize blood loss and create a bloodless surgical field. The surgeons should discuss this with you before the case starts, but if they don't and you get asked this question in the middle of the case, you need to know why. It falls under your job description to maintain a lower mean arterial pressure (MAP), but it also falls on you to know if the patient is an appropriate candidate for hypotensive anesthesia, and if not, be prepared to discuss this with the surgeon and explain why it isn't appropriate for that patient.

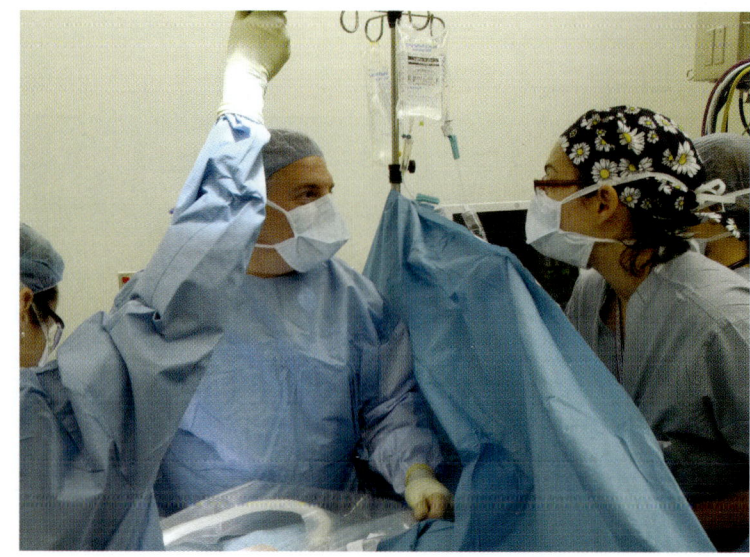

FIGURE 53-1 Even when there is a lot of chaos (or apparent chaos), it is critically important to communicate across the drape

- One of my favorite stories is of an attending anesthesiologist who was repeatedly asked to maintain the systolic blood pressure at less than 100 in a patient with baseline hypertension. She, of course, was uncomfortable with this, but despite discussion, the surgeon failed to budge on his request. Her solution? Take a piece of tape, write "99" on it, and place it over the blood pressure reading on the monitor facing the surgeon. The point being, if hypotensive anesthesia is not appropriate for the patient, then the technique should be avoided.
- Contraindications to hypotensive anesthesia include the following:
  - Congenital heart disease
  - Severe anemia
  - Coronary artery disease
  - Congestive heart failure
  - Poorly controlled hypertension
  - Increased intracranial pressure
  - Significant cerebrovascular disease
  - Low flow states to the liver or kidney

Surgeon: Is the patient types and crossed? Can you give the patient a unit of blood?

- Ideally, you will be well aware of ongoing blood loss during the case and have a good handle on when the patient needs to be transfused, but studies have shown that the calculation of estimated blood loss (EBL) in the operating room is inaccurate. Prior to starting a case, it is a good idea to determine your threshold for transfusing the patient and calculate how much blood can be lost prior to transfusion. This is easily enough determined by using transfusion guidelines of hemoglobin of 6 to 7 for otherwise healthy patients and hemoglobin of 9 for patients with cardiovascular disease. Then, to determine how much blood can be lost before you reach that hemoglobin, use the equation:

$$EBL = (Blood\ volume) \times \frac{Hgb\ starting - Hgb\ acceptable}{Hgb\ starting}$$

- Ideally the surgeons should allow you to determine when to transfuse a patient, but all too often you will hear them escalate the blood status of the patient. This can mean one of two things. First, it can mean they are losing a lot more blood than you think they are. But it can also mean that their idea of when the patient needs to be transfused is different from yours. In either case, it is a cue for you to do a few things. First, discuss with the surgeons why they are escalating the blood status. Second, try to obtain a blood sample so you can get an actual hemoglobin level. Third, determine if the patient needs to be transfused. If there truly is a great deal of blood loss and the patient needs blood, then give it. But it is also part of your job to treat the patient safely, and if the hemoglobin is 9.9 and the surgeons just think the patient needs blood because "she is a little old lady," then it is your job to discuss with them why transfusing the patient may not be necessary.
- On the flip side of this, beware of surgeons who don't want you to transfuse because they are sure they haven't lost that much blood (surgeons tend to severely underestimate the blood loss). Have your facts ready (e.g., hemoglobin, vital signs, amount of blood currently present in the suction canisters) to back up your plan.

Surgeon: We are going to lose a little blood here in the next few minutes. (Or: Can I get a second suction set up?)

Chapter 53 DECODING SURGEON SPEAK

Anesthesiologist (into phone): Can I please get a rapid transfuser.
- If the surgeons specifically tell you they are going to lose blood (even "a little blood"), they are doing so to give you time to get ready for it. You will most often hear this from surgeons who frequently do cases involving a lot of blood loss, such as large spinal fusions, certain orthopedic procedures, and liver resections. They are well aware that the high volume of blood they may lose can have serious implications on the patient's outcome, and they want to keep you in the loop throughout the surgical procedure.
- Usually, there is very good communication between the surgeons and anesthesiologists during these cases. It is a cue to you to make sure you have everything in the room ready to give the patient large amounts of blood fast.
- Beware of the normal sounds of suction going silent. Either someone stepped on the tubing, or there will be a solid column of blood being transfused from the patient to the canister.

Surgeon: Rotate the table toward me. Keep going. Keep going. Keep going.

The senior author has a good friend who, during one of her first anesthetics, couldn't figure out why the surgeon kept looking at her and asking for the table position to be changed; apparently someone forgot to inform her that while not necessarily in the job description, this does fall in the hands of the anesthesiologist. Most of the time bed positioning involves only a simple up and down to achieve a height that is comfortable for the surgeon, but in certain procedures, you will be asked to move the table to a position that you are certain will cause the patient to slip right off and on to the OR floor. Lessons to be learned from this:
- Double check that the safety strap is fastened before the patient is prepped and draped.
- Watch the patient and your lines during any repositioning of the table. The last thing you need is for the little old lady with poor IV access to have her 22-gauge IV pulled out when the table is being moved.
- After the table has reached the new position, check all pressure points again and repad as necessary, as it is possible the patient has shifted along with the table.

In addition to the above issues, you need to remember that patient position can have implications on your anesthetic as well. Familiarize yourself with the hemodynamic changes associated with different patient positions. Also beware of the following:
- The Trendelenburg position, especially if it is severe, will cause multiple issues for you. First, the pushing of the abdominal contents on the diaphragm can cause difficulty ventilating the patient. Second, if left in that position for a long time, gravity will take its course and dependent edema of the face will ensue. This can involve the vocal cords.

Surgeon (at the end of the case while closing fascia): I want zero twitches.
- This is a classic example of surgeons knowing a little about anesthesia, but not everything, and the knowing anesthesiologist can improve the situation without delaying wake-up (which will just proceed to irritate the surgeon).
- Having good relaxation while closing fascia actually does create improved surgical conditions, and the surgeons can tell if the patient isn't very relaxed during this part of the case because the unrelaxed patient will start to "push their bowels out," which the surgeons will be sure to tell you about.
- If the patient really only has one twitch during closure and isn't attempting spontaneous ventilation, the placebo effect can work for you. Inform the surgeon that you just gave more muscle relaxant, and more often than not the surgical field will magically become optimal again. Do make sure that the patient is actually deeply anesthetized before trying this.
- Most of the time, if the patient is truly beginning to move or "push their bowels out," deepening the anesthetic will provide ample relaxation. There are ways to do this other than muscle relaxant, namely propofol or narcotic. Resist the temptation to placate the surgeon and give large doses of muscle relaxant so close to the end of the case. This will result in one of two things: a very long wake up, which won't make anyone in the room happy, or having to take a patient intubated to the recovery room, which won't teach the surgeon a lesson; it will only punish the patient.

Surgeon (at the beginning of the case while using electrocautery on muscle): This patient is not relaxed! Get your attending in here!

As you recheck your twitch monitor and find that the patient really has no twitches, check in with your knowledge of neuromuscular blockade. Where does a neuromuscular blocking drug work? Yep, the neuromuscular junction. And where is the electrocautery stimulating the muscle? Yep, directly on the muscle fibers. Spine surgeons are especially prone (no pun intended) to this complaint. You can try bringing up a PowerPoint presentation on the OR computer, but it'll be a tough audience. Go ahead and let your attending back you up on this one.

Surgeon: Can you extubate the patient deep?
- It can be irritating at the end a case to have the surgeon tell you how to wake the patient up. When the surgeons ask you to extubate deep, it is because

they don't want the patient bucking on wake up. Unfortunately, this is a natural reaction to having a large piece of plastic shoved down your throat. For most patients, while the bucking isn't ideal, it won't necessarily hurt them. However, in certain patient populations, namely neurosurgery and certain ENT cases, bucking on wake-up can cause bleeding from the surgical site, and this can have severe consequences, especially in neurosurgery.
- If this request is made, you do NOT need to honor it if the patient isn't a candidate for deep extubation, but do explain to the surgeons why you made this decision and do your best to execute a smooth emergence.
- If you do decide to honor it, be sure you're aware of the risks and are 100% sure that you will be able to safely and effectively mask ventilate the patient through emergence.

Cardiac surgeon: I'm going to be pushing on the heart for a minute.
- If you hear these words, perk up and pay attention. Believe it or not, this is a statement aimed directly at the anesthesiologist, and will frequently be heard during off-pump coronary artery bypass graft (CABG). Basically, when surgeons push on the heart, they are dropping the preload to nothing. Nothing in = nothing out = MAP in the teens = iatrogenic PEA.
- The surgeons want you to be aware of this for two reasons: first, you aren't going to treat this with a large bolus of pressor, as it won't do much good; second, it is your job to tell them when the pressure is too low. At that point, they will take their hands off the heart and allow the hemodynamics to recover before repeating the maneuver. If you aren't ready for this or aware of what they are trying to tell you, be prepared for your own sympathetic response, because it is a scary how low the blood pressure will drop.

Surgeon: I need to clamp the IVC.

This won't often be spoken directly to the anesthesiologist, but if you hear these words, you again need to be prepared for a drop in the blood pressure. When the IVC is clamped, you are going to lose about half of your preload, meaning the blood pressure is going to tank, and unlike the above scenario, this time you will need to treat it.

Surgeon: Turn off the music.
- Universal for "things aren't going the way I planned," especially if a minute ago they were singing along with the music. This can mean any number of things, from they got into a vessel, to there is cancer everywhere in the abdomen, to the exposure just sucks.

- Often, things will look great at your end, but it is a good time to step back and reevaluate. First, it is probably a good idea to figure out the source of the frustration. If it is a difficult exposure, then it won't affect you as much, but if it is that they got into a bleeder, then you need to know about it.
- Second, figure out if there is anything you can do from an anesthetic perspective to help them, or at least not hinder them further. This isn't the time to realize the patient is light because it is only going to make the surgeons more upset. Basically, run through a mental checklist of everything. Are the vitals okay? Is the patient well anesthetized? Is the patient paralyzed (if appropriate)?

Surgeon: Closing music please.
- Ah, it's the end of a successful nephrectomy and the closure has begun. At that point of the procedure the surgeons are feeling triumphant and want some triumphant music, at the very least something loud and upbeat.
- Remember, though, that like induction, the emergence is a risky part of the anesthesia, and you're now like a pilot bringing an airplane in for a landing. Maintain friendly but firm control of the operating room environment.
- Start by complimenting the surgeons on the amazing beauty of their closure (if this is a plastics case, you will get some serious mileage from making that observation).
- Make the team aware of any items of concern you have.
- And always, always, make sure you can hear the pulse oximeter above the ambient noise in the room.

Surgeon: What is the CVP?
- This is commonly heard during liver surgery, especially liver resections. Elevated central venous pressure (CVP) causes hepatic congestion, which increases bleeding during the resection. Thus, the surgeons like to keep the CVP low, usually less than 8, often less than 6, and some even ask for 0, during these cases.
- Usually they will discuss this with you before the case starts so that a balance can be struck between optimum surgical conditions and optimum everything-else conditions.

Surgeon: The patient is awake!
- To most surgeons, there are only two planes of anesthesia: awake and asleep. Thus, any time they detect even the slightest movement, they will feel the need to inform you that the patient is "awake" (never mind that you are probably already dealing with it). This is a common scenario at the beginning of a case when you have only used short-acting muscle relaxant and you are running the patient in a lighter

plane of anesthesia to maintain hemodynamics while the patient is begin prepped. When the surgery starts, the patient will often move slightly with the stimulation of surgical incision. You can prevent this by paying attention, and when the surgeons go to scrub, deepen your volatile anesthetic and give a little narcotic in preparation for the incision.
- This is also a common thing to hear at the end of the case when you have the patient spontaneously ventilating; reassure the surgeons that, indeed, the patient is not awake but simply breathing on his/her own.
- It is very common to hear this comment during a sedation anesthetic. Most surgeons don't truly understand the concept of sedation anesthesia and will tell you every time the patient moves instead of realizing that maybe they need to provide a little more local anesthetic to anesthetize the area. In this scenario, it may, in fact, behoove you to point out (nicely) that this isn't a general anesthetic and some more local (but not too much local; you should give them a maximum) would be prudent.

Surgeon: Call the office and tell them to cancel my clinic.
- This is an ominous phrase, frequently heard in peripheral vascular cases. It means the case is running much longer than anticipated and it is not nearing an end any time soon. Make sure your volatile anesthetic is filled to the top and settle in for a long day.

Surgeon (during laparoscopic cases): Gas on (or, insufflate please).
- During laparoscopy, CO_2 is used to fill (or "insufflate") the abdominal cavity in order to create good exposure for the surgeons. Knowing when insufflation occurs, and to what pressure, is important to the anesthesiologist as many physiologic alterations occur as a result of insufflation of the abdomen.
- These physiologic changes include:
  - Elevated peak airway pressures
  - Increased E_TCO_2
  - Hemodynamic derangements that can include hypotension secondary to decreased preload and hypertension in response to the laparoscopy
  - Decreased urine output
  - Subcutaneous emphysema
  - Air embolus
- If you aren't aware that insufflation occurred, you may look at your patient's vital signs and wonder whether you should start giving dantrolene, as the changes can be quite significant.

Surgeon (during a tracheostomy): We are going to be entering the airway shortly.
- Tracheostomy requires a great deal of cooperation between the surgeons and anesthesiologists. While generally a quick procedure, it has many complications, the two most dangerous of which are airway fire and losing the airway. Thus, the surgeons will let you know when they will be entering the airway.
- This is your cue to decrease your FiO_2 as low as possible to prevent airway fire, especially if the surgeons are using electrocautery. It also lets you know that you are going to lose the ability to deliver positive pressure ventilation, as the hole in the trachea causes a massive leak in your system. If you aren't aware of these things, there could be serious implications.

Surgeon (during any "scope" case): We're opening.
- Any time a surgical procedure is performed with a scope (laparoscopic, arthroscopic, thoracoscopic), the surgeons will always consent the patient for an open procedure as well. Scopes are wonderful minimally invasive tools, but in cases that turn out to be more complex than anticipated, they will often convert to an open procedure in order to facilitate surgical exposure.
- This means two things for you: first, it is likely to be a much longer than the originally anticipated case and also that the patient is going to have more issues with postoperative pain control secondary to the much larger incision. The major implication here is that you may need to consider a postop epidural for pain control in that patient.
- Furthermore, with an open procedure, you will have increased insensible fluid loss from exposure as well as the possibility of increased blood loss. Alter your anesthetic appropriately.

Surgeon: Scalpel. Stapler. Irrigation.
- While you don't need to know the use of every single surgical instrument, it is important to be aware of some of them, as they can give you clues to where exactly in the procedure the surgeons are. "Scalpel" generally means they are ready to make incision. It is your cue to make sure the patient is deep enough and has some narcotic on board. Being aware of this will help prevent the dreaded "the patient is awake."
- "Stapler": anytime you hear this, be aware that this closure is going to be fast. Essentially, you should become familiar with the steps to closure in many types of cases. In an abdominal case, just because they have started closing fascia (deep layers) doesn't mean they will be done soon. But it is a cue to you to start getting ready for the end of the case. If you are familiar with what layers need to be closed, you won't be miffed when you turn the gas off and the patient "wakes up" and there is still 30 minutes left

in closure. On the flip side, once that stapler comes out, you have about 3 minutes until that incision is completely closed.
- Finally, be aware of how much and how often irrigation is being used. It gets suctioned into the same canister as the blood, and it isn't uncommon for the newbie anesthesiologist to think that the 2000 mL in blood-tinged fluid in the canister is all blood. Ask the scrub tech how much irrigation has been used and it will guide you to your actual blood loss.
- Of note, for some odd reason, surgeons have a tendency to call irrigation "irritation." I don't know why, but if you hear them say "irritation" and then they dump a bunch of saline into the belly, that is why.

Surgeon: Tourniquet down.
- The tourniquet is a beautiful thing in that it greatly helps minimize blood loss in orthopedic procedures. It can, however, occasionally be the bane of the anesthesiologist's existence.
- Tourniquets that are left inflated for more than 1.5 to 2 hours start to cause a great deal of pain, resulting in tachycardia and hypertension that doesn't always respond very well to narcotics. For this reason alone, the words "tourniquet down" are music to your ears (that and the fact that closing, along with the requisite closing music, will soon follow).
- You also need to be aware of the physiologic implications of the tourniquet. The entire time the tourniquet has been up, that extremity has been undergoing anaerobic metabolism, meaning there is a buildup of CO_2, lactic acid, and other by-products of metabolism in that extremity, and when the tourniquet comes down, these will all wash into the systemic circulation. This will cause an elevation in the patient's E_TCO_2 as well as a drop in the blood pressure. You can offset this by increasing minute ventilation and volume loading shortly before the tourniquet comes down.

Surgeon: I'm going to go talk to the family.
- Surgeons only operate on one patient at a time, and frequently leave the room well before the patient emerges. Therefore, not only is it part of the culture, but it's also much easier for surgeons to make time to speak with patients' families. No matter how admirable this may be, it may be impossible for us to leave patient care to do the same on a routine basis.
- However, if there has been an untoward event or complication, whether or not it was related to the procedure or the anesthetic, think about finding a way to go with the surgeon to speak with the family. It allows for the family to hear from their team of doctors, and may allow you to take a moment to debrief with your colleague on the way.
- Now, if something really bad happens, make sure to call whatever support mechanism your hospital has set up to help you.

CONCLUSION

While this is by no means an all-encompassing list of the things you will hear during your career as an anesthesiologist, it is a start, and a good collection of phrases that you will hear frequently and what the meaning behind them is. At times, the things the surgeons tell you will make it seem as though they are micromanaging your anesthetic, or are, indeed, a better anesthesiologist than you are. During these times, a good sense of humor and a heavy dose of sarcasm can be your friend!

Surgeon (bent over his liver transplant): Why is the K so high? Haven't you been following it?

Anesthesiologist: No, we just sit back here all day, twiddling our thumbs.

SUGGESTED READING

Duke J. *Anesthesia secrets.* Philadelphia: Mosby; 2006, pp 484–487.
Chapter on deliberate hypotension focuses on how to manage the technique and also contraindications to the technique.

Fleischer L. *Evidence based practice of anesthesiology,* 2nd ed. Philadelphia: WB Saunders; 2009, pp 156–162.
Discusses thresholds for transfusion and summarizes various clinical trials done on the morbidity and mortality related to blood transfusion.

Lee J-W, Cassorla L. Positioning and associated risks. In: Stoelting RK, Miller RD, eds. *Basics of anesthesia,* 5th ed. Philadelphia: Churchill-Livingstone; 2007, pp 291–303.
Discusses basic implications of common patient positions in the operating room.

Practice guidelines for perioperative blood transfusion and adjuvant therapies: an updated report by the American Society of Anesthesiologists Task Force on Perioperative Blood Transfusion and Adjuvant Therapies. *Anesthesiology* 2006;105:198–208.
Comprehensive report by the ASA regarding guidelines for the use of blood products in the perioperative period.

Weingram J. Laparoscopic surgery. In: Yao F-S, Fontes M, Malhotra V. *Anesthesiology: problem-oriented patient management.* Philadelphia: Lippincott Williams & Wilkins; 2008, pp 848–880.
Discusses the anesthetic implications of laparoscopic surgery.

PART IX

FAR FROM THE MADDENING CROWD

CHAPTER 54

PREADMISSION TESTING

MARK SLOMOVITS
STEVEN H. GINSBERG

The calamity that comes is never the one we had prepared ourselves for.

Mark Twain

INTRODUCTION

Preop clinic. Preanesthesia testing. PATs. The "clinic." Call it what you will, but short of the 500 lb, bearded, combative, Down syndrome patient with a bowel obstruction, nothing strikes as much fear into the anesthesiologist's heart as covering the preoperative clinic. While many anesthesiologists delight in spending every day dealing with patients who are, well, anesthetized, others may occasionally appreciate having an actual conversation with a fully awake and vigorous individual. Although the preanesthetic evaluation is regarded by many anesthesiologists as anathema, it remains vitally important to our successful daily provision of anesthetics.

The preanesthesia evaluation is intended to lay the groundwork for a safe and successful flight sans turbulence (especially that which is unexpected) as well as a smooth takeoff and landing. The anesthesiologist, upon assessing the patient's history, examination, and other objective data, will then create a plan for the administration of anesthesia that is customized for that patient's unique situation. The skill required for a meaningful preoperative assessment includes being shrewdly suspicious, understanding the appropriate questions to ask, and knowing which diagnostic paths to pursue. A tremendous variety of diagnostic tests of all shapes and sizes lie at your fingertips, but knowing which one is appropriate to acquire for your patient is a skill. This chapter provides a model of how a typical preanesthesia evaluation should proceed and discusses some of the reasoning behind the decision making that you will likely be faced with in the dreaded clinic. (Figure 54-1)

"WHAT SURGERY ARE YOU HAVING PERFORMED?"

They always taught us in medical school to start the interview with open-ended questions, but this one sounds pretty narrow. On the contrary, this question allows one to gather information about the patient's knowledge and insight regarding his or her condition and pending operation.

- Knowledge of the procedure being performed is vastly important. Nominally, it allows one to consider the location of the surgical site and laterality. The anesthetic plan will begin to take shape as you consider the likely positioning of the patient and the inherent risks that may be involved. Consider:
  - The patient with previous cervical spine fusion who can't turn or extend the neck for laryngoscopy
  - The steep Trendelenburg position necessary for a robotic surgery that may result in significant facial and airway swelling thus reducing the chance for postop extubation
  - What kind of vascular access will be required and whether it will be accessible following positioning and surgical prep and drape. Perhaps there is an active arteriovenous (AV) fistula in the only exposed extremity.
- The anesthesiologist should also begin to contemplate the actual complexity of the surgery and the complications inherent to it. These facts

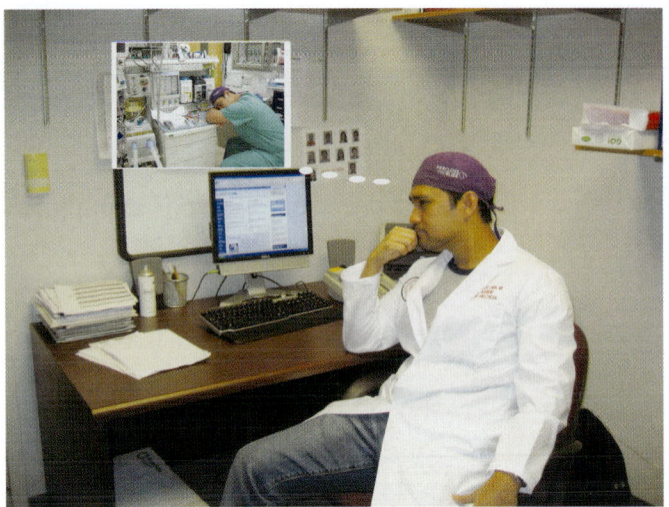

FIGURE 54-1 Dr. DeLara undoubtedly loves the PAT clinic, but dreams of working hard in the OR.

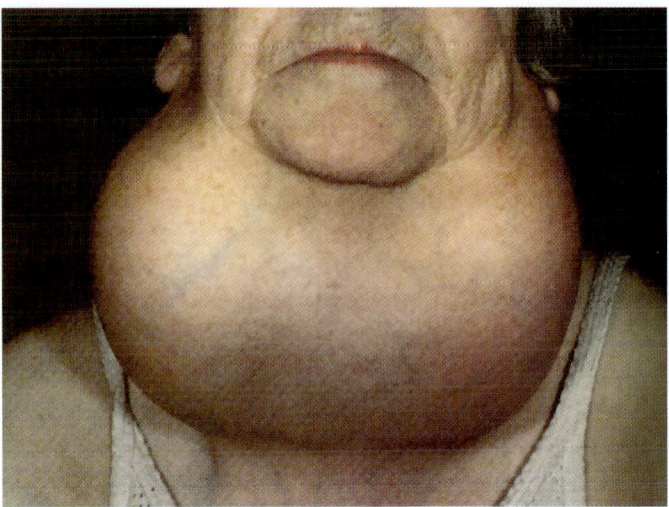

FIGURE 54-2 Would you like to intubate this one? Please, be my guest, it'll be a great learning experience!

assist you in risk stratifying the patient and should guide all additional questioning and decision making required for obtaining or bypassing further diagnostic testing.

- Tying it all together, an example: a patient presenting with a large neck mass[1] for resection should set you on a specific path of thinking (Figure 54-2):
  - There may be a need for additional central access for excessive bleeding and the subsequent need for transfusion, but the neck may not be the ideal site for this because of the location and sheer enormity of the tumor.
  - Multiple structures exist in the neck that may be relevant to the anesthesiologist, one of which is the recurrent laryngeal nerve. The possibility of its transection may affect your decision to extubate the patient at the surgery's conclusion for fear of airway obstruction.
  - Lastly, a neck mass will most certainly set off alarms for difficult intubation and thus a chest x-ray or neck CT scan may be necessary as well.

"DO YOU HAVE ANY MEDICAL CONDITIONS?"

Now we get open-ended with our questions. We provide the patient with a soapbox and say, "Go!" As the patient rattles off their various maladies, you should be considering how each one can affect your developing anesthetic plan.

- How grave or controlled is the patient's disease process?
  - Will the uncontrolled hypertensive develop a skyrocketing blood pressure following intubation and rupture a brain aneurysm?
  - Will the hypovolemic, recently dialyzed renal failure patient become profoundly hypotensive following induction?
  - Will the emphysematous patient on mechanical ventilation burst a bulla and develop a pneumothorax after coughing?
  - Will the chronic diabetic with undiagnosed gastroparesis aspirate during an intubation attempt?
- We could certainly go on, but creating an exhaustive list would be *(ahem)* exhausting. The clinical information you gather will be critical in managing each of the patient's existing conditions during the perioperative period. It will also be relevant in classifying the patient's risk, which will help guide whatever further objective information will be needed.

The common theme forming here is that it all relates back to patient risk stratification and optimization. In a sense, we expect the worst and plan for the worst too.

"WHAT SURGERIES HAVE YOU HAD PREVIOUSLY? HAVE YOU HAD ANY PROBLEMS WITH ANESTHESIA?"

Perish the thought, but sometimes we anesthesiologists have to put on our surgeon's cap and think about the patient like our colleagues on the other side of the drape.

- The length and complexity of the surgery is important to our planning and we must consider whether this procedure will be a simple sprint or a complex marathon.
    - Is this a new umbilical hernia or is it a redo ventral hernia?
        - The patient having an initial herniorraphy may tolerate deep sedation with local anesthesia.
        - The patient undergoing a repeat hernia repair following previous mesh insertion will likely appreciate having a plastic tube placed in their trachea.
    - The point you must realize is that repeat operations may have extensive scar formation and the consequent difficult dissection will complicate not only the procedure but the anesthetic management as well.
- Another consideration is the presence of devices and foreign bodies such as pacemakers, automatic implantable cardioverter-defibrillators (AICDs), nerve stimulators, etc.
    - Knowing about the patient's past history of congestive heart failure may hint at the presence of an internal defibrillator. This may lead you to consider disabling it using a magnet or by contacting a company rep. It might also be a good idea to have an external defibrillator in the operating room and to place defibrillator pads on the patient prior to induction.
- Along similar lines, it should be requested of the patient to remove all jewelry. This includes from locations where you'd never think to ask.
    - Jewelry carries the potential to cause burns when electrocautery is in use near it.
    - Also, expect intraoperative fluid shifts leading to swelling that can be dangerous to tissue near the jewelry.
        - A long unmoved wedding ring can lead to ischemia of the digit when that finger swells during a long procedure.
- Now, consider the possibility of difficulty with past anesthetics. These may be isolated incidents or may be critical events that should be contemplated prior to all further anesthetic administrations.
    - A previous intubation where the patient went home with a chipped tooth is unfortunate and will certainly increase the care with which you intubate to avoid it happening again. Although you may devote more attention to your airway exam, this incident will likely have little effect on your overall plan.
    - On the other hand, the patient who had profound nausea and vomiting after an appendectomy may require some modification of the planned anesthetic management. You may consider avoiding inhalational agents and will likely administer a combination of antiemetics as well, but just so long as you're preparing for it ahead of time.
- Last, but far from least, is the need to obtain knowledge about past airway difficulties. Your own airway exam is critical towards planning your induction and intubation, but significant findings are often subtle and overlooked.
    - Identifying a Mallampati class 2 airway with a normal thyromental distance may comfort you until you notice the healed tracheostomy scar that the patient then reveals is left over from some previous surgical catastrophe. Thus it may occur to you that perhaps it would be a good idea to have some extra airway equipment on hand when putting this patient to sleep, if you choose to put the patient to sleep at all.

"WHAT MEDICATIONS DO YOU TAKE?"

The medications that a patient takes will play a central role in the administration of anesthesia. Some anesthetics may be augmented by prescribed medications and others diminished by them, while other drugs may create hemodynamic instability. Knowing the effects of the patient's medications will assist in creating the anesthetic plan.
- You may want patients on clonidine to continue taking it so they don't exhibit any rebound hypertension, yet patients on losartan may exhibit intraoperative hypotension if they continue it. By convention, we prefer that patients continue taking their antihypertensives on the day of surgery[2] (with a mere sip of water, of course.)
- A specific medication issue arises for the majority of the diabetic population involving the need for NPO status on the day of surgery. It would be unwise for these patients to continue taking their hypoglycemic meds when they don't intend to eat anything. These are typically stopped before surgery to prevent dangerous hypoglycemia.
- On the other hand, insulin dosing is continued (albeit usually at a reduced dose) to prevent profound hyperglycemia and its inherent complications. These adjustments should be made with consideration for the patient's surgery start time and its expected duration.
    - If patients are scheduled for a brief procedure to be done first thing in the morning, then their typical regimen should be continued since they can be up and eating relatively soon postoperatively.

- If the case is longer, more complex, and begins later in the day, then the insulin regimen should be reduced by 30% to 50%[3] or otherwise you may have to administer that candy bar in a vial known as D50.
- A frequent issue that will arise in the preop clinic is that of anticoagulant medications. These are most commonly identified in patients who have received valve replacements or who have been stented previously.
  - The quandary lies in balancing the need to maintain stent patency and thus life and limb versus uncontrollable bleeding in the OR. The presence of these on the medication list should lead you to address your concern over its discontinuation or continued administration, but the decision should ultimately be left up to the surgeon or prescribing physician.
    - A cardiologist may be comfortable with stopping the Plavix for a few days, but the cardiac surgeon may prefer that the patient receive a heparin infusion in the hospital prior to the surgery.
- As a general rule, if patients are taking some medication or supplement that is not critical for their continued functioning or health, they should discontinue it. Logically, this would reduce their risk of unanticipated interactions and side effects and would also improve their overall NPO status.
  - We encourage patients to take their morning dose of metoprolol to control their blood pressure, but adding that enormous fiber tablet to the mix is unnecessary and can only increase their risk for aspiration.
  - A caveat to this rule involves patients on anti-anxiolytics. The necessity of anxiolysis to a patient's overall health can be argued, but continuing to take them on the day of surgery can only assist the anesthesiologist and prevent potentially crippling patient anxiety and stress prior to induction.
    - Furthermore, the prescribed dose that the patient typically takes on the morning of surgery is unlikely to be enough to interfere with obtaining adequate surgical and anesthesia consent.
- Lastly, although technically not a medication, a continuous positive airway pressure (CPAP) device used at home to counteract obstructive sleep apnea should undoubtedly be revealed to the anesthesiologist.
  - These patients are known to have multiple comorbid conditions such as coronary artery disease, cerebrovascular disease, congestive heart failure, etc. Even more relevant is the fact that they suffer increased adverse perioperative events.[4]

Patients' unique attributes can all be identified using a history, physical exam, and observation skills. This is the first step to take toward optimizing their condition and reducing their overall surgical risk.

"DO YOU HAVE ANY ALLERGIES TO MEDICATIONS OR MATERIALS?"

What could be more embarrassing than administering a prophylactic dose of cefazolin to someone who is allergic to it? Your face will certainly be red after that, maybe not as red (and swollen) as the patient's but red nonetheless.

- Identifying patients' allergies goes beyond what they are allergic to, including also what actually happens to them when they become exposed. Itching, swelling, and redness are all indicators of allergic reactions, yet hemodynamic or airway collapse may indicate far more dire consequences.
- A latex allergy is something that anesthesiologists often have to address and prepare for in the perioperative period. Aside from simply questioning the patient regarding an allergy to latex-based products there must also be a logical thought process concerning the patient's risk factors.
  - Patients with spina bifida, urologic anomalies, and those with multiple surgeries during childhood are often predisposed to latex sensitivity.
  - The same holds true for health care workers and those who are otherwise frequently exposed to latex products.
  - A history of unexplained anaphylaxis in a surgical or medical setting may also raise suspicion of latex hypersensitivity.[5]
- The presence of these factors should lead anesthesiologists to communicate their concerns to the surgical team and to prepare themselves for a latex-free anesthetic environment. Furthermore, plan B should be prepared in case of an incidental exposure to latex and the inevitable physiologic consequences that will develop.
- Drugs eliciting allergic responses in patients should be avoided, obviously, but sometimes it may involve medications that are critical to the planned anesthetic. A reluctance to administer a certain drug may significantly compromise the ability to perform the ideal anesthetic plan for patients, thus exposing them to unwarranted risks.
  - Consider patients who have previously undergone oral surgery and received an incidental injection of lidocaine and epinephrine solution intravascularly,

subsequently becoming severely tachycardic. The experienced practitioner certainly would not constitute this as a true allergy, but the patients may refuse to receive this drug again for fear of their heart exploding in their chest. This scenario could potentially preclude these patients from receiving lidocaine in the future despite how urgent it may be.
- A similar logic applies to patients who report drowsiness, nausea, or even generalized pruritus in response to narcotics such as codeine or morphine. These patients are likely experiencing isolated drug side effects rather than having an allergic reaction but may insist on avoiding these drugs anyway.

The preanesthetic evaluation is thus the ideal forum to sift out misconceptions and to educate patients about what medications they should or should not receive. Lastly, if the patient exhibits symptoms of a true allergy and the drug in question is absolutely necessary, then formal allergy testing may be indicated, but an alternate plan avoiding that drug should be prepared nonetheless.

"DO YOU SMOKE? DO YOU DRINK ALCOHOL? DO YOU USE ANY DRUGS?"

- The so-called "toxic habits" can certainly affect your anesthesia administration.
  - The lifelong smoker may have a consistent obstructive pattern on mechanical ventilation.
  - The chronic alcoholic may require larger doses of anesthetics to achieve appropriate anesthetic depth.
  - The OxyContin addict may scream bloody murder in pain at the conclusion of a minor, relatively painless procedure.
- The onus rests on the interviewer to put patients at ease and to assure them of the importance of full disclosure. Patients should be made aware of the potential effects that their substance use can have on them while under anesthesia and thus you should implore them to speak truthfully about their habits.
- Smokers should be encouraged to stop smoking prior to surgery regardless of the procedure or when it is scheduled for. Multiple studies have delineated the benefits toward reducing overall surgical complications following perioperative smoking cessation.[6]
- In keeping with NPO guidelines, smoking should also be prohibited immediately prior to surgery because of the increased production of airway secretions and the reduced clearance by chronically paralyzed cilia.

"ARE YOU ABLE TO WALK UP A FLIGHT OF STAIRS? CAN YOU CARRY GROCERIES DOWN THE BLOCK?"

Assessing physical and mental limitations is critical to the preop evaluation, as these will guide the ordering of further diagnostic tests, the creation of an intraoperative management plan, and the ability of patients to appropriately consent for their procedure.
- Patients with low intelligence or with psychiatric illness may not be able to fully comprehend the scope of what they are having done to them and thus may not be able to legally consent for their surgery and the associated anesthesia.
  - A guardian is often present with these patients to begin with, but occasionally you will need to make your own judgment regarding the patients' capacity to grasp what they are consenting for and then perhaps seek out a third party.
- A patient's level of exercise tolerance or functional capacity is vitally important for most presurgical evaluations.
  - Minor surgical procedures may not necessitate million dollar workups, but if a patient experiences angina upon walking to the store, then red flags should be raised.
- Anesthesia is used to reduce the physiologic stress of surgery, yet it may not be enough to preclude disastrous consequences in patients with tenuous physiology.
  - Patients with advanced coronary artery disease may be undiagnosed if they've never seen a cardiologist, but their symptomatology may give you reason to be concerned.
    - Instead of chest pain they may experience dyspnea with light activity. This might lead you to wonder whether their problem has a cardiac or pulmonary etiology.
  - Further testing is certainly appropriate in these situations and particularly for complicated and high-risk procedures. As a rule of thumb one must consider whether any further testing (and resultant surgical delay) will actually modify the outcome of the surgery or anesthesia.
    - It is likely that coronary revascularization will improve a patient's chances of getting through a hip replacement but may not be necessary to survive a melanoma excision.
- Thus cardiac risk stratification is where we get to the real meat of this topic. The elements of this decision making can be confusing and convoluted but will contribute greatly to doing the right thing for your patient's safety.

Table 54-1 Levels of Risk Factors for Surgery

Risk Factor	Symptom/Characteristic	Surgery
Major/High	MI within 1 month	Emergent
	Decompensated CHF	Aortic
	Unstable angina	Major peripheral vascular
	Severe valvulopathy	Major blood loss
	High-grade AV block	Major fluid shifts
	SVT with uncontrolled ventricular tachycardia	
	Symptomatic ventricular arrhythmias	
Intermediate	Stable angina	Orthopedic
	Compensated CHF	Prostate
	Past MI	Carotid
	Q-waves on ECG	Head/Neck
	Diabetes	Intrathoracic
	Renal insufficiency	Intraperitoneal
Minor/Low	Past stroke	Cataract
	Uncontrolled hypertension	Breast
	Poor exercise tolerance	Skin
	Non-sinus rhythm	Endoscopy
	Abnormal ECG	
	Age >65	

- The initial step begins with identifying patient risk factors and classifying them into major, intermediate, or minor on the scale of predictors.
  - Evaluate Table 54-1 and keep in mind that the presence of the major risk factors will play the foremost role in your decision making.
- The next consideration is the complexity and risk affiliated with the pending surgery.
  - Low-risk procedures typically have a cardiac risk of less than 1% and rarely require further testing.
  - The intermediate-risk procedures carry a cardiac risk of between 1% and 5%.
  - The high-risk procedures carry a greater than 5% cardiac risk and frequently require further cardiac evaluation.
- Within the high-risk category, emergent procedures likely provide the highest pound-for-pound cardiac risk to the patient. Despite this, the procedures are emergent and very likely need to proceed without the benefit of any further testing.[7]
- The ECG is the simplest and most commonly ordered diagnostic cardiac test, but before ordering an ECG one should consider whether the information that it provides will actually contribute to changing your overall anesthetic plan.
  - An ECG is relevant for a patient that exhibits any of the symptoms or characteristics shown in Table 54-1, but there are many other germane factors to consider. Thus we must synthesize all of the obtained information into a plan for further evaluation.

- The presence of major risk factors (especially unstable angina and decompensated heart failure) is an indication for immediate cardiac evaluation likely via invasive intervention (e.g., coronary angiography).
- Other patients become a little harder to classify. The existence of two out of three of the following factors is a signal for further cardiac evaluation:
  - Present intermediate-risk factors
  - Poor functional capacity
  - High surgical risk
- Fulfilling these criteria requires the patient to move on to noninvasive testing of cardiac function.
  - Exercise stress testing is reserved for those patients with a normal ECG who can actually exercise, because a treadmill stress test may not be the ideal setting for a lower extremity amputee.
  - Pharmacologically induced stress tests can achieve the same diagnostic endpoints in the patients who cannot use the treadmill. These include dipyridamole, adenosine, or dobutamine stress tests and often incorporate echocardiography or nuclear imaging to actually visualize perfusion defects in the stressed heart.
- Diagnostics such as echocardiography and stress tests can be costly and time consuming and may delay the planned surgery. Diagnostic serum tests, on the other hand, appear to be harmless, which lead us to consider getting them.
  - Fight the urge to order every blood test under the sun because the more you order, the more likely you are to discover false positives that may be irrelevant to the procedure at hand but that must now be further investigated.
  - A patient with chronic obstructive pulmonary disease (COPD) who is pending lung reduction surgery likely needs a preoperative chest x-ray. The healthy 17-year-old with the torn anterior cruciate ligament (ACL) probably won't benefit from a chest x-ray since we don't expect any significant pulmonary effects during or after the surgery.
  - When there is an expectation of significant blood loss then it is reasonable to get a hemoglobin level to establish a baseline. Further, if a type and screen is done preoperatively it will be appreciated when blood needs to be rushed into the OR emergently.
  - A relatively healthy patient who is not taking blood thinners probably will not benefit from checking a set of coagulation factors.
  - A patient on Synthroid with chronic hypothyroidism may benefit from thyroid function tests to identify abnormalities, while a normal healthy patient will not likely gain anything from this test.
  - If the patient is a female of child-bearing age, then a pregnancy test is always a good idea. Certain anesthetics can cause a plethora of in utero problems, especially in the first trimester, so testing may be performed for reassurance.

In any event, if you order a test, you should actually follow it up; otherwise, you probably didn't really need it in the first place. Always recall that the tests you order are intended to improve the outcome of your surgery in some way; will the obtained data modify your management at all? Do you expect it to affect the patient's postoperative morbidity and mortality? (Figure 54-3)

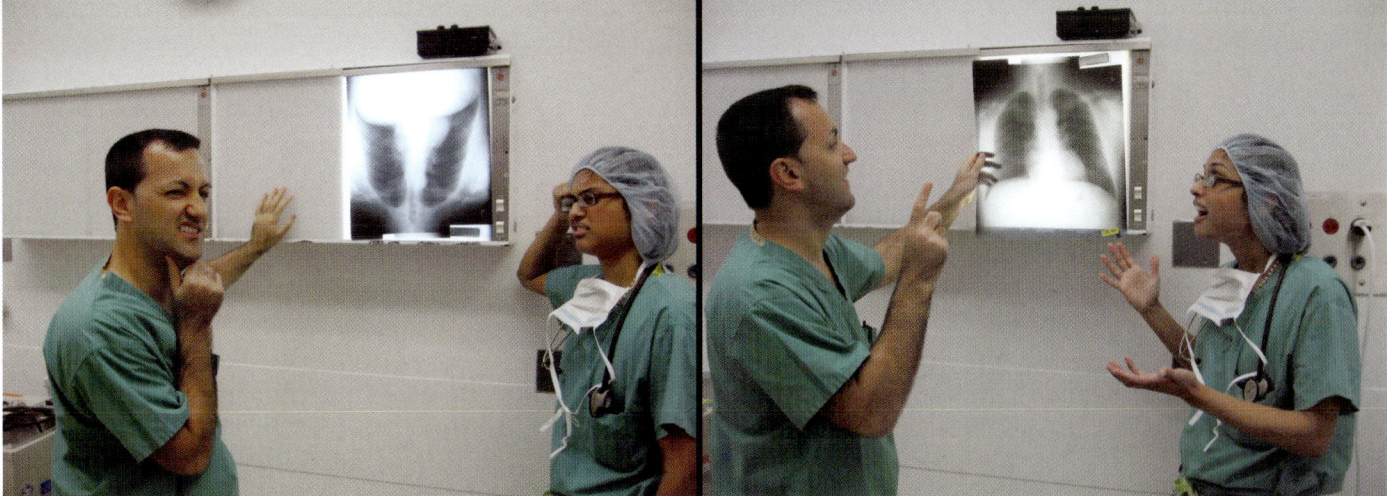

FIGURE 54-3 Dr. Slomovits and Dr. Mathew demonstrate that, with a little effort, anesthesiologists can interpret chest x-rays too.

"THIS WON'T HURT. I'M JUST GOING TO PERFORM A BRIEF EXAMINATION."

Enough with the talking, let's do some doctor-like stuff. What is the patient's baseline? That might just be something you'd wish you knew after the patient wakes up and can't feel his or her left pinky.
- Depending on the type and complexity of the surgery, a new physical finding may be evaluated further or addressed after the procedure. In either case it should be documented so there is no question as to whether it was present prior to the operation.
- Similar thinking applies to any surgeries on the brain, carotid artery, spine, or peripheral nerves. A thorough neurologic exam is critical to establishing the patient's baseline status so as to evaluate their improvement or deterioration after the procedure. In the same vein, the patient's sensorium is easily assessed simply by speaking with them.
    - If they don't know what year it is today, then it's probably not the anesthesiologist's fault if they think it's 1942 postoperatively.
- Finally, the airway exam is paramount in the preoperative setting, as many problems may arise during induction and intubation. Appropriately assessing the patient's ability to be easily intubated cannot be downplayed. An unanticipated difficult intubation may create an unsafe situation for the patient where one was not otherwise necessary.
- An easy to intubate airway and an extremely difficult to intubate airway are somewhat easy to spot, but those in between fall into a somewhat gray area to the inexperienced eye.
- A thorough assessment of the patient's mouth, palette, neck, throat, and dentition (do they actually have any teeth?) is vital. (Table 54-2)
    - How likely is laryngoscopy to be successful?
    - Will a fiberoptic scope be necessary?
    - Does it seem that you will be able to manually ventilate the patient or will he or she need to keep breathing spontaneously?
- The final step is to prepare patients for the various techniques that may be attempted for achieving adequate airway control. Their cooperation in the actual act of fiberoptic intubation cannot be underestimated, and educating them to the procedure and its purpose will allow them to mentally prepare for the process.

"ARE YOU WILLING TO CONSENT FOR THE ANESTHETIC PLAN?"

Now that you've obtained all the necessary data and prepared patients to undergo further testing, it's time to tell them exactly what you plan to do and to obtain their permission for it.
- A plan should be in place for all further preop testing that is yet to be obtained.
- All medication stoppages or continuations should be arranged.
- A strategy for induction, intubation, and maintenance, as well as awakening and extubation

Table 54-2 Airway Features to Check for Preoperatively

Airway Feature	Run for the Hills If You See...
Upper incisor length	Long
Maxillary and mandibular incisor relation during closure	Prominent overbite
Maxillary and mandibular incisor relation during protrusion	Mandible reaches anterior to maxilla
Maxillary and mandibular incisor relation during opening	>3 cm
Uvula visibility	Mallampati class 3 or 4
Palatal shape	Narrow or arched
Compliance of submandibular space	Stiff, indurated, noncompliant
Thyromental distance	<3 finger breadths
Neck size	Short and thick
Head/neck range of motion	Poor extension or flexion

versus continued mechanical ventilation should already exist.
- The patient can thus be informed of the anesthetic technique you intend to use and why you chose that particular method.
  - A knee arthroplasty done under spinal or regional anesthesia may seem the obvious choice for the initiated, but a patient may be concerned about the concept of "being awake" for the surgery.
- There are of course many toys that anesthesiologists often play with in the OR that may become necessary during certain surgeries. The value or disadvantage of these tools should be considered.
  - It is reasonable to start a lower extremity vascular bypass with good peripheral IV access, but should there be excessive bleeding a central line may become necessary.
    - Furthermore, the patient should be informed of the possibility and the likelihood, in your estimation, of the occurrence of substantial bleeding that may require a transfusion.
  - Some surgeries can call for an epidural being placed prior to induction but with the purpose of augmenting pain control postoperatively.
    - Patients should be led to understand that the epidural is not actually the anesthesia method, which may be a source of confusion for them.
  - Other anesthesia adjuncts that patients may become intimately familiar with if things take a turn for the worse in the OR include arterial lines, Swan-Ganz catheters, transesophageal echocardiography, etc. Patients should always be made aware of the possibility of these devices being used.

Communicating the risks and benefits of the intended anesthesia method is central to obtaining consent and to putting the patient at ease with the plan. Finally, if you do not expect to be the anesthesiologist on the day of surgery then communicating your objective and subjective findings as well as your tentative plan to the anesthesia team is the final essential step. An appropriate handoff punctuating your concerns and how you would address them is crucial to ensuring that all of your efforts on the patient's behalf aren't for naught.

Now that you have exhausted all of your questioning (and the patients hopefully have as well) and evaluated all necessary diagnostic tests, you can send them off to have their surgery. You should rest assured that you have done due diligence to ensure that the patient can safely undergo anesthesia and wake up comfortably at the end.

Pat yourself on the back, but don't hurt yourself, there are more patients to be seen.

REFERENCES

1. http://wendyusuallywanders.files.wordpress.com/2008/04/goiter.jpg
   Have you ever seen a neck like this before? It seems that every anesthesiologist should know that patients like this DO exist out there in the ether.
2. Prys-Roberts C. Should antihypertensive medications be continued through the perioperative period? In: Fleisher L, ed. *Evidence-based practice of anesthesiology*. Philadelphia: Saunders; 2004, pp. 68–76.
   This is an excellent discussion of the benefits and drawbacks of hypertensive medications in surgical patients.
3. Afifi E, Rosenbaum S. Does perioperative hyperglycemia increase the risk of postoperative complications? In: Fleisher L, ed. *Evidence-based practice of anesthesiology*. Philadelphia: Saunders; 2004, pp 172–180.
   A review of the need and techniques for modifying hypoglycemic regimens in the perioperative period.
4. Chung F, Yegneswaran B, et al. STOP Questionnaire: a tool to screen patients for obstructive sleep apnea. *Anesthesiology* 2008;108:812–821.
   Patients with obstructive sleep apnea are becoming increasingly common in the OR due to the progressive obesity epidemic in America. This article applies to the perioperative physician because it discusses a simple way to assess for the presence of sleep apnea.
5. Holzman R. What is the optimal perioperative management for latex allergy? In: Fleisher L, ed. *Evidence-based practice of anesthesiology*. Philadelphia: Saunders; 2004, pp 111–117.
   What do you do differently for a latex-sensitive patient? How do you identify those at risk for latex-sensitivity? Look no further than this treatment of the issue.
6. Findlay J. Is there an optimal timing for smoking cessation? In: Fleisher L, ed. *Evidence-based practice of anesthesiology*. Philadelphia: Saunders; 2004, pp 57–61.
   Smoking has multiple negative effects on the body and there may potentially be an exacerbation of these effects if one stops smoking at the "wrong" time. Patients should be encouraged to quit regardless of the circumstances and as soon as possible, but the effects will differ if it is 2 months, 2 weeks, or 2 days preoperatively.
7. Fleisher L, Beckman J, et al. ACC/AHA 2007 guidelines on perioperative cardiovascular evaluation and care for noncardiac surgery. *J Am Coll Cardiol* 2007; 50:e159–e242.
   The guidelines set forth describing the strategy for perioperative cardiac risk stratification and optimization.

CHAPTER 55
OFF-SITE ANESTHESIA

CHRISTIAN ALTMAN

Travel is glamorous only in retrospect.
Paul Theroux

Editors' note: The content of this chapter is similar to that of the MRI and catheter lab chapters, but the concepts are worth repeating, as offsite work is very anxiety provoking, and thus worth another look.

INTRODUCTION

Let's face it: more and more procedures requiring anesthetics are being performed in off-site locations (GI lab, interventional radiology, CT/MRI, electrophysiology lab, and cardiac cath lab, to name a few). While many of the procedures scheduled in remote locations are considered "low-risk" surgeries, problems can arise quite quickly. In a 2009 U.S. closed claims analysis of anesthesia complications, airway management was the most common reason for malpractice claims against anesthesiologists. The occurrence of respiratory complications in an off-site venue was twice that of operating room locations (44% vs. 20%). Of the off-site locations, the GI suite comprised one third of the malpractice claims, with monitored anesthesia care (MAC) being involved in 82% of these cases.[1]

Although it might be reassuring to think that all patients scheduled for procedures in remote areas of the hospital are a pristine picture of health, this just isn't the case. Many of these patients are even more complicated than the ones we routinely care for in the main OR.

For example, let's take a case I had in the GI lab a couple of weeks ago. The patient was an 81-year-old woman who had undergone a left mandibulectomy/fibular free flap reconstruction with radiation and chemotherapy for squamous cell cancer 10 years earlier. Having a complaint of dysphagia, she came to the GI lab for an esophagogastroduodenoscopy (EGD) and esophageal dilation. As you can imagine, her mouth opening was severely suboptimal, especially when you remember that the GI practitioners need to put a scope down the patient's throat after I put her to sleep. To complicate matters, this patient also had limited neck mobility and atrial fibrillation with severe mitral regurgitation and severe tricuspid regurgitation.

Before giving you more juicy details about this off-site adventure, let's look at some of the salient points for anesthetic management in the most distant locales in the hospital.

Be Prepared

Set up your space as you would for a general anesthetic in the main OR, even if you are planning MAC for your patient. You never know what you may need during the procedure (Figure 55-1).

- Machine: equipment check, backup oxygen tank, suction
- Monitors: electrocardiogram leads, blood pressure cuff, pulse oximetry, E_TCO_2, temperature (in the MRI suite, these need to be MRI-compatible)
- Medications: sedatives, narcotics, induction agents, muscle relaxants, maintenance anesthetic (IV vs. inhaled anesthetics, depending on your hospital's gas scavenging setup), muscle relaxant reversal, adjuncts (e.g., antacids, antiemetics)
- Mask ventilation: masks, oral airways, nasal airways (with lubricant), tongue blades, mask strap
- Intubation: laryngoscope handles and blades, endotracheal tubes, stylets
- Other: nasal cannula with E_TCO_2 port, extension tubing for IV lines, phone number to main anesthesia desk

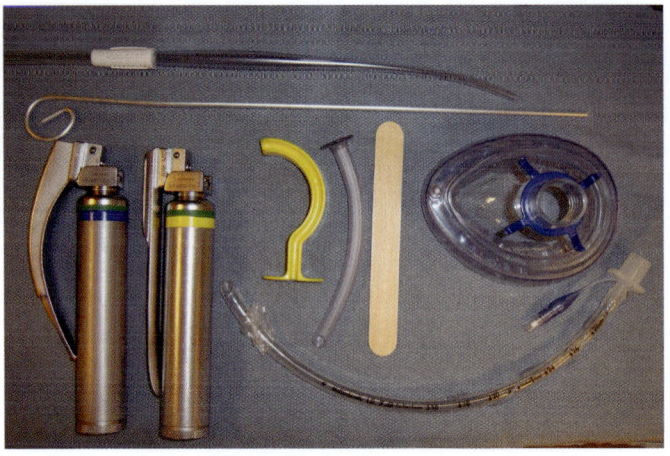

FIGURE 55-1 Normal airway setup.

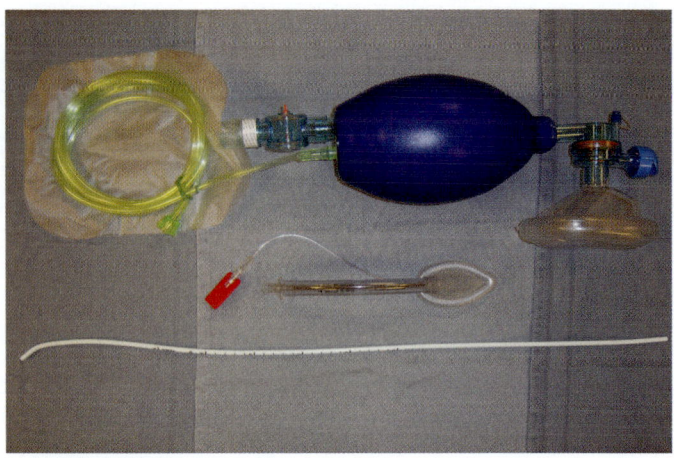

FIGURE 55-2 Airway resuscitation equipment.

Be More Prepared

Even if you're anticipating a routine induction and intubation, be ready for hemodynamic and airway complications. Always have the following, at a minimum (Figure 55-2):

- Resuscitation medications: inotropes/pressors (e.g., ephedrine, phenylephrine, epinephrine, atropine, calcium); antihypertensives (e.g., esmolol, labetalol, hydralazine, nitroglycerin); IV fluids
- Airway rescue equipment: laryngeal mask airway (LMA) of various sizes, Eschmann stylet, Ambu bag
- Backup medications: determine what quantity of medication you think you might need (propofol, fentanyl, muscle relaxant, etc.) and then get more. Get a lot more! Those cerebral aneurysm coiling cases booked for 3 hours can easily extend to double that time or more.

Deal with Real Estate

While setting up your room, you will probably figure out that you have less space in an off-site setting than you do in the typical OR Figures 55-3 and 55-4:

- You may not have a lot of room to maneuver once the procedure starts, so have things organized from the beginning. If you will be geographically separated from the patient (i.e., in the MRI suite), hook up extension tubing to your IV line so you'll have a way to give the patient medications during the procedure. If you're planning to run an infusion for anesthetic maintenance, you may need extension tubing for that medication to minimize IV dead space and deliver the infusion as close to the patient as possible.
- The MRI suite also requires special nonmetallic monitors and laryngoscopes that are not affected by the magnet in the MRI machine. For general anesthesia,

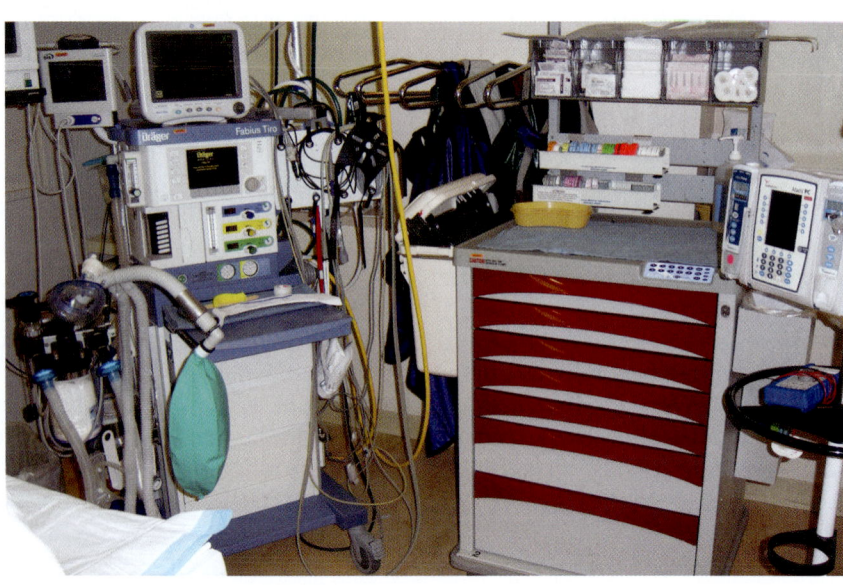

FIGURE 55-3 Off-site anesthesia area, demonstrating space limitations.

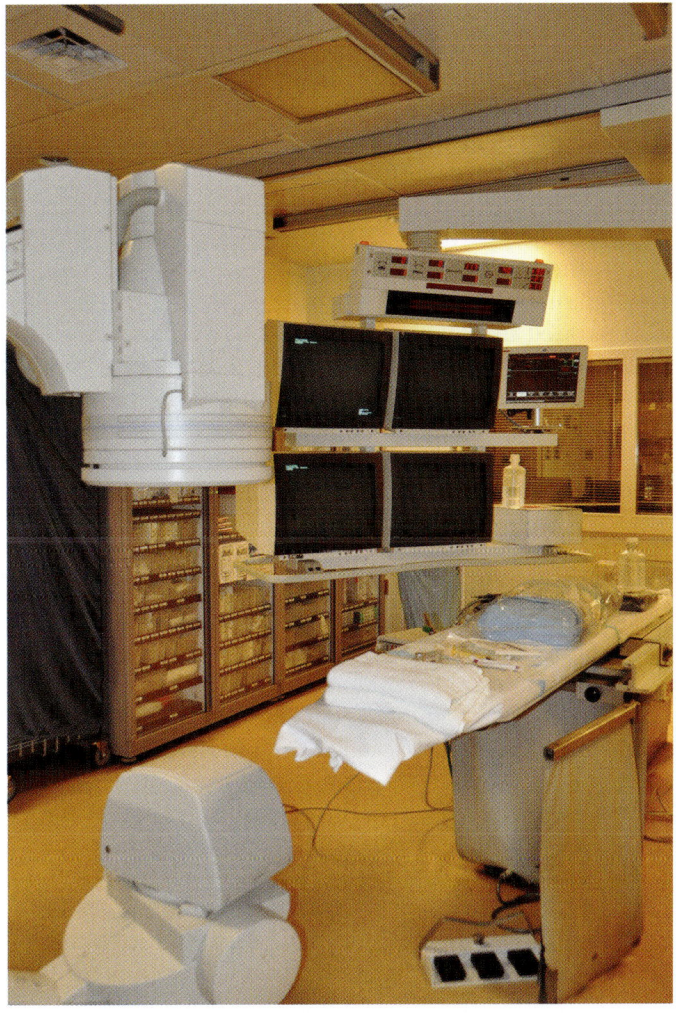

FIGURE 55-4 The anesthesia machine and monitors are placed behind a bank of screens.

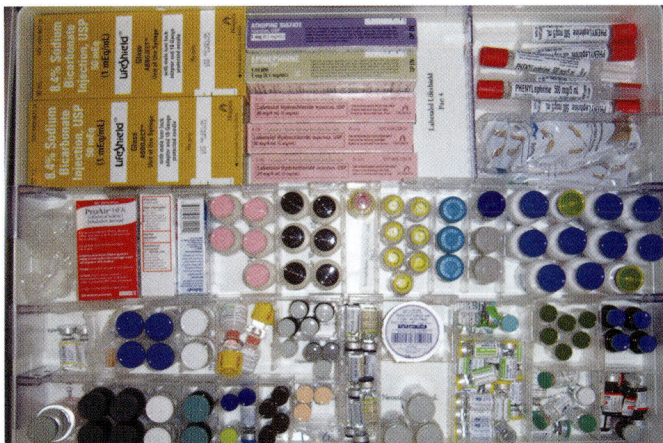

FIGURE 55-5 Anesthesia medication drawer.

the patient can be connected to the ventilator through breathing circuit extension tubing if the anesthesia machine will be located distantly from the patient.
- One more tip about your general setup: don't forget about your suction equipment! Often the suction canister is located in the most inconvenient spot in the room, making this crucial piece of apparatus easy to overlook. If you don't see it, ask someone to help you.

Know What's in Your Toolbox

Make sure you have a handle on the organization of your pharmaceutical armamentarium (Figure 55-5).
- Not knowing this crucial piece of information will put you at risk for making a drug error in an emergency situation or in cases with suboptimal lighting conditions (for instance, interventional radiology procedures). You may be lucky and have an off-site anesthesia cart that has the same supplies and layout as the carts in the main OR.
- Other hospitals use a different setup, such as an off-site medication "tool box" that is stocked by the pharmacy and takes up less space in the procedure suite. Whatever your situation, make sure you know what medications you have before you need to use them! (And if you're missing something, go grab it before the procedure starts.)

"It's Just a 15-Minute Procedure; Can I Just Do an Abbreviated Preop?"

- Now that we've got some basic equipment set up in the room, it's time to preop the patient. While many off-site procedures are considered low risk on the American College of Cardiology (ACC)/American Heart Association (AHA) cardiac risk algorithm, don't write them off as entailing routine anesthetics. You will want to interview the patient just as thoroughly as you do your patients in the main OR. This includes past surgical history, prior anesthetic complications, allergies, medications—you get the idea. I heard a story of a colleague who once ran into a cath lab just in time to ask, "Any anesthetic problems?" The patient looked up and said (I kid you not), "Yes, I have Malignant Hyperthermia (MH)."
- Once you finish asking the patient all of these questions, don't forget to look at the airway! Remember: planning a safe anesthesia is an all-important part of surviving an off-site anesthesia day.
- Is the patient at risk of needing a blood transfusion? A radiofrequency ablation of a lung lesion might not seem like a risky procedure, but in a sick, anemic patient with hepatic failure who unexpectedly bleeds, you might not be able to get emergency *anything* as smoothly as you would in the main operating room. Your threshold for obtaining at least a type and screen should be adjusted accordingly.

"It's Just a 15-Minute Procedure; The Anesthetic Shouldn't Be a Big Deal, Right?"

- After seeing the patient, it is time to put together your anesthesia plan. For some off-site cases, a MAC technique may be appropriate. (But don't forget that general anesthesia, with a secure airway, is the backup anesthesia for any sedation case!)
- For MAC cases in a "shared airway" situation (such as upper endoscopy in the GI suite), topicalizing the posterior pharynx with Cetacaine spray works well. This technique helps patients tolerate the passage of the scope, and it helps you to avoid oversedating the patient during this stimulating part of the procedure. But don't be too generous with the Cetacaine spray, as there is a risk of methemoglobinemia!
- For other cases, you will need to deliver a general anesthetic. Always remember to think about the practical aspects of securing the airway. For instance, will there be a "shared airway" situation during the procedure? If so, an LMA probably isn't a sensible option. Will the patient be prone for the procedure? Again, you would want to consider a cuffed endotracheal tube in that situation.
- No matter what your anesthetic preference, always have contingency plans A, B, and C, and probably D—especially since working in a remote location falls outside your normal comfort zone.

A Few Words About the Difficult Airway

- If you come across a patient who may pose an airway challenge, take a few minutes to put together your very best management strategy. (No, this does not mean you fake an illness and head home for the day.) When formulating your plan, make your first approach your best one. Consider what resources you can utilize to safely take care of the patient. Maybe you have a more experienced colleague who can come and give you a hand.
- In a more complicated situation, you may need a few minutes to topicalize the patient for awake fiberoptic intubation, which also requires time to get the fiberoptic scope from the main OR.
- Finally, don't forget to utilize the procedure suite staff. The nurses there often have lots of experience, and they should be able to help you with specific tasks if you ask them. But remember: they may not be entirely attuned to anesthesia issues and jargon, so they may need more explicit communication than operating room personnel.

Getting the Procedure Done

- Once you get the patient into the procedure room, you will want to hook him or her up to your American Society of Anesthesiologists (ASA) standard monitors. This includes E_TCO_2, which sometimes requires a bit of creativity and jerry-rigging, depending on your traveling anesthesia machine and monitors. During a MAC case, the E_TCO_2 waveform may be the first indication that the patient needs assistance (e.g., chin lift, nasal trumpet) in maintaining a patent airway. The E_TCO_2 is equally important during a general anesthesia case.
- Vigilance is crucial. In the MRI suite, you will be separated from your patient by quite a distance and will not be able to see if the endotracheal tube becomes disconnected from the breathing circuit. In the interventional radiology suite, there may be a giant bank of monitors between you and the patient. (Anesthesiologists are forever hitting their heads on these, so maybe we should start wearing helmets.) In some environments the patient may be prone or may be facing 180 degrees away from you. In short, never start an anesthetic without an E_TCO_2 monitor! And don't forget the suction! Finally, these patients are particularly vulnerable to injuries related to positioning. Be vigilant of these and other basics that are easy to take for granted in the main operating room.
- Even with the most thorough planning, sometime during your career you will encounter an airway that doesn't behave the way you expect it to. For these situations, you will want to know the ASA difficult airway algorithm backward and forward. When you are in this predicament, keep a level head. Herein lies the importance of keeping the phone number to the main OR handy. Call for help right away if you are having problems, but bear in mind that it may take longer for assistance to arrive, depending on how remote you are in your off-site location. In the meantime, ask for help from your procedure-room friends. Instructed well, a nurse or other staff member can give good jaw thrust or cricoid pressure to aid in mask ventilating or intubating a difficult patient. Now is not the time to be a superhero and try to do everything yourself. Keeping the patient safe is your number-one priority.

CASE EXAMPLE

So how did we handle the complicated airway patient in the GI lab? During the preop interview, we consented the patient for an awake nasal fiberoptic intubation. After the anesthesia tech brought the fiberoptic scope down from the main OR, we gave the patient one spray of Neo-Synephrine spray in each nare as well as midazolam 0.5 mg IV. We took the patient to the procedure room and hooked her up to the basic monitors, including a nasal cannula with an E_TCO_2 port in the patient's mouth. To add a little more sedation, we administered ketamine 10 mg IV and began a low-dose remifentanil infusion of 0.02 µg/kg/min. We began topicalizing the patient's right nare with 4% lidocaine on cotton swabs, adding one at a time to gently dilate the nasal passage. Once the patient was safely sedated and topicalized, we were able to easily pass the fiberoptic scope. Luckily, her thin body habitus worked in our favor and her vocal cords popped right into view. We sprayed the cords with 4% lidocaine and then passed the scope into the trachea. The nasal RAE tube smoothly passed through the nose and into the trachea, confirmed with a view through the fiberoptic scope. We attached the circuit, confirmed an E_TCO_2 waveform, and gently anesthetized the patient with propofol. The procedure went quickly, and we successfully extubated the patient once the GI docs were finished.

CONCLUSION

- Airway/respiratory complications are more common during off-site anesthetics than during anesthetics in the main OR.
- Always be prepared for a general anesthetic even if you are planning MAC/sedation.
- Be familiar with medications you have available for your anesthetic as well as for resuscitation.
- Have airway rescue equipment available; you never know when you may need it.
- Don't skimp on the preop; this will help you put together the safest anesthetic plan for the patient.
- Have multiple backup plans for every off-site anesthetic you administer.
- Don't be afraid to call for help.

REFERENCE

1. American Society of Anesthesiologists. Practice guidelines for management of the difficult airway. *Anesthesia* 2003;98:1269–1277.
   The ASA difficult airway algorithm can be found here. For the most current practice guidelines, you can always visit the ASA Web site.

SUGGESTED READING

Metzner J, Posner KL, Domino KB. The risk and safety of anesthesia at remote locations: the US closed claims analysis. *Curr Op Anaesth* 2009;22:502–508.
Respiratory events are the top risk of anesthesia in remote locations and occur twice as often in off-site areas than in the main operating room.

CHAPTER 56

TRANSPORTING A PATIENT, OR DON'T GET CAUGHT IN THE ELEVATOR UNPREPARED

SARAH OLSON HECK
CHRISTINE PARK

Death and sorrow will be the companions of our journey.

Winston Churchill, House of Commons Speech, October 8, 1940

INTRODUCTION

Consider the following case: It's 4 AM and you are finishing an emergent cesarean-hysterectomy for postpartum hemorrhage in a patient who had an unknown placenta accreta. The case started 6 hours ago when the patient suddenly bled over a liter and a half and she became unstable with a systolic blood pressure in the 50s. She was then emergently taken to the OR for a cesarean section that turned into a hysterectomy secondary to uncontrolled bleeding. She had a difficult airway, requiring a GlideScope after three unsuccessful attempts at direct laryngoscopy (DL); she received 13 units of blood product, and is now in diffuse intravascular coagulation (DIC). Although she has been stable for the past 2 hours, she has nonetheless bought herself a bed in the ICU—the ICU that is a quarter mile away through an underground tunnel between the hospital you are currently in and its affiliated institution where the ICUs are harbored. You are exhausted and your mind starts drifting toward the few hours of precious sleep you are hoping to catch after you drop her off in the ICU.

At the end of a case like this, it is easy to start thinking ahead to the next step (the next case, lunch, sleep, heading home), but one of the most tenuous portions of the case still lies ahead of you: transporting her to the ICU.

You may be asking yourself why transport is such a stressful period for the anesthesiologist when the surgical procedure is already completed. The answer arises from some basic principles that are paramount to anesthesiology:

1. When a situation arises where you need more hands, call for help.
2. The safest place for a sick patient is in the OR or the ICU.
3. Have everything you could possibly need for plans A to Z prepared and set out before your case starts.

The period when you are transporting patients essentially violates every single one of these rules. First, you are trucking critically ill patients through hallways and elevators (violating principle number 2), where your access to resources such as equipment, drugs, and personnel is severely limited (violating principles 1 and 3).

So, given that it seems everything is working against you while transporting patients to the ICU, it can be (and is) done safely every day. The key to getting the patient to the ICU unscathed is simple: be prepared.

Let's reconsider the case presented at the beginning of the chapter. Suppose you were the anesthesiologist. There are many issues facing you while you are transporting her. How are you going to make sure she gets to the ICU safely? She has previously been hemodynamically unstable and has the potential to again become unstable. You have a very long way to transport this patient, increasing the amount of time during which any host of problems could arise.

Smooth patient transport begins with having a plan in place before you leave the operating room. You should prepare any emergency equipment and drugs that you might need and make sure that equipment is working and easily accessible throughout transport (Figures 56-1 and 56-2).

What exactly do you need to prepare for transport? Basically, you need to think about four broad categories: airway, drugs, monitors, and IV access.

AIRWAY

Going back to the scenario presented at the beginning of the chapter: we have a patient who required special airway equipment for intubation and who has now received a large volume of fluid, possibly leading to upper airway edema. The last thing you want is for this patient to extubate herself during transport. And if she does extubate herself, you need to be prepared to handle that.

The most crucial step here is to make sure she doesn't become extubated in the first place.

1. Check that your endotracheal tube (ETT) is properly secured and in the correct position before leaving the OR. Recall where the ETT was taped at the start of the procedure. If it has migrated appreciably, check the position and move it if necessary. Double check that the patient still has bilateral breath sounds. If the tape job is questionable, take the time to retape it. You will thank yourself later.
2. Ensure that the patient will be adequately sedated throughout transport. We will consider this further in the next section, which discusses drugs.
3. Say the worst-case scenario does occur and the patient becomes extubated during transport. As long as you are prepared to mask ventilate, oxygenate, and reintubate the patient, this won't be a disaster.
4. Bring along the following items, and you will be able to achieve these goals:
   - Oral/nasal airways
   - ETT, styleted and balloon checked

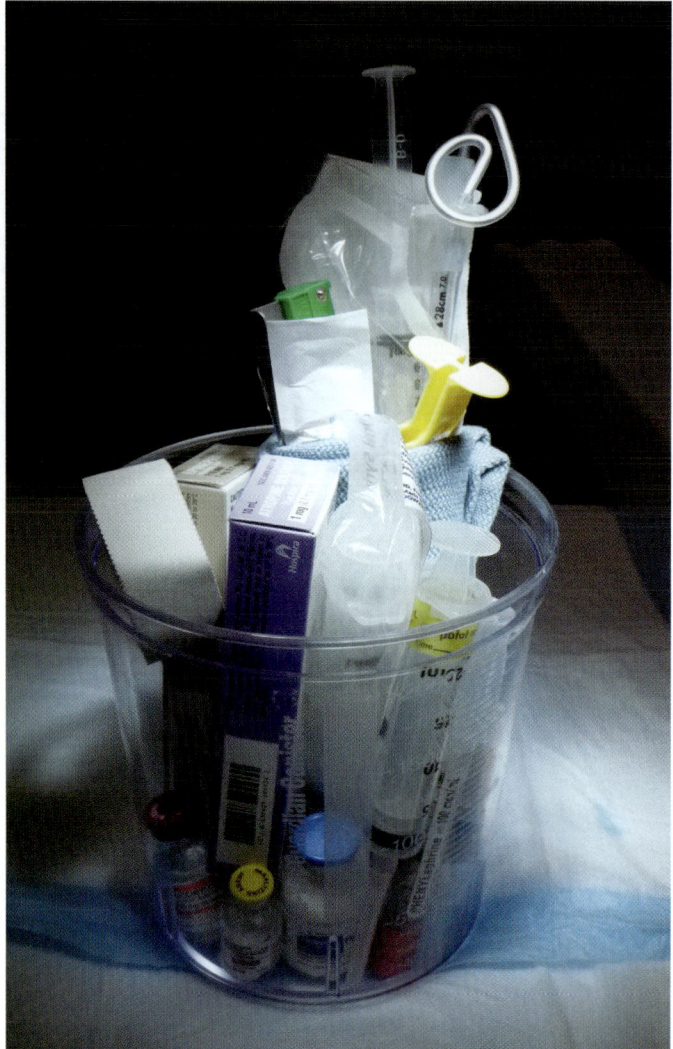

FIGURE 56-1 Transport armamentarium version 1.

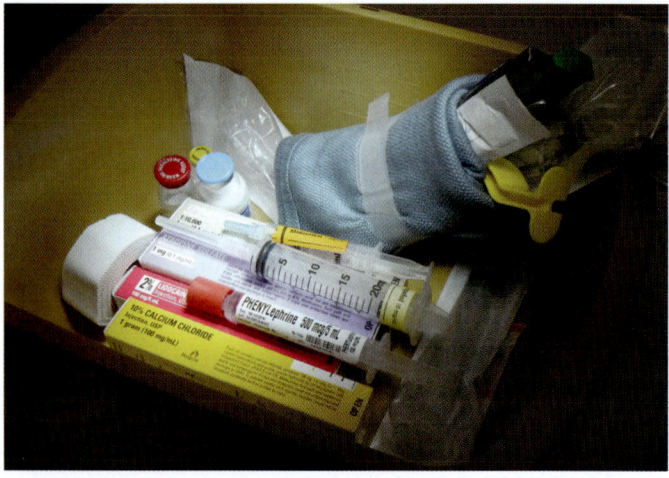

FIGURE 56-2 Transport armamentarium version 2.

- Laryngoscope handle with working light and appropriate blade (i.e., the same one the patient was successfully intubated with at the start of the case)
- Ambu bag and appropriately sized face mask
- Drugs (see below)
- Oxygen tank with adequate supply of oxygen

Any time you transport a patient, intubated or extubated, you need to check that you have an oxygen tank. These are usually already present on the patient's bed, but it is your responsibility to make sure it's not only there but also has an adequate supply of oxygen to get you to your destination (and then some). The tank is of no use to you if it is empty, or will be shortly. How long will the tank last, you ask? Good question!

A full E cylinder of oxygen is under 2000 mm Hg psi and contains 660 L of oxygen. The amount of oxygen in the tank is proportional to the psi. Thus, if the tank has a psi of 1000 mm Hg, you have 330 L of oxygen.

If the tank has a psi of 250, how much oxygen remains?

$$\frac{2000 \text{ mm Hg}}{660 \text{ L}} = \frac{250 \text{ mm Hg}}{x}$$

To solve for x,

$x = (250)(660)/2000$
$x = 82.5 \text{ L}$

Now you know how much oxygen remains in the tank, but you need to know how long that will last. This depends on the amount of oxygen the patient is requiring. To figure this out, all you need to do is divide the amount of oxygen remaining in the tank by the flow you have the patient on. Say you want to transport your intubated patient on 10 L/min of oxygen and you have 1000 psi remaining in the tank. From the calculation about, we know that there is 330 L of oxygen in the tank:

$$\frac{330 \text{ L}}{10 \text{ L/min}} = 33 \text{ min}$$

DRUGS

When in the operating room, you have your entire armamentarium of drugs available to you at a moment's notice. You will need to streamline this for transport, as it isn't necessary or efficient to bring your entire drug box with you. To determine what is necessary, consider your patients' needs, and anticipate what emergency drugs you may need during transport. There are essentially three categories of drugs you will need:

1. Sedation (midazolam, propofol, narcotic)
2. Vasoactive agents (phenylephrine, ephedrine, ± epinephrine, esmolol, nitroglycerine)
3. Airway (propofol, succinylcholine)

Sedation
- A properly sedated patient will make your transport much smoother. Just before leaving the operating room, you will need to liberate the patient from the inhaled anesthetic. Unfortunately, this does mean that at some point the patient will wake up, and we all know that when patients wake up, they tend to become hypertensive, tachycardic, and reach for their ETT; you don't want this happening in the middle of that long hallway.
- So you need to figure out how to keep the patient sedated during your journey to the ICU. Agents such as midazolam and propofol are probably your best bet as they are easily titrated and fast acting.
- Narcotics are also a good choice, as pain is a powerful stimulant that can cause agitation in the postop patient, and they will also help the patient tolerate the ETT better.
- Monitoring the vital signs will help you determine if the patient requires more sedation. A patient who is becoming more hypertensive and tachycardic during transport is likely in pain or a light plane of anesthesia, and requires a dose of something to deepen sedation.

Vasoactive Agents
- On the flip side of the patient not being sedated enough are too much sedation, residual anesthetic, and lack of surgical stimulation, which can cause the patient to become hypotensive during transport, and you need to be prepared to treat this as well.
- Many patients who had an otherwise uncomplicated anesthesia will still become hypotensive when surgical stimulation ceases. Phenylephrine and ephedrine are usually sufficient to treat this, and thus these drugs should always be with you during transport.
- Patients who had hemodynamic instability during the procedure will require more preparation, but here are a few basic rules:
  - If at anytime during the case the patient required a drip of any vasopressor, bring the drip with you on transport, even if it is no longer running.
  - Any agent out of the normal that you frequently needed during the case (e.g., esmolol, nitroglycerine, epinephrine) should come with you during transport.
  - If you have a high suspicion of the patient arresting or becoming very unstable during transport, epinephrine is your friend.
  - The idea is to streamline what drugs you bring with you, but still make sure you are prepared to treat the patient.

Airway

- If you properly sedate the patient, as outlined above, hopefully you won't need these drugs, but you always want to have them with you.
- Essentially, you need an induction agent and a muscle relaxant. If you are already bringing propofol with you for sedation, this can easily be used for induction, if necessary. The muscle relaxant of choice in this situation is succinylcholine (unless contraindicated) because of its fast onset of action.

MONITORS

1. Any patient going to the ICU needs to be transported with full monitoring, including pulse oximetry, ECG, and blood pressure.
2. Make sure there is a transport monitor on the bed and that it is fully charged and working. Just prior to leaving the room, switch the OR monitors over to the transport monitor.
3. Confirm that you can see the monitor and that the alarms and pulse oximeter sound are turned on. A monitor that you can't see or hear is of no use to you (Figures 56-3 and 56-4).

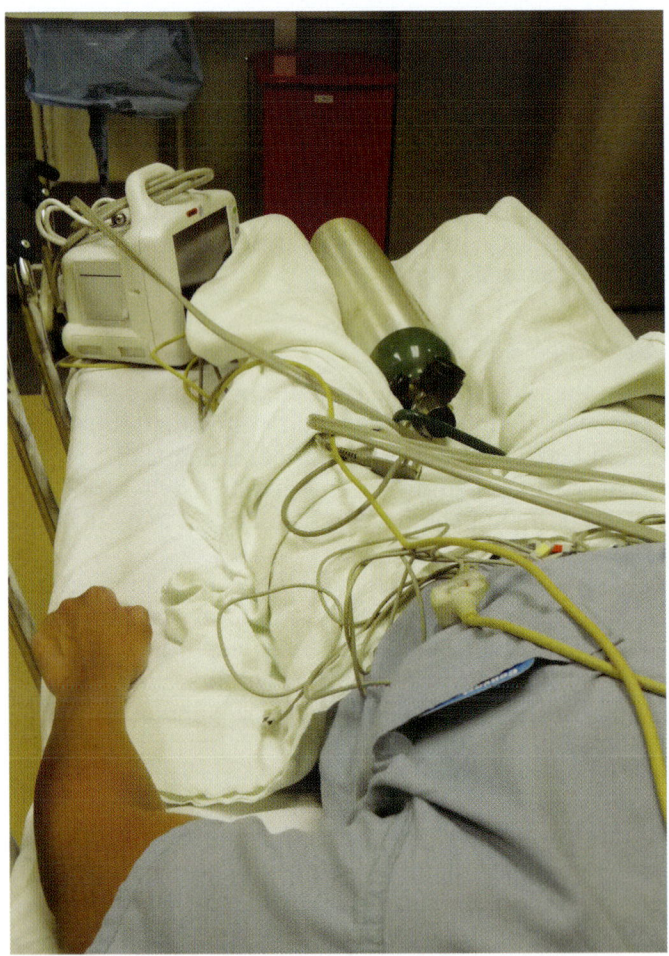

FIGURE 56-3 Not only is this monitor partially blocked, it's also difficult to see the monitor at this angle.

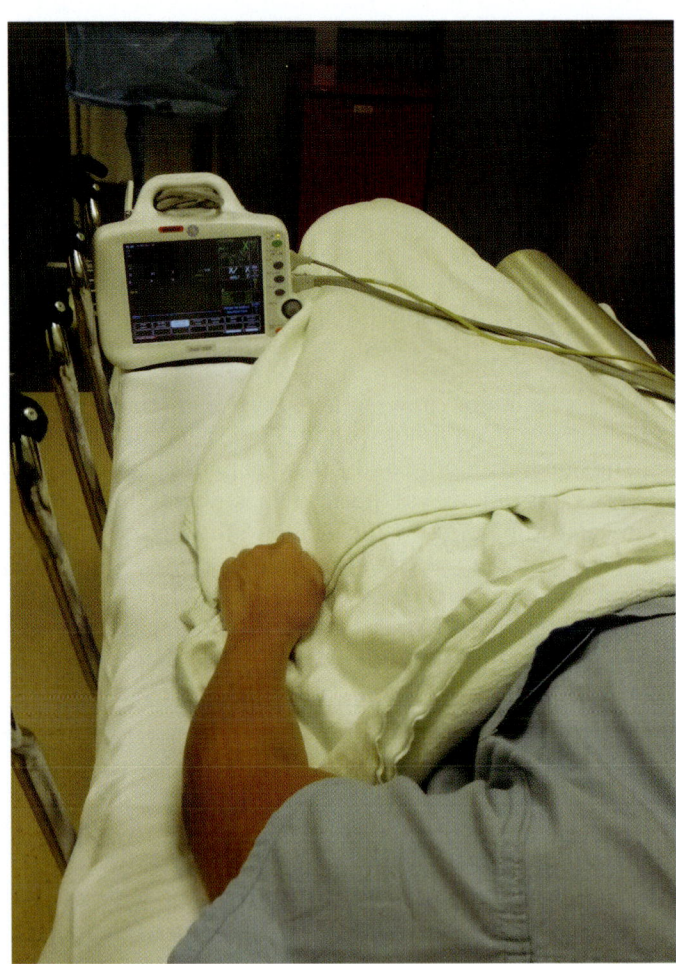

FIGURE 56-4 Monitors are now in clear view of anesthesiologist at the head of the bed.

IV

The last thing to check before rolling out of the room is that you have a readily accessible, freely running IV.

1. Dedicate one of your IV lines for pushing drugs during transport. This IV should be at the head of the bed and run freely.
2. Make sure you know what line you are using and hook up any drugs you think you might need to the stopcocks before leaving the OR.
3. Have in line a normal saline (NS) flush so the drugs can be rapidly administered.

HOW TO BE A TRANSPORT ROCK STAR

The above things will help you keep the patient alive and stable from the OR to the ICU. If you really want to be a rock star, you will have considered all of this prior to the end of surgery, so everything is in the room and prepared, your IV lines and monitors are untangled, and the minute the drapes come down you will be ready to move the patient to the transport bed and roll to the ICU.

1. When the surgeons start closing deep layers, start preparing the above-mentioned items. Place them in an accessible place that you can place at the head of the bed during transport.
2. Ask your circulating nurse to check outside the room to make sure the patient's bed is there and equipped with a transport monitor and full tank of oxygen.
3. Untangle the monitor and IV lines as best you can. Unhook anything that isn't necessary (e.g., if you have an arterial line, you can remove the noninvasive blood pressure cuff; if you have a central line, you can heplock peripheral IVs that aren't necessary). This way there are fewer things to move and thus a lower risk of lines being pulled out. At the same time, check that you have enough slack on your lines for moving the patient to the ICU bed.
4. Once the drapes are down, double-check the patient's airway. Is it in the proper position and securely taped?
5. Transfer the patient to the transport bed in a move that you lead and coordinate.
6. After transferring the patient, recheck that the airway is secure (e.g., do you have end-tidal CO_2).
7. Find an IV line and position the ports near you. Make sure it runs and flushes.
8. Make sure the patient is properly sedated.
9. Move your monitors over to the transport monitor once you have ensured that the patient is stable.
10. Check your oxygen tanks to make sure you have enough oxygen to get you to your destination. Hook the Ambu bag to the oxygen tank and make sure the bag inflates.
11. Begin ventilating the patient with the Ambu bag.
12. Turn off your volatile anesthetic.
13. Transport the patient to the ICU.

CONCLUSION

The most important thing is to prepare ahead of time and don't allow yourself to be rushed. The surgeons will be anxious to get to the unit at the end of a long procedure, but don't let them push you around. They took their time and operated in a safe manner, so now it is your job to get the patient to the ICU in a safe manner. If this means telling them to hold up for a minute while you find a dedicated IV line, then it is your prerogative, and duty, to do so.

SUGGESTED READING

Miller R. Neuromuscular blocking drugs. In: Stoelting RK, Miller RJ, eds. *Basics of anesthesia,* 5th ed. Philadelphia: Churchill-Livingstone; 2007, pp 135–154.
Discusses contraindications for the use of succinylcholine and other neuromuscular blocking agents.

Mort TC. Complications of emergency tracheal intubation: immediate airways related consequences, part II. *J Intensive Care Med* 2007;22(4):208–215.
Discusses morbidity and mortality related to emergency intubation occurring outside of the operating room.

Roth PA, Howley JE. Anesthesia delivery systems. In: Stoelting RK, Miller RJ, eds. *Basics of anesthesia,* 5th ed. Philadelphia: Churchill-Livingstone; 2007, pp 185–206.
In-depth discussion of anesthesia delivery systems, including how to determine what gas is contained in a canister and how to determine the amount of compressed gas remaining in the tank.

CHAPTER 57

INTENSIVE CARE UNIT

NISHANT GANDHI
THERESA L. HARTSELL

It's a matter of taking the side of the weak against the strong, something the best people have always done.
Harriet Beecher Stowe
All I care about is life, struggle, intensity.
Emile Zola, My Hates (1866)

INTRODUCTION

You're about to face your first (or at least your first as an anesthesiologist) rotation in the critical care unit! Despite many of us choosing anesthesiology in part because of interest in critical care, it's amazing how we get comfortable taking care of one patient at a time in a setting that we control. Before we teach you everything there is to know about critical care medicine (just kidding!), let's step back and answer a few basic questions:

- Why is rotating through the ICU important?
  - The ICU is a terrific physiology lab, where you have an up close and personal opportunity to understand critically ill patients (or at least their cardiac, pulmonary, and renal physiology) in ways that you can apply to the operating room.
  - You'll enhance your role as a perioperative physician. You'll remember (or relearn) diagnostics and therapeutics from general medicine, and gain experience with postoperative physiology past what you'll see in the recovery room. Remember, the surgical stress response isn't over just because the skin is closed! You might just start fine-tuning your anesthetic plan with that in mind.
  - With an increasingly aging population and the changing frontiers of surgery, you'll absolutely be seeing more critically ill patients in the future, and your anesthesia group may be called upon to manage aspects of ICU care by the hospital. Even if not, they'll show up in your OR!
  - It's an important subspecialty of anesthesia (that is, it's on your exam!).
  - You may actually get to know and enjoy your fellow residents of the surgical persuasion!
- How is the ICU different from the operating room?
  - You need to manage many patients instead of just one (prioritize!).
  - You need to remember more data on each patient (across more patients!).
  - You need to follow patient trends over a longer period of time.
  - You now care about renal, hematology, infectious disease, nutrition, etc.
  - There are often more team members and/ or stakeholders, so more emphasis on communication and potentially less autonomy.
  - You're not the one responsible for the pumps/vents, so get used to delegating instead of doing yourself.
- How is the ICU the same as the operating room?
  - Pharmacology and physiology are still pharmacology and physiology!
  - Sometimes you do need to focus intensely on just one patient.
  - Communication and teamwork are key!
  - We can say, "Hours of boredom; moments of terror!"

HOW TO PREPARE (THINGS TO DO BEFORE YOU START)

- Know your unit! Are you rotating in a medical, surgical, or mixed med-surg unit? Or possibly a subspecialty unit for care of cardiac, neuro, trauma, or burn patients? Pediatrics? This will give you an idea as to how to focus your reading ahead of time. Think about the common diseases or procedures that you'll see and think about how to manage them or what the postop complications might be. Some pre-rotation reading topics may jump to mind.

- Know your patients! You wouldn't head to the OR without doing a thorough preop evaluation, so neither should you show up for the ICU without doing a basic chart review on at least the patients who have been in the unit for a while. A little bit of effort the day before you start can go a long way toward hitting the ground running.
- Remember your passwords! You may need to access medical information systems that are different from those in the OR, so be sure to check out whether you need additional permissions/passwords or that you remember the ones you previously used.
- Check out the syllabus, and set some learning goals. Be sure you understand what you're expected to learn, and checking this out will help you identify areas you need to focus on quickly in order to take care of your patients (whom you know from your chart review!)
- Do your laundry and grocery shopping. Seriously! You will be working hard and need to be sure you have what you need to keep life moving along! If you don't know your hours or call schedule, be sure to ask in advance.
- Finally, know when to report and be sure you know the dress code! Sounds simple, but being late for rounds in a highly organized unit is not the way you want to start. Neither is walking in wearing scrubs if rounds are a formal "professional dress and white coat" affair. Consider yourself warned!

ON THE FIRST DAY (PAY ATTENTION TO THESE THINGS)

- Take a tour. Where is the emergency equipment (code cart, emergency airway, etc.)? Where can you find supplies for procedures? Is there a "line cart" or other mobile storage area? Find out where the call rooms are, where the bathrooms are (not always obvious!), and where you can find or store food and drink. Also find out where you should be when you're not actively involved in a patient room (nurses need to know where to find you, and may assume you're "hiding" if you're not accessible).
- Meet your team. How many layers of providers are there, and what are your lines of supervision? Some ICUs have 24/7 in-house attending intensivist coverage; others may have fellows who are directly involved with team supervision as well. Are your attendings and fellows all from anesthesia, or are some from surgery or medicine or pulmonary training? Are your fellow residents all from anesthesia, or will you work alongside residents from other disciplines (a terrific thing as you can learn a lot from each other)? Are you expected to teach junior residents or medical students? Are there mid-level providers such as nurse practitioners and physician assistants? If so, how do they integrate into the team?
- Get to know the nurses and other specialist providers. ICU nurses have a reputation for being fierce patient advocates and rightly so. Keep in mind that they've been doing this longer than you have, but that it's in their best interest as well as yours for there to be a good relationship. They can help you quite a bit, and help the patient even more. Make the effort to introduce yourself to the charge nurse and bedside nurses so that they know you, and work toward mutual respect. Similarly you may find pharmacists (some of whom may be critical care specialists with doctorates and residency training), respiratory therapists, physical and occupational therapists, critical care technicians, social workers, chaplains, etc., all of whom can help you get the right care for your patients (Figure 57-1).
- Find out the "stakeholders" for unit patients. Is this an "open" unit, where you're taking care of patients under the auspices of their primary physician who may or may not have ICU experience? In this case you may work closely with a number of consultants who can teach you about their specific area and you'll need to communicate with all? Is it a "closed" unit, where the ICU team is the exclusive primary team? Or in-between (may be called "semi-open," "semi-closed," or "mandatory consult"), where the ICU team manages all of the patients in coordination with their admitting team? In these cases you'll work closely with an intensivist who is trained to provide specialty organ-specific care while balancing needs across multiple systems. There may be some degree of shared decision making with other teams and some degree of limitation as to who can write orders for the patient as well, so it is important to know what level of communication with other teams is expected.
- Learn the order sets. Are there specific forms, either paper or on the computer, that are used for admissions, progress notes, rounds, or data maintenance? Most units also have common issues addressed with protocols, pathways, care bundles, and order sets, so it's important to find out about these also. It's easier for you not to reinvent the wheel, and although care may need to be individualized, these usually reflect the collective agreement of many parties. Knowing what exists will save you from doing something completely off

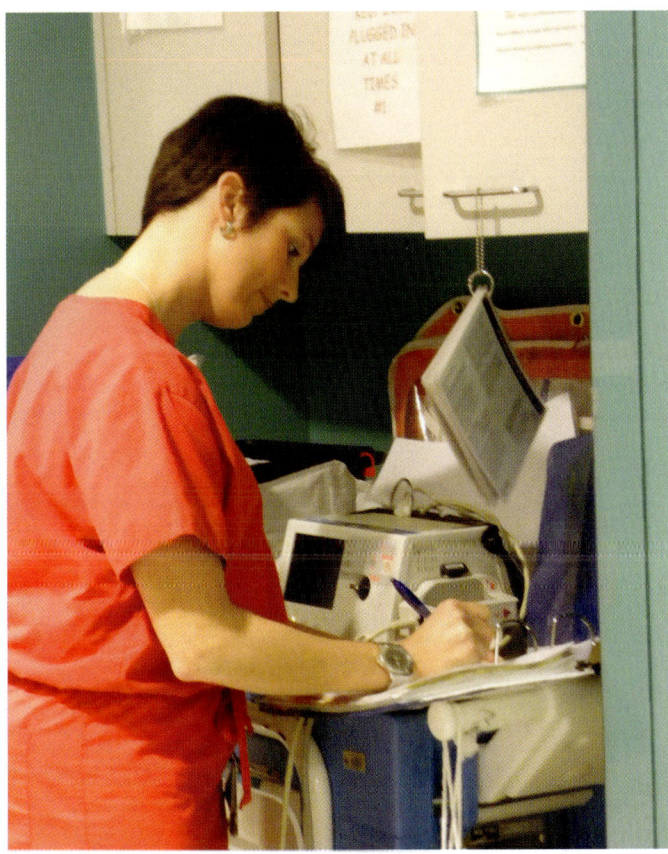

FIGURE 57-1 Make friends with the nurses; trust us on this one!

the wall without even knowing it! Not to mention saving you from forgetting something important!

DAILY ICU LIFE

Rounds

Often referred to as "shifting dullness," rounds usually occur in the morning and possibly the afternoon/evening, and do actually serve some purpose. Since a great deal of your ICU life may be spent rounding, and certainly a great deal of your evaluation, let's spend some time on what rounds accomplish and how you can excel.

- Taking care of the patient: Duh. This one is obvious. But especially for us, we are so used to the focused care of one patient at a time (in the OR), that the big picture for multiple patients can get lost. Don't forget why you are here! Take the opportunity to focus on how the patient is doing, what's going on, and whether the patient responded to your treatment. Be sure you've examined the patient and have up-to-date labs; if not, cue someone to look them up while you're talking. You'll also be appreciated if you ask the patient (if appropriate) and the bedside nurse if they have any pressing issues you need to address (it avoids them correcting you while you talk, if things have changed since you pre-rounded).

- Handing off care: Yeah, it's 8 AM. You've been up all night. It's time to go home. Well, someone has to take care of the patient once you leave, right? Usually it will be a colleague at or near your level. Think about what you would want him/her to know about what happened last night. Obviously you won't forget about a patient you had to intubate, or somebody that had a major operation. But just as important is the family meeting that happened, or maybe a new positive blood culture, or an important discussion with the surgeon. You don't want the team, after you leave, to be wondering about things and feeling that they have to call you to get details. Be specific about where you think the patient is heading and what issues you think might occur. Try hard, also, to use your best stage voice and be sure that everyone can hear (except the family in the next room; that's a Health Insurance Portability and Accountability Act [HIPAA] violation!). But seriously, if the entire group can't hear you, it's just a waste of time!

- Setting daily goals: You've just discussed the assessment and plan on rounds, but does anyone really understand or remember what's supposed to happen? It's easy to make nebulous plans ("Let's wean the vent, and see if we can diurese the patient"), but if they're not brought into operational language ("Let's change the vent to a pressure support mode and wean with a plan to assess for extubation midafternoon; we'll give a dose of furosemide and plan to redose if needed to reach a net −2 L balance, if tolerated"), you may find that you don't make any real progress. Our aim is to get patients better and out of the unit, so setting specific, operational goals can make that happen. It also can make sure that everyone (the sleepy intern, the bedside nurse) understands what's expected. Your unit may use a "daily goals sheet" to facilitate this, so that everyone can be "on the same page" with the plan, and if not, consider using one yourself (Figure 57-2).

- Ensuring "best practice": With each patient having many caregivers, and so much focus on unstable critical illness that we often forget the housekeeping items, a careful review on rounds can catch the things we know each patient should have. These are the things we call "best practices" and include things like aspiration precautions (head of bed greater than 30 degrees), daily wake-ups for patients on sedation, daily screen for vent weaning/extubation, deep venous thrombosis (DVT), peptic ulcer prophylaxis,

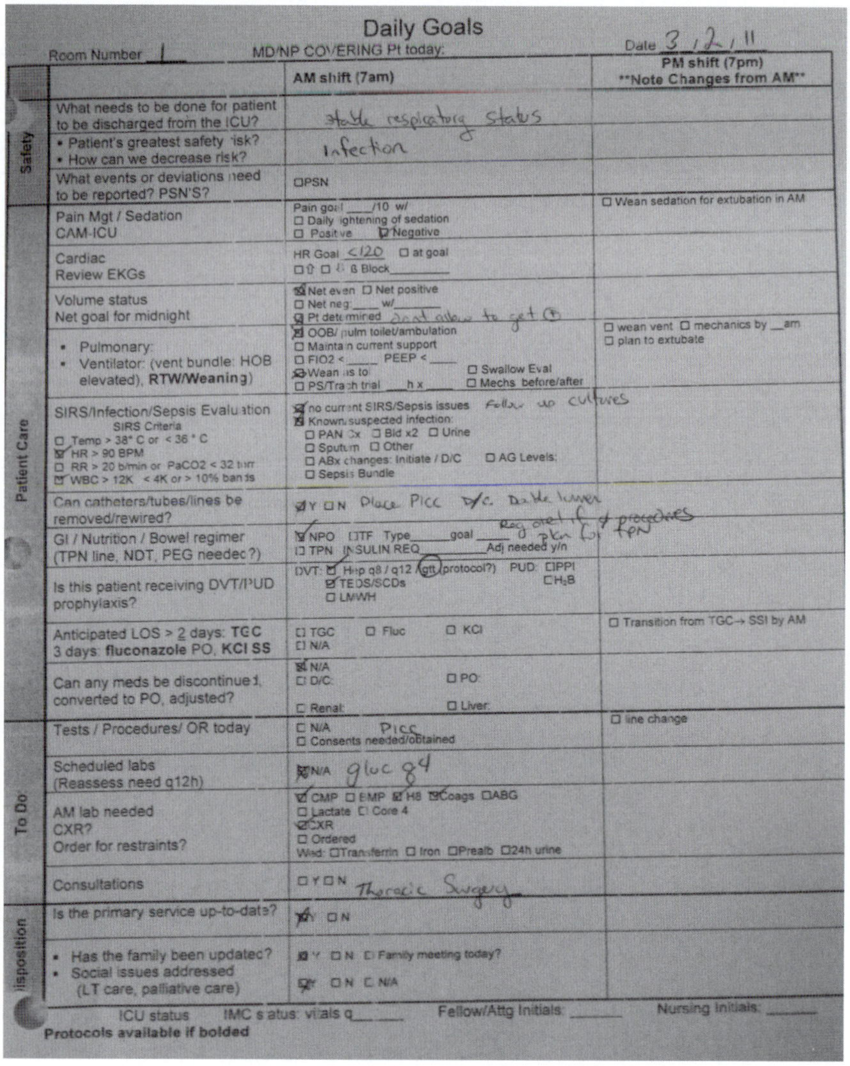

Daily Goals

Room Number 1 MD/NP COVERING Pt today: Date 3/2/11

		AM shift (7am)	PM shift (7pm) **Note Changes from AM**
Safety	What needs to be done for patient to be discharged from the ICU?	stable respiratory status	
	• Patient's greatest safety risk? • How can we decrease risk?	Infection	
	What events or deviations need to be reported? PSN'S?	☐PSN	
Patient Care	Pain Mgt / Sedation CAM-ICU	Pain goal ___/10 w/ ☐ Daily lightening of sedation ☐ Positive ☑ Negative	☐ Wean sedation for extubation in AM
	Cardiac Review EKGs	HR Goal <120 ☐ at goal ☐⇧ ☐⇩ ß Block______	
	Volume status Net goal for midnight	☒ Net even ☐ Net positive ☐ Net neg:___ w/___ ☒ Pt determined	
	• Pulmonary: • Ventilator: (vent bundle: HOB elevated), **RTW/Weaning**)	☒ OOB/ pulm toilet/ambulation ☐ Maintain current support ☐ FIO2 < ___ PEEP < ___ ☒ Wean as tol ☐ Swallow Eval ☐ PS/Trach trial ___h x ___ ☐ Mechs before/after	☐ wean vent ☐ mechanics by __am ☐ plan to extubate
	SIRS/Infection/Sepsis Evaluation SIRS Criteria ☐ Temp > 38° C or < 36° C ☑ HR > 90 BPM ☐ RR > 20 b/min or PaCO2 < 32 torr ☑ WBC > 12K < 4K or > 10% bands	☒ no current SIRS/Sepsis issues Follow up cultures ☒ Known/suspected infection: ☐ PAN Cx ☐ Bld x2 ☐ Urine ☐ Sputum ☐ Other ☐ ABx changes: Initiate / D/C ☐ AG Levels: ☐ Sepsis Bundle	
	Can catheters/tubes/lines be removed/rewired?	☑ Y ☐ N Place PICC	
	GI / Nutrition / Bowel regimen (TPN line, NDT, PEG needed?)	☑ NPO ☐ TF Type____ goal____ ☐ TPN INSULIN REQ______ Adj needed y/n	
	Is this patient receiving DVT/PUD prophylaxis?	DVT: ☐ Hep q8 / q12 / gtt (protocol?) ☑ TEDS/SCDs ☐ LMWH PUD: ☐ PPI ☐ H_2B	
	Anticipated LOS > 2 days: **TGC** 3 days: **fluconazole** PO, **KCl SS**	☐ TGC ☐ Fluc ☐ KCl ☐ N/A	☐ Transition from TGC→ SSI by AM
	Can any meds be discontinued, converted to PO, adjusted?	☒ N/A ☐ D/C: ☐ PO: ☐ Renal: ☐ Liver:	
To Do	Tests / Procedures/ OR today	☐ N/A PICC ☐ Consents needed/obtained	☐ line change
	Scheduled labs (Reassess need q12h)	☒ N/A gluc q4	
	AM lab needed CXR? Order for restraints?	☑ CMP ☐ BMP ☑ H8 ☑ Coags ☐ ABG ☐ Lactate ☐ Core 4 ☑ CXR ☐ Ordered Wed: ☐ Transferrin ☐ Iron ☐ Prealb ☐ 24h urine	
	Consultations	☐ Y ☐ N Thoracic Surgery	
Disposition	Is the primary service up-to-date?	☒ Y ☐ N	
	• Has the family been updated? • Social issues addressed (LT care, palliative care)	☒ Y ☐ N ☐ Family meeting today? ☒ Y ☐ N ☐ N/A	

ICU status IMC status: vitals q____ Fellow/Attg Initials: ____ Nursing Initials: ____

Protocols available if bolded

FIGURE 57-2 The dreaded goal sheet. It may seem like an unnecessary pain, but take the time to fill it out; the nurses will love you and it may save you some day!

and glycemic control. Medications not needed should be stopped, and each day a review of whether antibiotics can be tailored or stopped and lines can be removed is important. Make a point of covering these items as a checklist as part of your assessment and plan or daily goals discussion, and you'll never miss them.

- Explaining your reasoning and getting feedback: Rounds are your chance to shine. Present the data in an organized fashion, and try to save your thoughts and ideas until the end. Be sure you know what you did and why, and how the patient's exam, labs, and studies support your conclusions. There may be some pieces of the puzzle that don't fit; it's appropriate to mention them along with your thought process, and it's definitely OK to mention if the patient's response to treatment caused you to change your hypothesis about what's going on. If an interesting disease process popped up during the day, be prepared to discuss it, maybe even have a relevant study to quote, or better yet, have copies for everyone. Be open to suggestions and comments about your management, as that's how we learn (Figure 57-3).
- Learning from bedside, case-based teaching: Often in the OR there's not time to focus on extended bedside teaching, so rounds can often be a terrific opportunity for a structured, case-based discussion led by your fellow or attending. Think of each patient as an oral-boards question; the pathophysiology of the patient and your decisions regarding it will be a good prep, and the opportunities for this type of learning may be more common in the ICU than in the OR, so take advantage of it. Nurses, respiratory therapists, pharmacists, nutritionists, and social workers may contribute a great deal to rounds, and your goal is to learn what you can from all of them, as well as use their suggestions to formulate an ideal plan for your patients for the day (Figure 57-4).

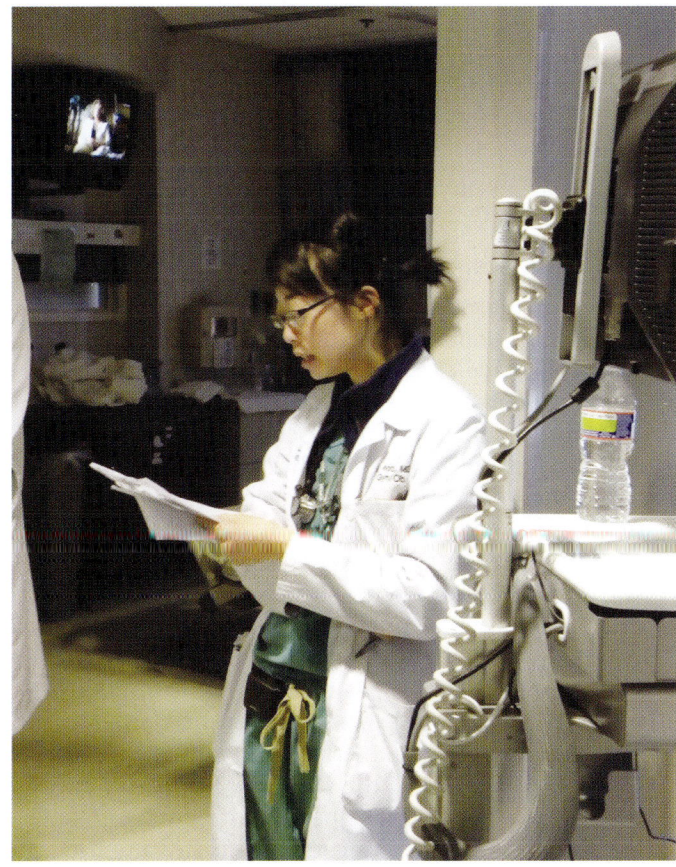

FIGURE 57-3 To truly succeed while presenting, organize yourself! Using the SOAP format is quite helpful.

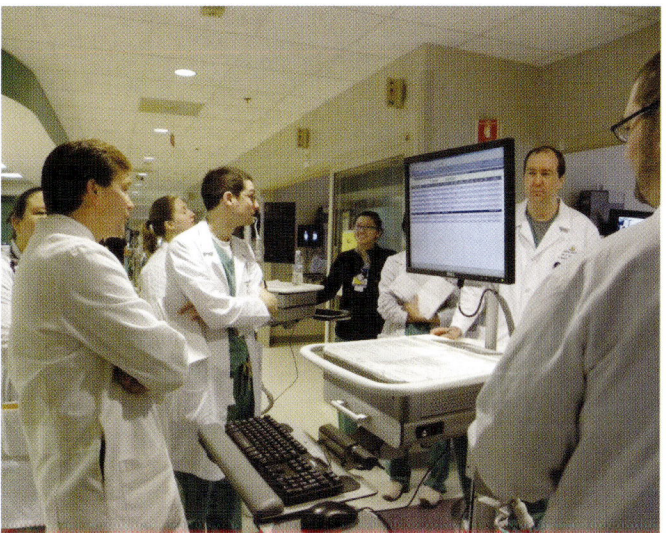

FIGURE 57-4 ICU rounds don't have to be painful, as long as you understand what the goals are?

- Organizing your thinking: Although you'll likely have a presentation structure specific to your institution/unit, here's one that's good for a general organ-system based approach:
  - Significant interval events or studies
  - Neuro
    - Glasgow Coma Scale (GCS), neuro exam
    - Richmond Agitation Sedation (RAS score)/analgesic medications
    - Delirium Confusion Assessment Method (CAM-ICU)
    - Sleep-wake cycle
  - Respiratory
    - Lung exam, presence of secretions, etc.
    - Amount of oxygen required, and how this has changed; or
    - Ventilator status, weaning parameters and how these have changed
    - Arterial blood gas (ABG), chest x-ray (CXR)
  - Cardiovascular
    - Cardiac exam, monitor rhythm, vital signs (VSs) trends, invasive monitoring data
    - Cardiac meds, including vasoactives with trends
    - 12-lead ECG if concern/surveillance for ischemia
  - Renal/fluids/lytes
    - Input/output (I/O), net fluid balance, weight if available
    - Urine output and response to interventions
    - BUN/Cr and any trends (need to renally dose meds?)
    - Electrolytes and any trends
  - GI/nutrition
    - Abdomen exam
    - Source of nutrition, calorie/protein counts, nutrition labs
    - Glycemic control, insulin regimen
    - Peptic ulcer disease (PUD) prophylaxis
    - Pertinent labs
  - Heme
    - Active bleeding?
    - Hb/Hct, platelets, coags and transfusion or anticoagulant therapy
    - DVT prophylaxis
  - Infectious Diseases (ID)
    - WBC and trends, fever curve
    - New and/or important positive/negative cultures
    - Antibiotics: agent, days of projected course, organism treating
    - Lines: days, and whether still needed
  - Psychosocial issues for patient or family
  - Assessment: be sure to include your assessment of what is going on to explain all of those factoids, if the patient is improving/worsening, what you anticipate the patient's issues will be, the trajectory of their illness today. Any safety concerns?

- Plan: operationalize, operationalize, operationalize. Talk about using a daily goals sheet. Think about what has to be done for the patient to leave the unit. How tight a watch do you need to keep on this patient today? How does this patient's "scut list" items rank in priority to other patients'?

Post-Rounds Discussion

Immediately after rounds the team for the day should meet and make sure that all tasks from the "scut" or daily goals sheets are assigned. Items that need to be done immediately can be identified, and other work flow can be determined.

Procedures

- Typically procedures should be done as early in the day as possible so as not to hold up further care or patient transfer, and to free up caregivers for other tasks that may develop later in the day. In fact, it may be worth doing some of these overnight if things are calm and quiet, to improve efficiency during the day.
- Common ICU procedures are the same as in the operating room and so are discussed elsewhere in this book. However, if you're on a team with residents from other specialties, take advantage of the different skill sets. Let the surgical resident take the airway management, but ask if you can do the subclavian lines and chest tubes, for example.
- Keep in mind that sterile technique and maximum barrier precautions are equally if not more important than in the OR when placing or changing invasive monitoring lines. Lines placed in the ICU are commonly present for days (or longer) and catheter-related bloodstream infections are a large source of nosocomial morbidity/mortality.
- ICU patients are also more likely to have had previous lines and/or issues that make them "difficult," so take advantage of nursing and physician help to troubleshoot and be an extra pairs of hands.
- Procedure notes are also key, so be sure not to forget to do these once the procedure is done.

Patient/Unit Maintenance

- Keep rounding! The successful ICU resident will never stop rounding. Literally. Do laps around the unit, each time checking on patients for issues, labs that have come back, progress toward goals. This is a great time to have short discussions with patients and families for updates, and talk with the nurses about their concerns. You'll never miss a brewing problem, and if the nursing staff knows that you're attentive, they're more likely to come find you early with problems. And they won't need to come interrupt you with routine order requests because you'll have already done them on the last lap!
- Repeat labs/studies. Speaking of routine order requests, part of your plan/goals set on rounds should be what parameters you'll want to follow throughout the day and how often. Be sure that these get ordered, and likewise be sure that frequent labs are stopped when no longer needed. Pay attention to routine daily labs as well; not every patient needs every lab every day, but make a rational decision (if patients aren't anticoagulated, they likely don't need daily coags, unless you're following their liver function, for example). Chest x-rays aren't needed for every patient every day, but may be necessary to help evaluate fluid status or an elevated WBC. If you get one, or an ECG to look for ischemia, be sure to look at it! (Figure 57-5).

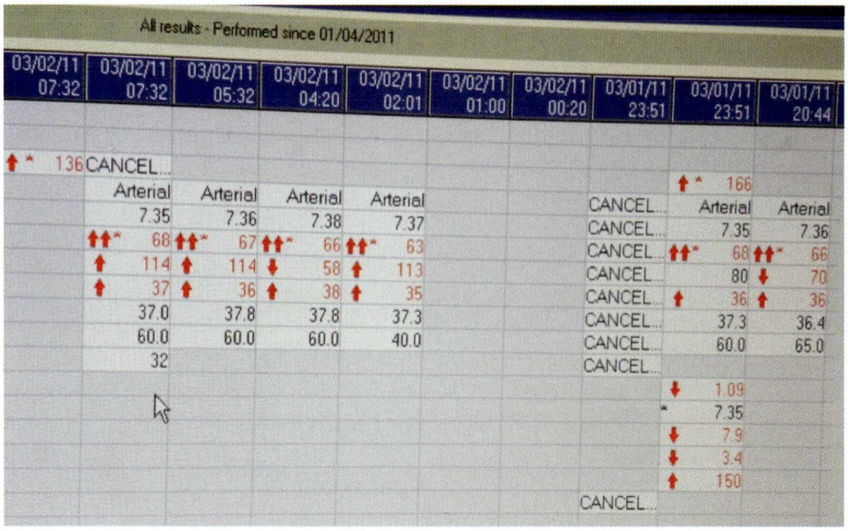

FIGURE 57-5 Looking at the patient's labs over a few days and trying to find trends will be helpful with management.

- Volume status: Particularly if you are in a surgical unit, every patient needs attention paid to volume status every day, and frequently throughout the day. Part of the surgical stress response includes capillary leak that resolves as the inflammatory state subsides; your goal is to give the patient fluid when needed, stop when no longer needed, and often to help diurese when the perioperative volume begins to mobilize. Medical and surgical patients with cardiac, pulmonary, and renal issues make fluid management more complex and often more deleterious when neglected. When you think of your plan/goals for the day, always include volume status. (And don't forget your own volume status too; be sure to remember to stay hydrated!)
- Nutritional status: Patients can go for days without nourishment, but issues like wound healing, protein synthesis, and gut mucosal integrity make this an important area for the critically ill. Be sure to have a plan each day for nutrition (even if the plan is to reevaluate the following day) and if you are using parenteral or enteral supplementation, have a plan for assessing adequacy (weekly prealbumin, iron studies, and urinary nitrogen excretion, for example). Although you may rely on nutrition support services, be sure that you know how many calories and how much protein your patients are receiving, and whether that's enough. Always use the enteral route when possible.
- Electrolyte management: Critical illness and many of our therapies can change the levels of electrolytes. Some of these are symptomatic and don't need to be treated; others are more important and should be addressed, particularly if there are daily trends. Be sure you know what you're measuring. (For example, a total calcium measurement reflects protein levels more than calcium levels, so be sure you know how that correlates with an ionized calcium. A serum magnesium doesn't reflect total body magnesium stores at all since it's mostly intracellular, and the test is expensive, so you're better off just repleting if you're concerned, since it takes a lot of magnesium to cause symptoms from hypermagnesemia). Recognize what derangements are truly the result of patient processes, and what you've done yourself (through parenteral nutrition supplementation, for example). Pay attention to daily trends in sodium (may reflect volume status) and phosphate (may reflect nutrition and/or refeeding, and definitely can contribute to weakness or failure to wean from the ventilator). Serum bicarbonate, while manipulated by many things we do, can often be a sensitive marker of patient well-being; if your patient's serum bicarb drops suddenly, even if the level is still normal, be alert for acidosis and brewing shock!
- Glycemic control: Not too long ago, there was a trend toward "tight" glycemic control. We now know that this may have more risk than benefit. Remember that stress/inflammation causes insulin resistance, though, and so often your patients will trend toward hyperglycemia even if not diabetic at baseline. Why do we care? Even short-term hyperglycemia is detrimental to patients with neurologic dysfunction, and is correlated with both surgical site infection and poor wound healing. Plus, it's tough to grasp someone's fluid status when the urine output is artificially elevated from osmotic diuresis. So find out what your unit's convention is about glucose control and follow it, keeping in mind that patients with significant tissue edema may not absorb subcutaneous insulin well and may need intravenous administration.
- Review medications: Be sure each day to review the list of medications each patient is receiving. You may be surprised! Make sure everything has a therapeutic purpose (stop things that need to be stopped). Be sure that needed medications are being given, as often things are held because a patient isn't taking PO or may have vital sign derangements. In addition, be sure you know how often prn medications are given; the "every hour prn anxiety" lorazepam that is actually given every single hour may be contributing to your patient's delirium! Don't forget to change dosing if creatinine clearance changes (Figure 57-6).
- Discharge/transfer planning: Your ultimate goal is to get every patient out of the unit. To achieve this, you need to keep discharge planning in mind every day. Be sure you know the levels of care within the hospital: what types of monitoring or nurse/patient ratios are available in step-down units or on the floor, and what therapies can or can't be given. Pay attention to fluid management, medications in drip form (insulin gtt, furosemide gtt, pressors) that likely can't be given on the floor and given consideration to transitioning in a timely manner. Some forms of lines (sheath introducers, arterial lines) may not be appropriate for the floor.
- Communication: While you're paying attention to all of the above, responding to urgent issues, and trying to read, be sure that you pay attention to lines of communication. Members of your own team, as well as other stakeholders in the care of the patient (primary care providers, surgical teams) may need to know about changes in a patient's condition or if the plan for care has changed. It can be burdensome to keep everyone in mind when you're actively treating the patient, but if you think about what you'd expect if you were in their shoes, it may guide your practice. Find out who the appropriate contact people are, and be sure to catch as many as possible when they arrive personally on the unit to see their patients.

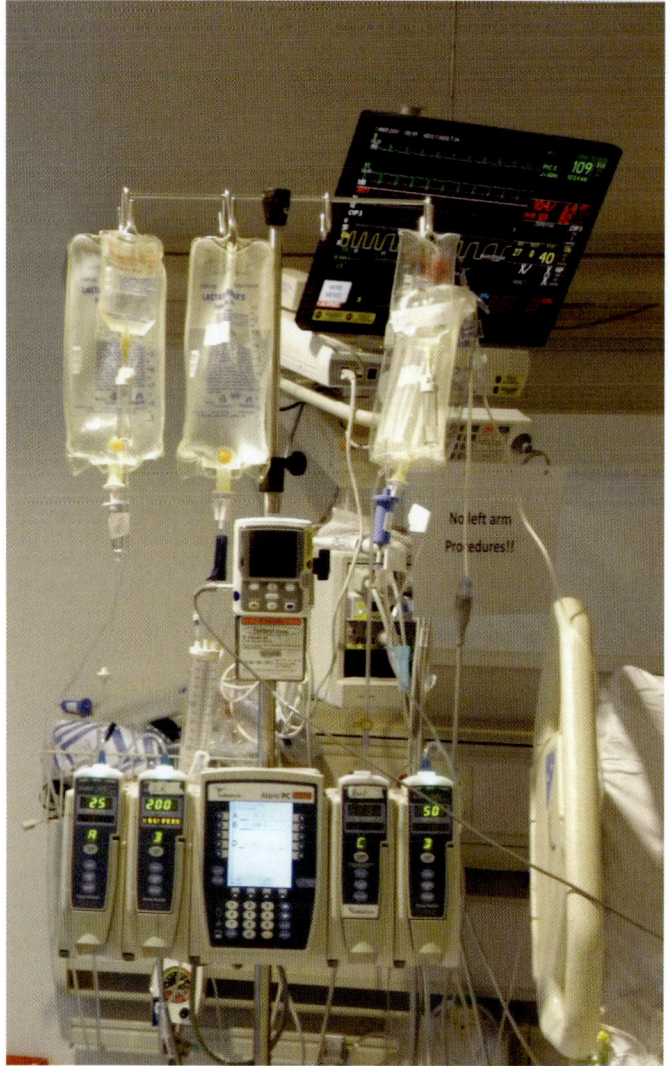

FIGURE 57-6 Not an uncommon sight with a critically ill patient: multiple meds means multiple problems. Remember, you know how this stuff works, you use the same things in the OR, so don't get intimidated.

Admissions

- Whether your patients are arriving from the emergency room, the floor, or a procedure area, their arrival is likely the most important part of your day. In some units, admissions can be predicted (elective OR cases) or at least arrive with some warning; for others this may be less so, particularly if you are not the one authorizing the admission. Regardless, if you're responsible for admitting patients, you should arrive at the bedside at the same time that they do.
- First and foremost: ABCs! Airway, breathing, circulation. Transport is a time when many patients decompensate (or have IVs closed down to avoid running bags dry, or are hypoventilated because you

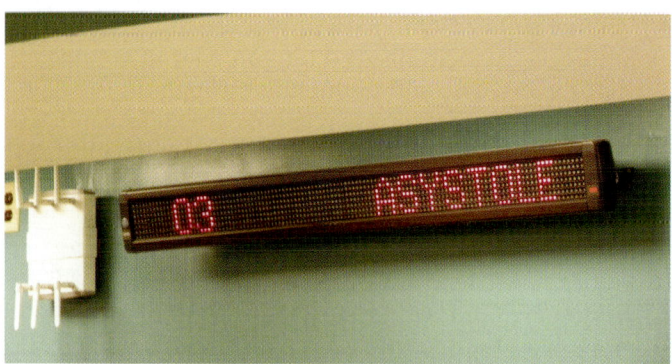

FIGURE 57-7 Just as in anesthesia, patients can go south pretty quickly in the ICU. The key when facing scary words like the above are to maintain your composure and remember your ABCs.

can't reach the Ambu bag easily). Do a quick visual inspection, and if possible, touch their hand or foot looking for temperature. Check vitals or a quick pulse, with full exam to follow later (Figure 57-7).
- Listen carefully during handoff, and ask any questions you have. What are the major concerns for this patient? Are there expectations for ongoing care or items that need to be completed? Be sure responsibility for ordering labs/tests/procedures and especially any communication to family or other physicians is clearly assigned, if not already done. Be sure you understand any previous operations or comorbidities that may impact care.
- With your team, including the patient (if appropriate) and bedside nurse, develop a plan for care. Decide if immediate intervention or lines/procedures are needed. Follow up on any labs. Make sure everyone understands the issues and priorities, as well as what tasks are their responsibility.
- Once the patient is settled in, think about what you expect their illness trajectory will be. How much direct attention will be needed? How often will you follow up? How will you know if the patient is responding appropriately to therapy? Are there issues that you think might develop? If you can assess and predict what a patient will do, you're less likely to allow them to reach a life-threatening state. You'll also know when it's appropriate to communicate with others or ask for help—when the patient falls off the expected trajectory.
- Surgical stress response: If your patients are arriving from the operating room, part of predicting their illness trajectory is to estimate the degree of their surgical stress response. Most postoperative patients develop some degree of systemic inflammatory response syndrome (SIRS), the magnitude of which is determined by the type/site of surgery and other factors. Be aware of sympathetic stimulation

(tachycardia), possible febrile response (tachycardia, vasodilation), capillary leak (requiring fluid resuscitation), antidiuretic hormone production (oliguria), and insulin resistance (hyperglycemia) and how you intend to address each given the patients' other issues.

Discharges

- Don't you hate it when your patient is crashing on the floor, and you call the ICU fellow or charge nurse, only to hear, "Sorry, we don't have any beds!" followed by a click. Then there you are, sitting at the bedside of a sick patient, not able to go anywhere, because you can't transfer the patient where he needs to go most.
- Well, this is why utilization matters. If we kept patients in the ICU indefinitely, nobody else would ever be able to come here. This seems like a silly point, but it needs to be emphasized. It would be impossible to keep operating rooms or medical wards running without somebody making daily decisions on who needs to be in the ICU. And you can't even get to that point without addressing the reasons why a patient should be in the ICU in the first place. Here are some thoughts to get you started:

1. Mechanical ventilation: this is a no-brainer. If patients can't be liberated from the ventilator, in the majority of institutions, they will not qualify for a floor bed (Figure 57-8).
2. Unstable hemodynamics: that guy with the blood pressure of 70/30 on two pressors can't leave the unit.
3. Anything that needs to be measured frequently (neuro checks, urine output, blood sugar); if it has to be done every hour, you can't expect the floor nurse who may have up to 10 patients to be able to get to it.

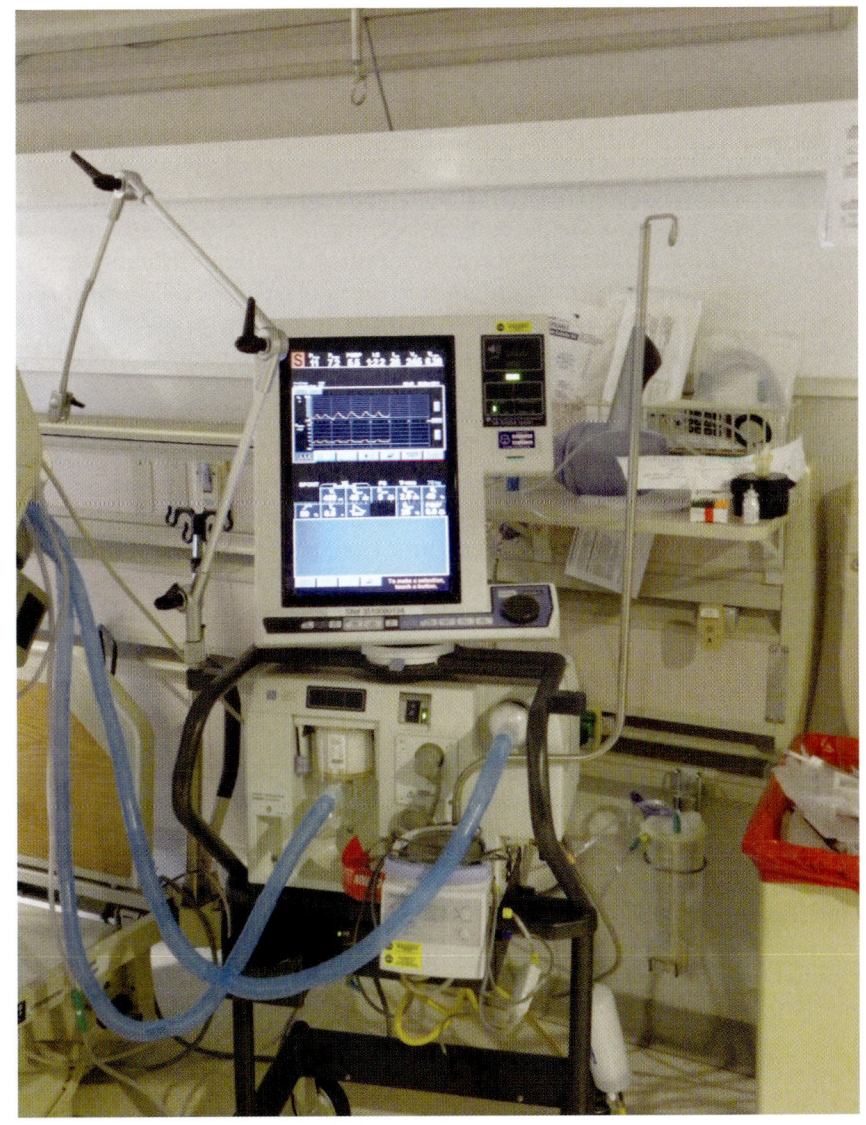

FIGURE 57-8 This crazy machine can be your worst enemy. Spend the time to learn the settings and it can be your best friend instead. Use your friendly neighborhood respiratory therapists; they are a great resource!

- Although discharges may happen most frequently in the mornings, you'll be thinking of discharge planning throughout the day. You may be tasked with writing a formal transfer note in the chart. Whether or not you do, you should be sure to speak with whomever will be caring for the patient on the ward so that they understand ongoing therapies and concerns. One of the most common reasons for patients to return to a surgical ICU is because fluid management plans weren't followed on the ward, which could be remedied by a simple page or phone call.

Patient and Family Interactions

- Patient- and family-centered care is now emphasized more and more, even in the often harsh, impersonal atmosphere of the intensive care unit. Unlike your role in the OR, where your patient/family interactions are often limited to focused pre- and postop conversation, in the intensive care unit you will find more opportunities and expectations for conversations.
- Many intensive care units are moving toward expanded visiting hours or even 24-hour visiting, which may include family presence on rounds or at certain procedures or resuscitation attempts. Find out your unit culture and be aware of how this may impact you (watch what you say!).
- Plan to speak with each patient or family briefly at least once each day; that's your role as their physician, and frequent updates not only help you avoid misunderstandings, but also may help you find out key pieces of information. In addition, when and if the time comes for making complex decisions, you will have already laid both the relationship groundwork and some understanding of the situation in place.
- Given the complexity of patients who are critically ill, everyone admitted to the unit for more than 5 to 7 days probably deserves a sit-down family meeting to be sure all questions are answered and a joint understanding of expectations is formed. This may be time-consuming, but it will save time and effort in many ways down the road! You may or may not be expected to lead or be part of such a meeting; take the opportunity if you can to observe those who are skilled at leading such discussions. If you are leading one for the first time, it's often useful (after introductions) to begin by asking those present about their understanding of the patient's illness; this lets you focus your comments in the correct area and at the correct level of understanding as you begin to guide the conversation.
- At some point you will have a patient who does not have a survivable illness, and it may fall to you both to explain circumstances to the patient and family and to help them understand what choices they have in deciding the goals of care. Too often this is approached as "Do you want to sign a DNR order?" which takes a complex value judgment and decision process and boils it down to a yes-or-no question. Although it's appropriate to feel uncomfortable in such conversations—most of us are used to being in a curative role—this is an excellent opportunity to watch how others (not only physicians) interact to provide comprehensive supportive care. You'll also realize how important those daily interactions are, as such conversations are much easier if the family already knows you.

CONCLUSION

Many residents have described the ICU as "the toughest job you'll ever love." This is a place where you may have lots of patients, you may have very sick patients, and frequently you'll have lots of very sick patients. You'll work hard and sometimes you'll end the day remembering the things you could have done differently more acutely than the things that you did well. However, you'll also have a sense of accomplishment as you tackle complex problems as part of a team and support patients and families through difficult times. Moreover, when you return to the OR, you'll be amazed at how much you've learned. Take advantage of the ICU to actively solicit feedback and apply what you learn to your next patient.

Be sure to be kind to yourself while you work hard in the ICU. This is a place where work-life balance is essential; you can't take care of others unless you are able to take care of yourself. You may find yourself with more hours or call shifts than usual, so be sure to get plenty of sleep, stay hydrated, and keep up with those things that keep you motivated and strengthened: exercise, social life, or quiet time. Often you'll develop close friendship with residents from other disciplines, unit staff, or other specialists. These can be a source of enjoyment and also give you key contacts for later on (put your ICU pharmacist on speed-dial!). And who knows, you may even discover an exciting subspecialty career!

SUGGESTED READING

American Society of Critical Care Anesthesiologists' Resident's Guide to the Learning in the ICU. www.ascca.org.
This publication is only available by download for a fee from the Web site. Look for the link on their home page. The Web site contains case-based ICU learning modules with reading lists developed by anesthesiologists.

American Thoracic Society (ATS) Reading List. http://www.thoracic.org/education/career-development/residents/ats-reading-list.

A comprehensive reading list for the resident rotating in adult critical care, including articles on critical care procedures. The Web site also includes career development resources and guidelines, although they are geared toward the pulmonary intensivist. Look in the education section for some basic primers on hemodynamics, acid-base interpretation, and mechanical ventilation.

Cassell J. *Life and death in intensive care.* Philadelphia: Temple University Press; 2005.

This easy-to-read book, which has become a classic in critical care circles, investigates the many aspects of end-of-life care and how our cultural definitions and values influence that care in the surgical ICU.

Critical Care Medicine Tutorials. www.ccmtutorials.com.

Developed by Dr. Patrick Neligan, an intensivist in the University of Pennsylvania, specifically for anesthesia residents rotating in the surgical ICU. This site includes a problem-based approach to critical care and a number of very practical tutorials in basic areas like mechanical ventilation and sepsis.

Pronovost P, Berenholtz S, Dorman T, Lipsett PA, Simmonds T, Haraden C. Improving communication in the ICU using daily goals. *J Crit Care* 2003;18(2):71–75.

Describes one example of a daily goals form for use in the ICU.

The Pulmonary Artery Catheter Education Project. www.pacep.org.

A collaborative effort of eight professional organizations (including the American Society of Anesthesiologists and the SCCM) that offers interactive modules on Swan-Ganz catheter placement and interpretation of waveforms/numbers.

Society of Critical Care Medicine Learn-ICU initiative: www.LearnICU.org.

The Society of Critical Care Medicine (SCCM) has a wide variety of learning resources for adult and pediatric ICU on their newly remodeled LearnICU Web site. Included are current hot topic journal and review articles, professional guidelines, learning modules, self-assessments, and podcasts arranged both by type of resource and subject area.

Society of Critical Care Medicine Resident ICU Curriculum. www.LearnICU.org/Fundamentals/RICU.

Link directly, or via the SCCM's Learn-ICU site, to this set of 39 fundamental learning modules on the basics of adult critical care or a parallel curriculum for pediatric critical care. Access is free; register with your email address to access pre- and posttest assessments, or have your rotation director register the residency as a whole.

CHAPTER 58

HIGHWAY TO THE DANGER ZONE: HAZMAT

JAMES A. ROTHSCHILD
BRADFORD WINTERS
KELLY BRENAN-ROTHSCHILD

"It's classified. I could tell you, but then I'd have to kill you."

Maverick, *Top Gun*
(screenplay by Jim Cash and
Jack Epps, Jr., 1986)

INTRODUCTION (FIGURE 58-1)

You spend so much time concentrating on your patients, we think it's high time you start thinking about yourself for once. The goal here is to be able to identify the major sources of danger in the operating room and to understand the protective measures available to avoid pain, injury, or worse... We'll go over a few, but just remember that vigilance is the key to success as disaster lurks with every needle, every turn of that vaporizer dial, and every press of the x-ray button. Here we go.

DO YOU SMELL SOMETHING? THE VOLATILE GASES (FIGURE 58-2)

Did you know that less than 5% of the volatile gases are actually metabolized by the patient? The rest are exhaled by the patient and either blown directly into our faces, or preferably taken away by operating room scavenging systems.

The one "take-away" point here is that, if you can smell the vapor, then it's way above allowed concentrations. The National Institute for Occupational Safety and Health (NIOSH) has come up with a set of standards for keeping the operating room atmosphere "gas free" (insert favorite surgeon joke here). They are as follows:
- Nitrous oxide alone = 25 parts per million (ppm) for an 8-hour time-weighted average
- Volatile anesthetic alone = 2 ppm over 1 hour
- Volatile gas with 25 ppm of nitrous = 0.5 ppm over 1 hour

THE RISKS

Back in the 1970s, when our attendings were busy wearing bell bottoms and preaching about free love, a couple of key studies came out that claimed that repeated daily exposure to volatile anesthetics may place female anesthesia providers at increased risk of miscarriage and birth defects. Now we know that these studies were critically flawed, and the research since then has been conflicting at best, but these important studies raised the issue (and fears) surrounding long-term occupational exposure to the volatile anesthetics.

Other potential long-term exposure risks include:
- Cognitive and behavioral impairment
- Possible increase central nervous system effects
- Sevoflurane and compound A: nephrotoxic in rats, no reported cases in humans
- Animal evidence of increased apoptotic cell death in early infancy (although corresponding human equivalent age is approximately 26 weeks of gestation)

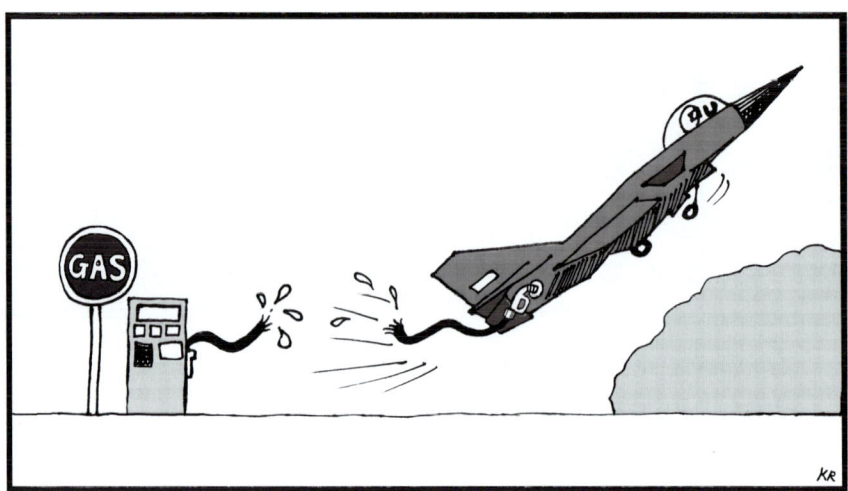

FIGURE 58-1 Before taking off to the danger zone, make sure you remember the basics.

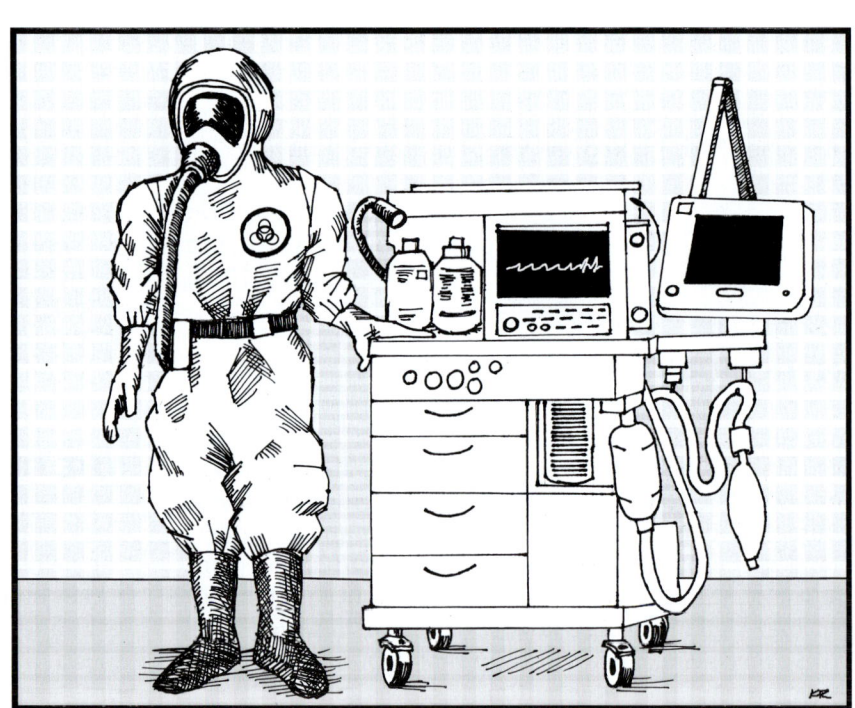

FIGURE 58-2 We work in a toxic place.

WHERE'S THAT SMELL COMING FROM?

The repeat offenders:
- Circuit disconnects
- Mask inductions
- Laryngeal mask airways
- Uncuffed endotracheal tubes

WHAT CAN BE DONE?

1. Air exchange system: One study found that by exchanging operating room air 10 times per hour, the ambient concentration of anesthetic gases was reduced by 75%. For operating rooms in the United States, the current requirement is to undergo 15 to 21 complete room air exchanges per hour, with at least three of these being with the outside air.
2. Use an appropriate scavenging system (40 to 60 L/min capacity).
3. Use low flows: 2 L/min or less.
4. Minimize mask induction/anesthesia: pediatrics is the biggest offender here!
5. Be constantly vigilant for circuit leaks/disconnects.
6. Since we don't really know the harm, keep exposure to a minimum.

HISTORICAL TRIVIA

Notable side effects of the volatile gases of days gone by:
- Diethyl ether, cyclopropane: flammable
- Chloroform: hepatotoxicity and fatal arrhythmias
- Trichloroethylene: hepatotoxicity and fatal arrhythmias
- Halothane: malignant hyperthermia, type 1 hepatitis = transient, reversible, 1:3 to 1:20; type 2 = fulminant, 30% to 70% mortality, 1:37,000 (requires repeat exposure)
- Methoxyflurane: nephrotoxic due to excessive plasma fluoride concentrations

THE OLD GUY ON THE BLOCK: NITROUS OXIDE (FIGURE 58-3)

He may smell like sweaty gym shoes, but boy has he managed to stick around. Nitrous was discovered in 1772 and first used by dentists in 1844, two years before William Morton's famous ether anesthesia debut at Massachusetts General.

Nitrous comes with its own set of unique risks with prolonged exposure, so much so that many anesthesiologists question whether or not we should continue to use this classic standby. These risks include:
- Reduction in antioxidant activity in plasma cells and erythrocytes
- Reduced vitamin B_{12} activity, leading to decreased bone marrow function
- Inhibition of neutrophil apoptosis, leading to prolonged inflammatory reactions
- Increased DNA breaks/mutations
- Teratogenicity in animals, but only when used at much higher concentrations than we would ever see in the operating room
- Increased homocysteine levels, which may increase cardiovascular risk over the long term
- Potential to damage the ozone layer: N_2O is considered a "greenhouse gas" and has a half-life long enough to make some fear that it may be contributing to global warming (in contrast to the volatile agents whose much shorter half-life in the stratosphere makes them far less significant threats to the ozone layer).

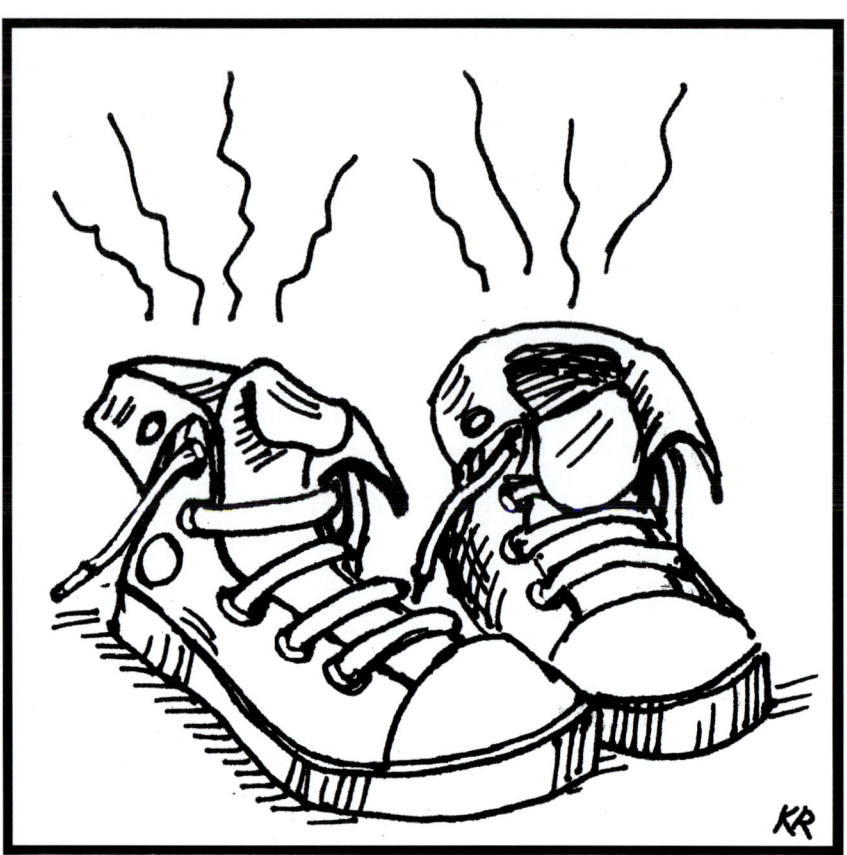

FIGURE 58-3 Toxic locker room material.

SOMETHING ELSE TO THINK ABOUT

- The postanesthesia care unit (PACU) can be another source of ambient volatile gases. As patients off-gas their slumber cocktails, they release significant quantities of anesthetic into the atmosphere. Furthermore, since recovery units tend to not have as robust air circulation systems, PACUs can be really intoxicating venues (U.S. requirement is six air exchanges per hour, with two being with outside air). In fact, many studies have reported gas levels higher than the previously stated allowable maximums in recovery units.
- Many anesthesiologists argue that decreased greenhouse gas emission is yet another reason for the expansion of total intravenous anesthesia (TIVA). But did you know that propofol is a phenol-based chemical that is passed largely unchanged into human excrement? And since phenol happens to be a potent poison to ocean wildlife, some speculate that if TIVA replaced inhalational anesthetics, we might poison our aquatic friends with patient feces. Gross!

RADIATION EXPOSURE (OR WHY AM I GLOWING?) (FIGURE 58-4)

Radiation safety poses an interesting paradox when it comes to operating room safety. As our imaging devices become more advanced, they are able to emit less radiation in order to produce the same quality of images. On the other hand, we are constantly inventing more radiation-emitting technologies as we push the envelope of our diagnostic and therapeutic advances in the field. This means as anesthesia providers, we are likely being exposed to more, and not less, ionizing radiation in the operating room.

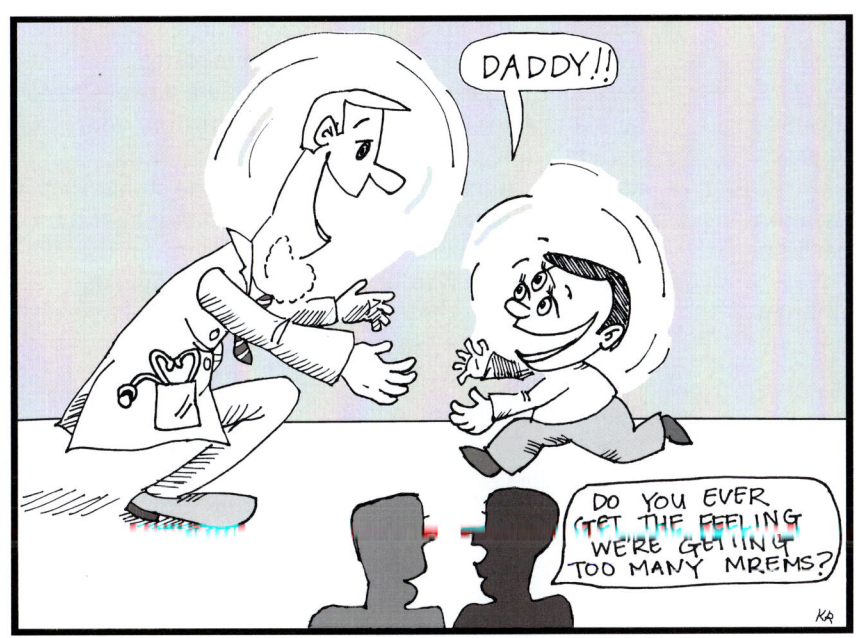

FIGURE 58-4 Radiation safety is no joke!

SAVE YOUR UNBORN CHILDREN

- Increase your distance! Scatter radiation levels are inversely proportional to the square of the distance from the source. This means that doubling your distance cuts your exposure to one quarter. It also means that exposure is minimal beyond 36 inches. Put another way, 6 feet of air is the equivalent of 9 inches of concrete when it comes to protecting your progeny.
- Wear your lead! Lead aprons 0.5 mm in thickness attenuate 97% to 99% of scatter. Don't forget your thyroid shield.
- Know your limits. Annual occupational exposure limit is 5 rem/year (5000 mrem) to the torso and 50,000 mrem to the hands. Incidentally, radiology personnel rarely absorb 10% of this in a year. The pregnancy limit is 500 mrem throughout the course of the pregnancy.
- Know when to run. Fluoroscopy machines are the biggest offenders.
  - Posteroanterior (PA) chest x-ray = 35 mrem
  - Hip x-ray = 500 mrem
  - Dental survey x-rays = 450 mrem
  - Three-view mammogram = 510 mrem
  - Barium enema = 4550 mrem
  - Cardiac catheterization = average 100,000 mrem for a 50-minute procedure
  - Regular C-arm = 1200 to 1400 mrem per minute!
  - Mini C-arm = 120 to 400 mrem/min
- Understand the C-arm. The x-ray generating tube should be placed as far from the patient as possible and the image receptor should be as close to the patient as possible in order to minimize scatter, thereby protecting our loved ones. You should also stand on the side opposite the beam generator if given the choice.
- The mini–C-arm emits only 10% of the scatter as compared with the full-sized version. Unfortunately, it requires the surgeon and operator to be closer to the source.
- Use the ALARA principle. No matter what the recommended limits are, always attempt to keep exposure *a*s *l*ow *a*s *r*easonably *a*chievable (ALARA).

OTHER IMPORTANT RADIATION TRIVIA

- Increased patient body habitus = increased scatter = increased gonadal exposure for us. In fact, for every 3 cm of tissue thickness that the beam has to penetrate, scatter radiation doubles.
- There are two kinds of radiation: ionizing and nonionizing. Ionizing is the bad stuff. Nonionizing is laser, ultrasound, MRI, etc.
- The biggest hazard from nonionizing is probably thermal injuries from generated heat.
- There are two categories of damage from ionizing radiation: deterministic and stochastic. Deterministic damage occurs slowly enough and falls below a given threshold so that cells are able to repair themselves. Stochastic effects, however, are cumulative and permanent over our lifetime.
- The average exposure of the public to ionizing radiation is 360 mrem per year, with 300 mrem being

from "natural" sources (cosmic ionizing radiation, microwaves, food, water, etc.) and 60 mrem from diagnostic radiographs.
- Average exposure to ionizing radiation from cosmic rays to 24 mrem per year at sea level. This increases by 1 mrem per 1000 feet above sea level.
- A 5-hour airplane flight averages 2.5 mrem. Aviation personnel can average as high as 600 mrem per year depending on flight hours and aircraft type.
- We receive an average internal exposure of 40 mrem per year from things like food and water, which can contain isotopes of potassium and radon gas!

HAVE YOU SEEN MY KEYS?: THE MRI MACHINE (FIGURE 58-5)

True, MRIs produce nonionizing radiation, so the risk of true radiation damage is negligible. However, MRIs have their own set of potential risks:
- MRIs can turn ferrous surgical instruments, fire extinguishers, etc. into dangerous projectiles.
- MRIs can heat up cables and electrodes, causing thermal injury to both you and your patient, particularly if the cables are left coiled. Always make sure all cables and lines hang straight from your patient while in the scanner.
- MRIs can "quench," which refers to the sudden loss of magnetic field as the cryogens that cool the machine's magnets escape into the room (in the event of a breach from, say, that fire extinguisher now turned missile), displacing all available oxygen. RUN! (with your patient, of course).
- Finally, don't discount the sound that these monstrous electromagnets produce. The sound pressure produced by the gradient coil impacting the mounting structure can easily exceed the occupational limit of 100 dB. Hearing protection is mandatory!
- A wheelchair once found its way into one institution's MRI scanner. For a short time they had the world's first "sitting MRI"!

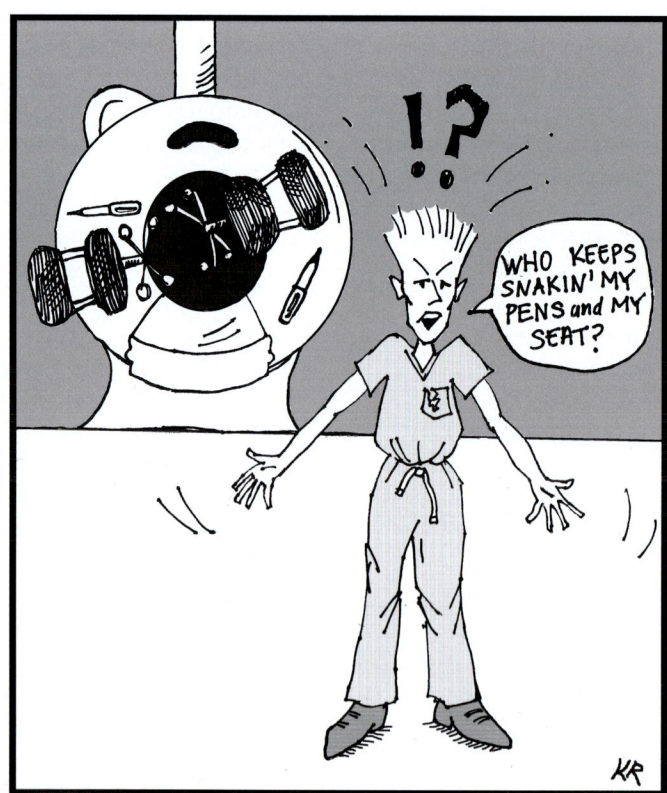

FIGURE 58-5 MRI safety is also no joke!

ELECTRICITY: A SHOCK TO THE SYSTEM (FIGURE 58-6)

Since 40% of hospital electrical accidents occur in the operating room, we felt it prudent to highlight electricity as yet another potential source of danger. Fortunately, the people who build our workplaces have come up with some really nifty ways of protecting both us and our patients.

- Operating room power is isolated from the utility company by an isolation transformer, which can be found in each OR. What these separate transformers do is prevent a grounded system. You might be thinking, why would you want to prevent grounding? What this means is that our systems require two separate faults before a circuit can be completed, thereby injuring the patient or the operator: the first fault grounds the system with the utility company, and the second fault completes the circuit and causes the shock.
- Each electrical appliance in the operating room is prone to some small amount of leakage current. This leakage current must be kept below a certain threshold (10 µA) in order to prevent the first fault, or grounding of the operating room.
- The other advantage of an isolation system is that it prevents the use of breakers (like the kind you have in your house). You can imagine that having the OR go dark because we "blew a breaker" might be problematic.
- The ORs also have line isolation monitors (LIMs; also called ground fault detectors), which detect short circuits in the OR and alarm if the cumulative leakage current from our appliances exceeds 2 to 5 mA (the range where shock can occur across intact skin—so-called macroshock).
- The problem with LIMs is that they measure and detect only in a range far above what can cause a shock to the patient who has indwelling catheters like central lines (so-called microshock). You may be protected but your patient may not be.
- The allowable leakage current from any single piece of equipment in the OR is 10 µA.
- If a LIM alarm sounds, the correct course of action is to unplug pieces of equipment one at a time until the offending piece is identified and can then be removed from the room.

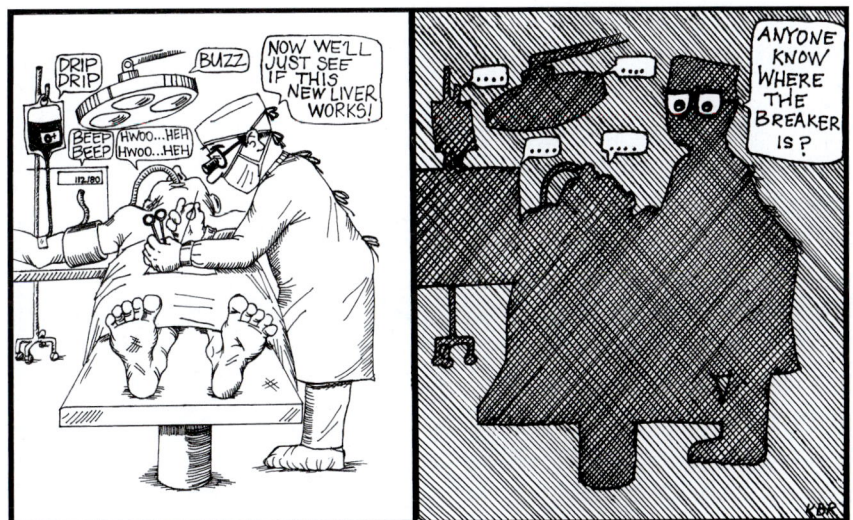

FIGURE 58-6 Be ready for a power outage.

A REALLY STICKY SITUATION: AVOIDING NEEDLESTICK INJURIES (FIGURE 58-7)

The risk of needlestick injuries is real, and it's no laughing matter. The rates of needlestick injuries are largely unknown, but estimates range from 600,000 to 1,000,000 needlestick injuries occurring each year in health care workers, with less than 30% of these actually being reported. This means that at least 15% of surgical procedures involve some form of cut or needlestick injury. Surgeons sustain approximately 59% of these injuries, followed by scrub nurses at 19% and anesthesiologists at 6%. Aside from constant vigilance, appropriate use of sharps disposal containers, and fatigue management, we have little to add that's not glaringly obvious. Needlestick injuries can potentially be some of the most devastating of any mentioned in this chapter. Just to drive the "point" home a bit, think about the following statistics:

- Hepatitis C: May remain infectious for up to 16 hours in dried blood on environmental surfaces. Seroconversion rate after needlestick is 1.8% to 3%. There is no postexposure prophylaxis (PEP) available. Test immediately after exposure and then again in 6 months. Hep C results in chronic hepatitis in 85% of people infected; 20% progress to cirrhosis and 3% to hepatocellular carcinoma.
- Hepatitis B: Can be infectious for up to 14 days in dried blood on environmental surfaces. Seroconversion rate is 27% to 62% if patient is HBeAg positive and 23% to 37% if source is HBeAg negative (remember that HBeAg is the marker for active disease). If the provider is vaccinated and a confirmed responder, no postexposure treatment is necessary. If not vaccinated, immediate immunoglobulin treatment is recommended.
- HIV: Seroconversion rate is approximately 0.3% after needlestick and 0.09% with mucous membrane exposure. Risk of transmission is increased by high patient viral titers, hollow-bore needles, and percutaneous exposure. PEP should be instituted immediately, but definitely within 24 hours of exposure, and continued for 4 weeks. Retest at 6 weeks, 12 weeks, and 6 months.
- For seroconversion rates, remember the rule of 3's: 30% for Hep B, 3% for Hep C, and 0.3% for HIV.

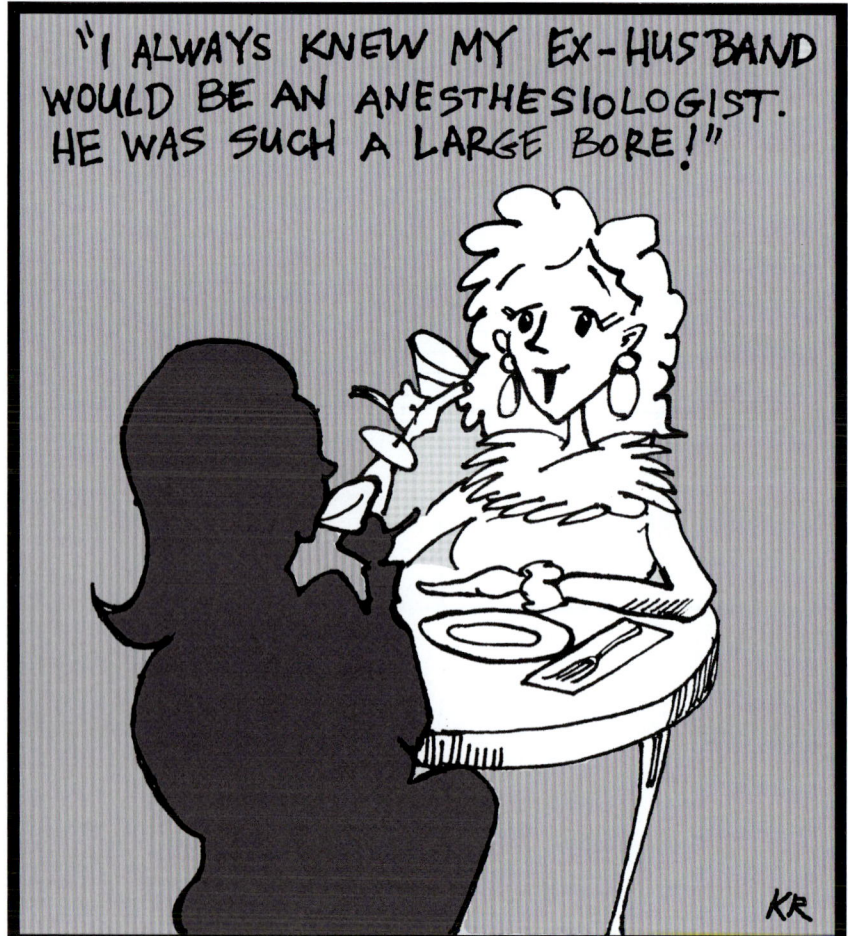

FIGURE 58-7

SUPER GLUE FOR BONES: METHYLMETHACRYLATE (MMA)

Despite its rather pungent odor, studies have shown that this bondo for bones is actually relatively safe over the long term. Granted, it does carry acute warnings for skin and eye irritation, bronchospasm, chemical burns, headache, and anaphylaxis, but if you can get by all of that, it's really relatively benign stuff over the long term. Seriously, long-term studies have failed to show any evidence of permanent toxic or carcinogenic effects from MMA under normal conditions of use. Here are some quick facts that may help this stuff "stick" in your memory:

- The Occupational Safety and Health Administration (OSHA) recommended exposure level (REL) is 100 ppm over 8 hours. Scavenging devices and air circulation in operating rooms are able to reduce airborne concentrations by over 75%.
- Airborne concentrations over 170 ppm for over 8 hours have been associated with chronic liver, lung, and kidney damage in laboratory animals.
- Preparation of MMA involves an exothermic reaction with a maximum temperature of 70° to 110°C, so watch your fingers.
- Uses for MMA include ortho bone cement, ophthalmology intraocular lenses, maxillofacial reconstruction, plastic surgery, dental prostheses, and podiatry orthotics.
- All personnel handling MMA should use proper personal protective equipment to include face shields and protective eyewear. All handling should also be performed in a well-ventilated location.
- Keep in mind that MMA does carry an increased risk for hypotension and embolic events in the patient, likely secondary to interference with calcium mobilization.

WATCH YOUR STEP: ACCIDENTS AND OTHER MISCELLANEOUS HAZARDS

The operating room is teeming with opportunities for provider self-harm. Cords and wet floors can present significant trip hazards. Fires and explosions are constant threats; all operating room personnel should be trained in the proper use of fire extinguisher equipment. Lasers are being increasingly used in surgical procedures, and providers should be aware of the proper eye protection for use with each individual laser type. Cytotoxic chemotherapeutic are increasingly being infused in the operating room under hyperthermic conditions and pose direct threats to health care workers both through direct skin contact and vaporization/inhalational injuries. As such, knowledge of appropriate personal protective equipment is a must.

The bottom line is that the list goes on and on. Further, as we continue to make advancements in our diagnostic and treatment capabilities, these risks are only likely to increase. The responsibility of protecting yourself comes down to one person: you! Proper knowledge of personal protective measures and appropriate emergency safety protocols and procedures are an essential part of our job. As the anesthesiologist, it is our responsibility to know how to protect ourselves, our patients, and other staff members. As the ORs have become increasingly dangerous places to work, our job has expanded from internist, pediatrician, or pharmacist to toxicologist. Good luck!

SUGGESTED READING

Barash PG, Cullen BF, Stoelting RK, Cahalan MK, Stock MC. *Clinical anesthesia*, 6th ed. Philadelphia: Lippincott Williams & Wilkins; 2009, pp 58–73, 165–185.

Berguer R, Heller PJ. Preventing sharps injuries in the operating room. *J Am Coll Surg* 2004;199(3):462–467.

Bovill JG. Inhalation anaesthesia: from diethyl ether to xenon. *Handb Exp Pharmacol* 2008;(182):121–142.

Byhahn C, Wilke HJ, Westpphal K. Occupational exposure to volatile anaesthetics: epidemiology and approaches to reducing the problem. *CNS Drugs* 2001;15(3):197–215.

Irwin MG, Trinh T, Yao CL. Occupational exposure to anaesthetic gases: a role for TIVA. *Expert Opin Drug Saf* 2009;8(4):473–483.

Kettenbach J, Kacher DF, Kanan AR, et al. Intraoperative and interventional MRI: recommendations for a safe environment. *Minim Invasive Ther Allied Technol* 2006;15(2):53–64.

Leggat PA, Smith DR, Kedjarune U. Surgical applications of methyl methacrylate: a review of toxicity. *Arch Environ Occup Health* 2009;64(3):207–212.

Singer G. Occupational radiation exposure to the surgeon. *J Am Acad Orthop Surg* 2005;13(1):69–76.

Vetter RJ. Medical health physics: a review. *Health Phys* 2005;88(6):653–664.

CHAPTER 59

SIMULATION

CHRISTINE PARK
OLYA POLISHCHUK

There is no disguise which can for long conceal love where it is or simulate it where it does not.
— Francois Duc de la Rochefocould,
Reflections (1678)

INTRODUCTION

So, you have graduated medical school and somehow survived another year of rounding during your intern year, and now you are ready to start your residency to become the world's greatest anesthesiologist.

Right before the start of your residency, you realize that you know nothing about anesthesia. Though You've spent at least 4 years of your life learning medicine, suddenly it seems like anesthesia knowledge comes from medical school. Questions run through your head: How does the machine work? How do I set up the room? How do I start an IV or an arterial line? How do I zero the transducer? How do I start an infusion of propofol? What do I do if the patient desaturates or the endotracheal tube comes out? And so on. All these unfamiliar things in a very new environment but with real patients trusting you. Scary!

Though eventually all these things will be learned in the OR, one of the safest and the least intimidating way to learn is in the simulator lab. The simulator lab provides ample opportunity to learn and practice all things anesthesia! There is a lot of energy and focus on simulation research for education right now, not only for novice residents but also for maintenance of certification in anesthesiology, and the ACGME now requires some kind of simulation experience every year during residency training.

In this chapter we will discuss:
- Simulator types
- Applications
- Pitfalls
- The educator's role
- Sample scenarios

SIMULATOR TYPES

- First, let's make a distinction between simulators and simulation.
- *Simulator* is a generic term referring to a physical object, device, situation, or environment where a task or a series of tasks can be realistically and dynamically represented.
- *Simulation* is a process or event that presents problems authentically. The participant is required to respond to the problems as he or she would under natural circumstances. After the simulation is over, the participant usually receives performance feedback in a structured debriefing.
- Simulators and simulation run the gamut of fidelity, from high to low, and each has its own particular benefits.
- Simulation is a fairly ancient concept. For example, there was a full-body obstetrical mannequin made several hundred years ago in France in order to teach labor and delivery. To help with realism, the mannequin has her hand to her forehead to simulate great pain.
- The first full-body mannequin as we think of it today was developed in the 1960s by the anesthesiologist Dr. Stephen Abrahamson. This mannequin could actually do things our current mannequins cannot, like fasciculate after administration of succinylcholine, and "buck" on the endotracheal tube.
- High-fidelity mannequins: Today's high-fidelity mannequins include adult, obstetric, child, and infant models. Some models can be transported to in-situ environments. Their "vital signs" are controlled by a remote computer (Figure 59-1), and they have physical features such as reactive pupils, eye blinking, chest rise and fall with breathing, pulses (at least carotid and radial), and

a range of heart and lung sounds. IV placement is possible in some, as is placement of a chest tube, needle thoracostomy, and even central line placement. The "patient" can talk to you if there is a microphone planted in the mannequin. Or sometimes the voice of the patient will simply be transmitted over speakers. With a creative genius for a technician, many, many more special effects can be created (Figure 59-1).

- Standardized patients: More than likely, you've interacted with standardized patients in simulated patient encounters. Unlike every other modality of simulation, you are interacting with real people.
- Surgical simulators: Full-body mannequins just don't have the level of fidelity needed for most surgical procedures. There is a wide array of surgical simulators available to teach procedures like laparoscopy, arthroscopy, and endoscopy.
- Part-task trainers: In many situations part-task trainers are the best devices to teach specific skills. There are IV arms, intubation heads, regional anesthesia trainers, transesophageal echocardiography trainers, and many others.
- Screen-based simulation: There is a whole virtual world of screen-based training and simulation systems available. Most of the time the fidelity is nothing compared to the gaming technology, probably because your average gamer is not beating down the doors for medical educational simulation.
- Role-play or oral examination: Continuing down the fidelity spectrum, role-playing and oral examinations are a kind of low-fidelity simulation. Although the environment and props are usually completely lacking reality, the instructor may attempt to create real-time interactions and decision making in order to make his or her point.
- Written examination: Now we're really stretching it, but the argument can be made that written exams are indeed a very low fidelity kind of simulation. By presenting hypothetical situations, you may imagine yourself in that situation as you think about your "next best step."

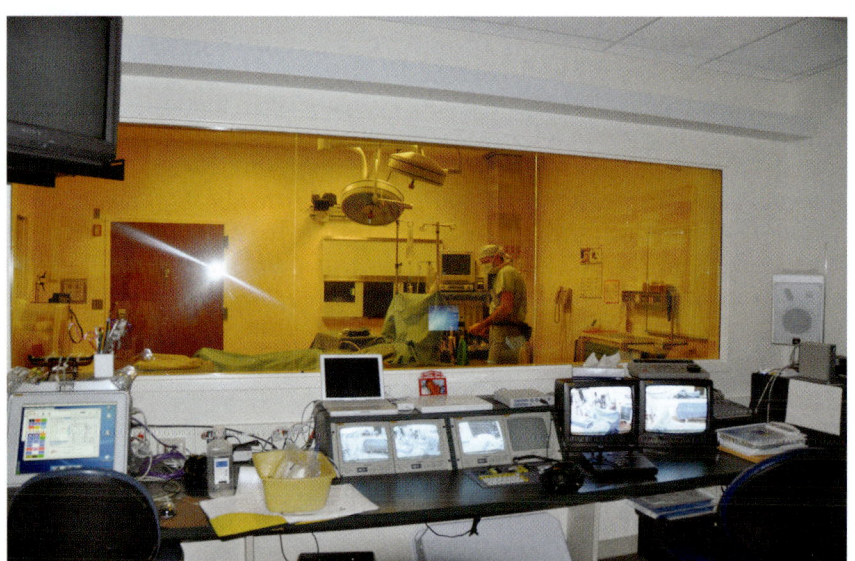

FIGURE 59-1 A behind-the-scenes look of the simulated operating room from the control room.

APPLICATIONS

- Procedural training: Plenty of procedures can be practiced using simulation. For anesthesia, for example there are airway management, line placement, and regional anesthesia technique part-task trainers.
- Simulation of straightforward cases from induction to extubation: Sure, once you get the hang of things, this will become second nature, but when you're first starting, everything is foreign! How do patient's vital signs change with various induction agents? Can you mask ventilate and how do you place oral airways or do jaw thrust? How will you secure the airway? There are 45 minutes left in the case, do you re-paralyze? How will you extubate this craniotomy patient after an aneurysm clipping?
- Simulation of acute events. Practically any vital sign perturbation can be simulated. The mannequin's BP, heart rate and rhythm, end-tidal CO_2, temperature, and breath sounds can be altered alone or in any combination. You can be provided with central venous pressure (CVP) and pulmonary arterial pressures if you "place" the relevant lines. Some trainees will wait months before seeing a true intraoperative emergency and some might see it on day one but be too overwhelmed to really learn much. The simulator lab is a safer if not less nerve-wracking way to experience your first (and second, and third) incident of autonomic dysreflexia, or high spinal, or crash cesarean delivery under general anesthesia.
- Simulation of crises: These can be cardiac arrest scenarios or mass casualties. Here is where the ABCs and the advanced cardiac life support (ACLS) protocols can be learned, practiced, and reinforced. When the adrenaline in you is pumping, you can get tunnel vision or you can freeze. Sure, it's easy to say what an algorithm is when you're answering a multiple-choice question, but much more difficult when chaos is running in real time. Simulation can improve communication and resource management skills while in crisis, too. How many times have you been to a code where no one knows who is performing which role? A call for epinephrine is given and several people administer it? Or no one?
- Communication mechanics: Have you ever listened to the communications between air traffic control and the pilot as your flight gets ready to take off? Closed-loop communication is a very important technique to ensure that communication is correctly interpreted and confirmed by both parties. Using people's names rather than generically calling out "we need a unit of blood in here," is an incredibly effective way to get someone's attention and get what you need. Yet it's alarmingly rare in day-to-day communication in the perioperative environment. Simulation is a great strategy to introduce people to good technique and to practice it until people feel less self-conscious and adapt it to real life (Figure 59-2).
- Communication systems: The OR, PACU, ICU, off-site airways, and OB are all places where we rely on our colleagues to provide important, accurate, yet succinct information about one or several dozen patients. Did you find out the patient's potassium prior to giving succinylcholine for an emergent airway on the floor? Did you get a handoff about this patient's severe preeclampsia prior to placing an epidural?
- Low-frequency, high-consequence events: Here we're not just talking about malignant hyperthermia scenarios, although that's important too. We're also talking about learning how to have difficult conversations with patients and their families, whether it's dealing with an irate patient, or discussing withdrawal of care, or disclosing an unforeseen outcome. Your own hospitals will also have support systems set up to help you, and simulation is a natural adjunct.

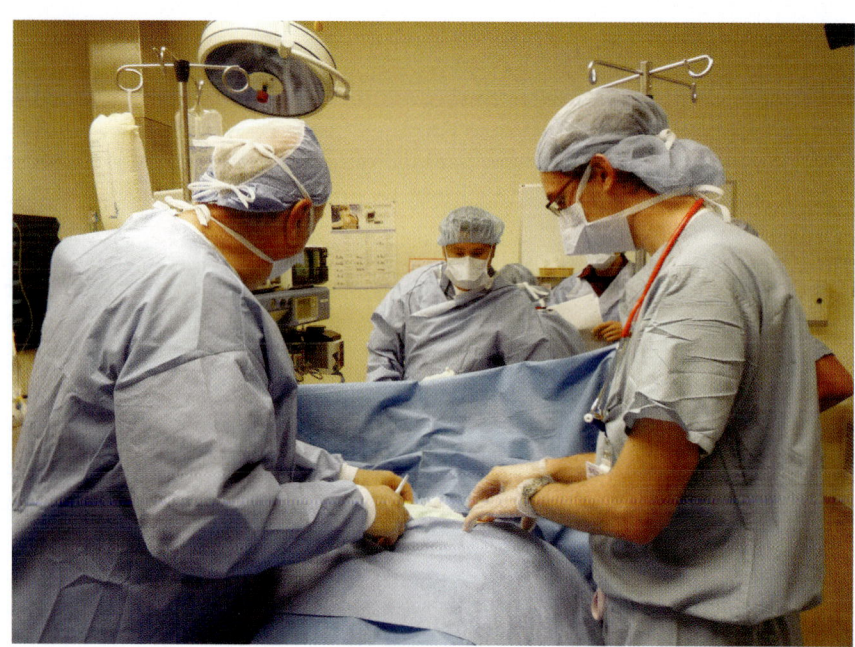

FIGURE 59-2 People experience real emotions and tensions during simulations that can be amplified in team scenarios.

CHALLENGES

- Airway fidelity: Simulators are just that—they simulate. There are many aspects of real patient care that are difficult to simulate. Unfortunately, airway is one of them. Mask ventilation on a mannequin seems so, well, plastic. The vocal cords look so, well, plastic. Get your basics down with simulation, so that you are well prepared to learn how to deal with the secretions, blood, coughing, and patient movement that just can't be simulated well.
- When you are working with the simulator, remember to articulate all your thoughts and actions. Most of the time, someone is sitting in the other room watching you. The only way you are going to learn from the experience if that person can analyze and give you feedback on your thought process.
- Time in the simulator lab is not equivalent to time in reality. In the simulator lab, when you call for help, it can be there in a blink of an eye; when you call for blood, someone gets it to you momentarily; when you send off specimens to the labs, the results are generally given to you within seconds. Just remember that in real life everything takes time. An arterial blood gas result will not be available to you for what seems like an eternity and you may need to make a decision by using clinical judgment with little laboratory evidence. If someone is helping you start an IV or an arterial line, it may take that person several minutes, which makes him or her unavailable to you for that precious time.
- Simulator mannequins are not real people, and though we can make their vital signs go up and down, it is hard to add emotions or other physiologic responses to stress. A simulator can't shiver, flush, blush, sweat, or vomit, although you could check out your local gag store and pick up some fake rubber vomit. These are physical findings that, if noted in a patient, could serve as important diagnostic tools. So if, for example, an allergic reaction case is being practiced, it may need to be stated that a patient has urticaria.
- When following a script in the simulator lab, it is easy to oversee perfect learning opportunities. Unless a strict script needs to be followed (e.g., for a research project), let your mind wander and let each scenario unfold. As an example, while running a simulation scenario on endobronchial intubation and hypoxemia, the students correctly identified the problem and pulled back the endotracheal tube to the appropriate position. In the process, the simulator instructor recognized that the student did not inflate the endotracheal tube balloon. So, despite continued 100% FiO_2 hand ventilation, the patient continued to desaturate. We were now in the midst of a completely different scenario: circuit leak and hypoxemia!
- Unless your facility has a fancy simulator with capability to read bar codes and identify medications that are being administered, you will have to verbalize what and how much of each medication is being given. This way the simulator controller can change the physiologic parameters in response to your actions.

THE EDUCATOR'S ROLE

The simulator is only as good as the instructor running it. You may have the best simulator in the world with the latest and greatest high-tech functions. But in the end it is up to the instructor to decide how to use the simulator, what scenarios to run, and how to engage the participants. Instructors should consider the following suggestions:

- Start easy and basic. Teach the students the simple things first: airway management, code algorithms, charging the defibrillator, paddle placement, etc.
- As the students advance, start adding more complex tasks with multiple decision branches. The patient is hypotensive and also hypoxic. Patient is hypotensive and has ECG changes.
- Another layer of complexity includes adding scenarios where teamwork and crisis resource management are necessary. Crisis resource management is an attempt to create functional teamwork from the chaos that usually ensues in hectic and emergent situations.
- In medical settings, most mistakes that occur can be traced back to communication breakdown, and thus it is important to educate medical providers about how to manage critical situations with many people. The term *crisis resource management* may sound abstract to you now, as you read this from the comfort of a seat in a café, but a poorly handled critical event is a terrible thing to witness. Teams don't function poorly because they don't care. They care sometimes to the point that their own emotions become an obstacle. Using simulation, teams can learn how to operationalize leadership, followership, communication, management of resources, and avoidance of fixation.
- Tailor the scenario to each student and situation. Try not to follow a very strict script, but instead modify the scenario as you go along. You will be amazed what excellent teaching opportunities pop up.
- Take advantage of the simulator to create some rare yet important medical events. One may never see a case of malignant hyperthermia or thyroid storm in their career. A simulator is the perfect place to introduce students to these rare cases. And if then your students happens to be unfortunate enough to witness a true case of malignant hyperthermia, they will be certain to come back and thank you (Figure 59-3).
- Finally, be prepared for the participants to do everything but the actions you expected to see! Your learning objectives may change dramatically if you thought this was going to be a scenario about troubleshooting a patchy nerve block but the participants induce general anesthesia and give succinylcholine in a patient with renal failure. When participants do things differently from what you anticipated (and they often, if not usually, do), you must be ready to talk about it in the debriefing.

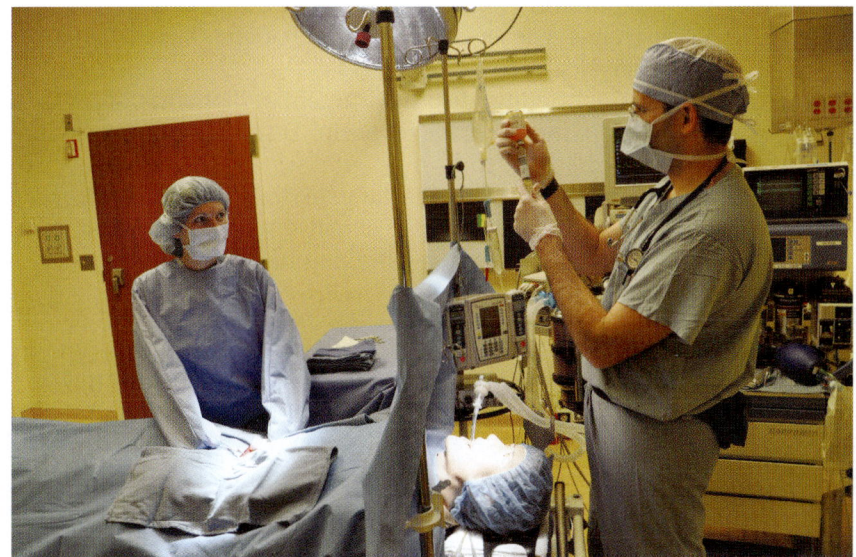

FIGURE 59-3 A resident practices drawing up Dantrolene.

DEBRIEFING

- The key for any educator in the simulator is the debriefing session, which should occur at the end of any scenario. Preferably, debriefing should occur immediately postscenario while the case is fresh. First, the students evaluate and respond to their performance. Then the debriefer ensures everyone's understanding of the event. Finally, take-home messages are summarized for each scenario.
- Refrain from jumping to conclusions, and ask open-ended questions to discover what the framework of thinking was. Instead of asking, "So, why is labetalol the wrong drug to give?" ask the students what their thought process was when they chose to administer the drug. Did they have the correct information needed? Did they have a different priority than yours? Did they know the risks involved? Did they make a drug error?
- Refrain from lecturing. Remember, what the participants have just been through is an experience with layers of complexity. During debriefing you want to explore what happened and why. By all means, augment the debriefing with facts and literature, but don't overshadow the simulation experience with PowerPoint.
- If you're teaching a course in which there is the valuable opportunity to go back and repeat the scenario, the benefits of a good debriefing can be immediately appreciated.
- Use of video: Videos are valuable and can be used for immediate playback so that participants can objectively see themselves in action. Do two participants disagree about whether the blood pressure fell first or whether the patient desaturated first? Does one participant claim they told the other about latex allergy, but the other claims they didn't? Roll the tape!
- There are several levels of debriefing:
  - Facilitator-led. Here the instructor has the knowledge and leads the participants. This type of debriefing is common.
  - Peer-led, facilitator-guided. Here both the participants and the instructor collectively have the knowledge. This type of debriefing is more difficult to learn how to do. It requires a high level of engagement by both instructor and participant. This type of debriefing is, in general, the desired target, since even novice residents already have quite a lot of knowledge and skills.
  - Peer-led and guided: This level of debriefing is fairly rare. In this case, the participants are highly skilled in the debriefing process, and essentially run the debriefing without instructor guidance.

CASE SCENARIOS

Simple Scenario 1

- Resident walks up to a simulator, and the monitor shows ventricular fibrillation.
- Resident recognizes the problem and calls for help and initiates basic life support (BLS).
- Resident instructs help to continue chest compressions and begins to ventilate the patient with Ambu bag.
- Resident instructs help to apply paddles, charge to 200 and synchronize, and shock.
- Nothing happens.
- Resident instructs to increase to 360 and shock again.
- Nothing happens.
- Someone says, "Wait, should that be asynchronous?"
- Shock in asynchronous mode and the simulator returns to sinus rhythm.
- In debriefing, look over the video and compare the performance to ACLS protocol.

Simple Scenario 2

- Resident takes over a case in the operating room.
- Sign out is given.
- Patient begins to desaturate.
- Resident puts the patient on 100% FiO_2, auscultates the lungs.
- Resident acknowledges wheezing and high peak airway pressures, and proceeds to treat bronchospasm by deepening the anesthetic and administering albuterol.
- Patient does not improve.
- Resident calls for help while administering more albuterol.
- Help suggests you check the patient's history and physical.
- In debriefing, discuss differential diagnosis of hypoxia and bronchospasm. Discuss appropriate time to call for help.
- Emphasize the importance of looking at the history and physical exam. Resident discovers that patient was allergic to penicillin and had received cefazolin preoperatively.

Scenario 3: Learn When Not to Intervene

- Resident is doing an ENT case and the surgeon injects lidocaine with epinephrine and starts the case.
- Resident recognizes hypertension and tachycardia, and suspects they are due to pain because the case just started.
- Resident administers fentanyl and deepens the volatile agent.
- Patient continues to be hypertensive and tachycardic.

- Resident administers labetalol to treat hypertension.
- Five minutes later the patient is now hypotensive.
- Resident opens up fluids and gives a 500-mL bolus.
- Patient develops ectopy.
- Now the *resident* is hypertensive and tachycardic.
- Instructor stops the scenario before the resident becomes a patient.
- During the debriefing, the resident reviews events.
- Did the resident realize that epinephrine was administered? Does the resident understand the transient actions of epinephrine?
- Resident learns each treatment created a new problem and that the best course of action is not always immediate reaction.

Scenario 4: Managing Your Resources

- PACU resident gets called by a nurse to evaluate a hypertensive patient.
- Another nurse calls the resident to evaluate someone with hypoxemia.
- Resident looks the first patient over, sees that the patient is stable, and says that he will be back shortly. Instructs the nurse to notify him if anything changes.
- Resident goes to evaluate the second patient. Patient is intubated, hypoxemic, and hypotensive.
- Resident correctly identifies that the endotracheal tube has been displaced.
- Resident calls for help immediately, takes the endotracheal tube out and starts mask ventilating the patient. Help arrives with intubating equipment.
- Meanwhile, the first patient's nurse calls out that the patient is having ST changes.
- Resident identifies someone in the help group to evaluate the patient while she continues to manage the airway of the second patient.
- During the debriefing, the team discusses the problems with managing more than one crisis at a time: how you triage needs and how you divide up skilled personnel.

Scenario 5: Managing Family Members

- PACU resident is called to evaluate a patient with chest pain and shortness of breath.
- Resident comes to the patient's bay and is immediately approached by a family member screaming at the resident to do something because the patient is feeling awful.
- Resident gives a cursory acknowledgment to the family member but focuses his attention on the patient and the nurse who is giving him factual information.
- Meanwhile the family member keeps anxiously asking the resident about what he is going to do and keeps asking the patient if she is OK, repeatedly.
- Resident does a quick history and physical.
- Family member continues to raise his voice. Resident is trying not to raise his voice.
- Resident makes the decision to ask the family member to step out for a few minutes while he evaluates the patient. The family member is resistant but eventually complies.
- In debriefing, the team discusses strategies to manage difficult conversations and to maintain tactful control of a situation.

Scenario 6: Difficult Surgeon

- The resident takes over a case. Patient is intubated and under general anesthesia.
- Hand-off is given, "Patient is having a liver resection. We have an 18-g IV for induction. I was going to put in another IV after."
- A "surgeon" is across the drape.
- You look at the upper extremities and see no viable candidate for a bigger IV.
- You say, "I think I need a central line for adequate access, in case we need to resuscitate."
- Surgeon says, "No. There will be minimal blood loss."
- You hear the suction sounds and slowly the patient's BP is dropping.
- A second surgeon in the field says, "We are losing some blood."
- The resident opens up the IV fluids and says, "I need more access." Surgeon yells back, "Just make sure the CVP stays at zero."
- BP drops to 70; patient is tachycardic and has ST depressions.
- Resident calls for help and orders blood in the room stat. Gets the Cordis kit out and sends off an arterial blood gas (ABG).
- ABG comes back with Hgb 6.3, pH 7.17.
- In the debriefing, concentrate on the art of talking to difficult people and standing up for what you believe to be the safest action for the patient.
- Resident and "surgeon" have a discussion. The resident learns that the "surgeon" had some issues with central lines in the past and now almost always opposes them. There was no discussion prior to the case about the anesthesiologist's concerns and surgeon's concerns.

Scenario 7: Off-Site Airway Case 1

- ICU resident gets called to an airway.
- Patient is on the floor, obtunded, face mask on, saturating 83%, other vital signs looks good.
- Resident examines the patient. Patient doesn't respond to a deep sternal rub.
- Resident asks others present in the room for patient's history and quick review of recent events.

- Resident learns that patient has stage IV breast cancer was admitted with fevers, was doing well until about 20 minutes ago when she started experiencing labored breathing and became hypoxic and eventually unresponsive.
- Resident identifies the need for securing an airway and gathers the necessary equipment.
- Respiratory therapy is at bedside with a ventilator.
- Resident skillfully intubates the patient and verifies the position of the endotracheal tube.
- As resident is securing the endotracheal tube, a person in street clothes runs into the room, yelling, "What are you doing to my mother? She is DNR!"
- Everything stops and there is utter silence.
- In debriefing, the instructor and students go over the indications for intubation. How to manage an off-site airway, what information to gather from other team members, what equipment do you need, what medications you need, do you need medications in an obtunded patient?
- Resident did everything appropriately except check the patients DNR status.

Scenario 8: Off-Site Airway Case 2
- ICU resident called for an airway.
- Resident arrives in the patient room and is met by the "nurse" and the "primary service fellow."
- The "fellow" says, "Patient is desaturating, you need to intubate him."
- Resident looks over the patient. Patient is saturating 90% on room air, somewhat tachypneic, other vitals are normal.
- Resident approaches the patient and puts a face mask on the patient prior to anything else. Patient's saturation improves to 99%. Resident asks for the patient's medical history. Patient notes that he feels much better.
- Fellow says, "Well, he was doing well before and he is going to IR in the morning for an aneurysm coiling, can't you just intubate him now? He will need it tomorrow anyway."
- Resident downgrades the patient to a nasal cannula and patient continues to do well.
- Resident that has a discussion with the fellow about the downside to intubating the patient there and then.
- In debriefing, instructor and the students discuss how the resident skillfully handled the situation.

Scenario 9: Can't Intubate, Can't Ventilate
- Resident sets up to do a standard induction.
- Routine patient for a hernia repair.
- Patient develops trismus (if the mannequin can't develop a tight jaw, it can be taped).
- Resident tries to mask ventilate but can't.
- Saturation starts to drop.
- Resident starts down the difficult airway algorithm, after unsuccessful mask ventilation, and tries to place an oral airway unsuccessfully. Resident tries a laryngeal mask airway (LMA), also unsuccessfully. Resident eventually arrives at cricothyrotomy.
- In debriefing, go over the difficult airway algorithm.
- Discuss trismus, does it mean malignant hyperthermia?

CONCLUSION

The scenarios listed above are just a sampling of what kinds of elements can be thrown into simulator sessions. The goal of any scenario is the same: shake up the student a bit, and then make sense of it in the debriefing.

Ideas for other scenarios are endless; just let your mind wander, then go to your friendly neighborhood simulation lab and try one out! (Figure 59-4)

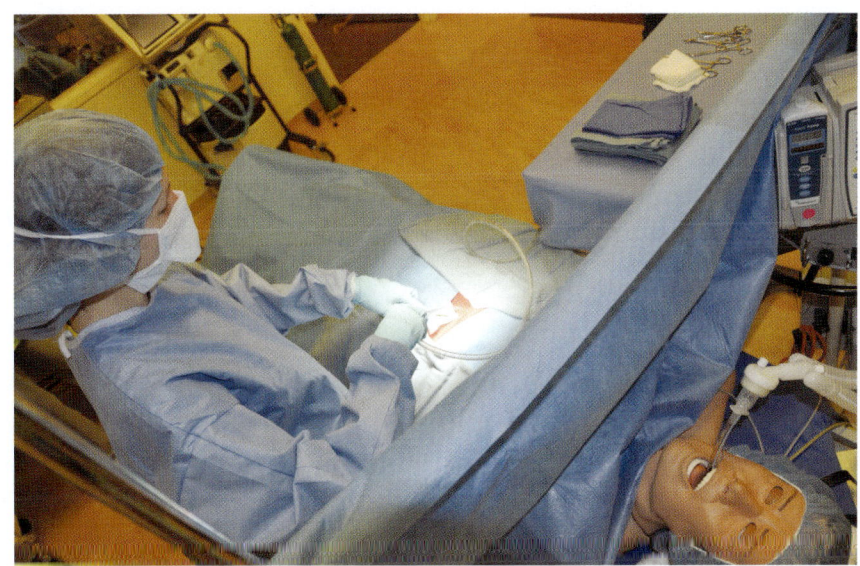

FIGURE 59-4 Remember, a simulator is the technology. You make simulation come to life by what you put into it.

SUGGESTED READING

Cooper JB, Taqueti VR. A brief history of the development of mannequin simulators for clinical education and training. *Qual Saf Health Care* 2004;13(Suppl 1):i11–i18.

An informative overview of simulators and simulation strategies used in medical education.

Denson, Abrahamson. A computer-controlled patient simulator. *JAMA* 1969;208(3):504–508.

The landmark article describing SimOne, the prototypical high-fidelity mannequin simulator.

Gaba DM. Crisis resource management and teamwork training in anaesthesia. *Br J Anaesth* 2010;105(1):3–6.

This article describes the past and current landscape of simulation for team training, as adapted from Cockpit Resource Management in aviation.

Gallagher CJ, Tan JM. The current status of simulation in the maintenance of certification in anesthesia. *Int Anesthesiol Clin* 2010;48(3):83–99.

This article addresses the use of simulation for practicing anesthesiologists, for whom participation in simulation in mandatory to obtain specialty recertification.

Park CS, Rochlen LR, Yaghmour E, et al. Acquisition of critical intraoperative event management skills in novice anesthesiology residents by using high-fidelity simulation-based training. *Anesthesiology* 2010;112(1):202–211.

The investigators created and tested a simulation-based curriculum to teach novice residents how to manage critical intraoperative events.

Rudolph J, Simon R, Rivard P, et al. Debriefing with good judgment: combining rigorous feedback with genuine inquiry. *Anesthesiol Clin* 2007;25(2):361–376.

This article describes a model for debriefing to improve reflective practice.

CHAPTER 60

FIGHTING AN UPHILL BATTLE: ANESTHESIA FOR THE OBESE PATIENT AND WEIGHT-LOSS SURGERY

EMMETT WHITAKER
OWEN HALLORAN

"You want me to do WHAT?"
David, on first seeing Goliath

INTRODUCTION

The World Health Organization (WHO) has found that more than 50% of adults are overweight, with at least 10% of those being obese. We won't even get started on children. As obesity continues to burgeon as an epidemic, we can expect to see many overweight and obese patients in the operating room. In addition, more and more obese patients are pursuing surgical options for weight loss. These patients represent a cohort with their own set of anesthetic risks. As perioperative physicians, we need to be ready and able to manage these patients.

Let's talk a little bit about obesity itself. Overweight patients can be classified by body mass index (BMI):
- Overweight (BMI 25–30)
- Obese (BMI 30–35)
- Morbidly Obese (BMI 35–45)
- Superobese (BMI >45)

To determine your patient's BMI, divide weight in kilograms by height in meters squared. You find as you gain experience as a clinician that there ain't no mountain high enough when it comes to BMI and obesity.

Often, obese patients are unable to make lifestyle changes necessary to lose the weight they have accumulated. Therefore, many patients are choosing the surgical route to lose weight. Indications for weight loss surgery have changed over the years, but to simplify, surgery should be considered as a treatment option for patients with a BMI >40 and those with a BMI >35 who present with obesity-related comorbidities such as hypertension, diabetes mellitus, hyperlipidemia, and obstructive sleep apnea.[1] As our population becomes more obese, it stands to reason that more patients will be eligible for weight loss surgery and will pursue it.

SURGICAL TECHNIQUE

In terms of surgical technique, there are currently three options for surgical dieting: laparoscopic or open gastric bypass, gastric sleeve resection, and laparoscopic band application.
- The old standby, of course, is *gastric bypass*. Make sure that when you interview patients and they

say they are having a "bypass" that you ask which kind! Clinicians sometimes assume patients mean the coronary artery variety, which of course would indicate a different clinical scenario. The gastric bypass is usually done via a minimally invasive approach. Usually, the surgical result is a smaller functional stomach pouch, and a secondary "remnant" pouch, both of which are still connected to the intestine. Just as you bypass a blockage in coronary artery surgery, the idea here is to reroute the alimentary tract such that a portion of the stomach and a large section of the intestine's absorptive mucosa is "bypassed" by the food.
- Though less common, gastric bypass is still occasionally done as an open surgical procedure. This is usually due to the patient's surgical history or a failed attempted at minimally invasive technique. This is a higher degree of difficulty for optimizing the patient's postoperative ventilatory function given the longer operation with a more painful incision.[2]
- Another technique commonly used is a *sleeve gastrectomy*, also known as a gastric sleeve. The goal here is to create a smaller functional stomach, forcing the patient to eat less by way of early satiety. This is typically done with a minimally invasive procedure.
- Finally, some patients may opt for the adjustable gastric band, more commonly known as the *lap band*. In this procedure, the surgeons go in laparoscopically (hence the "lap" part of the name) and place an inflatable silicone band around the loop portion of the stomach. This creates a small pouch in the upper stomach that quickly fills with food, leading to early satiety. As a patient loses weight, the band can be adjusted. Very recently, the Food and Drug Administration (FDA) loosened its restrictions on who can have this surgery. This means millions more patients will be eligible for weight loss surgery in upcoming years!

This is relevant for licensing purposes too as it's likely that you are going to encounter an obese patient on your oral board exam. Staying true to form, let's attack this from a preop-intraop-postop perspective.

PREOPERATIVE CONSIDERATIONS

What makes anesthetizing these patients difficult? Is it even difficult, or is it just different? We would argue that some of the pathophysiologic changes in overweight patients makes them unique, and puts them at higher risk for complications. The main challenge to these patients, as alluded to earlier, is defending their postoperative ventilatory function against numerous pre-, intra-, and postoperative threats. Remember: "Defend the lung volumes!" Basically you don't want to be reintubating the patient later in the postanesthesia care unit (PACU), or, even worse, in the OR before you leave the room. This is both embarrassing for you and an unnecessary danger for the patient. Don't worry, the rest of this chapter is devoted to showing you how NOT to be in that situation.

Let's first address a few common comorbid conditions that we see in obese patients:
- As you already know, obesity predisposes patients to numerous comorbidities. The most common conditions include obstructive sleep apnea (OSA), hypertension, diabetes mellitus, dyslipidemia, coronary artery disease, and osteoarthritis. Some patients may have even suffered a myocardial infarction or developed pulmonary hypertension and heart failure.
- Many obese patients have multiple cardiovascular risk factors: smoking, hypertension, dyslipidemia, and vascular disease to name a few. Beware of early coronary artery disease! Typically, if these patients have decent exercise tolerance (they can walk a distance without chest pain or shortness of breath) they aren't in imminent danger of dying in the operating room. You need to be able to risk stratify based on history! Be familiar with the American College of Cardiology (ACC)/American Heart Association (AHA) guidelines on perioperative cardiac risk (see Suggested Reading, below).
- A full discussion of all these comorbidities is outside the scope of this chapter, so we will concentrate on a common condition in this patient population that is important to anesthesiologists: OSA.
- OSA is caused by obstruction of the upper airway during sleep, leading to chronic hypoxia. It is often accompanied by snoring.
- Preoperative candidates for weight loss surgery should be given an OSA questionnaire[3] prior to weight loss surgery. If the questionnaire is positive, they are referred for a sleep study. If the sleep study is positive for sleep apnea, the patient is started on continuous positive airway pressure (CPAP) at night. This can help to reverse some of the effects that chronic hypoxia can have on the patient's other conditions including hypertension and pulmonary hypertension. There are data that suggest that this treatment decreases the length of ICU stay after weight loss surgery.[4]
- Patients with OSA are typically exquisitely sensitive to narcotics. We'll talk more about this later.
- A common fallacy is that obese patients always have difficult airways. This, of course, is not necessarily true. We've all seen that thin woman that was

impossible to intubate and that 350-pound patient who was a cinch. You should, of course, do a complete airway exam, assessing the patient's airway as you would any other. The trick here is to be prepared for anything. Of course, a red flag is always raised when a patient says, "They told me last time they couldn't get the tube in."

- You can also tell a lot about an obese patient's airway based on the distribution of their fat. Obese patients tend to have two basic body shapes: apple and pear. Large neck circumferences (>43 cm) in obese patients have been shown to be associated with difficult direct laryngoscopy.[5] If you are not able to tell by driver's license photos that patients are obese, they are probably pear shaped, and will probably be easier to intubate as they have less fat distribution in the head and neck. Conversely, patients with an apple shape, meaning they are thick throughout their body, head, and neck, may be harder to intubate.
- You always want to assess for the possibility of difficult ventilation as well. Obese patients tend to be more difficult to mask ventilate if they have a history of snoring, if they are edentulous, or if they have facial hair.[6]
- Despite all of these warnings, you're still not likely to have big trouble with the airway if on examination you find a Mallampati class I, good thyromental distance, and good neck extension. Oh, and the data back this up too.[7]
- You are probably understanding by now that you're not likely to need to do an awake fiberoptic intubation in these patients unless they have other conditions, but it may be considered from time to time, particularly in the superobese. While this is true, many clinicians like to have the fiberoptic/difficult airway cart available. If you do encounter a difficult intubation, we recommend immediate placement of a laryngeal mask airway (LMA). You can then intubate fiberoptically through this device once you have established stable ventilation.
- Of course, you'll use standard American Society of Anesthesiologists (ASA) monitors for these patients. In the operating room you'll place a pulse oximeter, an appropriately sized noninvasive blood pressure cuff, and electrocardiogram leads.
- It turns out that invasive monitors rarely, if ever, add anything to the management of these patients. Of course, there are situations in which one might feel compelled to place an arterial or central line. It can be tricky finding the right-size blood pressure cuff to place on an extremity, it's the old cylinder over a pyramid problem; however, it is a very rare necessity to have to place an arterial line due to lack of reliable cuff pressures.
- In some instances, obtaining reliable peripheral intravenous access can be difficult or impossible in obese patients. In such cases, central venous access may be compulsory for safety reasons. Like many decisions you will make in the operating room, you'll have to evaluate your patients on a case-by-case basis to determine the safest course of action. For open cases we like to have two reliable peripheral IVs. If we can't get two, then we place a central line, because if you can't get two lines as anesthesiologist in the OR, then somebody caring for that patient later on that evening when the single line gets pulled out will definitely not be able to get one, and thus it becomes a safety issue headed off by the responsible anesthetist in the OR.

INDUCTION

The induction phase is a potentially dangerous period for these patients. You need to make sure that you have as much time as possible to work through a difficult airway algorithm should you need to, and it is much more pleasant to do that with SpO_2 ticking along at 100%. In order to maintain this pleasant work situation, your mantra for induction should be: maximize apneic oxygenation, minimize apneic time, ommmmmm.

- These patients have a significantly decreased functional residual capacity (FRC). In addition, what little FRC they have is displaced and squished in the supine position. For these reasons, they have very little reserve, and prudent anesthesiologists will always have this in the back of their mind when dealing with obesity.
- Proper positioning is crucial for these patients and should be prepared in advance of bringing the patient into the room. You need to create a 30-degree head-elevated ramped position using blankets or a commercial product (Figures 60-1 and 60-2).
- "Ramping" serves two important purposes. First, it creates a head elevated, neck extended sniffing position that is important for intubation. The goal is to horizontally align the patient's external auditory meatus with the sternal notch. In other words you want the trachea pointing up at you, and you want space between the sternum and the chin to fit the laryngoscope handle. When you see these patients lying flat you will see what we mean. Second, taking the weight off the patient's chest using the ramp improves the patient's FRC and is one of the two ways we can improve apneic oxygenation.[8]
- The other way we can improve apneic oxygenation is to preoxygenate with pressure support. Patients may not like this, or in fact they may be used to this

from their home CPAP machine, but reassure them it is for their safety. You can do this with an advanced ventilator with pressure support (PS) mode, or simply have the patient breath against a partially closed adjustable pressure limiting (APL) (popoff) valve.
- When choosing induction agents, remember the other half of your mantra: minimize apneic time. We perform a rapid induction with fast-acting agents such as propofol and succinylcholine. This is not the same as a rapid sequence induction, which is usually performed to prevent aspiration. The rapid induction is done to provide rapid intubating conditions such that in an emergency we can move on to plan B more quickly. In addition, the shorter duration of apnea will help prevent the development of atelectasis.
- We attempt to ventilate early and often. Once again, this is not a traditional rapid sequence intubation for aspiration prevention; this is a rapid intubation, period.
- Propofol should be dosed at 2 mg/kg total body weight (TBW). In general, lipophilic drugs are dosed on TBW. This will ensure an adequate depth of anesthesia. Most studies suggest a dosage cap of 350 mg and you should always be prepared with phenylephrine.[9] Succinylcholine should also be dosed as 1 mg/kg TBW.[10]
- Remember to consider early placement of an LMA if intubation proves difficult.
- No matter how well you have done "defending the lung volumes," there is bound to be some degree of atelectasis immediately after intubation; we recommend a recruitment maneuver immediately after intubation: apply 30 cm H_2O manually and hold it for 30 seconds, as tolerated.
- Remember that you'll need to remove your ramp when you are done intubating in order to position and pad the patient correctly. The ramp can cause injury if left in for the duration of the case, and it would make operating quite difficult for the surgeons.

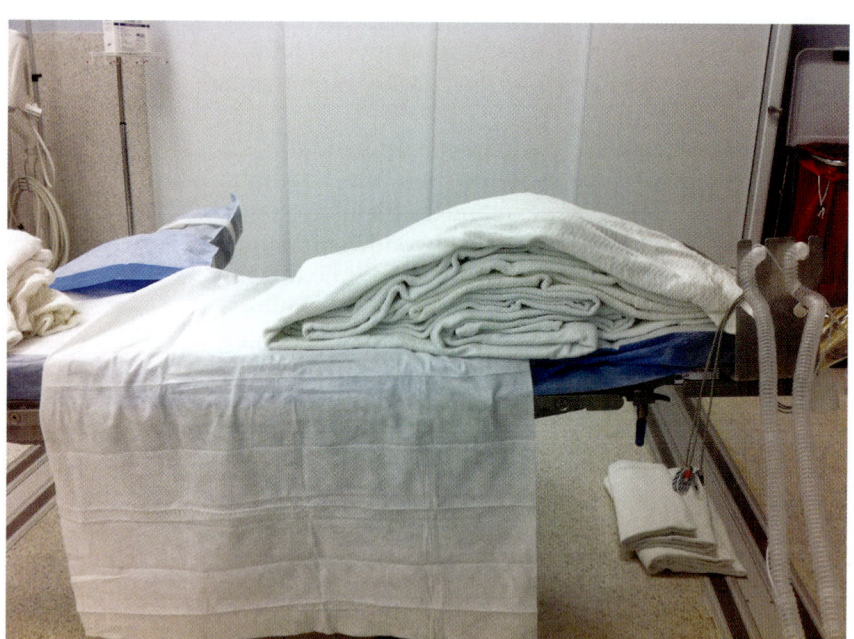

FIGURE 60-1 A ramp created with blankets.

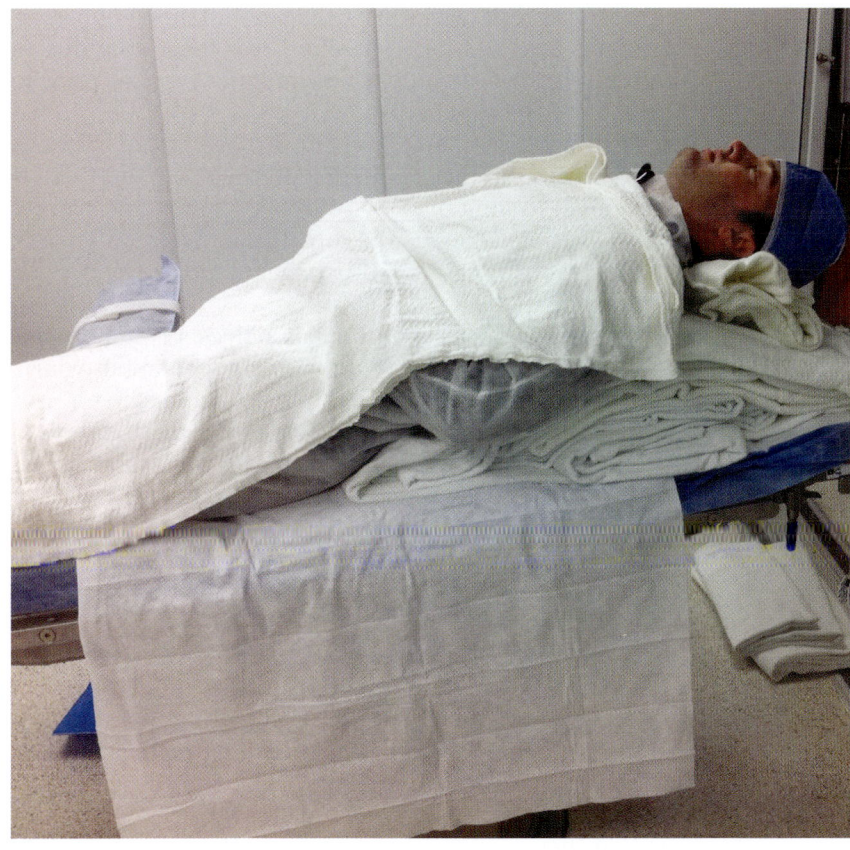

FIGURE 60-2 How to position a patient on the ramp.

MAINTENANCE

Now that you've successfully secured the patient's airway, you can relax. Actually, no you can't; you need to continue to work to keep your patient as optimized as possible! The goals of the maintenance phase, other than to keep the patient alive, is to continue defending the lung volumes in order to ready your patient for a safe extubation at the end of the case. Remember, this patient's body habitus AND your friend general anesthesia are working against you!

- Before we get too deep into this, remember (and this is important): do not put anything in the mouth that has not been discussed with the surgeon and communicated appropriately. The biggest concern to the surgeon is anastomotic leak. This is a grave danger to the patient should it develop. From time to time, the surgeon will unsuspectingly staple across a phantom nasogastric (NG) or orogastric (OG) tube, or an esophageal or nasopharyngeal temperature probe that has fallen down into the stomach; it is a huge detriment to the anastomosis that requires an immediate revision. During the safety time-out, it is important to communicate what you have in the patient's mouth. You should consider using a temperature-sensing Foley catheter or skin temperature probe for temperature monitoring.
- All your normal positioning concerns apply here, and more. For laparoscopic procedures, the patient will be placed into the steep Trendelenburg position, so take great care in securing the arms to the arm boards in such a way that they don't fall off while minimizing the potential for nerve injury.
- Intraoperative threats to the lung volumes: supine positioning with a heavy abdomen pressing against the lungs, general anesthesia, insufflation of the abdomen during laparoscopic procedures, and inadequate ventilation.
- Your ventilatory strategy (you guessed it): defend the lung volumes! Perhaps *the most important thing* you can do for these patients is to give them physiologic tidal volumes with positive end expiratory pressure of 7 to 10 cm H_2O.[11]
- We also recommend relative hyperventilation with an end-tidal CO_2 goal of approximately 30 prior to insufflation of the abdomen. This allows for some accumulation if you run into problems ventilating the patient once the surgeons insufflate.
- Volume control is the appropriate ventilator mode for these patients; using pressure control for a case

in which the intrabdominal pressure can vary widely is tantamount to turning off the high-pressure alarm. You don't want to turn around and notice the CO_2 is 65 because you have been getting 200-cc tidal volumes without realizing it. If you are getting a high-pressure alarm, consider increasing the patient's inspiratory time in combination with dropping the positive end-expiratory pressure (PEEP) slightly, as you are in fact increasing the patient's mean airway pressure, which is important for preventing postoperative atelectasis.
- We maintain general anesthesia with a balanced technique consisting of small doses of narcotic and a short-acting volatile anesthetic (desflurane). Using desflurane appears to lead to faster awakening and extubation in these patients.[12] We typically don't go above 1 minimum alveolar concentration (MAC) with a balanced approach; this will lead to a prolonged washout time and a groggy patient at the end of the case. We often switch to nitrous oxide during the closure period at the end of the case to begin the washout of desflurane sooner, leading to a faster, crisper awakening at the end of the case.
- With regard to neuromuscular blockade, it's not what you choose, it's how you use it. Of course, patients coughing and bucking during surgery not only annoys the surgeons, it threatens your precious lung volumes and makes you look bad. We recommend rigorous checking of twitches and titration of neuromuscular blockers to a maximum of two twitches. If you're easily distractible, consider an infusion of neuromuscular blocker. You should dose nondepolarizing neuromuscular blockers on ideal body weight, like most other hydrophobic drugs.
- To calculate ideal body weight:
  - Men: 50 + 2.3 kg per inch over 5 feet
  - Women: 45.5 + 2.3 kg per inch over 5 feet
- Fluids, fluids, fluids. These patients, if insufflated, behave as though they have temporary abdominal compartment syndrome. Titrate crystalloid appropriately according to the patients' underlying disease.[13] A good rule of thumb is to keep them well hydrated (they need that intravascular volume) but don't overdo it (defend the lungs, as pulmonary edema is a bad thing).

EMERGENCE/POSTOPERATIVE CONSIDERATIONS

As you can imagine, obese patients are at a considerably increased risk of postextubation obstruction and desaturation.[14] In addition, if the cumulative detriments to the patients pulmonary function have not been sufficiently counterbalanced, this could lead to the downward spiral of postoperative atelectasis, hypoventilation, hypercarbia, and desaturation. Therefore, we must continue to carefully address a number of important issues prior to extubating these patients:
- Postoperative analgesia: pain management can be very tricky in these patients; on the one hand there is a threat to lung mechanics from splinting and pain; on the other there is the threat from oversedation, airway obstruction, and hypoventilation from over narcotization.
- For these reasons multimodal analgesia is important. After communicating with your surgeon about your plan, consider ketorolac. Bariatric patients given ketorolac after surgery have an earlier discharge from the PACU and better outcomes in general.[15] This makes everyone happy! Furthermore, if you've ever had surgery, you may know what a huge help surgical-site local anesthesia can be. Communicate with the surgeons; ask them to put in a long-acting local at the end!
- Remember: in the setting of OSA, these patients are exquisitely sensitive to narcotics. Though the data supporting this finding come primarily from the pediatric population and this finding has not been demonstrated in adults, most anesthesiologists choose to be on the safe side and treat them as if they are sensitive to opioids. We typically do not give more than 2 mg of hydromorphone intraoperatively to narcotic-naive patients while they are anesthetized. One should consider waiting until the patient is awake to give additional doses.
- Epidural analgesia has also been used successfully in these patients and certainly should be considered for open cases. However, epidural placement can be technically challenging and time-consuming, with a higher failure rate in these patients.
- Always administer full neuromuscular blockade reversal and verify the presence of four strong twitches prior to extubation.
- It is not recommended to have these patients spontaneous ventilating in the supine condition with the ventilator off. This is destroying all of the hard work that you have done defending the lung volumes. Extubate the patient from a minimal pressure support setting to preserve as much of the lung volumes as you can. Avoid the supine position as much as possible.
- Not surprisingly, these patients should be fully awake and on 100% oxygen prior to extubation. This is where the use of desflurane comes in handy. We also encourage the use of nitrous oxide. If you haven't walloped them with a lot of narcotic, they should wake up readily.
- Remember, leaving the patient intubated is ALWAYS an option. Better to extubate in the PACU or ICU

than to have an unplanned reintubation flail in the hallway.
- Always give supplemental oxygen immediately after extubation, and anticipate some desaturation despite its presence.[14] If the patient was on CPAP before surgery, strongly consider its use after surgery. Of course, surgeons fear an anastomotic leak more than anything, and may balk at the use of CPAP in the PACU. There is good evidence that the use of CPAP does NOT increase the risk of an anastomotic leak,[16] but in the interest of playing nice in the sandbox, you should discuss CPAP with the surgeon in advance.
- CPAP may actually improve outcomes and definitely improves lung function in the immediate postoperative period.[17]
- PACU discharge is similar to the discharge of other patients. Essentially, the patient's got to be back to his or her baseline mental status and vital signs. Oxygenation and ventilation should be adequate.[18] Pain control should be satisfactory, and nausea and vomiting, if present, should be controlled.
- ICU care is sometimes appropriate, but, if you've done your job defending the lung volumes, not very often.

CONCLUSION

Caring for obese patients isn't easy, but it isn't hard if you've continued to be vigilant about preserving their pulmonary function throughout the entire perioperative period. In the cases we've seen at our center requiring unplanned postoperative reintubation, some common themes occur: PEEP was not used intraop, desflurane was not used, large doses of narcotics were used, the patient was not fully reversed from neuromuscular blockade, or the patient was extubated prior to being fully responsive. There is nothing groundbreaking here; just be as diligent as you always are. The induction period can be made safer by doing a few extra things, like building the ramp and using pressure support preoxygenation, and working rapidly so in the rare instance you can quickly move on to plan B. In addition, you need to be creative with your postoperative analgesia plan other than relying solely on narcotics. How about nonsteroidal antiinflammatory drugs (NSAIDs) or local anesthesia? Some centers are even using dexmedetomidine. And postoperatively you should probably resume the patients' CPAP if they have OSA. Inevitably, you will encounter obese patients in your practice, and you may even end up providing anesthesia for bariatric surgery. And given the alarming trends in our society in terms of obesity, this skill set is an increasingly important aspect of each anesthesiologist's training.

REFERENCES

1. Snow V, Barry P, Fitterman N, Qaseem A, Weiss K. Pharmacologic and surgical management of obesity in primary care: a clinical practice guideline from the American College of Physicians. *Ann Intern Med* 2005;142(7):525–531.
2. Adams TD, Gress RE, Smith SC, et al. Long-term mortality after gastric bypass surgery. *N Engl J Med* 2007;357(8):753–756.
3. Chung F, Yegneswaran B, Liao P, et al. STOP questionnaire: a tool to screen patients for obstructive sleep apnea. *Anesthesiology* 2008;108:812–821.
4. Hallowell PT, Stellato TA, Petrozzi MC, et al. Eliminating respiratory intensive care unit stay after gastric bypass surgery. *Surgery* 2007;142(4):608–612.
5. Gonzalez H, Minville V, Delanoue K, et al. The importance of increased neck circumference to intubation difficulties in obese patients. *Anesth Analg* 2008;106:1132–1136.
6. Kheterpal S, Han R, Tremper KK, et al. Incidence and predictors of difficult and impossible mask ventilation. *Anesthesiology* 2006;105:885–891.
7. El-Ganzouri AR, McCarthy RJ, Tuman KJ, et al. Preoperative airway assessment: predictive value of a multivariate risk index. *Anesth Analg* 1996;82:1197–1204.
8. Collins JS, Lemmens HJ, Brodsky JB, et al. Laryngoscopy and morbid obesity: a comparison of the "sniff" and "ramped" positions. *Obes Surg* 2004;14:1171–1175.
9. van Kralingen S, Diepstraten J, van de Garde EM, et al. Comparative evaluation of propofol 350 and 200 mg for induction of anaesthesia in morbidly obese patients: a randomized double-blind pilot study. *Eur J Anaesthesiol* 2010;27:572–574.
10. Cheymol G. Effects of obesity on pharmacokinetics implications for drug therapy. *Clin Pharmacokinet* 2000;39:215–231.
11. Cadi P, Guenoun T, Journois D, et al. Pressure-controlled ventilation improves oxygenation during laparoscopic obesity surgery compared with volume-controlled ventilation. *Br J Anaesth* 2008;100:709–716.
12. Strum EM, Szenohradszki J, Kaufman WA, Anthone GJ, Manz IL, Lumb PD. Emergence and recovery characteristics of desflurane versus sevoflurane in morbidly obese adult surgical patients: a prospective, randomized study. *Anesth Analg* 2004;99(6):1848–1853.
13. Holte K, Kehlet H. Postoperative ileus: a preventable event. *Br J Surg* 2000;87:1480–1493.
14. Ahmad S, Nagle A, McCarthy RJ, et al. Postoperative hypoxemia in morbidly obese patients with and without obstructive sleep apnea undergoing laparoscopic bariatric surgery. *Anesth Analg* 2008;107:138–143.
15. Govindarajan R, Ghosh B, Sathyamoorthy MK, et al. Efficacy of ketorolac in lieu of narcotics in the operative management of laparoscopic surgery for morbid obesity. *Surg Obes Relat Dis* 2005;1:530–535.
16. Huerta S, DeShields S, Shipner R, et al. Safety and efficacy of postoperative continuous positive airway pressure to prevent pulmonary complications after Roux-en-Y gastric bypass. *J Gastrointest Surg* 2002;6:354–358.

17. Neligan PJ, Malhotra G, Fraser M, et al. Noninvasive ventilation immediately after extubation improves lung function in morbidly obese patients with obstructive sleep apnea undergoing laparoscopic bariatric surgery. *Anesth Analg* 2010;110:1360–1365.
18. Benumof JL. Obesity, sleep apnea, the airway and anesthesia. *Curr Opin Anaesthesiol* 2004;17:21–30.

SUGGESTED READING

2009 ACCF/AHA Focused Update on Perioperative Beta Blockade Incorporated into the ACC/AHA 2007 Guidelines on Perioperative Cardiovascular Evaluation and Care for Noncardiac Surgery. http://circ.ahajournals.org/cgi/reprint/CIRCULATIONAHA.109.192690.

INDEX

A

abdominal surgery, nerve blocks, 301–307
  abdominal visceral-sensory innervation, 301–302
  abdominal wall innervation, 301
  field blocks, 307
  intraabdominal local anesthetic irrigation, 307
  regional anesthesia techniques, 302
    dermatomes, 302
    ilioinguinal/iliohypogastric, 306
    intercostal, 304–305
    neuraxial anesthesia, 302
    thoracolumbar paravertebral, 302–304
    transversus abdominis plane block, 302
  spinal nerves, 301
ABG. *See* arterial blood gas (ABG)
Accreditation Council for Graduate Medical Education (ACGME), 551
acetaminophen, 252
ACL. *See* anterior cruciate ligament (ACL)
acromegaly, 114
adjustable pressure limiting (APL), 564
advanced cardiac life support (ACLS) protocols, 553, 556
AI. *See* awake intubation (AI)
AIMS. *See* anesthesia information management systems (AIMS)
air exchange system, 543
airway
  exam, 514
  features to preoperatively check, 514
  fidelity, 554
  management equipment, 260
  oral, 91
  resuscitation equipment, 518
alcohol wipe, 336
allergy testing, 511
alopecia, 462

ambu bag, 87, 120, 183, 219
American College of Cardiology (ACC), 519, 562
American Heart Association (AHA), 519
  guidelines, 562
American Society of Anesthesiologists (ASA), 520, 563
  difficult airway algorithm, 101, 119, 150
anatomic variant, 119
anesthesia, 536. *See also* anesthesia information management systems (AIMS)
  ablations, 409–410
  administration of, 507, 509
  aicd placement/testing, 408
  for cardiac catheterization lab, 407–412
  in cath lab, 411
  control room, 410
  full-wrap lead shielding, 411
  generator
    pocket placement, 408
    subsequent tests of, 408–409
  Hall's laws of, 236
  HME filters, 179
  hybrid catheterization lab, 410
  to larynx and trachea, 123
  lead screen, staff, 409
  machine, 519
  magnetic resonance imaging (MRI), 447–450
  maintenance, 251
  medication drawer, 519
  monitors, 408, 519
  postanesthesia care unit (PACU), 93
  radiation safety, in catheterization lab, 410–412
  regional, 251
  spinal, 197–205
  stereotactic catheterization lab, 410
  value-added anesthesiologist, 449
anesthesia information management systems (AIMS), 491–496

  anesthesia record, evolution of, 491–492
  benefits of, 492
  charting, 495–496
  definition of, 492
  drawbacks of, 492–493
  equipment, 493
  modus operandi of, 493
  SOAPMIT method, basic room setup, 494
  type of, 494
  use of, 494–496
anesthesiologists, 9, 23, 27, 101, 103, 119, 142, 150, 176, 185, 186, 197, 215, 231, 251, 257, 261, 335, 499
anesthesiology, 3, 523
Anesthesiology News, 87
anterior cruciate ligament (ACL), 513
anterior superior iliac spine (ASIS), 75, 77, 286, 306, 324
antibiotic therapy, 9
anticholinergic, 252
antiinflammatory agents, 252
antisialagogue, 121
aortic arch, 390
APL. *See* adjustable pressure limiting (APL)
apparent chaos, 500
Arrow™ Femoral Arterial Line Catheterization Kit, 78
  contents, 78
arterial blood gas (ABG), 532, 554, 557
arterial hemorrhage, 337
arterial line insertion. *See also* radial A-line
  secured, 62
  through-and-through technique for, 63
arterial puncture, 27
arteriovenous (AV) fistula, 3, 507
arthritis, 114
aseptic technique, 233

ASIS. *See* anterior superior iliac spine (ASIS)
as low as reasonably achievable (ALARA)
  principle, 545
aspirin, 208, 231
asthma, 104, 105, 170
ataxia, 233
atropine, 310, 518
automatic implantable cardioverter-defibrillators (AICDs), 509
autonomic nervous innervation, 301. *See also* nerve blocks
awake intubation (AI), 119
  advanced preparation, 120
  aspiration prophylaxis
    intravenous hypnotics, 122
    sedation, 122
    supplemental oxygen, 122
  bad, 119–120
  common difficulties, 126
  difficult airway, 119
  extubation of, 127–128
  flexible fiberoptic bronchoscope equipment, 121
  further preparation, 121
  good, 119
  physiology, 127
  preoperative dialogue, 120
  preoperative visit, 120
  remedies, 126
    awake trach, 127
    LMA/LMA, 126
    retrograde wire, 127
  secretions, 121–122
  strategy, 120–121
  surgical opposition, 127
  technique, 122
    atomizer, 124
    chin lift, 125
    fiberoptic, 125
    fiberoptic with tape, 125
    FOB, 124
    nasal intubation, 123
    nebulizing, 124
    oral or nasal route, regardless of, 123–124
    OR bed, 125
    topicalization devices, 123, 124
    Williams airway, 124
  troubleshooting, 126
  ugly, 120

B

back up right pressure (BURP), 116
balloon inflation, 397, 398
basic life support (BLS), 556
beat-to-beat blood pressure monitoring, 57
benzodiazepine, 252
beta-blocker, 436
betadine, 248, 337
biopsy. *See* lung biopsy
bladder exstrophy
  anesthesia maintenance, 251
  caudal epidural blockade
    technique, 248–249
    use of, 248
  congenital disorder, 247
  fluid management
    blood loss, 251
    driving blind, 250
    maintenance, 250–251
    preoperative deficit, 251
    third space loss, 251
  neonatal airway, 247–248
  opioids, side effects, 252
  postoperative, 251
    anticholinergic, 252
    antiinflammatory agents, 252
    benzodiazepine, 252
    narcotics, 252
    regional anesthesia, 251
  tunneled caudal catheter placement of, 249–250
  withdrawal, 252
blood patch. *See also* epidural blood patch
  PDPH incidence, 231
blood, pus, oxygen and water (BPOW), 347
body mass index (BMI), 561
BPOW. *See* blood, pus, oxygen and water (BPOW)
brachial A-line, 67
  angiocath, 71
    uses, 68
  arterial tracing, 72
  brachial artery, palpate, 69
  complications
    neuronal/adjacent structure injury, 73
    thrombosis, 73
  contraindications, 67
  equipment, 67
  indications, 67
  philosophy, 67
  red pulsatile blood flow, 70
  Seldinger technique, 70
  sterile fashion, prep/drape, 69
  syringe, uses, 68
  technique, 67–72
  tubing/transducer, 72
  typical femoral arterial line kit, 68
  visual of wire, 71

brachial arterial line. *See* brachial A-line
brachial plexus (BP) blocks, 257. *See also* upper extremity block
  anatomy of, 258
bronchodilator, 122
Bullard scope, 117
bupivacaine, 249, 251
  in peripheral nerve catheters, 314
BURP. *See* back up right pressure (BURP)

C

calcium, 251, 518
cannulation, 19
capnography, 117, 171, 190
carboxyhemoglobin, 172
cardiac anesthesiologist, 9
cardiac disease, 398
cardiac pacemaker. *See* pacemaker
cardiac risk stratification, 511
cardiopulmonary bypass, 350
carina, 353
carotid artery, palpating, 330
carotid puncture, 19
caudal catheter
  insertion of, 249
  tunneling of, 250
caudal epidural block
  analgesia, 239
  angiocath, 241
  epidural kit, 240
  equipment, 240
  20-G catheter, 241
  local anesthetic doses, 243
  placement, 239–242
  technique, 248–249
  tegaderm, tape barrier, 242
  thread, 242
  use of, 248
cefazolin, prophylactic dose, 510
Centers for Disease Control and Prevention (CDC) guidelines, 31
central venous access, in pediatric patient
  anesthesia, 29
  central line catheter sizes and length, 30
  complications of, 29–30, 40
  contraindications, 29
  femoral vein
    advantages and disadvantages, 39
    anatomy of, 39
    femoral line placement, 40
    landmarks, 40
    placing, 40
    procedure and approach, 39–40

INDEX

troubleshooting, 40
indications, 29
internal jugular
  advantages and disadvantages, 30
  anatomy of, 30
  blood flows towards probe, 34
  equipment, 32
  kiddies, ultrasound, 34
  nicking the skin, 33
  placing dilator, 33
  positioning the patient, 32
  procedure and approach, 31–35
  squishable, 34
  sterile drapes, 32
  sterile dressing, 33
  vessels, ultrasound image of, 34
  watching the needle, 35
  watching the wire, 35
subclavian
  advantages and disadvantages, 36
  anatomy of, 36
  complications, 38–39
  dressing, 38
  landmarks, 36
  needle placement, 38
  placement extraordinaire, 38
  procedure and approach, 36–38
  suprasternal notch, 36
troubleshooting, 35–36, 38
central venous pressure (CVP), 553
  causes, 502
  monitoring, 249
cerebral ischemia, 233, 428
cerebral oximetry, 439
  accuracy, 441
  advantages, 441
  contraindications, 440
  disadvantages, 441
  equipment, 440
  indications, 440
  near-infrared monitor
    display, 442
    sensor pad placement, 443
    spectroscopy, 442
  numbers, interpreting, 440–441
  studies, 441
  technique, 440
cerebrospinal fluid (CSF), 329, 427–428
  density of, 199
  leaks, 149
cesarean, 302, 523, 553
Cetacaine spray, 520
chest x-rays (CXR), 513, 532
chronic obstructive pulmonary disease (COPD), 513
chylothorax, 20
closed-loop communication, 553
coagulopathy, 10, 15, 24, 149, 184, 197

Cohen® tip-deflecting blocker, 358
communication, 535
  mechanics, 553
  systems, 553
continuous positive airway pressure (CPAP) device, 93, 510, 562, 564
  use of, 567
COPD. See chronic obstructive pulmonary disease (COPD)
coronary artery bypass graft (CABG), 502
coronary artery surgery, 562
coronary revascularization, 511
CPAP device. See continuous positive airway pressure (CPAP) device
cranial nerve, 232, 233, 340, 428
Crawford needle, insertion of, 249
CREST syndrome, 329
cricoid cartilage, 11, 248, 267, 268, 329
cricoid pressure, 87, 105, 110
cricothyroid membrane (CTM), 127, 153, 154
crippling patient anxiety, 510
crisis resource management, 555
critical care medicine, 529
critical care technicians, 530
CSF. See cerebrospinal fluid (CSF)
C-spine, 464
CTM. See cricothyroid membrane (CTM)
cuff perforation, 354
Cushing's triad, 426
C5 vertebra, 267
C6 vertebra, 267
C7 vertebra, 225, 267
CVP. See central venous pressure (CVP)
cytomegalovirus (CMV), 251

D

danger zone highway, 541–542, 549
  accidents and hazards, 549
  block nitrous oxide, old guy on, 543
  electricity, 547
  historical trivia, 543
  MRI machine, 546
  radiation exposure, 544
  radiation trivia, 545–546
  risks, 541–542
  smell coming from, 543
  sticky situation, 548
  super glue for bones, methylmethacrylate (MMA), 549
  unborn children safty, 545
  volatile gases smell, 541
dantrolene, drawing up, 555

debriefing, levels of, 556
deep venous thrombosis (DVT), 531
delirium confusion assessment method, 533
dexmedetomidine, 310
dextran, 233
diaphragmatic paralysis, 264, 270
diffuse intravascular coagulation (DIC), 523
diphenhydramine, 407
direct laryngoscopy (DL), 523, 563
dizziness, 123
Doppler scan
  continuous-wave, 383
dorsalis pedis (DP) artery, 81
dreaded goal sheet, 532
drugs, 525–526
  airway, 526
  armamentarium of, 525
  eliciting allergic responses, 510
  sedation, 525
  vasoactive agents, 525
DVT. See deep venous thrombosis (DVT)
dyspnea, 511

E

echocardiography (ECG), 512, 513
efficiency
  airway equipment, 456, 457
  beware of, 456
  common glitches, 456
  contraindications, 453
  drugs, 457
  indications, 453
  IV line setup, 457
  machine, 454
  monitors, 455, 459
  OR table, 458
  people, help, 460
  philosophy of, 453
  preoxygenating, 459
  ready for induction, 459
  stuff, in margins
    mnemonic for pregame, 456
    obligatory anesthesia, uh, fool around time, 456–458
  suction, 457, 458
  teamwork, 453–454
  technique, 455
  typical start, 458–459
electrocardiogram, 517
electrolyte management, 535
elevated intracranial pressure. See intracranial pressure (ICP) monitoring
embolization, 50, 73, 83

EMLA cream, 66
endotracheal intubation, 103
endotracheal tube time (ETT), 98–99, 524, 525
end tidal CO_2 (E_TCO_2) detector, 183
   waveform, 520, 521
ephedrine, 310, 518
epidural analgesia, 566
epidural blood patch
   anesthesia, Hall's laws of, 236
   appropriate position and tourniquet, 234
   contraindications, 232
   equipment needed, 234
   history and physical examination prior, 233
   indications, 232
   mechanism of action, 232
   philosophy/alternatives, 232–233
   sterile blood draw, 236
   sterile field, 235
   technique, 235
   venipuncture site prepped sterilely, 234
   what if, 236
epidural hematoma, 204
epidural(s)
   actual stick, 220
   airway preparation, 219
   beware, 208
   cervical, 220–221
   common glitches, 219
   contraindications, 207
   dosing, 220
   equipment, 208
   history and physical, 208–209
   indications, 207
   loss of resistance (LOR)
      air vs. saline, 215
   philosophy, 208
   sitting/side position, 210, 219–220
   spinous process, 215, 217–218
   spots, marks, 216
   technique, 209–214
      catheter, 212–214
      glass syringe/LOR technique, 212
      securing catheter with tegaderm, 214
      sitting position, 210
      spinous processes, 211
      tuohy needle, in supra/interspinous ligament, 211
   thoracic, 220
   ultrasound guidance, 215–218
   uses, 207
epiglottis, 106, 110, 114–116
epinephrine, 310, 518, 556
Eschmann stylet, 518
esmolol, 518

esophagogastroduodenoscopy (EGD), 517
estimated blood loss (EBL), 500
etomidate, 372
ETT. See endotracheal tube time (ETT)
excessive bleeding, 515
external jugular (EJ), 4
extinguisher equipment, 549
extracorporeal membrane oxygenation (ECMO), 350

F

facial hair, 90, 563
family-centered care, 538
fatigue, 123
femoral arterial catheterization, 75–80
   anatomy, 75, 76
   anesthetize, area, 79
   artery, locate, 79
   bony landmarks, 77
   complications, 76
   contraindications, 76
   equipment, 78
   on the floor, 79
   indications, 75–76
   procedure, 79
   pulsatile flow, 79
   technique, 76–77
   troubleshooting, 80
femoral line. See also femoral venous access
femoral vein
   advantages and disadvantages, 39
   anatomy of, 39
   complications, 40
   femoral line placement, 40
   landmarks, 40
   placing, 40
   procedure and approach, 39–40
   troubleshooting, 40
femoral venous access, 43–47
   advancing wire, 46
   contraindications, 44
   equipment, 44
   femoral line history and physical, 44
   femoral lines, philosophy of, 44
   guidewire, in femoral vein, 47
   indications, 43–44
   numb and number, 46
   sterile, 45
   technique, 44–47
fentanyl, 199, 229, 251, 252, 259, 310, 318, 407
fiberoptic bronchoscope (FOB), 102, 104, 105, 110, 117, 120, 121
   flexible, 121
   injection port of, 123

   intubation, 150
   LMA size, 104
   SGA, 105
   wire-guided by, 351
fluoroscopy machines, 545
FOB. See fiberoptic bronchoscope (FOB)
Food and Drug Administration (FDA), 562
foreign body removal, 130
FRC. See functional residual capacity (FRC)
freely running IV, 527
full-body mannequin, 551
functional residual capacity (FRC), 563

G

gaming technology, 552
ganglion block. See stellate ganglion block
gastric bypass, 562
gastric sleeve. See sleeve gastrectomy
getting started. See efficiency
Glasgow Coma Scale (GCS), 533
glycopyrrolate, 121, 172
ground fault detectors, 547. See also line isolation monitors (LIMs)

H

handoff, operating room, 479–483
   in aviation, 479
   benefits of, 480
   definition of, 479
   example of, 481
   face to face, 482
   information needs, 480–483
   in PACU, 483
   recovery room, 483
   risks of, 480
   solution, 480
   standardized, 485–489
      cardiac ICU, 488
      recovery, 486
      recovery room, 487
      surgical intensive care unit (SICU), 487
      talk intraoperatively, 485–486
      verbal, 489
headache, 123
Health Insurance Portability and Accountability Act [HIPAA] violation, 531
hematoma, 197, 204, 208, 225, 243, 259, 267, 270
   formation/compartment syndrome, 58
hemodialysis, 9, 23
hemodynamic instability, 525

hemoglobin, 40, 92, 251
  transfusion guidelines, 500
hemorrhage, 298, 337, 342
hemothorax, 20
high-fidelity mannequins, 551
HIV, 548
hoarseness, 19, 270
Horner's syndrome, 271
hydralazine, 518
hyperalimentation, 9, 29, 49, 249
hypercarbia, 105, 566
hypotensive anesthesia
  contraindications to, 500
hypovolemia, 23, 197, 207, 376
hypoxemia, 127, 350, 554

I

ibuprofen, 204
ICP monitoring. *See* intracranial pressure (ICP) monitoring
ICU. *See* intensive care unit (ICU)
ideal body weight, 566
IJ line. *See* internal jugular (IJ) line
image receptor, 545
IM medications, 4
induction agent, 526
infection, 58
  at the site of entry, 23
inovent system, 362
intended anesthesia method, 515
intensive care unit (ICU), 521, 523, 524, 529–538
  advantage of, 538
  aspects of, 529
  daily ICU life, 531–538
    admissions, 536–537
    discharges, 537–538
    patient and family interactions, 538
    patient/unit maintenance, 534–536
    post-rounds discussion, 534
    procedures, 534
    rounds, 531–534
  electrolyte management, 535
  on the first day, 530–531
  nurses, 530
  vs. operating room, 529
  patient's labs, 534
  preparation for, 529–530
  resident, 557, 558
internal defibrillator, 509
internal jugular
  advantages and disadvantages, 30
  anatomy of, 30
  blood flows towards probe, 34
  equipment, 32
  kiddies, ultrasound, 34
  nicking the skin, 33

placing dilator, 33
positioning the patient, 32
procedure and approach, 31–35
squishable, 34
sterile drapes, 32
sterile dressing, 33
vessels, ultrasound image of, 34
watching the needle, 35
watching the wire, 35
internal jugular (IJ) line, 9–20
  anatomy, 10
    at 45 degrees, 18
    at 90 degrees, 18
  CMS rules, 20
  complications, 19–20
    carotid puncture/cannulation, 19
    chylothorax, 20
    hemothorax, 20
    hoarseness, 19
    phrenic nerve injury, 19
    pneumothorax, 19
  contraindications, 10
  pay-for-performance (P4P) initiatives, 20
  procedure and approach, 10–19
    advancing the wire, 14
    anatomical landmark approach, 11–15
    angiocatheter, advancing, 14
    blood return, 15
    catheter and kit selection, 11
    finding the vessel, 14
    patient preparation, 10–11
    skin nick, making, 14
    US-guided approach, 15–19
  relative anatomy of, 17
  right internal jugular (RIJ), 9
  trocar needle, 18, 19
  ultrasound anatomy, 17
  ultrasound machine, 17
  ultrasound probe, 17
  used for, 9
  US-guided central line insertion, 20
interscalene groove, 267
intraaortic balloon pump (IABP), 75
intracranial hypertension (IC-HTN), 428
  treatment of, 435–437
intracranial pressure (ICP) monitoring, 427
  cerebral autoregulation, 428
  cerebral perfusion pressure, 428
  cerebrospinal fluid (CSF), 427–428
  Codman™ external drainage device, 433
  complications of, 432
  herniation syndromes, 429
  increased, consequences of, 428–429
  indications for, 430

intracranial hypertension (IC-HTN), 428
  measures to control, 436
  treatment of, 435–437
intracranial pressure monitoring, 430–435
  intraventricular catheter setup, key elements of, 432
  left frontal ventricular catheter, 433
  Monro-Kellie doctrine, 427
  pressure-volume curve, 428
  types of, 431
  waveform, 434
invasive techniques, 562
ischemia monitoring, 385
IV catheters
  dilator, 15
  large-bore central, 14
  secure, 15
  transducing, 14

J

Jehovah's Witness patient, 403
jugular veins
  anterior, 162
  bleeding, 162
  compression of, 473
  internal, 36
  vascular injury of, 329
  wire seen, 416

K

ketamine, 310, 372
kiddie airway, 145
  anatomy and implications for management, 145–147
  chest x-ray, 147
  complications of, 152
  cricoid cartilage, 147
  difficult airway in kids, 150–152
  equipment, 148–150
  ETT, ultrathin bronchoscope, 151
  Frova® intubating, 151
  larynx
    infant, 147
    view of, 151
  LMA sizes, 149
  mask
    sizes, 149
    ventilation and intubation, 146
  Miller/Mac blade sizes, 149
  physiology and implications for management, 148
  sharing with surgeons, 152
  thyroid cartilage, 147
knee arthroplasty, 515

L

labetalol, 518
laparoscopy, 503
  procedure, 499
lap band, 562
laryngeal mask airway (LMA), 101–110, 182, 518, 558, 563
  AirQ, 102
  classical, 102
  cobra PLA, 102
  contraindications, 103
  endotracheal tube, 108–109
  indications, 103
  insertion technique, 106
  intubating LMA (ILMA), 102, 108
    factors affecting, 110
    insertion of, 106–107
    intubation technique, 106–108
    removal of, 108–109
    troubleshooting, 110
  patients examples, 103–105
  placement of, 564
  specific recommendations for, 104
  supraglottic airways (SGAs)
    bowls of, 110
    types of, 101–102
  supreme, 102
  tips/tricks, standard and disposable, 105–106
laryngoscopes
  blades, 181
  image, 192
  insertion, 116
  video, 117
laryngoscopy, 113–118
  equipment, 113
  glidescope, 117
  history and physical examination, 114–115
  indications, 113
  laryngoscope insertion, 116
  laryngoscopic methods, 115
  Macintosh/Miller, 129
  mallampati I, 114
  mallampati IV, 115
  nasotracheal laryngoscopy, 117
  orotracheal intubation
    access and positioning, 115
    technique, 115–116
    tube position, verification of, 117
  scissor-like maneuver, 116
  sniffing position, 116
  thyromental distance, 114
  video laryngoscopes, 117
laryngotracheal anesthesia (LTA), 170
latex allergy, 510, 556
lidocaine, 123, 124, 155, 158, 160, 171, 251, 556
ligamentum flavum, 228
limb ischemia, 57
line isolation monitors (LIMs), 547. *See also* ground fault detectors
LMA. *See* laryngeal mask airway (LMA)
lobectomy, 348, 350
loss of appetite, 233
lower extremity nerve blocks. *See* nerve blocks, lower extremity
lower extremity surgery
  isobaric solutions, 204
Ludwig angina's, 114
Luer-lock syringe, 357
lumbar epidural. *See* epidural(s)
lung biopsy, 348
lung isolation, 347
  absolute contraindications, 348
  absolute indications, 347–348
  achieving options, 351–352
  airway, difficulties, 350
  Arndt® bronchial blocker, 354, 358
  Arndt *vs.* Cohen tip-deflecting blockers, 358–359
  carina, 353
  Cohen® tip-deflecting blocker, 358
  double-lumen ETT, 353
  equipment, 348–349
  EZ Blocker®, 352, 359–360
  Fugi Uniblocker®, 352, 359
  history/physical examin, 350
  intercostal block, 361–362
  maneuvers, 361
  nitric oxide delivery device, 362
  one-lung oxygenation tips, 360–361
  philosophy of, 350
  relative indications, 348
  techniques
    double-lumen endotracheal tube, 354–356
    univent, 356–358
  Univent®, 354
L1 vertebra, 199, 293

M

Macintosh blade, 117
macroshock, 547
Magill forceps, 191
magnetic resonance imaging (MRI), 445
  anesthesia, 447–450
  characteristics of, 446
  dangers of, 445–446
  infusion pump, 450
  iron oxygen tank, 449
  machine, 546
  principles of, 445
  produce nonionizing radiation, 546
  quench button, 446
  resuscitation equipment, 450
  safety, 546
  suite, 518
malignant hyperthermia (MH)
  scenarios, 519, 553, 555
mask induction, for pediatric patients, 95–99
  airways
    pediatric/adult, 99
    setup, 96
  blood pressure cuffs, different size, 98
  emergency drugs, 96
  endotracheal tube time, 98–99
  hug the kiddie, 98
  IV setup, 96
  laryngospasm, 99
  mask, holding, 98
  NPO guidelines, 97
  pediatric patient arrives, 97–98
  placement, 98
  premedication, 97
  preoperative assessment, 97
  room setup, 95
mask ventilation, 87, 554
  anesthesia, 90
  claustrophobic patient, 92
  common glitches, 90
  continuous positive airway pressure (CPAP)
    on floor, 93
  contraindication, 87
  equipment, 87–88
  escape, 90
  face strap, 92
  facts, 93
  history, 88
  indication, 87
  induction, 89–90
  laryngospasm, 93–94
  Mapleson circuit, 88
  oral airway, 91
  oxyhemoglobin dissociation curve, 92
  perfection, 93
  philosophy of, 88
  physical, 88
  pictorial, 90–91
  reverse trendelenburg, 92
  rhinoplasty patient, 93
  technique, 88–89
  two-handed, 91
mastoid process, 318
mean arterial pressure (MAP), 499
meperidine, 407
methadone, 252
methemoglobinemia, cause, 123
methylmethacrylate (MMA), 549
  preparation, 549

midazolam, 310, 407
midthoracic, 224, 227
minimum alveolar concentration (MAC), 566
mitral regurgitation (MR), 385, 388, 403
monitored anesthesia care (MAC), 517
monitors, 526
monoethylglycinexylidide (MEGX), 251
Monro-Kellie doctrine, 427
morphine, 252
MRI. See magnetic resonance imaging (MRI)
MTB. See Mycobacterium tuberculosis (MTB)
mucosal atomization device, 123
multimodal analgesia, 566
Murphy's eye, 126
muscle fasciculations, 372
musculocutaneous nerve
  on axillary ultrasound, 276
Mycobacterium tuberculosis (MTB), 175–179
  filtering facepiece, 176
  heat and moisture (HME) filters, 178
  intraoperative, 178–179
  postoperative, 179
  powered air-purifying respirator (PAPR), 177
  preoperative, 176–178
  tuberculin skin test (TST), 175
myoclonic movements, 372

N

naloxone, 252
narcotics, 252
  infusions, 219
nasogastric tube (NGT), 189–193
  coiled inside mouth, 192
  complications, 189
  contraindications, 189
  equipment, 189–190
  indications, 189
  laryngoscope image, 192, 193
  positioning of head, 191
  procedure, 190–191
  troubleshooting/clinical pearls, 191–193
National Institute for Occupational Safety and Health (NIOSH), 541
nausea, 252, 257, 293, 301, 428, 509
NAVEL, 44
NAVY, 44
neck, anatomical landmarks, 163
needle's angle, 224
needlestick injuries, 548
neo-synephrine spray, 520

nephrectomy, 502
nerve blocks, kiddie, 317–324
  axillary block, 319–320
  block of Arnold, 318
  dorsal penile nerve block, 324
  femoral nerve block, 322
  ilioinguinal/iliohypogastric nerve block, 324
  infraclavicular nerve block, 322
  lower extremity blocks, 322
  pediatric population, special considerations, 317–318
  popliteal nerve block, 323
  sciatic nerve block, 322–323
  supraclavicular block, 320–322
  trigeminal nerve blocks, 318
    Maxillary division, 318–319
    ophthalmic division, 318, 319
  upper extremity blocks, 319
nerve blocks, lower extremity
  ankle block, landmarks for, 290
  block selection for, 280
  continuous peripheral nerve block (CPNB), 280
  femoral block, 282–283
    landmarks, 282
    ultrasound guided, 283
  lateral popliteal, 284
    ultrasound-guided, 285
  lumbar plexus block, 281–282
    landmarks, 281
    needle insertion and orientation, 281
    responses, 282
  patient setup, 280
  popliteal block, 284–285
  posterior popliteal, 284
  sciatic nerve block, 286–289
    anterior sciatic landmarks, 289
    complication, 286
    indications, 286
    Labat landmarks, posterior classic approach of, 286, 287
    parasacral approach, 286
    Raj approach, 286, 288
    subgluteal, 286
    subgluteal approach landmarks, 289
  selection, 279
  single shot vs. continuous infusion, 279–280
  ultrasound vs. nerve stimulation, 279
nerve damage, 58
neuraxial anesthesia, 198, 295
neuromuscular blocker, 566
NGT. See nasogastric tube (NGT)
nitroglycerin, 66, 518, 525
noninvasive blood pressure
  cuff, 527

monitor, 80
noninvasive technique, 391
nonsteroidal antiinflammatory drugs (NSAIDs), 567
normal airway setup, 518
normal saline (NS) flush, 527

O

obese patient
  anesthesia for, 561–567
  comorbid conditions, 562
  emergence/postoperative considerations, 566–567
  induction phase, 563–565
  maintenance, 565–566
  preoperative considerations, 562–563
  surgical technique, 561–562
obesity-related comorbidities, 76, 561–563
  diabetes mellitus, 561
  hyperlipidemia, 561
  hypertension, 561
  obstructive sleep apnea, 561
obligatory anesthesia, uh, fool around time (OAFAT), 456
obstructive sleep apnea (OSA), 562
Occupational Safety and Health Administration (OSHA), 549
off-site anesthesia, 517–521
  area, 518
  case example, 520–521
  deal with real estate, 518–519
  difficult airway, 520
  procedure, 519–520
  toolbox, 519
operating room (OR)
  fires, 141–144
    core elements, 141
    fire extinguishers, 144
    fuel sources, 141
    ignition sources, 141
    laser fire, 142–143
    laser surgery, guidelines, 143
    principles of, 143–144
    remote fires, 143
    toxicants, 142
  handoff, 479–483
    in aviation, 479
    benefits of, 480
    definition of, 479
    example of, 481
    face to face, 482
    information needs, 480–483
    in PACU, 483
    recovery room, 483
    risks of, 480
    solution, 480

operating room (OR) *(Continued)*
  intubations, outside, 181–187
    advanced airway supplies, 182
    assessment of situation, 184–186
    code box, 181, 182
    endotracheal tubes, 181
    end tidal CO_2 (E_TCO_2) detector, confirmation, 183
    equipment, 187
    headboard, 187
    laryngoscope/blades, 181
    optimizing environment, 186–187
    oral airways, 181
    syringes/needles, 181
    tube exchanger, 184
ophthalmic anesthesia, 335
  akinesia, 342
  chemosis, 342
  conjunctiva, 339
  contraindications, 335–336
  equipment, 336
  eye, needle angle, 339, 340
  indications, 335
  inferior oblique/rectus muscle, 339
  iodine solution, 342
  local anesthetic, 338
  Muller's muscle, sympathetic blockade of, 341
  needle insertion point, 339
  oculo-compression device, 343
  optic nerve, 338
  philosophy, 335
  subconjunctival hemorrhage, 342
  surface anatomy, examine, 338
  technique, 336–343
  ultrasound, 337, 338
opioids, side effects, 252
OR. *See* operating room (OR)
organ-specific care, 530
orogastric (OG) tube, 565
ovassapian airways, 121, 124
overweight patients, 561. *See also* obese patient
  classification of
    by morbidly obese, 561
    by obese, 561
    by overweight, 561
    by superobese, 561
  pathophysiologic changes in, 561
oxybutynin patch, 252
oxygenation, 360–361
oxygen insufflation, 137, 151
oxyhemoglobin dissociation curve, 92

P

pacemaker, 365
  anatomy/function, 366
  coding system, 367
  impact on surgery, 368–371
    channels, 371
    failure to capture, 369
    failure to output, 368–370
    malfunctions, 368
    runaway, 369, 371
    tachycardia, 369, 370
    undersensing, 369
    Wenckebach phenomenon, 370–371
  indications, 365
  intraoperative management, 372–373
  magnets, 368
  overview/history, 365
  pacing codes, 367–368
  preoperative management, 371–372
pain blocks, chronic, 325
  anterior lumbar epidural space, lateral fluoroscopic view of, 328
  epidural kit, 326
  epidural steroid injections (ESIs), 325
    complications, 326–328
    contraindications, 325
    indications, 325
    procedure, 325–326
  fluoroscopically guided lumbar foraminal injection, 326
  left carotid artery, palpating, 330
  lumbar sympathetic block, 332
    anterior fluoroscopic view of, 334
    complication, 334
    contraindications, 332
    indications, 332
    lateral fluoroscopic view of, 333
    needle, placing, 333
    patient positioning, 332
    procedure, 332–334
    radiographic contrast, injection of, 327
  stellate ganglion block
    complications, 329–331
    contraindications, 329
    fluoroscopic image of, 331
    indications, 328–329
    procedure, 329
    ultrasound-guided, 330
palpate brachial artery, 69
palpate vessel, 82
pancuronium, 247
part-task trainers, 552
patient-centered care, 538
patient controlled epidural analgesia (PCEA), 314
patient positioning techniques. *See* positioning techniques
patient transportation, 523–527
  airway, 524–525
  drugs, 525–526
    airway, 526
    sedation, 525
    vasoactive agents, 525
  freely running IV, 527
  monitors, 526
PDPHs. *See* postdural puncture headaches (PDPHs)
pedal A-line
  absolute *vs.* relative contraindications, 81
  anatomy of, 81–82
  complications, 83
  dorsalis pedis artery, 82
  equipment, 81
  foot, anatomy of, 82
  indications, 81
  posterior tibialis artery anatomy, 83
  technique, 82–83
PEEP. *See* positive end-expiratory pressure (PEEP)
penile block
  in child, 243–245
  dorsal nerve, injecting, 245
  equipment, 243
  paraurethral, ventral injection, 244
  penis, intradermal/subcutaneous ring weal, 244
peripheral intravenous (IV) access, 3–7
  anesthetic, 6
  antecubital fossa, 7
  equipment, 5
  external jugular (EJ), 4
  IV 101, 3
  pediatrics, 4
  saboteurs, 4–5
  tape, applying, 7
  technique, 4
  Y/X configuration, 6
peripherally inserted central catheter (PICC) lines, 5
  comments, 50–53
  complication, 50
  contraindications, 49
  equipment, 49
  flushing recommendations, 51
  indications, 49
  inserted into peelaway sheath, 53
  IV catheter, 52
  kids, 50
  peel-away sheath with a dilator, 52
  pertinent history/physical examination, 49
  placement by x-ray, 53
  technique, 50
  vein
    cannulation of, 51
    selection, 50

peripheral nerve catheters, 309–315
    American Society of Regional
            Anesthesia Pain Resource
            Center, 314
    complications, 314–315
    indications, 309–314
        anesthesia techniques, 309
        choice of drugs, 314
        contraindications, 310
        equipment, 310
        history and physical
                examination, 311
        patients dislike, 310
        technique, 311–314
    in-plane ultrasound technique, 312
    placement needle, 314
    sterile prep/drape for placement, 312
    ultrasound in-plane view, 313
phantom nasogastric (NG) tube, 565
pharmaceutical armamentarium, 519
phenol, 544
phenylephrine, 104, 123, 280, 310, 499,
        518, 564
phrenic nerve injury, 19
PICC lines. *See* peripherally inserted
        central catheter (PICC) lines
placebo effect, 501
pneumonectomy, 348, 350, 396
pneumothorax, 4, 9, 15, 19, 23, 271,
        396, 508
polyvinyl chloride, 142
port access surgery
    arterial line, 422
    atrial-SVC junction, 422
    benefits, 414
    cardiopulmonary bypass (CPB),
            initiation of, 423
    complications, 413
    coronary sinus, 418
        catheter, 417
        catheter ports, 417
        inserting, 418–419
        and IVC, 419
        view of, 418
    echo, 415
    EndoClamp, 423
    11F coronary sinus introducer, 416
    indications, 413
    insertion of neck lines, 415–417
    internal jugular vein, wire, 416
    lines needed for, 415
    lung isolation, 415
    mini-aortic valve, 420, 421
    mini-sternotomy, 420
    monitor with five pressures, 414
    preliminary lines, 415
    pulmonary vent, 417
        catheter, floating, 419–421
        tip, 419
    right internal jugular (RIJ), 415
    setup, 414
    superior vena cava (SVC)-atrial
            junction, 422
    surgery, 423
    surgical lines, 421–423
    table setup, 414
positioning techniques, anesthetized
        patients, 471–478
    arms, 472
    beach chair, 478
    case report, 478
    head prone, 474
    head side view, 475
    hips and knees, 476
    lateral decubitus/park bench
            position, 474–475
    leg, lateral knee, 477
    legs padded on side, 475
    lithotomy, 476–477
        front view, 476
        side view of, 472, 476
    prone, 473–474
    sitting/beach chair position, 477–478
    supine, 471–472
positive end-expiratory pressure
        (PEEP), 566
postanesthesia care unit (PACU), 93,
        544, 562
    resident, 557
postcardiopulmonary bypass period, 67
postdural puncture headaches
        (PDPHs), 204
posterior pharynx, 356
posterior superior iliac spine (PSIS),
        286
posterior tibial (PT) artery, 81
posterior tibial nerve, 290
postexposure prophylaxis (PEP), 548
postextubation obstruction
    risk of, 566
postoperative analgesia, 566
preadmission testing, 507–515
    alcohol intake, 511
    allergies to medications/materials,
            510–511
    brief examination, 514
    consent for anesthetic plan, 514–515
    drugs intake, 511
    medical conditions, 508
    medications takeing, 509–510
    previous surgeries, 508–509
    problems with anesthesia, 508–509
    surgery perform, 507–508
preanesthesia evaluation, 507
preanesthesia testing (PATs), 507
pregnancy, 294, 411

preoxygenation, 88, 92, 247, 494, 567
pressure support (PS) mode, 564
procedural training, 553
propofol, 310
pseudoaneurysm/thrombosis, 58
PSIS. *See* posterior superior iliac
        spine (PSIS)
pulmonary arterial pressures, 553
pulmonary artery catheter, 395
pulmonary hypertension, 396, 562
pulse oximeter, 10, 80, 526, 563

Q
Quincke needles, 231

R
radial A line, 57–66
    Allen's test, 58
    anatomy of
        radial artery, 58
        vs. ulnar artery cannulation, 58
    artery, compress, 62
    catheter over wire, 61
    indications, 57
        beat-to-beat blood pressure
                monitoring, 57
        blood gases/activated coagulation
                time (ACT) monitoring, 57
        complications, low rate of, 57
    insertion methods, 58–66
        anterograde artery cannulation, 66
        direct cannulation, 58–62
        localization with EMLA cream, 66
        secure, 65
        subcutaneous nitroglycerine, 66
        techniques for neonates, 66
        through-and-through technique,
                63–64
        US-guided technique as rescue, 65
    landing zone with chlorhexidine, 59
    needle, 61
    risks/complications, 57–58
    sterile gloves, 60
    transducer holder, 65
    tubing, catheter attaching, 62
radial arterial line catheters. *See*
        radial A-line
radiation-emitting technologies, 544
radiation exposure, 544
radiation safety, 545
    in catheterization lab, 410–412
radiation trivia, 545–546
RAE tube, 521
ramping, 563, 564
    patient position, 565
Raynaud's syndrome, 329

recommended exposure level (REL), 549
resident approaches, 558
respiratory therapy, 558
resuscitation, 450, 518
retroperitoneal bleed, 39, 40
retroperitoneal hematoma, 40
Richmond Agitation Sedation (RAS score), 533
rocuronium, 247
roomsmanship, 461–470
  body mechanics, 464
  chest rolls, comparison, 465
  documentation, 468–469
  drip, 470
  E_TCO_2, 470
  hextend vs. mannitol bag, 463
  line maintenance, 466–467
  moving patients, 464–465
  neat anesthesia records, 469
  patient positioning, 461–462
  pen vs. sharpie, 469
  professionalism, 468
  prone view, mock-up of, 465
  rapid transfuser, setting, 468
  sabotaged, 470
  steep trendelenburg position, 462
  stopcocks, labeled, 467
  surveillance, 463
  transporting patient, 466
  troubleshooting, 468
ropivacaine, in peripheral nerve catheters, 314

S

sacrococcygeal ligament, 248
saphenous nerve, 290
scavenging system, 543
scissors, 447
scleroderma, 119
screen-based simulation, 552
sedation anesthetic, 503
Seldinger technique, 127, 350
shifting dullness rounds, 531
simulated operating room, 552
simulation, 551–559
  applications, 552–553
    case scenarios, 556–558
    challenges, 554
    of crises, 553
    debriefing, 556
    definition, 551
    educator's role, 555
    people's experience, 554
    simulator types, 551–552
simulator
  advantage, 555
  fiberoptic, 120
  mannequins, 554
  types, 551–552
skin temperature probe, 565
skyrocketing blood pressure, 508
sleep-wake cycle, 533
sleeve gastrectomy, 562
smooth wake up procedures, 169
  capnograph, 171
  complications, 172–173
  lidocaine, 171
  technique, 169
    anesthetics, 169–170
    ETT cuff, 170–172
    spontaneous ventilation, recovery of, 169
    suctioning, 170
SOAP format, 533
spasm, 66, 83
spinal anesthesia, 197–204
  complications, 204
  contraindications, 197
  CSF, 203
  equipment/personnel, 197–198
  25-G needle, 201
  history/physical examination, 198
  indications, 197
  introducer needle, 201, 202
  kit, typical contents, 198
  L3-4 interspace with thumbs, 200
  needle
    insertion, 202
    tip, 203
  paresthesia, 204
  philosophy of, 198
  redirecting, hitting bone, 203–204
  side effect, 204
  small-gauge needle, 201
  spinous processes, sterile gloves, 200
  technique
    anatomy, 199
    drugs, choose, 198–199
    lateral position, patient, 203
    patient seated, 199–203
spinal cord, 199, 223, 224
spinal-epidural anesthesia. See spinal anesthesia
spinal hematoma, 197
Standard American Society of Anesthesiologists (ASA) monitors, 247
steep Trendelenburg position, 565
stellate ganglion block
  complications, 329–331
  contraindications, 329
  fluoroscopic image of, 331
  indications, 328–329
  procedure, 329
  ultrasound-guided, 330
stenosis, 325, 381, 383, 385, 387, 404
sternal notch, 563
sternocleidomastoid muscle (SCM), 268
sternomastoid muscle, 10
stylet
  Eschmann intubating, 518
subclavian
  advantages and disadvantages, 36
  anatomy of, 36
  complications, 38–39
  dressing, 38
  landmarks, 36
  needle placement, 38
  placement extraordinaire, 38
  procedure and approach, 36–38
  suprasternal notch, 36
  troubleshooting, 38
  vein catheterization, 23–28
    absolute vs. relative, contraindications, 23–24
    advance, 27
    anesthesia, 26
    complications, 27
    equipment, 24
    identification, 26
    indications, 23
    internal jugular (IJ) vein for central access, 23
    patient selection, 23
    patient's history, 24
    physical, 24
    position the patient, 25
    preparation, 24
    skin incision, 27
    subclavian vein, 26
    technique, 24–27
    thread the guidewire, 26
    troubleshooting, 27–28
    workspace, 25
succinylcholine, 372
sufentanil, 199
super glue for bones, methylmethacrylate (MMA), 549
superior laryngeal, 123, 124, 152
superior vena cava (SVC)
  atrial junction, 422
  syndrome, 23, 44, 398
supine position, 31
suprasternal notch, 36
sural nerve, 290
surgeon speak decoding, 499–504
  surgeons and anesthesiologists relationship, 499
surgery levels, of risk factors, 512
surgical airway, 153
  anatomical landmarks, 163
  Arndt Cricothyrotomy Kit, 158
  catheter positioned on skin, 160

contraindications, 153
cricothyroid membrane (CTM), 154
dilator/catheter, 160
dilator/guidewire, 159
   removal of, 167
dilator, trach loaded on, 165
equipment, 154
excision tracheal ring/hook elevation, 164
18-G needle and saline-filled syringe, 159
historical neck picture, 162
indications, 153
jet ventilator, 157
location, 154
neck positioning, 163
percutaneous dilational cricothyrotomy, 157–160
percutaneous tracheostomy, 165–168
surgical cricothyrotomy, 160–161
technique, 154
thyroid cartilage, 154
trach/dilator, insertion of, 167
tracheal dilatation, 167
tracheal exposure, 164
tracheal guidewire, insertion of, 166
tracheal hook, application of, 164
tracheal ring, excision of, 166
tracheostomy, 161–164
   airway fires/bleeding, complications, 168
   transtracheal catheter ventilation, 154–157
   wire reinforced catheter, 156
surgical cricothyrotomy, 155, 160–161
surgical dieting, options for, 561
surgical simulators, 552
surgical-site local anesthesia, 566
surgical technique
   for obese patient, 561–562
   for weight-loss surgery, 561–562
SVC. See superior vena cava (SVC)
Swan-Ganz catheter, 395
   anatomy, 398
   complications, 396
   contraindications, 396
   equipment/personnel, 396–398
   expert advice, 403–404
   indications, 395–396
   inserting, Swan, 398
   normal values, 404–405
   pressure tracings, illustrations, 402
   pulmonary artery catheter
      examples, 398
      sheath, threading, 400
   right jugular vein, introducer sheath, 397
   sheath, slide, 402

sterile flushing, 400
techniques, 399–402
   of placing, 401
   troubleshooting, 403
sympathetic blocks
   lumbar sympathetic ganglion block, 332
   Muller's muscle, 341
syringes
   glass, 212
   18-G needle and saline-filled, 159
   intubations, outside, 181
   Luer-lock, 357
   tuberculin (TB), 3
   uses, 68
systemic inflammatory response syndrome (SIRS), 536
systolic blood pressure, 500

T

tachycardia, 123
Taylor approach, 258
TB protection. See *Mycobacterium tuberculosis* (MTB)
TEE. See transesophageal echocardiography (TEE)
temperature-sensing Foley catheter, 565
temporomandibular joint pathology, 119
tetracaine, 198, 336
thoracic epidurals, 223–229
   benefits, 223
   considerations for pain service, 229
   contraindications, 223
   dosing, 228–229
   harpoon preparation, 226–227
   indications, 223
   ligamentum flavum, 228
   low-down, 224
   medications, 225
   midthoracic level, 227
   needle
      angle, 224
      feeling, 226
      insertion site, 225
   paramedian technique, 227
   preparation, 225
   risks, 224
   setup, 226
thrombosis, 58, 73, 531
through-and-through technique, 63–64
thyroid storm, 555
tongue depressor, 89, 121, 124
topicalization devices, 121
total body weight (TBW), 564
total intravenous anesthesia (TIVA), 544
tourniquet, 234, 504
toxic locker room material, 544

toxic place, 542
tracheal cuff, 353
tracheal dilatation, 167
tracheal exposure, 164
tracheal ischemia, 148
tracheal perforation, 36, 39
tracheostomy, 503
transducer, 65, 67, 72, 78, 79, 81, 261, 262, 265, 268, 274, 296
transesophageal echocardiography (TEE), 375–393
   abdominal aorta, transabdominal ultrasound, 393
   aortic valve (AV), views of, 387
   aortic wall dissection, 382
   ASE/SCA 20 standard views
      aortic valve, 385
      left ventricle, 384–385
      mitral valve, 385
      tricuspid/pulmonic valve, 385–389
   cardiac cycle sequence, mid-esophageal four-chamber view, 388
   complications, 377
   continuous-wave Doppler (CWD) scan, 383
   contraindications, 377
   ejection fraction (EF), calculation of, 387
   epiaortic ultrasound (EAU), 390–391
      examination, 390
   epicardial (EUS) ultrasound, 390–391
   equipment
      probe manipulation, 379–381
      proper probe insertion, 378–379
   handle and controls, 380
   indications, 377
   lateral view of, 379
   left ventricle (LV)
      segment model, 386
      transgastric middle short axis view, 386
      transgastric view of, 376
   midesophageal four-chamber view, 384, 389
   probe, 377–378
   probe tip in lateral/anterior view, 380
   RV/LV, transgastric middle short axis view of, 389
   systole, mid-esophageal four-chamber view, 388
   thoracic aorta, 383
   transthoracic echo, 392
   transthoracic echocardiography windows, 391
   transthoracic ultrasound, 391–393
   ultrasound machine, 378
   ultrasound physics, 381–384

transfering of patients, 404, 464
transport armamentarium
  version 1, 524
  version 2, 524
transvenous cardiac pacing, 9, 29
transversus abdominis plane (TAP) block, 293
  anatomy, 293–295
  blind/landmark-guided technique, 296
  catheter insertion, 298
  complications, 298
  dosage, 298
  equipment, 296
  in-plane ultrasound technique, 297
  live model surface anatomy, 296
  local anesthetic options, 298
  pediatric, special considerations, 298–299
  philosophy of, 296
  postoperative analgesia, 295
  problem solving, 299
  thoracoabdominal region, side profile of, 295
  transversus abdominis, 294
  ultrasound-guided technique, 296–297
  upper abdomen, 298
Trendelenburg position, 10, 11, 15, 24, 25, 31, 38, 134, 501
tuberculin (TB) syringe, 3
tumors, 114
Tuohy needle, 211, 226, 231, 248, 298, 313

U

ulnar nerve, 319, 471, 472
umbilical hernia, 509
uncontrollable bleeding, 510
uncontrolled hypertension, 508, 512
Univent®, 354, 356–358
unstable angina, 513
upper extremity block, 257. *See also* brachial plexus blocks
  anesthetic experience, 259
  axilla/proximally aim, 274
  axillary brachial plexus block, 273–276
  axillary ultrasound anatomy, 275
  block technique progression, 260–261
  contraindication, 259
  fascial sheath, 267
  Frankie say relax, 274
  infraclavicular brachial plexus block, 271–273

  infraclavicular landmarks, 271
  infraclavicular ultrasound anatomy, 273
  infraclavicular ultrasound-guided approach, 272
  in-plane needle/transducer orientation, 262
  interscalene area, ultrasound anatomy of, 270
  interscalene block, 269
  interscalene brachial plexus block, 267–271
  intralipid, 261
  local anesthetic toxicity, 259–260
  musculocutaneous block, 276
  needle, 261–263
  nice clavicle, 265
  out-of-plane needle/transducer orientation, 262
  points to avoid, 263
  pulse oximeter, 264
  setup, 263–264
    nerve block, 264
  studies, 258
  supraclavicular block
    in-plane approach, 266
    ultrasound anatomy of, 266
  supraclavicular brachial plexus block, 264–267
  time out, 260
  ultrasound, 261
  ultrasound-guided interscalene approach, 270
  ultrasound image, 263
  ultrasound physics, 261
urologic surgeries, 476

V

Valsalva maneuvers, 428
valvular stenosis, 381
vecuronium, 247
venous air embolism, 24, 25, 36
venous thrombosis, 27, 36
ventilatory strategy, 565
vertebral artery injection, 270
vertebral artery puncture, 36
video laryngoscopes (VLs), 129
  C-MAC™, 134–135
  contraindications, 130
  GlideScope® Cobalt AVL®, 131
  GVL® wide-angle anatomic larynx view, 131
  indications, 130
  indirect capability devices, 131
  King Vision™, 132

  McGRATH® MAC, 132
  Pentax AWS®, 133
  philosophy, 130–131
VLs. *See* video laryngoscopes (VLs)
volatile anesthetics
  exposure to, 541
volatile gases
  side effects of, 543
  smell, 541
vomiting, 88, 90, 170, 173, 233

W

weakness, 123
weight-loss surgery
  anesthesia for, 561–567
  emergence/postoperative considerations, 566–567
  induction phase, 563–565
  maintenance, 565–566
  preoperative considerations, 562–563
  surgical technique, 561–562
Whiz-Bang Intubation Gizmos, 129
  Bovie Aaron Surch-Lite™, 138–139
  case study, 135, 139
  cutting-edge gadget, 129
  lighted stylets (LSs), 138
  optical laryngoscope (OL), 135
    Airtraq®, 136
  optical stylets (OSs), 136
    Bonfils®, 136–137
    Clarus® video system, 137
    Levitan™, 137
    Shikani™, 137
    Video RIFL®, 137–138
  video laryngoscopes (VLs), 129
    C-MAC™, 134–135
    contraindications, 130
    GlideScope® Cobalt AVL®, 131
    GVL® wide-angle anatomic larynx view, 131
    indications, 130
    indirect capability devices, 131
    King Vision™, 132
    McGRATH® MAC, 132
    Pentax AWS®, 133
    philosophy, 130–131
William Morton's famous ether anesthesia, 543
World Health Organization (WHO), 561

X

x-ray generating tube, 545